JOSLIN'S DIABETES DESKBOOK

A GUIDE FOR PRIMARY CARE PROVIDERS

SECOND EDITION

D1506999

JOSLIN'S DIABETES DESKBOOK
A GUIDE FOR
PRIMARY CARE PROVIDERS

Second Edition

By
Richard S. Beaser, M.D.
and the Staff of Joslin Diabetes Center

ISBN: 1-879091-20-8
Published by Joslin Diabetes Center, Boston, MA
Web site: www.joslin.org

Joslin Diabetes Center
Publications Department
One Joslin Place
Boston, MA 02215

The publisher offers discounts on this book when ordered in bulk quantities.
For information, contact the Joslin Publications Department at
the address above or call 617-226-5815.

Joslin's Clinical Guidelines are independently developed and approved by Joslin
Diabetes Center through its Clinical Oversight Committee. Joslin accepts no
financial support for the development of its Clinical Guidelines.

About Joslin Diabetes Center

Dedicated to a world without diabetes and its complications

Joslin Diabetes Center is the world's largest diabetes research center, diabetes clinic, and provider of diabetes education. Joslin's concentrated focus on a single disease allows it to rapidly discover, create and distribute new knowledge about diabetes prevention, treatment options and research toward a cure.

Affiliated with Harvard Medical School, Joslin was founded in 1898 by a single physician, Elliott P. Joslin, M.D. Joslin today has three major divisions:

- Joslin Research, a highly collaborative team of more than 300 people with 40 faculty level investigators undertaking the largest research program aimed at preventing and curing type 1 and type 2 diabetes and their long-term complications.

- Joslin Clinic, the world's first and most respected diabetes care facility, which cares for 23,000 patients a year.

- Joslin Strategic Initiatives, which develops and markets innovative programs, products and services that expand the availability of Joslin knowledge and expertise to people with diabetes and the clinicians who care for them. One of these programs is Joslin's Professional Education program, which provides Continuing Medical Education (CME) programs for physicians, Continuing Education (CE) programs for non-physician medial professionals, and a program of education for corporate professionals for companies seeking to educate their staff. Educational programs are delivered through live seminars, in print, through CD and online.

For more information about Joslin and its activities, visit to www.joslin.org.

About Richard S. Beaser, M.D.

Richard S. Beaser, M.D. has held many roles during his 25-year tenure at Joslin Diabetes Center. His administrative posts include Section Chief of Joslin's Adult Diabetes Practice, Medical Director of the Diabetes Treatment Unit, and Director of Patient Education. Dr. Beaser has been an investigator in a number of clinical trials including the Diabetes Control and Complications Trial (DCCT). He has authored several books, including the *Joslin Diabetes Manual, 12th Edition; Outsmarting Diabetes;* and *The Joslin Guide to Diabetes.* Currently, he is the Medical Executive Director of the Professional Education Department. In this role, he has lectured extensively throughout the United States and abroad, and has appeared in educational teleconferences and video programs. Dr. Beaser holds an academic appointment as Associate Clinical Professor of Medicine at Harvard Medical School. He is a Boston native, and is married with 3 sons.

Contents

Chapter 1
Diabetes: Definition and Pathophysiology   1

Chapter 2
The Approach to Diagnose and Treatment of Diabetes Mellitus   **25**

Chapter 3
Monitoring Diabetes   **45**

Chapter 4
Adipose Tissue as an Endocrine Gland: A Possible Key in Understanding the Metabolic Mysteries 67

Chapter 5
Medical Nutrition Therapy and Diabetes 81

Chapter 6
Physical Activity for Fitness   **127**

Chapter 7
Type 2 Diabetes: Multiple Treatments for a Multicomponent Condition   153

Chapter 9
Using Insulin To Treat Diabetes — General Principles

Chapter 10
Designing a Conventional Insulin Treatment Program

Chapter 11
Physiologic Insulin Treatment Programs   325

Chapter 12
Educating the Patient   385

Chapter 13
Acute Complications 403

Chapter 14
Microvascular Complications 429

Chapter 15
Macrovascular Complications 459

Chapter 16
Diabetic Neuropathy   **481**

Chapter 17
The Foot: Clinical Care and Problem Prevention 505

Chapter 18
Surgical Management of
the Patient with Diabetes 521

Chapter 19
Gender-Specific Issues   541

Chapter 20
Pregnancy and Diabetes   573

Chapter 23
Psychological Issues in the   641
Treatment of Diabetes

Chapter 24
Diabetes in Culturally Diverse Populations:
Facing the Challenge in Clinical Practice   663

Authors and Reviewers by Chapter

Chapter 1 — Definition and Pathophysiology
By Richard S. Beaser, MD
> *Assisted by Elizabeth Blair, MSN, APRN, BC, CDE and Ramachandiran Cooppan, MD, FRCP(C)*

Chapter 2 — The Approach to Diagnosis and Treatment
By Richard S. Beaser, MD
> *Assisted by Elizabeth Blair, MSN, APRN, BC, CDE and Ramachandiran Cooppan, MD, FRCP(C)*

Chapter 3 — Monitoring Diabetes
By Richard S. Beaser, MD
> *Assisted by Catherine Carver, MS, APRN, BC, CDE and Elizabeth Blair, MSN, APRN, BC, CDE*

Chapter 4 — Adipose Tissue as an Endocrine Gland: A Possible Key in Understanding the Metabolic Mysteries
By Osama Hamdy, MD, PhD, FACE
> *Reviewed by Richard S. Beaser, MD and Amy P. Campbell, MS, RD, CDE*

Chapter 5 — Medical Nutrition Therapy
By Amy P. Campbell, MS, RD, CDE and Richard S. Beaser, MD
> *Reviewed by Osama Hamdy, MD, PhD, FACE*

Chapter 6 — Physical Activity for Fitness
By Edward S. Horton, MD; Catherine A. Mullooly, MS, RCEP, CDE; and Richard S. Beaser, MD

Chapter 7 — Type 2 Diabetes: Multiple Treatments for a Multicomponent Condition
By Richard S. Beaser, MD

Assisted by Om P. Ganda, MD; Elizabeth Blair, MSN, APRN, BC, CDE; and Ramachandiran Cooppan, MD, FRCP(C)

Chapter 8 — Pharmacotherapy for Type 2 Diabetes: Medications to Match the Pathophysiology
By Richard S. Beaser, MD

Assisted by Elizabeth Blair, MSN, APRN, BC, CDE and Ramachandiran Cooppan, MD, FRCP(C)

Chapter 9 — Using Insulin to Treat Diabetes — General Principles
By Richard S. Beaser, MD

Assisted by Elizabeth Blair, MSN, APRN, BC, CDE and Ramachandiran Cooppan, MD, FRCP(C)

Chapter 10 — Designing a Conventional Insulin Treatment Program
By Richard S. Beaser, MD

Assisted by William M. Sullivan, MD; Catherine Carver, MS, APRN, BC, CDE; Elizabeth Blair, MSN, APRN, BC, CDE; and Ramachandiran Cooppan, MD, FRCP(C)

Chapter 11 — Physiologic Insulin Treatment Programs
By Richard S. Beaser, MD; Osama Hamdy, MD, PhD, FACE; and Howard Wolpert, MD

Chapter 12 — Patient Education
Adaptation and revision by Elizabeth Blair, MSN, APRN, BC, CDE

Reviewed by Ramachandiran Cooppan, MD, FRCP(C) and Richard S. Beaser, MD

Chapter 13 — Acute Complications
By Ramachandiran Cooppan, MD, FRCP(C); Richard S. Beaser, MD; and Greeshma Shetty, MD
Reviewed by Elizabeth C. Bashoff, MD and William M. Sullivan, MD

Chapter 14 — Microvascular Complications
By Jerry D. Cavallerano, OD, PhD and Robert M. Stanton, MD

Chapter 15 — Macrovascular Complications
By Richard S. Beaser, MD and Michael Johnstone, MD
Assisted by Om P.Ganda, MD and Ramachandiran Cooppan, MD, FRCP(C)

Chapter 16 — Diabetic Neuropathy
By Roy Freeman, MD
Reviewed by Richard S. Beaser, MD

Chapter 17 — The Foot: Clinical Care and Problem Prevention
By Richard S. Beaser, MD and John M. Giurini, DPM

Chapter 18 — Surgical Management of the Patient with Diabetes
By Richard S. Beaser, MD and Elizabeth S. Halprin, MD
Assisted by Lyle Mitzner, MD and Ramachandiran Cooppan, MD, FRCP(C)

Chapter 19 — Gender-Specific Issues
By Julie L. Sharpless, MD; Peter N. Weissman, MD; and Kenneth J. Snow, MD, MBA
Reviewed by Richard S. Beaser, MD; Elizabeth Blair, MSN, APRN, BC, CDE; and Ramachandiran Cooppan, MD

Chapter 20 — Pregnancy
By Florence M. Brown, MD and Richard S. Beaser, MD
Assisted by Martin J. Abrahamson, MD and Suzanne Ghiloni, RN, BSN, CDE

Chapter 21 — Treatment of Children with Diabetes
By Elise Bismuth, MD and Lori M. Laffel, MD, MPH
Reviewed by Richard S. Beaser, MD

Chapter 22 — Diabetes in the Older Adult
By Medha N. Munshi, MD; Elizabeth Blair, MSN, APRN, BC,
CDE; and Ramachandiran Cooppan, MD, FRCP (C)
Reviewed by Richard S. Beaser, MD

Chapter 23 — Psychological Issues in the Treatment of Diabetes
By Barbara J. Anderson, PhD and Abigail K. Mansfield, MA
Reviewed by John Zrebiec, LICSW and Richard S. Beaser, MD

**Chapter 24 — Diabetes in Culturally Diverse Populations:
Facing the Challenge in Clinical Practice**
By Enrique Caballero, MD
Reviewed by Richard S. Beaser, MD

In addition, we wish to acknowledge the assistance and expertise of the following current and former Joslin staff members: Melinda Maryniuk, MEd, RD, CDE; Richard Jackson, MD; Elaine Sullivan, MD, RN, CDE; Joan Hill, RD, CDE, LDN; Lisa Bulduc, RN, CDE; Karen Chalmers, MS, RD, CDE; Maria Higgins Gallego, MEd, RD, CDE; Catherine Jarema, MS, RCEP, CDE; Satoka Hayakawa Porter, MS, RCEP, CDE; Mary Beth Kiley, RN, BSN, CDE; and Lauren Reynolds, MPH.

Authors and Reviewers

Martin J. Abrahamson, MD
Medical Director and Senior Vice
  President
Joslin Diabetes Center
Associate Professor of Medicine,
  Harvard Medical School

Barbara J. Anderson, PhD
Professor of Pediatrics
Baylor College of Medicine

Florence M. Brown MD
Co-Director, Joslin-BIDMC Diabetes
  in Pregnancy Program
Instructor in Medicine, Harvard
  Medical School

Elizabeth C. Bashoff, MD
Senior Staff Physician
Joslin Diabetes Center
Instructor in Medicine, Harvard
  Medical School

Elise Bismuth, MD
Research Fellow
Pediatric, Adolescent and Young
  Adult Section
Joslin Diabetes Center

Elizabeth Blair, MSN, APRN, BC,
  CDE
Adult Nurse Practitioner, Joslin
  Clinic
Joslin Diabetes Center

Enrique Caballero, MD
Associate Director of Professional
  Education
Director of the Latino Diabetes
  Initiative
Joslin Diabetes Center
Assistant Professor of Medicine,
  Harvard Medical School

Amy P. Campbell, MS, RD, CDE
Education Program Manager
Healthcare Services, Strategic
  Initiatives
Joslin Diabetes Center

Catherine Carver, MS, APRN, BC,
  CDE
Director of Education and New
  Program Development
Joslin Clinic, Joslin Diabetes Center

Jerry D. Cavallerano, OD, PhD
Beetham Eye Institute
Joslin Diabetes Center
Associate Professor, New England
  College of Optometry

Ramachandiran Cooppan, MD,
  FRCP(C)
Senior Staff Physician (Ret.)
Joslin Diabetes Center
Assistant Clinical Professor of
  Medicine, Harvard Medical
  School

Roy Freeman, MD
Director, Center for Autonomic and
    Peripheral Nerve Disorders
Beth Israel Deaconess Medical
    Center
Professor of Neurology, Harvard
    Medical School

Om P. Ganda, MD
Senior Staff Physician
Joslin Diabetes Center
Associate Clinical Professor of
    Medicine, Harvard Medical School

Suzanne Ghiloni, RN, BSN, CDE
Nurse and Diabetes Educator, Joslin
    Clinic
Joslin Diabetes Center

John M. Giurini, DPM.
Chief, Division of Podiatry, Beth
    Israel Deaconess Medical Center
Co-Director, Joslin-BI Deaconess Foot
    Center
Associate Clinical Professor of
    Surgery, Harvard Medical School

Elizabeth S. Halprin, MD
Staff Physician
Joslin Diabetes Center
Instructor in Medicine, Harvard
    Medical School

Osama Hamdy, MD, PhD, FACE
Medical Director, Obesity Clinical
    Program
Joslin Diabetes Center
Instructor in Medicine, Harvard
    Medical School

Edward S. Horton, MD
Vice President and Director of
    Clinical Research
Joslin Diabetes Center
Professor of Medicine, Harvard
    Medical School.

Michael Johnstone, MD
Director of Clinical Cardiology
Caritas St. Elizabeth's Medical
    Center

Lori Laffel, MD, MPH
Chief, Pediatric and Adolescent
    Unit
Investigator, Genetics and
    Epidemiology Unit
Joslin Diabetes Center
Associate Professor of Pediatrics,
    Harvard Medical School

Abigail Mansfield, MA
Clinical Psychologist

Lyle D. Mitzner, MD
Staff Physician
Joslin Diabetes Center
Instructor in Medicine, Harvard
    Medical School

Catherine A. Mullooly, MS, RCEP,
    CDE
Former Director, Exercise
    Physiology
Joslin Diabetes Center

Medha Munshi, M.D.
Director of Joslin Geriatric Diabetes
    Programs
Joslin Diabetes Center
Instructor in Medicine, Harvard
    Medical School

Julie L. Sharpless, MD
Clinical Assistant Professor of
  Medicine
University of North Carolina, School
  of Medicine.

Greeshma K. Shetty, MD
Endocrinology, Metabolism &
  Diabetes
Beth Israel Deaconess Medical
  Center
Joslin Diabetes Center
Instructor in Medicine, Harvard
  Medical School

Kenneth J. Snow, MD, MBA
Chief, Adult Diabetes
Director, Sexual Function Clinic
Joslin Diabetes Center
Assistant Professor in Clinical
  Medicine, Harvard Medical School

Robert C. Stanton, MD
Chief, Renal Section
Joslin Diabetes Center
Associate Professor of Medicine,
  Harvard Medical School

William M. Sullivan, MD
Senior Staff Physician
Joslin Diabetes Center
Instructor in Medicine, Harvard
  Medical School

Peter N. Weissman, MD
Associate Clinical Professor of
  Medicine and Endocrinology
Miller School of Medicine
University of Miami

Howard Wolpert, MD
Senior Physician, Section of Adult
  Diabetes
Director, Insulin Pump Program
Joslin Diabetes Center
Assistant Professor of Medicine,
  Harvard Medical School

John Zrebiec, L.I.C.S.W
Associate Director, Behavioral and
  Mental Health Unit
Joslin Diabetes Center
Lecturer in Psychiatry, Harvard
  Medical School

Acknowledgments

Although this book was by necessity written by a few, the contributions supporting the content have been provided by many.

The previous list of Authors and Reviewers acknowledges, by chapter, those who served either as authors or co-authors or provided the review or input that is essential to the accuracy of any comprehensive teaching endeavor. The time and counsel contributed by these individuals were essential. I would particularly like to thank Dr. Ramachandiran Cooppan, MD, FRCP(C) and Amy Campbell, MS, RD, CDE for reading and critiquing much of the text.

But there were other contributors. The authors of this book depend indirectly on contributions from the many physicians, nurses, dietitians, researchers, and other support staff that have made up the Joslin Diabetes Center and the Joslin Clinic in the over 100 years that it has been in existence. These individuals have all, in some manner, contributed to the body of knowledge that is reflected herein. Joslin Diabetes Center was led originally by Elliott P. Joslin himself, then by Dr. Howard Root, Dr. Alexander Marble, and, in the modern era, by Dr. Bob Bradley, Dr. Ken Quickel, Dr. Ron Kahn, and now, Ranch Kimball. Each of these presidents has promoted academic ferment and stimulated the intellectual atmosphere and clinical perspectives that have resulted in numerous publications and scientific and medical advances.

In addition, there are two physicians, now departed, whom I would like to cite for their professional and personal support. One is my father, Dr. Sam Beaser, and the other is my early mentor in education at Joslin, Dr. Leo Krall. These two physicians, although working at different institutions, were good friends and colleagues in research, and shared the spirit of clinical care and education that I have tried to embody in this book. Leo Krall represents the lineage of the giants of Joslin Diabetes Center. Leo was a personal mentor and friend from my first day as a fellow at Joslin to the time of his death. He not only taught me facts, but also guided my understanding of diabetes and the preeminent importance of teaching its treatment principles to others in order to ensure the progress of quality care and the improvement of outcomes. My father, Sam Beaser, was a diabetologist who first described combination oral therapy of type 2 diabetes while working at a neighboring institution, the Beth Israel Hospital. He provided me with fatherly guidance and a personal perspective on diabetes treatment that has been invaluable throughout my career. These two physicians together provided a tie to the continuum of progress in diabetes research and treatment that enhances our current ability to manage this condition and its complications.

I would like to express my deep appreciation to others whose roles at Joslin in Publications and Professional Education have been important to the institution as well as to the preparation of this book. In Publications, I would like to thank Susan Sjostrom, without whose tireless work this book would never have been published. Also, in Joslin's Professional Education/Continuing Medical Education Department I would like to acknowledge the superb work of Dr. Enrique Caballero, Sharon Garbus, Linda Baer, and the entire Professional Education staff in our Boston offices. I would also like to thank all of the faculty of the many Joslin education programs who have provided their skills and teaching expertise to help bring our programs to a level of excellence of which we can be proud. I would also like to thank those in industry whose support of our Professional Education programs over the years has been greatly appreciated.

Of course, acknowledgements would not be complete without expressing deep appreciation to my family. My wife Marguerite and my sons, Michael, Andrew and Daniel, tolerated many evenings with me at the computer. I hope that the benefits this book may bring to people with diabetes will serve as reward for their patience and understanding.

Finally, I would like to acknowledge the contribution of the millions of people who have diabetes. They, and only they, know first-hand what management of diabetes entails. They serve tirelessly and selflessly in research studies. They care for themselves and their diabetes every day of their lives, and, in doing so, they teach us a great deal about treating this condition, as educating is always a two-way street. If a healthcare provider cannot learn from his or her patients, he or she has not been exposed to the full curriculum of medicine. Those of us who deliver healthcare salute the patients that we serve.

Richard S. Beaser, MD
November, 2007

Foreword

Over 21 million people in the Unites States have diabetes mellitus, and this number continues to increase at the rate of about 1 million new patients diagnosed every year. In the United States, diabetes strikes every age group, ethnic group, and socioeconomic group. Diabetes creates an enormous economic burden on the nation, both in terms of direct healthcare costs and decreased productivity that is now estimated at over $140 billion annually. Diabetes not only remains the leading cause of blindness and renal failure in the U.S., but is growing to be an increasing proportion of the total number of cases. In addition, diabetes is associated with neuropathy, vascular disease leading to amputation, and markedly increases the risk of heart disease, birth defects and other serious problems. The World Health Organization has predicted a worldwide epidemic of diabetes over the next 25 years that will strike even harder at less-developed countries as they become more westernized.

What makes diabetes such a difficult and serious challenge? First, diabetes is not a single disease, but several complex disorders that share the major common features — elevated levels of glucose in the blood; abnormalities in lipid metabolism; and increased risk for long-term microvascular and macrovascular complications. About 1 million people in the U.S. have type 1 diabetes, an autoimmune disease in which the body's immune system turns against itself and destroys the insulin-producing beta cells of the pancreas. While traditionally the diagnosis of new onset type 1 diabetes was restricted to children and young adults, with increased immunological testing, we now recognize new onset cases of type 1 diabetes in all age groups. Indeed, 50% of new cases of type 1 diabetes occur in individuals over 21. While the adults with new onset type 1 diabetes may be slower to develop insulin dependence, all of these individuals are committed to a lifetime of insulin injections and careful glucose and dietary monitoring.

The most common form of diabetes and the major cause of the worldwide epidemic of the disease is type 2 diabetes. This form is closely linked to obesity and sedentary lifestyle, and both of these factors are increasing dramatically in the U.S. and worldwide. While type 2 diabetes used to affect primarily the elderly, it is now found in all age groups. In fact, the incidence of type 2 diabetes is rising fastest in children and young adults, due in large part to changing lifestyles. In major urban areas, between 20% and 45% of new cases of diabetes in children are type 2 diabetes. This is driven in part by a parallel epidemic — obesity in both children and adults. Since the risk of long-term complications of diabetes increases with duration of the disease, as more and more individuals develop diabetes at younger and younger ages, the medical community will be faced with a rapidly growing population of individuals at risk for the eye, kidney, vascular, and neurologic complications of diabetes. Unlike type 1 diabetes, which is due primarily to insulin deficiency secondary to beta cell destruction, type 2 diabetes is driven primarily by insulin resistance, which can affect multiple tissues of the body and eventually lead to relative insulin deficiency. Prevention of type 2 diabetes is possible for many people at risk by lifestyle and pharmalogical intervention.

Over the past few years, important clinical and research advances have begun to change our understanding of the fundamental abnormalities in diabetes, as well as our clinical approach to the disease. These studies have demonstrated clearly the important role of diet and activity on the rate of development of type 2 diabetes, and have shown how tight control of blood glucose can significantly decrease the risk of complications for patients with both type 1 and type 2 diabetes. To combat these problems, many pharmaceutical companies have now introduced genetically engineered forms of insulin with more desirable pharmacological properties, a variety of devices for monitoring diabetes control and new oral antidiabetic medications.

The primary care providers remain not only the first line of defense, but the major line of defense for the large majority of patients with diabetes. Most individuals with diabetes do not have access to highly specialized referral centers. Furthermore, since diabetes is a systemic disease and associated with many other common disorders, the challenge is often placed with the generalist to integrate the care of these complex patients.

The goal of *Joslin's Diabetes Deskbook* is to give primary care providers the necessary background information about the pathogenesis of diabetes mellitus and its complications, as well as the most up to date approaches to management and treatment of these patients. Keep in mind, however, that management of patients with diabetes is continually changing.

Clearly, as research begins to define the exact genetic and environmental factors leading to diabetes and begins to develop new therapies to treat, prevent or cure the disease, it will be up to the primary care provider to both manage these patients and direct them in appropriate channels to maximize their opportunities for optimal treatment. Indeed, even since the last edition of this textbook, a number of new agents have been introduced for the treatment of diabetes, including new insulins, new oral hypoglycemic drugs, new proteins and hormones that can stimulate the beta cell and new devices to monitor glucose and to inject insulin. We hope that *Joslin's Diabetes Deskbook* provides the central tool in your armamentarium for this goal, and that Joslin Diabetes Center itself can serve as the source for both specialty services and ongoing education and research about this challenging problem.

C. Ronald Kahn, M.D.
Vice Chair and Director, Joslin Diabetes Center
November, 2007

Introduction

The treatment of diabetes has come a long way in the last century! As we think back on the milestones in the treatment of this condition, we can appreciate how far we have come. While the "cure" is still elusive, effective management tools are better than ever before. Starting with the discovery of insulin in 1921, we have seen the development of antidiabetes medications; newer advances in insulin formulations and delivery, such as insulin pumps to help mimic normal secretory patterns; self-monitoring of blood glucose; the A1C measurement; and the many advances in prevention and treatment of the individual complications of this disease.

Yet, we are also seeing, right now, an epidemic of diabetes. Type 2 diabetes is increasing in numbers in both adults and children, due in part to sedentary life styles and dietary habits. And though we have a better understanding of the impact of type 2 diabetes on the risk of macrovascular disease, yet there are more and more people for whom these risks are unidentified and untreated.

Thus, the clinical challenges imposed by diabetes still remain, not just for the specialists in this area of practice, but for the primary care providers who provide care and counsel to over 90% of the people with this condition.

Joslin Diabetes Center has witnessed and, in fact, has been an integral part of many of these changes over the last century. Evolving from Dr. Elliott P. Joslin's practice, founded over 100 years ago, Joslin has been devoted to providing state-of-the-art diabetes care. Joslin has as its mission, beyond diabetes care, targeting basic and clinical research, and providing education for patients, practicing physicians, physicians-in-training, allied health professionals, and many others working together to control this condition. Throughout these many endeavors, the spirit of Elliott Joslin's original approach to patient care still shines through: involve the patient as part of his or her own healthcare team, and educate the patient to take as active a role as possible in self-care activities. This empowerment of the patient, long before the word "empowerment" was part of our common lexicon, has led to improved care, better outcomes, and a higher quality of life for patients with diabetes.

Joslin has always focused on the team approach to diabetes management. An integral part of this team, in addition to the patient and those medical professionals specializing in diabetes management, is the primary care provider. Particularly in this modern era with managed care and shared responsibilities, efforts to coordinate care among various providers are crucial in order to optimize health outcomes. Over the wide spectrum of care required by a person with diabetes, each provider, whether specialist or generalist, has a role to play. It is important to develop a comfort level with one's own role and the care that one is asked to provide; it is also important to be cognizant of the skills of other potential care-team members who may be called upon for their particular expertise when needed. It is really the reinforcement of this team approach that is at the core of Joslin's approach to diabetes management, and that is the philosophical backbone of this book.

With this philosophy in mind, *Joslin's Diabetes Deskbook* has been written for all members of the diabetes care team. Whether you are a primary care physician, a specialist, a nurse or nurse practitioner, physician's assistant, Certified Diabetes Educator, dietitian, exercise physiologist, patient with diabetes or someone close to a patient with diabetes, you are involved in the primary management of the care and treatment of a person with diabetes. And whatever your role, it is important that all the team members work together with common goals and methods.

At the core of diabetes management are treatment guidelines, both those promulgated by the American Diabetes Association (ADA) and those developed by Joslin Diabetes Center. The ADA, responsive to the needs of multiple constituencies of providers and patients, frequently publishes consensus statements and practice recommendations. In a supplement to Diabetes Care, published annually each January, the ADA updates all current, active practice recommendations.

Over the years, others, including Joslin, have published differing recommendations when there were disagreements with the ADA approach. However, recently, with many newer studies providing data with which to make better clinical decisions, the ADA has sought to establish guidelines that reflect a coalescence of opinion that most accept. This approach has largely succeeded, and the ADA is now generally recognized as the source of general clinical guidelines for the treatment of diabetes and related conditions.

However, by necessity so as to achieve widespread acceptance, guidelines and recommendations published by the ADA must be general in nature to be applicable to a broad spectrum of patients and practice settings. Each practitioner and institution must adapt these guidelines to the contingencies of its own diabetes practice. Readers of this book who care for people with diabetes are no exception.

In this light, Joslin Diabetes Center itself has a Clinical Oversight Committee, comprised of Joslin staff in all specialties and areas of expertise, which reviews clinical practice trends — those recommended by the ADA and others — and then develops its own specific Guidelines. These Guidelines are established after careful review of current evidence, medical literature and clinical practice. They are developed independently, without financial or other support from any outside entity. While these guidelines generally adhere to ADA recommendations, some may be more specific, detailed, or otherwise derived from Joslin's institutional practice or that of its Affiliates. Currently Joslin has developed the following Clinical Guidelines:

Clinical Guidelines for Adults with Diabetes

Clinical Guideline for Pharmacological Management of Type 2 Diabetes

Clinical Guideline for Inpatient Management of Surgical and ICU Patients

Guideline for Specialty Consultation/Referral

Guideline for Detection and Management of Diabetes in Pregnancy

Guideline for Management of Uncontrolled Glucose in the Hospitalized Adult

Clinical Nutrition Guideline for Overweight or Obese Adults with Type 2 Diabetes, Pre-Diabetes or Those At Risk for Developing Type 2 Diabetes

Guideline for the Care of the Older Adult with Diabetes

Both the ADA Guidelines and Joslin's Guidelines are available online and are regularly updated.

This book is written with the hope that it will help you provide your patients with the best treatment plans and clinical practices, individualized to accommodate patient needs and to focus on the whole patient — not just on the patient's glucose levels, but on other metabolic functions, and other medical and psychosocial issues as well. We hope *Joslin's Diabetes Deskbook* serves you and your patients well.

1

Definition and Pathophysiology

Richard S. Beaser, MD

Introduction

Diabetes Mellitus is not really a single disorder, but rather a constellation of abnormalities of glucose homeostasis that is associated with significant acute and chronic complications. The need to control glucose levels — to attempt to bring them back to as near normal as possible — stems from growing evidence that doing so will reduce the likelihood that the person with this condition will get these associated complications, which themselves carry considerable morbidity and mortality. Thus, the comprehensive treatment of diabetes calls upon multiple disciplines within an internal medicine practice, in addition to surgical, psychiatric, and allied health expertise as well.

The challenge to be successful in the treatment of diabetes is great because of the significant personal and economic costs of suboptimal therapy. People who have diabetes are hospitalized one and one-half to three times more often than people who do not have it. Their risk of atherosclerotic disease is two to four times greater. The highest incidence of adult blindness, chronic renal failure, and nontraumatic amputations occurs among the diabetic population. Thus, the goal of diabetes treatment is not measured only in terms of blood glucose levels, it is reflected in a more global effort: to prevent, or at least attenuate, the effects of the chronic complications of this disease.

Evidence has shown that comprehensive care, including early diagnosis, aggressive glucose control targeting normoglycemia as closely as possible, management of other metabolic risk factors, and continual screening for, and prevention and treatment of complications, can make the course of diabetes smoother and maximize quality of life for patients with this condition. Acquiring knowledge that can lead to better care is not a luxury, but a necessity. Although a physician or diabetes educator can offer guidance during office or hospital visits, the person with diabetes must live with it 365 days a year and be prepared to cope constantly with the problems diabetes brings to everyday life. It is the challenge of engaging the patient as an active participant in his or her own treatment program that makes diabetes all the more challenging to the healthcare professional.

The challenge of diabetes treatment, both from the standpoint of the professional and the perspective of the patient, must encompass this more global view of care as well. Treatment must transcend glucose control to target complication prevention and risk-factor reduction. Succeeding with these multiple goals requires patient involvement in self-management, both controlling glucose levels and seeking appropriate preventive care to reduce factors that may increase complication risk such as obesity, hypertension, dyslipidemia, neglected foot care, and cigarette smoking. Success, therefore, involves significant lifestyle changes.

While the common thread among all people with diabetes is that their blood glucose level is higher than normal, the causes for this elevation can vary. Therefore, in order to understand the clinical approach to diabetes, it is important to first appreciate the multiple pathophysiological events that can cause the condition. Understanding the etiology, and being able to assess which etiologic factors are predominant in a given patient, makes the decision about treatment a logical next step.

Therefore, while a book such as this must be general in nature, it must also be specific enough to provide useful suggestions to the healthcare professional — certainly with regard to medical treatment, but also with regard to how to help the patient learn to improve his or her self-care. Diabetes is a very personal disease, and through education, patients can acquire the knowledge that leads to self-management, which, in turn, will allow them to successfully cope each day with their condition. For the person with diabetes, knowledge and understanding are not a part of treatment — they *are* the treatment.

Normal Glucose Homeostasis

In a person who does not have diabetes, glucose is normally present in the blood before meals at a level between 60 and 120 milligrams per deciliter (mg/dl). Glucose is the major source of the body's energy. The source of this glucose can be exogenous dietary glucose, usually in the form of complex carbohydrates (starches) as well as simple sugars. Glucose is ingested and is absorbed through the wall of the gastrointestinal tract and enters the bloodstream and travels to cells throughout the body. For glucose to pass through the cell membrane and enter the cell to provide energy, insulin is needed. This hormone is produced by the pancreas and attaches to *insulin receptors* located on the outer surfaces of cells. It can also come from glucose stored in liver and muscle as glycogen; the presence of glucose from this source is modulated by glucagon, also made in the pancreas.

The presence of glucose in the blood stream, particularly rising glucose levels after ingestion, stimulates the production and release of insulin. The oral ingestion of food also stimulates the release of glucagon-like polypeptide -1 (GLP-1), a hormone made in the ileum and colon. Receptors for GLP-1 are present in the pancreatic islets, and GLP-1 stimulates the secretion of insulin and the suppression of glucagon in response to the incoming food. These hormonal changes also help maintain normal glucose levels in the post-meal state by properly utilizing the incoming glucose and shutting down endogenous glucose production. GLP-1 receptors are also present in the central nervous system, and GLP-1 helps trigger satiety after food is ingested.

During this postprandial time, the interaction between insulin and its receptors triggers the influx of glucose into cells. After that immediate post-meal time, energy needs are also present. Glucose is stored in muscle and liver, and the balance between insulin and glucagon secretion maintains adequate energy supplies and normal glucose levels.

Any interruption at a number of steps in this normal glucose homeostatic mechanism, such as interruption of the pancreas' ability to produce insulin, reduced GLP-1 action, or derangement of insulin's ability to signal the cells to allow the glucose influx, can lead to hyperglycemia.

The Pancreas

The pancreas, an endocrine gland situated below and behind the stomach, weighs about half a pound and resembles an elongated cone lying on its side. The broad part, or head, is located next to a curve of the duodenum, the part of the small intestine just beyond the stomach. The pancreas tapers off to the left in the direction of the spleen and left kidney and ends in a portion known as the tail. Within the pancreas, especially at the tail, are the insulin-producing clusters of cells known as the islets of Langerhans. A normal pancreas contains about 100,000 such islets. Of the cell types found in these islets, it is the glucose-sensitive β-cells that are key to glucose homeostasis. These cells are capable of measuring the blood glucose level within seconds with an accuracy to within 2 mg/dl and then of determining the quantity of insulin needed. Each islet contains between 1000 and 2000 β-cells, and these cells, in aggregate, can rapidly secrete the precise amount of insulin required based on their measurement of the serum glucose level.

The typical insulin secretory pattern occurs in two phases. Phase one, usually occurring during the first 15 minutes after food ingestion, represents the secretion of previously manufactured insulin that was stored within the β-cell. Subsequently, the second phase, a longer, more sustained but less acute secretory pattern, represents the release of newly manufactured insulin.

The islets of Langerhans also produce other substances. For example, α-cells produce and release glucagon, which, as noted above and in contrast to insulin, causes blood glucose levels to rise through mobilization of glucose stores in liver and muscle. This careful balance between insulin and glucagon secretion and action maintains normal blood glucose levels. Somatostatin, gastrin, vasoactive intestinal peptide (VIP), and pancreatic polypeptide (PP) are also produced in the pancreas. There is ongoing research into the roles of these substances and how they influence diabetes. Hormones from the pituitary, adrenal, and thyroid glands also play a role, with an anti-insulin effect. Thus, glucose control in a normally functioning body actually reflects a balance among the actions of various hormones.

Insulin Production

Insulin is a protein. It consists of two chains of 51 amino acids, the "A" and "B" chains, held together by two disulfide bridges. Within the β-cell, insulin is manufactured in a multi-step process. In the step just prior to the final emergence of the complete insulin molecule, the precursor molecule is called proinsulin and is made up of the 51 amino acids of the future insulin molecule, plus 31 amino acids of the "connecting peptide" (or "C-peptide"). In the final manufacturing step, this C-peptide is cleaved off, leaving the remaining A and B chains of the insulin molecule. Insulin and C-peptide, in equal amounts, are packaged in secretory granules within the β-cell, waiting to be used. The C-peptide itself is not thought to play a significant role in glucose homeostasis, but is released by the β-cells into the circulation. The major significance of C-peptide is its use as a "marker" for endogenous insulin production.

When the β-cell senses a rise in glucose levels, it releases insulin in two phases. During the first phase, which is very rapid and occurs within the first 10 to15 minutes after eating, it releases the insulin that was made earlier and is already stored within the secretory granules. The second stage follows. The continued increase in the postprandial glucose level signals the nucleus of the β-cell where DNA coded for insulin production is located. This DNA receives the message that the blood glucose level is rising and begins to reproduce its code onto messenger RNA, which, in turn, signals the production of more insulin. Insulin release into the blood can actually begin even before the blood glucose level becomes elevated.

Food entering the digestive tract stimulates the release of insulin from the β-cells. This release depends on the amount and the type of food eaten. Carbohydrates are the most effective stimulators. The combined effects of hormones from the digestive tract and the increasing blood glucose level sustain the release and formation of insulin. Protein can also function as an insulin secretagogue. GLP-1 is also produced in response to the presence of food in the GI tract.

In people who do not have diabetes, it is almost impossible to raise the blood glucose level above normal, regardless of what is eaten, because the insulin reserve is plentiful and is secreted in exactly the correct amount. In fact, if a person were to be given a slow intravenous infusion of a 5% glucose solution into an arm, the levels of glucose in blood drawn from a vein in the other arm would most often be normal. The person without diabetes can normally manufacture and release as much as 0.5 to 0.7 units/kg body weight per day.

Normal Metabolism and Insulin Function

Although digestion of food actually begins with digestive enzymes in the saliva, most of the digestive enzymes are found in the stomach. Digestive enzymes break down carbohydrate, protein, and fat into glucose, amino acids, and fatty acids, respectively. These basic components of the food then move through the gastrointestinal tract and are absorbed through the wall of the gut over the next hour or two. Once these components pass through the gut wall, they are absorbed into the bloodstream and circulate throughout the body. The rate of nutrient absorption impacts the rate and intensity of the postprandial glucose rise, which are important considerations in assessing glucose metabolic abnormalities and selecting treatment for people with diabetes. This subject will be addressed in this context later in the book. All three of these components — glucose, amino acids, and fatty acids — have the potential of being metabolically converted into energy.

The primary metabolic pathway for the production of energy is the Krebs cycle, named after the biochemist who first described it, Hans Krebs. This cycle is probably present in most cells of the body. The resulting energy fuels our daily activities and bodily functions, with waste products of this process, carbon dioxide and water, disposed of by way of the kidneys and lungs.

As noted, insulin is of key importance in the regulation of glucose availability and its influx into the cells. By interacting with *insulin receptors* located on the outer surface of cells, insulin triggers the cellular uptake and storage of glucose, thus controlling its use as an energy source. Insulin also inhibits the natural tendency of some tissues to make (gluconeogenesis) or remake (glycogenolysis) glucose that returns to the bloodstream and raises glucose levels. Insulin's major effect is on skeletal muscle, a major depot for glucose. However, it also regulates glucose intake and output of other cells, such as those in the liver.

The Body's Fuels

The two main fuels that the body relies on for energy are glucose from carbohydrates and fatty acids from fats. Protein can also provide an alternative source of energy if glucose is in short supply. Because humans eat episodically during the day, the fuel supply comes in sporadically. Mechanisms exist for the fuel to be stored for use between feedings. It is useful to review why each of these energy sources is needed and how it is used.

Carbohydrates

Carbohydrate is found in most foods (vegetables, pastry, bread, potatoes, pasta, etc.) and is the primary source of energy for the body. As food is consumed, the carbohydrate is digested into its basic constituent, glucose, and absorbed into the bloodstream. At this point, the glucose may be used to provide for either immediate energy needs or can be stored in muscle or peripheral tissues (primarily muscle) for later use.

When stored, carbohydrate is usually found within cells in the form of glycogen. Insulin is required for this storage process to occur. The largest depot of glycogen is in skeletal muscle, while the most accessible storage source is the liver, which provides glucose in the event that it is needed rapidly to raise the blood glucose level.

The availability of glycogen as a source of "quick" energy is quite important. Suppose someone with diabetes has taken too much insulin and as a result experiences a hypoglycemic reaction. Even if the person does not eat extra food immediately, the blood glucose level will usually rise subsequently. This is called "rebound hyperglycemia" caused by the release of glycogen from storage in the liver. This release is triggered by the body's hormonal "counterregulatory" mechanism made up of epinephrine (adrenaline) and glucagon. Although all people without diabetes, and most people with diabetes, have this ability to bring blood glucose levels back up to a safe range, people with diabetes still should treat low blood glucose reactions by consuming concentrated carbohydrates. They shouldn't depend on the usual automatic mechanism always functioning well enough to keep out of trouble, as a significant hypoglycemic event can overwhelm the counterregulatory function.

Glycogen is also released when muscular exertion requires it for energy. Long-distance runners often eat large quantities of carbohydrate prior to a race to "load" their glycogen stores for the long run. Unfortunately, while the available glycogen storage space in muscle and liver is limited, the *unlimited* storage depot for all of the excess glucose that is consumed is the adipose (fat) cells! Insulin is involved in this mechanism as well, helping promote the change of the excess glucose into fat, which is deposited for long-term storage. As a result, there is a myth among patients and some healthcare professionals that insulin injections make you fat. Insulin doesn't make you fat — excess calories make you fat. Insulin only helps by doing its job, and this underscores the importance of proper balance between insulin, food consumption, and activity.

Protein

Dietary sources of protein (e.g., meat, cheese, and fish) are digested into amino acids, which then enter the circulation. Circulating amino acids can also stimulate pancreatic insulin secretion. While proteins provide structural integrity and are part of important body constituents such as enzymes, they can also be metabolized into energy in a process similar to the metabolism of glucose. Amino acids, converted to glucose in the liver and stored as glycogen, can eventually provide energy, or can be stored as fat for later use.

Fat

The third fuel for the human metabolism is fat, (e.g., oils from corn, peanuts, and olives, as well as fat in meat, fowl, butter, and other dairy products such as milk, cream, and cheese). These foods are digested into fatty acids in the intestine and absorbed into the bloodstream where they are used by the body. Some fats are called "essential fats." The body needs these for metabolism and they must be in the diet. Most fats, however, are either used for energy or stored in cells as triglycerides for later use. When other fuels are in short supply, such as during prolonged fasting, the level of insulin in the blood falls. The reduced level of circulating insulin promotes the removal of the fat from the storage depots and helps its entry into the circulation, where it is accessible by muscle and other organs for use as energy.

Fat is a very efficient form of energy storage, providing 9.5 kilocalories (kcal)/gram of triglyceride, as compared to 4 kcal/gram of carbohydrates or proteins, either directly or from glycogen. The byproducts of fat metabolism are ketones (acetone).

The Pathophysiology of Diabetes

Diabetes occurs when the blood glucose level is too high as a result of a deficiency of available, effective insulin or insulin action. This lack of insulin can be absolute, seen when the pancreas does not produce enough (or produces none at all). Alternatively, a lack of insulin action might be a relative insufficiency as seen in type 2 diabetes with insulin resistance. In this situation, the pancreas may produce "normal" or even above normal amounts of insulin. However, for those with type 2 diabetes, the body needs even more insulin to overcome insulin resistance, which is the hallmark of type 2 diabetes. Some people may have insulin resistance, but if their pancreases are able to make the additional insulin needed to overcome that resistance and produce normoglycemia, they do not have clinically apparent type 2 diabetes. However, if the pancreas cannot produce enough insulin to overcome the insulin resistance, then hyperglycemia, and thus type 2 diabetes, results. This condition of hyperglycemia and type 2 diabetes occurs in this early stage in the natural history of this process in spite of the fact that the patient is making more than a "normal" amount of insulin, because this hyperinsulinemia is still insufficient to overcome the insulin resistance. We call this "relative insulin insufficiency."

As time passes and β-cell numbers decline, so too does the ability to produce insulin. The patient's pathophysiology evolves from a state of hyperinsulinemia but relative insulin insufficiency, to one of absolute insulin insufficiency. In this latter stage, insulin secretory capacity is below that of someone who does not have diabetes.

People with type 2 diabetes also have decreased GLP-1 production from the GI tract, which contributes to excess glucagon, particularly in the postprandial state, when it should be suppressed in the face of an incoming carbohydrate load. The lack of appropriate glucagon suppression also contributes to the hyperglycemia of type 2 diabetes.

Regardless of the exact etiology of the defects in insulin action and quantity, and, for type 2 diabetes, GLP-1 production and glucagon production, the net effect is that the cells lack fuel, and the body suffers from a lack of energy. People with undiagnosed diabetes or diabetes that is not optimally controlled complain of weakness and tiredness, and a usually active young child may be tired or listless. The body interprets this cell starvation as a need for more food and triggers a sense of extreme hunger, called polyphagia. The glucose level in the blood rises because it is not used. At the same time, needing energy, the body turns to stored fuels — glycogen, fat, and protein — to try to meet its needs. Thus, as the level of glucose in the blood continues to rise due to the deficiency of insulin effect, so does the blood level of fats.

Excess glucose is removed from the body by the kidney. Normally, as blood circulates through the kidney, glucose from the glomerular filtrate is retained, rather than lost in the urine. There is a level of blood glucose, however, known as the renal threshold, above which the reabsorption capacity of the kidneys is overwhelmed, and the excess glucose escapes into the urine. Once this level (usually 160 to 180 mg/dl) is passed, glucose spillage appears in the urine. With significant hyperglycemia, a significant proportion of the body's incoming calories — as much as 200 grams (800 calories) daily — can be lost as urinary glucose.

An interesting historical footnote is appropriate here. In his second edition of the textbook *Treatment of Diabetes* in 1917 during World War I, long before the discovery of insulin, Dr. Elliott P. Joslin wrote, "It is desirable in peace, but a duty in war, for every diabetic patient to keep sugar-free. The food which the untreated diabetic patient wastes in a week would feed a soldier for a day.'" (Indeed, 5600 calories would do it!) This appears a bit far-fetched today, but tells of the desperation of physicians in the pre-insulin days as they tried to save their patients.

The effect of renal clearance of excess glucose via the urine results in an osmotic diuresis that, in turn, results in the classic symptoms of diabetes: glycosuria (much urine glucose), polyuria (much urine), and, due to the fluid loss and dehydration triggering of thirst, polydipsia (much drinking). If the diabetes is the result of significant absolute insulin deficiency (type 1 diabetes), this insulin deficiency allows fat cells to release fat as an alternative energy source, with the metabolic end-product of ketones being produced. Left untreated, these acidic ketones result in the potentially fatal condition of ketoacidosis (see Chapter 13).

Types of Diabetes

As noted previously, there are two etiologies for most cases of the disease: 1) an absolute insulin deficiency that causes type 1 diabetes, and 2) a relative deficiency of insulin that causes type 2 diabetes. In early cases of type 2 diabetes, where there may be an absolute excess of insulin, it is still insufficient to overcome the degree of insulin resistance present. These two causes account for most of the cases of diabetes seen in clinical practice.

In 1997, a panel of international experts was convened by the American Diabetes Association to review diabetes classifications, as well as the diagnostic criteria for this condition. A focus of the panel's attention was the nomenclature for the two diabetes types. Previous terminology referred to type 1 diabetes as *insulin-dependent diabetes mellitus (IDDM)* and to type 2 diabetes as *non-insulin-dependent diabetes mellitus (NIDDM)*. Much confusion had arisen due to this terminology that implied *treatment* as the basis of classification, rather than the underlying pathophysiology. Clearly, patients who have the pathophysiology characteristic of type 2 diabetes — insulin resistance and relative insulin insufficiency — may need exogenous insulin treatment.

The expert panel recommended a number of changes in the classification system with the goal being to make the classification of diabetes clearer. (It also made revisions in diagnostic criteria in order to make the identification of people with diabetes easier, and, hopefully, to allow diagnosis to be made earlier in the natural history of the disease.) In the process of updating the diabetes classifications, a number of changes were made by that 1997 panel, and subsequently updated in 2004 (see Table 1-1). The numbering system now uses Arabic numerals for types 1 and 2, replacing the previously-used Roman numerals. A new classification has been created called Impaired Fasting Glucose (IFG) to accommodate the new focus on using the fasting glucose level as the basis of diabetes diagnosis. The definition of IFG was subsequently modified in 2004, reducing the lower value from 110 mg/dl to 100 mg/dl (see Table 1-1)

While the two major types of diabetes, type 1 and type 2, differ in their underlying pathophysiology, both result in elevated glucose levels and, ultimately, both increase, to varying degrees, the risk of developing the same long-term complications (see Table 1-2).

Type 1 Diabetes

Type 1 diabetes results from the destruction of the insulin-producing β-cells in the pancreas. This destruction is probably mediated by autoantibodies to these cells through a process referred to as autoimmunity.

TABLE 1-1.   1997 Diabetes Classifications

Type 1 Diabetes:	Autoimmune and idiopathic etiologies
Type 2 Diabetes:	Insulin resistance and an insulin secretory defect
Gestational:	Onset or recognition during pregnancy
Impaired Glucose Tolerance (IGT):	Based on an oral glucose tolerance test (OGTT), 2-hour Sample $\geq$ 140 mg/dl and < 200 mg/dl
Impaired Fasting Glucose (IFG):	Fasting glucose $\geq$ 110 mg/dl but <126 mg/dl

The immune system, carrying out a function essential to good health, normally directs antibodies and white blood cells against foreign substances such as viruses. In persons with type 1 diabetes, this is present due to an autoimmune etiology; the target of the immune defenses is part of the body itself — the β-cells.

Speculation varies on what triggers the onset of this autoimmune phenomenon, but many feel that it may be induced by a viral stimulus. Others have suggested chemical toxins. When initiated, the presence of autoantibodies may serve as markers of the ongoing autoimmune process that is leading up to the development of type 1 diabetes. These autoantibodies include islet cell autoantibodies ("ICAs," autoantibodies against the (β-cells), insulin autoantibodies ("IAAs," autoantibodies against the insulin itself), antibodies to glutamic acid decarboxylase ("GAD"), and antibodies to the tyrosine phosphatases (IA-2 and IA-2B). The presence of these antibodies may predate the clinical manifestation of type 1 diabetes by many years. Once fasting hyperglycemia is present, up to 90% of patients with autoimmune type 1 diabetes have at least one of these antibodies present. Over time, after the diagnosis of type 1 diabetes, these antibody titers often decline. Detection of such antibodies in people who do not yet carry the diagnosis of diabetes may be predictive of a future diagnosis, and such people should be especially vigilant for signs or symptoms of diabetes. Research to develop means to stop the diabetes from occurring is ongoing.

Type 1 diabetes may also be associated with other conditions having autoimmune etiologies, such as Addison's disease, Hashomoto's thyroiditis, Graves' disease, vitiligo, and pernicious anemia.

TABLE 1-2. Comparison of Type 1 and Type 2 Diabetes

Item	Type 1 Diabetes	Type 2 Diabetes
Percentage of people with diabetes	10%	90%
Former names	Juvenile diabetes, Brittle diabetes Insulin-dependent diabetes, type I diabetes	Adult-onset diabetes Stable diabetes Non-insulin-dependent diabetes, type II diabetes
Age of discovery	Usually below 40 years, but not always	Usually over 40, but not always
Condition when discovered	Usually moderately to severely ill	Often not ill at all, or having mild symptoms
Cause of diabetes	Reduced or absent insulin production	Insulin resistance and relative or absolute insulin secretory deficiency. Also, lack of glucagon suppression.
Insulin level	None to small amounts	Markedly elevated early — somewhat decreased later
Weight	Often thin or normal weight, often losing weight at diagnosis	Usually overweight, but 20% are normal weight
Acute complications	Ketoacidosis	Non-ketotic hyperosmolar hyperglycemic coma; Usually not prone to ketoacidosis
Usual treatment	Insulin, meal plan, exercise	Diet, exercise, if needed, antidiabetes medications, insulin

Other non-autoimmune causes of β-cell destruction can lead to type 1 diabetes as well. These include conditions associated with the destruction of the pancreas or its cells, such as pancreatic cancer, pancreatitis, or the removal of the pancreas by surgery. In addition, idiopathic diabetes, with no known etiology, can lead to significant insulinopenia and a risk of ketoacidosis. This form shows no evidence of autoimmunity, shows a strong inheritance pattern, and is more common in people of Asian or African origin.

Most often the person with autoimmune type 1 diabetes is young, and the clinical onset is fairly rapid — occurring over a period of a few days or weeks. However, some older individuals can also develop type 1 diabetes, though it usually has a much slower onset among this age group. In fact, type 1 diabetes in an older individual may initially resemble the clinical picture of type 2 diabetes. As aging can cause insulin resistance, and because the destruction of the β-cells occurs more slowly in an older person, an apparent misclassification on clinical grounds is common. Some have advocated performing tests to measure C-peptide in an attempt to more precisely gauge the degree of insulin secretory capacity that remains, and thus make the proper classification. However, in cases in which the classification is in doubt based on clinical characteristics, the C-peptide levels will usually be equivocal as well. Ultimately, the diagnosis should be based on clinical impressions. With regard to a patient for whom an incorrect classification is made — leading to a treatment that might ultimately be wrong based on the evolution of the underlying pathophysiology — clinical signs and symptoms will eventually make the true pathophysiology clear, leading the observant clinician to make the proper treatment adjustments.

While both types of diabetes can present with weight loss, people with type 1 diabetes tend to be at or below their "ideal" body weight at the onset of diabetes, and may lose even more weight rapidly with the onset of hyperglycemia. Nevertheless, obesity does not rule out the presence of type 1 diabetes. Ketonuria due to absolute insulin deficiency, accompanied by significant hyperglycemia, can be a clue that type 1 diabetes is the actual diagnosis. However, to further confuse things, some people present with ketoacidosis initially, but end up with a diagnosis of type 2 diabetes, treated with antidiabetes medications. This is referred to as "Flatbush Diabetes" as it was first described in Brooklyn. The best advice is to make the best diagnosis initially, treat accordingly, but watch carefully to make sure that you have not been fooled.

Type 2 Diabetes

About 90% of all people with diabetes have type 2 diabetes, which is, in reality, a spectrum of abnormalities involving glucose metabolism as well as other metabolic processes. Insulin resistance is the pathophysiologic hallmark of this condition, usually reflected primarily in liver and peripheral tissue (primarily muscle and adipose). With insulin resistance, increased amounts of insulin may be required to achieve a given hypoglycemic effect. Early in the natural history of type 2 diabetes, the pancreas may be able to produce this increased insulin quantity, and many people with this condition become hyperinsulinemic. Initially, the hyperinsulinemia may be able to compensate for the insulin resistance. Thus, some patients with insulin resistance may not meet the diagnostic criteria for diabetes because of this ability to compensate by secreting increased amounts of insulin. Over time, the numbers of β-cells often decline, and the hyperinsulinemia may be insufficient to overcome the insulin resistance, and clinical diabetes may be diagnosed. The natural history of this condition often leads to eventual hypoinsulinemia. Thus, insulin production in people with type 2 diabetes is referred to as "relative" insufficiency: the body does produce some insulin, sometimes quite a lot, but the need for insulin is so increased that production cannot keep up with the need. Further compounding things, of course, is the inability to suppress glucagon secretion, particularly in the postprandial state, which further promotes glucose production from muscle and liver. Succinctly described, type 2 diabetes represents insulin resistance accompanied by relative or absolute insulin deficiency, compounded by inadequate glucagon suppression.

A person with type 2 diabetes, therefore, has the potential for a variety of pathophysiologic abnormalities, ranging on the spectrum from predominant insulin resistance and relative insulin secretory insufficiency to predominant insulin secretory insufficiency with absolute reductions in insulin production, or anywhere in between. When pharmacologic treatment becomes necessary, selection will depend on the underlying predominant abnormality — insulin resistance would suggest certain antidiabetes medications, while insulin secretory insufficiency would suggest other antidiabetes medications that promote insulin secretion (and some may also help suppress glucagons), or perhaps insulin replacement therapy. However, in reality, when glucose metabolic abnormalities become manifest, insulin resistance, β-cell deficiencies, and abnormal glucagon suppression are all present. Thus, the current treatment trend is early combination pharmacotherapy to address these multiple defects.

However, type 2 diabetes should not be viewed only from the perspective of its impact on glucose metabolism. It is part of a constellation of abnormalities including hypertension, dyslipidemia, hypercoagulability, and abdominal obesity referred to as the "metabolic syndrome." This will be discussed further in Chapter 7.

People with type 2 diabetes are usually above their ideal body weight. Obesity itself contributes to insulin resistance, and, typically, the distribution of the obesity in patients with type 2 diabetes is abdominal. Chapter 4 will discuss in more detail the role of obesity and adipose tissue in the etiology of type 2 diabetes and the other metabolic abnormalities that contribute to increased vascular risk. Type 2 diabetes may present with the "classic" symptoms similar to those of the person with type 1 diabetes. Since some insulin is usually present, ketoacidosis is not usually present on diagnosis unless another significant precipitating stress or other circumstances complicate the presentation. The exception is the "Flatbush Diabetes" described in the previous section, where people present with ketoacidosis, but eventually turn out to have type 2 diabetes.

More commonly, however, people with type 2 diabetes are without symptoms altogether. It has been estimated that one-third of all people who actually have diabetes do not know that they have it because it has been asymptomatic and they have not been properly screened. Such people often have their diabetes diagnosed as a result of an elevated glucose level on a routine blood screening test, or, unfortunately, when they have a complication of diabetes as the initial, presenting finding.

Other Types of Diabetes

In addition to the two most common types of diabetes described above, the ADA's etiologic classification of diabetes mellitus lists other specific types (see Table 1-3). For example, while most people diagnosed as having type 2 diabetes are over age 40, there is an epidemic of obesity and therefore there is also type 2 diabetes among younger individuals. Some younger people also have what may seem clinically like type 2 diabetes, referred to as maturity-onset diabetes of the young (MODY), which represents one of the genetic defects of β-cell function. These patients tend to have impairment of insulin secretory response and relatively normal insulin action. Other genetic mutations leading to insulin secretory defects have also been described. Similarly, genetic abnormalities leading to insulin action defects can occur with varying degrees of clinical severity.

Other categories of diabetes include diseases of the exocrine pancreas, endocrinopathies (drug or chemical induced), infections, and other immune or genetic conditions.

Impaired Glucose Tolerance (IGT) and Impaired Fasting Glucose (IFG)

Historically, the category of impaired glucose tolerance (IGT) reflected what was often referred to in lay parlance as "borderline diabetes." In the revised classification system, these categories (IGT and IFG) represent stages between normal glucose homeostasis and diabetes. From an epidemiologic standpoint, these two conditions are not so much a "disease" as they represent increased risk for development of future diabetes, as well as being risk factors for macrovascular disease because of their association with the insulin resistance syndrome. Most individuals with IGT or IFT appear to be normoglycemic when tested routinely. Studies, particularly the Diabetes Prevention Program (DPP) for type 2 diabetes, are examining the exact nature and degree of risk conferred by IGT and IFT. Results announced in 2001 suggest that appropriate nutrition and exercise, as well as the drug metformin, can reduce the risk of progressing on to type 2 diabetes. There are phenotypic differences between these two abnormalities that will be discussed in detail in Chapter 2.

Gestational Diabetes Mellitus (GDM)

Gestational diabetes mellitus (GDM) represents any abnormality of glucose homeostasis that is diagnosed or has its onset during pregnancy. It may reflect a coincidental development of type 1 diabetes at the time of pregnancy, or the manifestation of a potential for type 2 diabetes that is made clinically apparent due to the physiologic stress of pregnancy. Clearly, for this latter group in particular, the glucose metabolic abnormality may have been present prior to pregnancy, but not detected. Six weeks postpartum, women should be reclassified as to the diabetes type present, IGT or IFG, or normal. A further discussion of GDM may be found in Chapter 20.

Epidemiology of Diabetes

There are multiple factors that can influence the risk of developing diabetes, and it is therefore not surprising that it is such a common disease. In fact, if one looks beyond those with diagnosed diabetes (most commonly type 2 diabetes) to all those with other manifestations of the insulin

TABLE 1-3. Etiologic Classification of Diabetes Mellitus

I. Type 1 diabetes* (β-cell destruction, usually leading to absolute insulin deficiency)
   A. Immune-mediated
   B. Idiopathic
II. Type 2 diabetes* (may range from predominantly insulin resistance with relative insulin deficiency to a predominantly secretory defect with insulin resistance)
III. Other specific types
   A. Genetic defects of β-cell function
      1. Chromosome 12, HNF-1α (MODY3)
      2. Chromosome 7, glucokinase (MODY2)
      3. Chromosome 20, HNF-4α (MODY 1)
      4. Chromosome 13, insulin promoter factor-1 (IPF-1; MODY 4)
      5. Chromosome 17, HNF-1β (MODY 5)
      6. Chromosome 2, *NeuroD1* (MODY 6)
   B. Genetic defects in insulin action
      1. Type A insulin resistance
      2. Leprechaunism
      3. Rabson-Mendenhall syndrome
      4. Lipoatrophic diabetes
      5. Others
   C. Diseases of the exocrine pancreas
      1. Pancreatitis
      2. Trauma/pancreatectomy
      3. Neoplasia
      4. Cystic fibrosis
      5. Hemochromatosis
      6. Fibrocalculous pancreatopathy
      7. Others
   D. Endocrinopathies
      1. Acromegaly
      2. Cushing's syndrome
      3. Glucagonoma
      4. Pheochromocytoma
      5. Hyperthyroidism
      6. Somatostatinoma
      7. Aldosteronoma
      8. Others
   E. Drug- or chemical-induced
      1. Vacor
      2. Pentamidine
      3. Nicotinic acid
      4. Glucocorticoids
      5. Thyroid hormone
      6. Diazoxide
      7. β-adrenergic agonists
      8. Thiazides
      9. Dilantin
      10. α-interferon
      11. Others
   F. Infections
      1. Congenital rubella
      2. Cytomegalovirus
      3. Others
   G. Uncommon forms of immune-mediated diabetes
      1. "Stiff-man" syndrome
      2. Anti-insulin receptor antibodies
      3. Others
   H. Other genetic syndromes sometimes associated with diabetes
      1. Down's syndrome
      2. Klinefelter's syndrome
      3. Turner's syndrome
      4. Wolfram's syndrome
      5. Friedreich's ataxia
      6. Huntington's chorea
      7. Laurence-Moon-Biedl syndrome
      8. Myotonic dystrophy
      9. Porphyria
      10. Prader-Willi syndrome
      11. Others
IV. Gestational diabetes mellitus (GDM)

*Patients with any form of diabetes may require insulin treatment at some stage of the disease. Such use of insulin does not, of itself, classify the patient.

resistance syndrome, including dyslipidemia, hypertension, and frank macrovascular disease, who have not yet developed glucose abnormalities, it may be even more prevalent than people realize.

Diagnosed diabetes affects over 7% of the population. However, the prevalence varies significantly according to racial and ethnic groups as will be discussed in more detail in Chapter 24. For example, based on data from the Third National Health and Nutrition Examination Survey (NHANES III), conducted between 1988 and 1994, among people aged 40 to 74 years, the prevalence of diabetes and undiagnosed diabetes, for key groups, showed:

	Diabetes	Undiagnosed Diabetes
• Non-Hispanic whites	8.7%	4.0%
• African Americans	13.3%	5.6%
• Mexican Americans	14.8%	6.6%

With respect to the "prediabetes" abnormalities, the prevalence of impaired fasting glucose and impaired glucose tolerance showed:

- 9.7% had impaired fasting glucose (fasting glucose 110–125 mg/dl)
- 15.6% had impaired glucose tolerance (fasting glucose β140 mg/dl, 2-hour glucose 140–199 mg/dl)

Considering the growing concern that these people may be at higher risk for both diabetes and its macrovascular sequellae than had previously been thought, clearly this condition may have wide-reaching implications.

As type 2 diabetes is the predominant form of diabetes, and aging is known to increase insulin resistance, it is not surprising that the prevalence of diabetes increases as people age:

- Age 18–44 years: 1.5%
- Age 45–64 years: 6%
- 65 years or over: 11%

Heredity

It has been known for a long time that heredity is involved in causing diabetes, as the familial prevalence of the disease is clearly evident. However, the risks of developing diabetes differ between type 1 and type 2. For example, the risk for developing concordance among identical twins runs about 90% with type 2 diabetes and about 50% with type 1 diabetes. Multiple genes probably play a role, as the pattern is inconsistent with single gene inheritance.

Studies have suggested a link between the development of type 1 diabetes and the presence of specific HLA types. (HLA, or human lymphocyte antigens, are found on chromosome 6, resulting in recognizable, unique cell surface markers that can be used to determine tissue types). Other antigens may also be involved. The picture is less clear for type 2 diabetes. From the perspective of the general population, the risk for developing type 1 diabetes is 0.3% at age 20, and 0.5% at age 50. Children of fathers with diabetes have a 6% chance of developing diabetes by age 20, while for offspring of mothers with diabetes, the risk is only 2%. Interestingly, for offspring of mothers who develop diabetes *after* the birth of the child, the risk is, as with fathers, 6%. Conversely, the risk to a child who has a mother with type 1 is less when the child is born after the mother is age 25. The risk of developing diabetes by age 50 if one has a sibling with type 1 is about 10%.

For *all* people getting type 2 diabetes, 20% of those people will develop it before the age of 40, 40% between the ages of 40 and 60, and 40% after the age of 60. People with parents having type 1 have about a 25% to 30% chance of developing type 1 and are more likely to develop it at a younger age. Making studies of the risk of developing type 1 more difficult, however, is the likelihood that other factors, particularly obesity, influence the incidence of diabetes beyond just genetic determinants. Offspring of two parents with type 1 may have a risk of developing diabetes that approaches 50% or more.

While studies of both types of diabetes in identical twins suggest a definite genetic link, it is not absolute. The current theory is that there are many factors that can predispose to diabetes, suggesting that multiple genes may be involved. Possibly a genetic trait making the individual susceptible to some external factor, such as a virus, might precipitate the development of diabetes.

One factor that makes study difficult is that we don't always know the details about our ancestors' medical problems. A study in Oxford, Massachusetts of all people with diagnosed diabetes showed that only 25% knew of relatives with diabetes at the start of the study, but after 15 years, because of an increased awareness of diabetes in the community, nearly 80% of them knew or had heard of some relative who had diabetes, either previously undiagnosed, simply unknown, or developed after the initial interview.

Viruses

The possibility that viruses may help cause diabetes has long been considered. In 1864, a Norwegian scientist reported that a patient developed diabetes following a mumps infection. More recently, a study reported that in Sweden the onset of diabetes following a mumps epidemic was greater than expected. English scientists have found in children a relationship between diabetes and a strain of viruses known as "coxsackie." Diagnoses of diabetes, along with virus infections, are more frequent during the winter months than summer. In studies of this diabetes/virus association, the British Diabetic Association reported an increased incidence of new cases of type 1 diabetes at about 4 to 5 years of age and even more at ages 12 to 13. It noted that at these ages the children received heavy exposure to various viruses as they started primary and secondary schools, respectively.

The mechanism by which viruses are involved in the onset of type 1 diabetes has been debated. They may trigger the autoimmune process itself in genetically predisposed individuals. However, for this to be the case, one would have to seek the exposure to the offending virus a number of years prior to the time of diagnosis, not just immediately preceding it. Indeed, some have suggested that the process may resemble that of HIV infectivity, with the diabetogenic virus initiating an autoimmune attack of a number of years' duration, in this instance on the β-cell.

Abdominal Obesity

Abdominal Obesity is a significant etiologic factor for type 2 diabetes. When superimposed on a hereditary predisposition for type 2 diabetes, as well as a hereditary predisposition for abdominal obesity itself, the additional pounds of adipose increase the insulin resistance that is a key pathophysiologic component. Of concern in recent years is that environment is further contributing to a tendency toward obesity — particularly in young people. The increasing preference of computer and video games over physical activities is resulting in an epidemic of obesity that extends into adulthood. The role of obesity in the etiology of diabetes will be discussed in more detail in Chapter 4.

Aging

Type 2 diabetes seems to be more common after age 40. In most people, glucose tolerance declines with aging. The relationship between diabetes and age will be discussed further in Chapter 22.

Diet

Diet has been discussed in many contexts: the changes in diets of many ethnic groups as they become "Westernized" can contribute to an increased incidence of type 2 diabetes, as well as to other related disorders. Higher caloric intake and the increased fat content of these meals are etiologic factors. Reduced fiber has also been suggested as a factor, as high-fiber diets seem to reduce the incidence of diabetes.

Hormones

Conditions leading to changes in the levels of various hormones, including the pituitary, thyroid, and sex hormones, can increase glucose intolerance. For example, excess pituitary growth hormone, as seen in acromegaly, counteracts insulin's effects and produces a diabetic-like state. Cortisol excess, as part of conditions such as Cushing's disease, has a similar effect. Glucagon-secreting tumors (glucagonomas) cause glucose elevations as well.

Circadian variations in hormone levels can affect glucose metabolism. An increase of growth hormone during the latter part of the sleep cycle results in a need for increased amounts of insulin just before awakening. This is known as the "dawn phenomenon" and causes difficulty in fasting glucose regulation of a person with either type of diabetes. This phenomenon is particularly noticeable in people with type 1 diabetes who are closely regulating their glucose control by using an intensive treatment program. Other hormones such as somatostatin can affect both insulin and glucagon levels.

Therefore, when treating patients with diabetes where the clinical setting suggests that these other conditions may be present, be sure to screen for them or even make aggressive efforts to rule them out.

Drugs and Medications

Many medications can also have adverse effects on glucose metabolism. While medications are not usually a true etiologic factor for diabetes, they can unmask less obvious glucose intolerance that had not yet been detected.

Diuretics are one type of medication that is commonly blamed for "causing" diabetes. When used for hypertension therapy in people with diabetes, they may cause worsening of glucose control, probably facilitated by a loss of potassium. Often, maintaining proper potassium replacement will ameliorate some of the diuretic-induced glucose intolerance. For a time in the past, the use of diuretics by people with diabetes declined due to concern over the problem of worsened glucose intolerance, but recently diuretic use, in moderate doses, and often in combination with other medications such as ACE-inhibitors, has returned as a reasonable tool in the treatment of hypertension in people with diabetes.

Other medications also can affect glucose metabolism or even unmask undiagnosed diabetes, but usually the importance of using them outweighs the concerns over glucose control, particularly if the glucose control medication can be adjusted to compensate. The medications that classically cause the worst deterioration of control are the corticosteroids, but fortunately such treatments are usually for finite periods of time.

Illness, Injury, and Stress

The stress resulting from illness or injury can result in elevations of glucose levels. The probable mechanism is an increase in insulin resistance brought on by the physical stress. Patients who are at high risk for diabetes should be carefully monitored during any illness or injury that could potentially lead to glucose intolerance.

As with medication use, the stress of illness or injury does not usually *cause* the diabetes to occur as a direct etiologic factor as much as it unmasks undiagnosed glucose intolerance. Those with litigious ideation following an accident, take heed! It is the rare accidental event that causes diabetes where it otherwise would not have been present. Note, too, that

the diagnosis of diabetes slightly earlier than otherwise would have occurred and the "burden" of needing therapy sooner may not necessarily
be such a bad thing. With the incidence of undiagnosed diabetes that is
nevertheless taking its toll on the development of macrovascular complications, the plaintiff should probably be thankful that, due to the "accidental" diagnosis of this condition, he or she was started on therapy
sooner rather than later!

Chronic mental stress probably does not cause much of a direct elevation in blood glucose levels, although it is often blamed. More often,
chronic stress is a distraction and is often an excuse or reason for not properly caring for the diabetes. Acute stress, such as the death of a loved one
or loss of a job, can unmask diabetes, but is not a direct cause.

2

The Approach to Diagnosis and Treatment

Richard S. Beaser, MD

Diagnosing Diabetes

The first challenge in treating diabetes is making the diagnosis. This may sound like an obvious statement until you realize that about one-third of all people who actually have diabetes have not yet been diagnosed. Most of these, of course, have type 2 diabetes, which can develop insidiously and have such subtle onset of symptoms that they are hardly noticed or are blamed on something else. Yet, by the time of diagnosis, the disease has had a head start in causing the chronic complications of diabetes. For this reason, the expert panel convened by the American Diabetes Association that reported revisions of the diagnostic classifications of diabetes in 1997 (discussed in Chapter 1) revised the diagnostic criteria for diabetes as well. The panel's goal was to make diabetes easier to diagnose, and thus more likely to *be* diagnosed. These diagnostic changes are based on epidemiologic data from the last several decades. The panel emphasized that using these criteria will not result in more people *having* diabetes, but it will result in more people who have the disease being discovered. The public health implications of complication reduction effected by early detection of diabetes and the initiation of effective treatment could be substantial.

Revised Diagnostic Criteria

The revised diagnostic criteria for diabetes are summarized in Table 2-1. The current recommended method for diagnosing diabetes is to use the venous fasting glucose level. Based on this measurement, **diabetes is defined as a glucose level >126 mg/dl, confirmed on repeat determination.** A "casual" (new terminology replacing "random") glucose level ≥200 mg/dl in the presence of classic symptoms would also make the diagnosis. The traditional oral glucose tolerance test (OGTT) is also still valid; however, as it is cumbersome to perform, it is not needed if a patient meets other criteria. Usually, an OGTT would be indicated if diabetes is strongly suspected and other test results are equivocal.

Fingerstick glucose measurement should not be used to diagnose diabetes. Also, urine testing should not be used to either diagnose or screen for diabetes. Blood glucose levels could be high enough to represent diabetes, but glycosuria may not be present due to a high renal threshold. Conversely, the presence of glucose in the urine without elevated blood glucose is not diagnostic for diabetes. Renal glycosuria, with the presence of urinary glucose but normal blood glucose levels, can be common in children. If glucose in the urine is detected, blood testing should be done.

Included in the ADA's 1997 recommendations were a revised listing of high-risk individuals and diabetes screening guidelines. Also included were new criteria for screening pregnant women (see Chapter 20). These guidelines will eliminate the need to evaluate women at low risk for gestational diabetes.

Screening

A patient suspected of having diabetes can be screened using the fasting plasma glucose test or an OGTT following a 75-gram glucose load (see Table 2-2). The ADA recommends using the fasting plasma glucose test because of its simplicity. A glucose value of ≥126 mg/dl after an 8-hour fast is diagnostic for diabetes if it can be confirmed by a similarly elevated value on a different day. The conditions of *impaired fasting glucose*

TABLE 2-1.   Categories of Diabetes Based on Diagnostic Criteria

Normal	Fasting plasma glucose <100 mg/dl (5.6 mmol/l) and Oral glucose tolerance test: 2-hour post-load glucose <140 gm/dl (7.8 mmol/l)
Impaired Fasting Glucose	Fasting plasma glucose ≥100 mg/dl (5.6 mmol/l) and <126 mg/dl (6.9 mol/l)
Impaired Glucose Tolerance	Oral glucose tolerance test: 2-hour post-load glucose ≥140 gm/dl (7.8 mmol/l) and <200 mg/dl (11.1 mmol/l)

Diabetes:	Symptoms of diabetes plus casual plasma glucose concentration ≥200 mg/dl (11.1 mmol/l). Casual is defined as any time of day without regard to time since last meal. The classic symptoms of diabetes include polyuria, polydipsia, and unexplained weight loss.
	      or
	Fasting plasma glucose ≥126 mg/dl (7.0 mmol/l). Fasting is defined as no caloric intake for at least 8 hours.
	      or
	2-hour plasma glucose ≥200 mg/dl (11.1 mmol/l) during an oral glucose tolerance test. The test should be performed as described by WHO, using a glucose load containing the equivalent of 75-grams of anhydrous glucose dissolved in water.
	
	A confirmatory fasting plasma glucose or two-hour glucose tolerance test should be done before the diagnosis is made.

NOTE: For diagnosis, do not use:
          Finger-stick blood glucose test or A1C

and *impaired glucose tolerance* are classified as "Pre-Diabetes" and are considered risk factors for future diabetes and for cardiovascular disease.

The benefits of community screening have also been debated for some time, with many arguing against the cost-effectiveness of this practice. In its position statement on Screening for Type 2 Diabetes, the ADA states that there is "insufficient evidence to conclude that community screening is a cost-effective approach to reduce the morbidity and mortality associated with diabetes in presumably healthy individuals. While community

TABLE 2-2.   How to Conduct an Oral Glucose Tolerance Test

For 3 days prior to the test, the patient should consume over 150 grams of carbohydrate daily, maintaining his or her usual amount of physical activity. (If carbohydrates are restricted or the OGTT is performed on a bedridden patient, the test may have a false-positive result.)

- The patient presents fasting, and a blood sample is drawn for determination of plasma glucose level. If the fasting sample is ≥126 mg/dl, then the diagnosis of diabetes is made and sampling at 2 hours is not necessary.
- The patient then consumes 75 grams of glucose in 250 to 300 ml of water over a period of 5 minutes. For children, the glucose load should be 1.75 grams/kg of body weight, up to a maximum of 75 grams of glucose.
- Blood samples should be collected at 2 hours post-glucose load in a tube containing sodium fluoride (6 mg/ml of whole blood) and centrifuged to separate out the plasma. Plasma should be frozen if the glucose measurement is not performed immediately.

To diagnose diabetes, a 2-hour OGTT is usually recommended. Table 2-1 lists the results that are normal, that diagnose impaired glucose tolerance, and that diagnose diabetes.

screening programs may provide a means to enhance public awareness of the seriousness of diabetes and its complications, other less costly approaches may be more appropriate particularly because the potential risks are poorly defined. Thus, based on the lack of scientific evidence, community screening for diabetes, even in high-risk populations, is not recommended." (ADA Position Statement; *Diabetes Care* 27 (Suppl 1):S13, 2004)

New Diagnostic Criteria vs. Old

The new diagnostic criteria are based on data suggesting that a fasting glucose ≥126 mg/dl is associated with an increased risk of microvascular complications, particularly retinopathy. Recently, however, concerns have been raised as to whether this pattern of glucose abnormality — the elevation of fasting glucose level — is really an appropriate means of

TABLE 2-3. ADA Criteria for Testing for Diabetes in Asymptomatic Adult Individuals

- Testing for diabetes should be considered in all high-risk individuals at age 45[†] years and above, particularly in those with a BMI ≥25 kg/m2*, and, if normal, should be repeated at 3-year intervals.
- Testing should be considered at a younger age or be carried out more frequently in individuals who are overweight (BMI ≥25 kg/m2*) and have additional risk factors:
  - Are habitually physically inactive
  - Have a first-degree relative with diabetes
  - Are members of a high-risk ethnic population (e.g., African-American, Latino, Native American, Asian American, Pacific Islander)
  - Have delivered a baby weighing >9lbs or have been diagnosed with GDM
  - Are hypertensive (>140/90 mm/Hg)
  - Have an HDL cholesterol level <35 mg/dl (0.90 mmol/l) and/or a triglyceride level >250 mg/dl (2.82 mmol/l).
  - Have Polycistic ovarian syndrome (PCOS)
  - On previous testing, had IGT or IFG
  - Have other clinical conditions associated with insulin resistance (e.g. PCOS or acanthosis nigricans)
  - Have a history of vascular disease

* May not be correct for all ethnic groups.

determining who is at increased risk for *macrovascular* disease, a significant complication seen in people with type 2 diabetes.

It is known that people with early type 2 diabetes lose their first-phase (early) insulin release. They also cannot suppress glucagon secretion, and thus have more glucose production from muscle and liver. These conditions contribute to a more pronounced postprandial glucose elevation early in the natural history of this multifactoral metabolic disease. Several studies such as the "DECODE" and "Funagata" studies have demonstrated that the presence of postprandial glucose abnormalities reflects a more significant risk for macrovascular disease. This postprandial elevation would reflect itself in the category of impaired glucose tolerance

(IGT), which was part of the old diagnostic categorizations, and not in the newer classification of impaired fasting glucose (IFG). Similarly, a casual glucose level obtained a number of hours postprandially might not reflect the degree of hyperglycemia that might be seen in the same patient during a formal OGTT. A normal casual glucose level could thus give false reassurance that diabetes, either current or future risk, or increased macrovascular risk are not present.

Since these new criteria were established, there has been much discussion about how to reconcile the fact that the new criteria may be easier to use for screening, but the OGTT and the older category of IGT may more effectively reflect macrovascular risk. Yet the argument has been made by members of that ADA expert panel that the risk for the microvascular complications of diabetes are more clearly associated with glycemic control *alone* and thus are a more appropriate yardstick against which to define the presence of diabetes. Hence, the new criteria are appropriate from this perspective.

Nevertheless, most acknowledge that macrovascular risk, while not as clearly and demonstrably related *alone* to hyperglycemia, clearly is *associated* with hyperglycemia, as well as with a number of other related and accompanying conditions such as dyslipidemia, hypertension, and hypercoagulability. Reducing the risk brought on by hyperglycemia as well as by those other metabolic conditions are all important objectives of a comprehensive treatment plan for type 2 diabetes. At the time of this writing, there is an ongoing discussion about refining the criteria for increased risk — the "metabolic syndrome" — and considering other factors such as abdominal adiposity in the consideration of risk stratification. Therefore, identification of people at increased risk for macrovascular disease, who thus may have any of the recognized risk factors present, is as important as diagnosing diabetes itself — which is just one on that list of risks.

Pending any revisions of the recommendations, it is clear that those with high-risk characteristics listed in Table 2-3 should not be ignored just because their fasting glucose is below 100 mg/dl. High-risk characteristics, regardless of glucose metabolic status, should trigger screening for other risk factors such as lipid disorders or hypertension, and antiplatelet therapy should be considered. Certainly, those patients who already have impaired fasting glucose (fasting plasma glucose 100–125 mg/dl), particularly if they have other high-risk characteristics, but even if they do not, should probably be considered for oral glucose tolerance testing to gauge the postprandial glucose pattern, and thus implicitly both the macro-vascular risk and the likelihood of progression on to true diabetes.

Symptoms of Diabetes

Diabetes has been referred to as "the great imitator," as it can present with varied symptoms and problems. **With significant hyperglycemia, however, the classic symptoms — including the "polys": polyuria (frequent urination), polydipsia (frequent consumption of liquids), and polyphagia (increased consumption of food), as well as weight loss, blurred vision, and fatigue — usually become manifest.** Onset of type 1 diabetes is usually more rapid than that of type 2 diabetes. Yet, the rate of beta-cell destruction can vary, tending to be more rapid in infants and children and slower in adults. Ketoacidosis may be present on presentation, particularly in those with rapid onset. However, in the adults, who may have residual beta-cell function for some time, this mode of presentation is much less likely. Extremely slow onset can lead to the mistaken assumption that the patient has type 2 diabetes.

Because type 2 diabetes usually develops more slowly, it may lead to insidious development of barely noticeable symptoms. The fact that one-third of all people who actually have diabetes have not yet been diagnosed is not surprising — these symptoms can often be missed. Therefore, it is important to be aware of signs and symptoms that might suggest underlying diabetes and thus lead to the proper diagnosis. Such symptoms themselves may develop gradually and often go unnoticed for considerable periods of time. Alternatively, with the rapid onset of type 1 diabetes, some signs and symptoms may appear abruptly and rapidly increase in severity. Either way, once symptoms are recognized, testing for the presence of diabetes should be performed and treatment, if the diagnosis is made, should begin.

Other signs and symptoms suggestive of diabetes include:

Skin Symptoms. Diabetes classically has been thought to produce itching of the skin, usually in the genital (especially vaginal) or anal areas. This can cause severe discomfort. Carbuncles, furuncles, and

difficulty in healing wounds also may be found. People with untreated diabetes may have very high levels of lipids in the blood,
which may cause small, raised bumps on the skin called xanthomas.
Usually, such symptoms represent significant elevations of glucose
levels that have been present for some time.

Gynecological Problems. Women with diabetes are prone to developing the fungal infections candidasis or moniliasis when their glucose
levels are not well-controlled. This may result in pruritis of the va-
gina, sometimes accompanied by a chronic discharge. Unfortunately,
it is not unheard of for a gynecologist to be the first to discover signs
of diabetes.

Impotence. Diabetes can lead to erectile dysfunction. While this is a
form of diabetic neuropathy that usually occurs after diabetes has
been present for some time, undiagnosed, and thus untreated, diabetes can hasten the development of this complication (see Chapter 19).

Testosterone Levels. The association of low testosterone levels in men
with type 2 diabetes and/or the metabolic syndrome has also been
described recently, and monitoring of testosterone levels may be warranted, with consideration of replacement therapy if indicated based
on symptoms and other safety considerations.

Neuropathies. The development of diabetic neuropathic symptoms
usually occurs after the disease has been present for a long period.
However, as seen with impotence, when the diabetes is present but
asymptomatic and therefore unrecognized for some time, signs of
nerve damage may be the first hint that diabetes is present. Typical
presenting symptoms include numbness, burning, tingling, or intense
sensitivity in areas of the skin such as the feet and legs. These symptoms are often worse at night, with characteristic nighttime leg
cramps being an example. Occasionally, facial nerve palsies may lead
to presentation with blurry or double vision that disappears when
one eye is closed. This usually disappears by itself in about 4 to 6
weeks. However, diabetes and neuropathy are not the cause of all
such symptoms, and, obviously, other causes should be sought if diabetes is not present.

Fatigue. While fatigue may be the earliest and most common symptom of diabetes, it is such a nonspecific symptom that the majority of

people with this complaint have developed it due to some other cause — or if it is caused by diabetes, it is frequently misdiagnosed. If the fatigue is due to diabetes, the fatigue usually disappears after treatment, though this might take some time.

Blurred Vision. Complaints of blurred vision are a classic presenting symptom of diabetes. Glucose accumulating in the lens of the eye causes changes in its shape and results in visual disturbances. Reduction and stabilization of glucose levels usually can correct this problem. However, this process may take 2 to 3 months, and it is recommended that ophthalmologic evaluation for corrective lenses be deferred until after the glucose control has been stabilized. If visual disturbances are really disruptive to the patient's lifestyle, then changes in corrective lenses during the process of initiating glucose control may be needed, but with the understanding that there may be a number of changes in prescription before the vision stabilizes.

If the clinician has a heightened index of suspicion when a patient presents with one of the symptoms described above, and if he or she recognizes the high-risk categories (see Table 2-3), there is an increased likelihood that the proper diagnosis will be made in a timely manner.

Standards of Care

In this era of managed care and disease management, the trend in the medical profession is to develop "standards of care" or "care guidelines." The motivation for preparing these documents varies depending on who is writing them. On one extreme, some focus on cost savings and limiting patients' access to expensive services, and on the other, some advocate extensive use of services, assuming that this approach will best ensure good health. The best approach is probably somewhere in between. Studies to determine optimal utilization of services, balancing cost against outcome, have been initiated in recent years.

The ADA publishes its standards of care annually in *Diabetes Care.* Based on these standards, other published data, and our own clinical experiences, the Clinical Oversight Committee of the Joslin Diabetes Center has developed its own Clinical Guidelines for Adults with Diabetes. These Guidelines can be found on Joslin's web site, www.joslin.org.

Keep in mind that clinical care guidelines are constantly changing based on new knowledge and clinical experience. The decision to publish such guidelines in a book of this nature is a "double-edged sword" in that parts of the recommendations are likely to have been changed long before the rest of the book is out of date. Yet the inclusion of this material provides an outline of what such standards should include. Readers who regularly care for people with diabetes are encouraged to keep abreast of the literature, so that they are aware of modifications in national standards of care that may affect these guidelines.

Treating Diabetes Aggressively

There are two main goals of the treatment of diabetes. One is to restore normal glucose homeostasis, thus preventing the effects of acute and severe variations in glucose levels; and the second is to reduce risk factors to prevent the long-term complications of this condition. Ultimately, these goals focus on establishing a balance between providing the means for the patient to live as "normal" a life as possible in spite of self-care requirements, and making the self-care effective enough so that the patient maintains optimal quality of life for the longest time possible. While these are not mutually exclusive, success requires involving the patient in treatment decisions and discussing and defining goals and objectives in terms that go beyond glucose numbers.

Unfortunately, some healthcare professionals, particularly in the past, developed a fatalistic attitude about diabetes. They felt that people with diabetes were inevitably going to develop complications of diabetes regardless of what glucose management treatment is prescribed. Why develop a complex treatment program that will only burden a patient's "good" years? Fortunately, with improved treatments and a better understanding of the etiology of complications, few clinicians take this approach today. However, even today, patients can live in denial. In the early years of their diabetes, they may feel well and see no need to become more aggressive with treatment. Others don't wish to make changes in their lifestyle, claiming "it is my choice to live as I want now, recognizing that I might not live as long." This latter statement invariably has overtones of denial: "*I* will escape those complications in spite of poor glucose control."

The Diabetes Control and Complications Trial (DCCT)

In the last decade, the literature has presented more evidence than ever before that aggressive control, based on the underlying pathophysiology and also encompassing risk factor reduction, *does* make a difference. The first of these landmark studies was the Diabetes Control and Complications Trial (DCCT) published in 1993. This was the first large-scale study that established conclusively that *aggressive diabetes control does reduce the risks of long-term complications.*

The study followed 1441 patients with type 1 diabetes for up to 9 years. All patients in the study received instruction in medical nutritional therapy and were given an exercise program. Approximately half of the patients in the study were randomly assigned to use *conventional* therapy. This therapy was based on the standard of care in the early 1980s, the time the study was initiated. Its approach included monitoring patients' glucose levels 1 to 2 times daily. Initially, urine testing was used, but as the standard of care evolved into blood glucose testing, the protocol was changed to include this latter monitoring method. However, the key was that the results were not used to adjust insulin treatment but rather to protect the patient from severe high and low glucose levels. The patient was treated with 1 to 2 doses of insulin daily, which were only adjusted to accommodate for significant variations in eating, activity, or timing. Hemoglobin A1c (A1C) levels, reflective of the average level of glucose control over a 2-to 3-month period, were measured quarterly. The patients and healthcare providers were blinded to the results, which were not used to routinely guide therapy unless the results were so excessively high as to indicate potential for acute danger.

Members of the other cohort were assigned to the "experimental" group: these patients monitored their glucose levels 4 or more times per day, and used *intensive therapy* (now called physiologic insulin replacement, see Chapter 11). Intensive insulin therapy (IIT) required that 3 or more daily insulin injections were given, and that an injection of regular insulin was administered before each meal. The doses of this regular insulin were adjusted by the patient based on self-monitoring of blood glucose (SMBG) levels. The goal was to target normal glucose levels. The results of monthly A1C tests were used to gauge treatment efficacy and to adjust the insulin regimen.

The experimental group of patients in the DCCT treated with IIT achieved an A1C level that was significantly lower than those patients who were assigned to the conventional approach, although values in the normal range were not always achieved. At the conclusion of the study, patients using IIT had a significant reduction in retinopathic, nephropathic, and neuropathic complications. They also, however, had a three-fold increase in severe hypoglycemia, although many investigators and patients will suggest that, as they became more skillful in using IIT, their ability to avoid significant hypoglycemia improved.

Of note was that there was no specific threshold level of A1C that a patient needed to reach to achieve significant complication risk reductions. Even patients who started with a very high A1C level and could only achieve modest improvements showed some reduction in complication risk. Therefore, an important conclusion of this study was that *any improvement in A1C reduces the risk of complications.* Thus if a patient cannot be aggressive enough in his or her efforts to achieve *optimal* diabetes control, *anything* that is done to improve the A1C level is worthwhile.

The Epidemiology of Diabetes Interventions and Complications (EDIC) is an extension of the DCCT. In 1994, 96% of the participants of the DCCT enrolled in this follow-up observational study of metabolic status and complication rates. Diabetes care was provided by the patients' usual physicians, and they were allowed to use conventional or intensive therapy or any combination thereof, regardless of their original cohort assignments. Most have used an intensive — now referred to as physiologic — insulin replacement program.

In this follow-up study, patients who were originally in the intensive treatment group had significantly fewer cardiovascular events (MI, coronary revascularization, and angina) as compared to patients assigned to the conventional group (0.4 vs. 0.8 events per 100 patient-years). Multivariable analyses demonstrated that the improvement in glycemic control during the earlier 6.5 years of the DCCT study was the key factor related to the reduction in macrovascular events. These study findings confirm that physiologic insulin replacement programs can reduce macrovascular risk in people with type 1 diabetes. Noteworthy is that early physiologic control has a pathophysiologic "memory." Even when the two cohorts' treatments were equalized, those who had been using physiologic replacement programs in those earlier years showed macrovascular benefits.

Type 2 Patients

It was the consensus among diabetes specialists and the ADA that the results and implications of the DCCT and EDIC extend to people with type 2 diabetes as well. Although the incidence of macrovascular disease in the relatively young population in the DCCT was too low to draw significant initial conclusions, the EDIC follow-up results are compelling with respect to macrovascular disease in the type 1 population. Further, studies in people with type 2 diabetes revealed some useful information regarding glucose control and complications.

From Japan came the Kumamoto Study, which paralleled the DCCT, but was conducted on insulin-requiring type 2 patients. This study showed that improvements in control comparable to those seen in the DCCT reduced the incidence of microvascular complications. This study also was able to draw conclusions on *macrovascular* disease, with similar, significant reductions in risk noted.

A study from Finland looked at cardiovascular endpoints in type 2 patients and demonstrated that reductions in both the number of events and the overall mortality occurred in patients who had lower A1C levels. Data from the Wisconsin Epidemiologic Study related glucose control, as measured by glycosylated hemoglobin, with endpoints such as progression to proliferative diabetic retinopathy, proteinuria, lower extremity amputations, ischemic heart disease, and overall mortality.

In 1998, the results of the two-decade-long United Kingdom Prospective Diabetes Study (UKPDS) were published. This was a complex study that followed large numbers of patients with type 2 diabetes over an average of 10 years. The goal was to determine whether glucose control using intensive pharmacotherapy resulted in clinical benefits and whether there were advantages or disadvantages of any specific treatment modalities. Specific glucose treatments included diet alone, oral therapy using the sulfonylureas chlorpropamide or glyburide or the biguanide metformin, or insulin injection therapy. The protocol included therapeutic crossovers and combinations. In addition, "tight" control of blood pressure was compared with "less tight" control with respect to outcome and advantages and disadvantages of specific therapies.

The results of this study suggested a number of conclusions that will be mentioned at various points in this book. Perhaps the most important conclusion was that, like the other studies reported earlier, aggressive control of diabetes and blood pressure *do* reduce the risk of long-term complications associated with diabetes.

Goals of Therapy

Most people today use the A1C as the primary yardstick of control, using a methodology whereby the range in people who do not have diabetes is 4% to 6%. Glucose goals are theoretically "normal" or "near-normal" levels that can be thought of as estimations of levels that would help achieve the desired A1C goals.

So what should be the goals of therapy? Many groups have their own perspectives on this question! And these perspectives have been evolving over the last few years, as we try to balance the ideal with the practical.

Table 2-4 outlines the current American Diabetes Association recommended goals of therapy. Since the ADA first published these treatment goals in the 1990's, the results of many other studies have further reinforced the recommendation that aggressive control should be the therapeutic goal for people with diabetes.

The new wording by the ADA — setting a general goal but stating that ultimately it should be individualized — is also reflected in the goals set by the Clinical Oversight Committee of Joslin Diabetes Center (Table 2-5). Joslin's goals also use the <7% A1C target as a practical level for patients using medications that may cause hypoglycemia to avoid the risk of that complication, but state that achieving normal blood glucose is recommended if it can be done practically and safely.

The European community has treatment goal recommendations (Table 2-6) that are two tiered, reflecting differences in goals to reduce macrovascular and microvascular risk. In 2001, the American Association of Clinical Endocrinologists (AACE) recommended targets for A1C of <6.5%, preprandial plasma glucose <110 mg/dl and a postprandial plasma glucose <140 mg/dl. While each association or institution may differ slightly from the others, the trends and implications are clear. Recommendations for target A1C are drifting downward based on assessment of newer data and buoyed by safer and more effective treatment tools. The target should be *at least* under 7%, perhaps lower based on the actual targeted recommendations by some, and an assessment of safety and practicality by others.

TABLE 2-4. **ADA Recommendations for Glycemic Control for Adults with Diabetes**

Glycemic Control	
A1C	• <7.0% for patients in general • For the individual patient as close to normal as possible without significant hypoglycemia[†]
Preprandial plasma glucose	90–130 mg/dl (5.0–7.2 mmol/1)
Peak postprandial plasma glucose[‡]	<180 mg/dl (<10.0 mmol/1)

* A1C normal range 4.0%–6.0%

[†] Less stringent treatment goals may be appropriate for patients with a history of severe hypoglycemia, patients with limited life expectancies, very young children or older adults, and individuals with comorbid conditions

More stringent glycemic goals (i.e., a normal A1C, <6%) may further reduce complications at the cost of increased risk of hypoglycemia

[‡] Postprandial glucose measurements should be made 1–2 h after the beginning of the meal, generally peak levels in patients with diabetes

Adapted from Table 6 — Summary of recommendations for adults with diabetes from Standards of Medical Care in Diabetes — 2007; *Diabetes Care 30:S10, 2007*

Achieving Individualized Goals

Clearly, any goal represents a standard of care that must then be individualized for each patient, balancing the risk of therapy against the benefit that the patient would receive from achieving this level of control. While trying to reach recommended goals of therapy is an important objective of therapy, for some people with diabetes doing so may be extremely difficult, impractical, or unsafe. However, because such goals may be unrealistic does not mean that the patient or healthcare professional should fail to be aggressive in their treatment approach. As noted above, studies such as the DCCT/EDIC suggest that *any* improvement in control is beneficial. Clearly, however, the obstacles to achieving ADA, Joslin, European or AACE goals should be reviewed among the healthcare providers and the patient and his or her family, and realistic alternative targets of therapy should be established. Keep in mind, also, that compromised goals at one point in time may be adjusted to be more aggressive in the future to

TABLE 2-5. Joslin Clinic Goals of Treatment for People with Diabetes

Biochemical Index	Normal	Goal	Initiation of Action Suggested
Average fasting plasma glucose (mg/dl) or preprandial level	<100	90–130	<80, >130
Average postprandial (2-hour) (mg/dl)	<140	<160	>160
Average bedtime glucose (mg/dl)	<120	110–150	<110, >160
A1C (%)[†] — sustained	<6	<7[‡]	≥7

* Laboratory methods measure plasma glucose. Most glucose monitors approved for home use calibrate whole blood glucose readings to plasma values. Plasma glucose values are 10-15% higher than whole blood glucose values. It is important for people with diabetes to know whether their meters and strips record whole blood or plasma results.

[†] A1C normal range 4.0%–6.0%

[‡] The true goal of care is to bring the A1C as close to normal as safely possible. A goal of <7% is chosen as a practical level for most patients using medications that may cause hypoglycemia to avoid the risk of that complication. Achieving normal blood glucose is recommended if it can be done practically and safely.

See the most current versions of Joslin's Clinical Guidelines on Joslin's web site, www.joslin.org

TABLE 2-6. European Diabetes Treatment Goals (1999)

Biochemical Index	Low Risk	Arterial Risk	Macrovascular Risk
Preprandial venous glucose (mg/dl)	<110	≥110	≥125
SMBG			
Fasting / preprandial (mg/dl)	<100	≥110	≥110
Postprandial peak (mg/dl)	<135	≥135	>160
A1c (%)*	≤6.5	>6.5	>7.5

* A1C normal range 4.0%–6.0%

IDF Europe. *Guidelines for Diabetes Care. 1999;16:716-730.*

accommodate changes such as improved patient attention to self-care, availability of others to help, or newer, safer or more physiologic therapies that allow lower glucose targets to be achieved safely.

The Tools for Treatment

The changes that have occurred in the treatment of diabetes since the first general use of insulin in 1922 have constituted one of the most exciting chapters in the history of medicine. Within just a few years, the outlook for people with diabetes changed from one of facing near starvation and mere survival to a life in which survival is taken for granted and the horizons are almost unlimited. Increasing numbers of people have lived for longer than 50 years following the diagnosis of diabetes — 50 useful and productive years.

Elliott Joslin used to say that the treatment of diabetes is more like a marathon than a sprint. Patients must adapt their lifestyles and self-care routines for the long haul. This is true, as the backbone of all diabetes treatments is nonpharmacologic — education, medical nutritional therapy, exercise, and self-monitoring. If these are not sufficient, *then* oral or injected antidiabetes medications , and/or insulin may be needed.

> *Education.* Education has been a vital part of diabetes management for decades. The DCCT and other recent studies have established it as crucial to the success of many, if not *most,* therapies. Yet there are no landmark studies that unequivocally document the direct benefit of education as a single component. This is probably because successful diabetes management and achievement of desired outcomes are often multifactorial. Many components of treatment contribute to successful outcomes, and education is clearly important to the efficacy of these components (see Chapter 12).

> *Activity.* Exercise is one of the original ways of controlling diabetes, used even before the introduction of pharmacologic interventions. Exercise alone is rarely enough to control diabetes, but it can improve the efficacy of other treatment components when used in combination with them. Exercise is beneficial because it improves general health and also reduces insulin requirements by reducing insulin resistance.

When designing a diabetes treatment plan, it is important to know the required level of activity of the individual. Exercise, to the extent that it is appropriate for the particular individual, can have multiple benefits.

Medical Nutritional Therapy. Regulation of nutritional intake is still crucial to the treatment of diabetes. As many people with type 2 diabetes retain some insulin secretory capacity, a properly designed nutrition program makes it easier for their insulin to be effective. The eating plan for people with type 1 diabetes is often less restrictive than that for a patient with type 2 diabetes, but it still will provide guidelines for more intelligent food choices and will coordinate nutrition with insulin and activity.

Oral and Injected Antidiabetes Medications. The spectrum of oral antidiabetes medications has widened considerably in the last decade. Previously there was one class of medications available in the United States, the sulfonylureas. This class, typically referred to as "oral hypoglycemic agents," works by sensitizing the beta-cells to more effectively secrete increased amounts of insulin in response to rising glucose levels. When they were the only available class, they were used with a "one size fits all" approach, regardless of whether or not the underlying pathophysiology in a given patient represented significant insulin secretory insufficiency.

Now, newer classes of medications can target specific pathophysiologic defects. Most are given by mouth, but injected medication is also being used for this purpose as well. Medications are available that increase insulin sensitivity, including the biguanides and the thiazolidinediones, which are very effective when either endogenous and/ or exogenous insulin is available. Medications in the class of α-glucosidase inhibitors can slow the gastrointestinal absorption of carbohydrate so that it is entering the circulation at the time that endogenous insulin secretion, lacking at the early "first-phase" release, is present. The familiar group of medications that stimulate insulin secretion, the sulfonylureas, has been joined by other medication groups that have similar effects, only focused primarily on the postprandial time frame. These medications include one from the meglitinide class and a member of the phenylalanine derivative class. A new group of medications restores incretin function. Incretins are hormones secreted by the gastrointestinal tract that communicate with the pancreas about incoming food, resulting in insulin secretion that is "glucose-dependent" (i.e., stimulated by the rising glucose levels rather than occurring independent of the insulin level), and suppression of glucagon secretion. One such type of medications, the GLP-1 agonists, are injected medications. Others, the DPP-IV inhibitors, are given by mouth.

Insulin. If the patient has either absolute or relative insulinopenia, then insulin therapy may be needed. Newer developments in available insulin include the development of synthetic human insulin and more recently the development of insulin analogs, including both rapid-acting insulin to cover incoming meals, and basal insulins to provide background insulin over a 24 hour period. These insulins have provided the tools to replace this hormone in a manner closer to normal insulin action patterns.

Using the tools described above, the essence of diabetes treatment is to develop a system of balances. The triad of variables — insulin or oral medications, food consumption, and activity — can all be adjusted by the treatment team, as well as manipulated as needed by a well-trained and skillful patient. Yet, there are also other factors — the "intangibles" that affect any treatment program. These intangibles are often imperceptible — daily variations in various factors such as stress, timing, food absorption, insulin absorption (from injections *or* inhalations), etc., that can also affect the diabetes. They are all factors that remind us that humans are not machines and do not live each day as if it were a carbon copy of the previous. However, the more attention that is paid to these variables, and the more we learn from them and about them, the more effective diabetes treatment can and will be.

Suggested Reading

Standards of Medical Care in Diabetes–2007, American Diabetes Association *Diabetes Care 2007 30: S4-41 (Updated annually — seek newest version)*

Diagnosis and Classification of Diabetes Mellitus, American Diabetes Association *Diabetes Care 2007 30: S42-47 (Updated annually — seek newest version)*

Diabetes Epidemiology: Collaborative Analysis of Diagnostic Criteria in Europe (DECODE). *Lancet* 1999; 354:617–621.

Tominaga M, et al. The Funagata Diabetes Study. *Diabetes Care* 1999; 22:920–924.

The DECODE study group. Glucose tolerance and mortality: comparison of WHO and American Diabetes Association diagnostic criteria. *Lancet* 1999; 254: 617–621.

3

Monitoring Diabetes

Richard S. Beaser, MD

We look at the discovery of insulin in 1921 as being the first milestone in the development of modern treatment modalities. The second milestone is the development of oral therapies in the 1950s. The third milestone is the development of tools to monitor diabetes treatment: the Hemoglobin A_1 ("glycohemoglobin") and the hemoglobin A_{1c} (now commonly referred to as HbA1c or A1C) measurements reflect overall control and risk of long-term complications; and self-monitoring of blood glucose (SMBG) charts the patterns of daily glucose levels. These two advances, both of which became available in the early 1980s, heralded the era of physiologic insulin replacement therapy. They also provided the tools to conduct such important studies as the Diabetes Control and Complications Trial (DCCT) and other epidemiologic and treatment studies that demonstrated that aggressive control does make a difference in long-term outcomes.

The Importance of Self-Monitoring of Blood Glucose and Glycohemoglobin Measurements

Overview

Self-monitoring (SMBG) is important for a number of reasons. A person with diabetes must always know his or her blood glucose value at any given time in order to prevent the potential dangers of acutely high or low levels. For those using physiologic insulin replacement therapy (in the past referred to as "intensive insulin therapy"), knowing the current level is essential if adjustments in insulin doses are to be made to target normoglycemia. In addition, for those patients using antidiabetes medication therapies, the glucose patterns can suggest the predominant underlying pathophysiology and thus lead to a more accurate medication selection. A further advantage: self-monitoring occurs during the patient's routine daily activities rather than in an artificial hospital setting as was the necessity just a few decades ago.

Perhaps equally important, but less obvious, is that SMBG more effectively engages the patient in his or her own self-care. **It is imperative that people who are self-monitoring know what to do with the results of their glucose checking so that they can take active steps to improve their control. They should be given instructions on how to interpret their results, what they can do themselves in response to the results, and when they should call for help.** Patient education is a critical component of every diabetes treatment plan. No patient should go in for a routine interval visit with a healthcare provider with a list of self-monitoring results that are significantly suboptimal, without having taken some corrective action during the interval between visits.

Goals of diabetes treatment need to be defined in terms of self-monitoring results. Ideal targets for fasting, prelunch and presupper, and postprandial glucose tests should be defined. Acceptable levels should also be determined, as not all values are likely to be ideal. In addition, the degree of variability should also be reviewed (see Chapter 2, Tables 2-4, 2-5, 2-6).

In sum, there are a few basic reasons why SMBG should be performed:

- to provide data about glucose patterns that can be used by the healthcare team, working with the patient, to make treatment decisions
- to provide data with which patients themselves can make daily decisions on treatment adjustments (in a physiologic insulin replacement program, for example)
- to provide feedback on how effectively the individual is adhering to daily self-care routines, including medical nutrition therapy, physical activity, and medication use

Glycohemoglobin, or A1C, goals are also a useful part of treatment monitoring beyond their obvious reflection of average glucose level and complication risk. These measurements can be reported to patients — providing positive feedback if the values reflect improvement or goals achieved, and conversely, indicating the need to strive for better control if they do not reflect improvement (see Chapter 2, Table 2-5).

These two means of monitoring diabetes, SMBG and glycohemoglobin or A1C measurements, are not meant to be used as a substitute for one another. They reflect different components of diabetes treatment and thus should complement one another.

The Glycohemoglobin Measurement (A1C)

One of the functions of the red blood cells is to carry oxygen to the cells throughout the body. Hemoglobin within the red blood cells is the substance that carries this oxygen. The most vital part of the hemoglobin molecule is a fraction called hemoglobin A.

Glucose binds to many molecules through a process referred to as "glycosylation." When the blood glucose level is elevated, more glycosylation occurs. Within red blood cells, the hemoglobin molecule becomes glycosylated. A small, measurable subfraction of hemoglobin A known as hemoglobin A1 forms when hemoglobin A is glycosylated. A further subfraction of the glycosylated hemoglobin A1 known as the hemoglobin A1c can also be measured. It is this fraction, the hemoglobin A1c, that is now most commonly measured as a reflection of glucose control. These glycosylated hemoglobin molecules are commonly referred to as "glyco-" (for glucose) hemoglobin: "glycohemoglobin." Technically, the term glycohemoglobin refers to hemoglobin A1, not hemoglobin A1c, although most use this term to refer to this latter measurement as well.

Recently, the ADA recommended shortening the terminology for the HbA1c to just "A1C" although the older terminology is still occasionally used. Both refer to the same entity, hemoglobin A1c. Further, most labs now measure the Hemoglobin A1c, and treatment targets are based on this measurement. Although methodology does still vary, the normal range in most labs for people who do not have diabetes is between 4% and 6% (or values very close to this range), making comparison easier. This number represents the percent of hemoglobin molecules that have been glycosylated. Alternatively, if the normal ranges of two values are quite different, one can calculate the percent above the upper limit of normal to make a crude comparison.

On average, red blood cells live for about 120 days, after which time they die and are removed from the circulation. New red blood cells are manufactured to replace them. At any given time, there are red blood cells that have just been born and those that are about to die. Thus, the average age for all the red blood cells present in the human body at a given time is about 2 months old, or half the total lifespan. Glycosylation occurs continually throughout the life span of the red blood cell. The amount of glycosylation of the hemoglobin depends on the level of blood glucose — the higher the blood glucose level, the more glycosylation will occur. Therefore, the glycosylated hemoglobin or A1C measurement is dependent on the average blood glucose level. As the average age of the total pool of red blood cells is 2 months, **the A1C measured represents predominantly the level of control during the previous 2-month period.**

The higher the result of the A1C level, the poorer the diabetes control during the past two months. (Tables 2-4, 2-5 and 2-6 in Chapter 2 show various groups' recommended goals for A1C levels.) As part of routine care, the American Diabetes Association recommends that the A1C level be measured 4 times per year for people with type 1 diabetes, and at least twice per year for those with type 2 diabetes, though more frequent monitoring is helpful to provide feedback to healthcare professionals and patients. **The target A1C is less than 7.0%, with anything 7.0% or higher suggesting the need for treatment adjustment** (see Chapter 2).

Conditions that May Cause Inaccurate Results

The A1C measurement, like many tests in medicine, is not perfect. People with unusual hemoglobin molecules, such as those with sickle cell anemia, may have invalid test results. It may also be in error in early stages of pregnancy because the fetus produces its own red blood cells. Also, be alert to patients who have recently had transfusions, as some of the hemoglobin that is being measured has not been in them for the requisite period of time. Anemias can render the glycohemoglobin measurement inaccurate as well, as the average age of a red blood cell is usually younger when some cause for premature red cell removal is present. Anything that causes red cells to live longer, such as a splenectomy, can also affect hemoglobin A1C measurement.

With respect to the testing methodology, when HPLC laboratory techniques are used to perform measurements, the number of things that can affect the test results is limited. Using this methodology, the most common factors that can affect A1C measurements are:

- Hemolytic anemias
- Carbamylated and acetylated hemoglobins (rare)
- "Fast" migrating hemoglobins, most commonly hemoglobins D, J, and N, can lower readings
- Fetal hemoglobin greater than 25% interferes with hemoglobin A1c measurement and cannot be corrected for
- True β-thalassemia will interfere with some HPLC methods, but the patient has to be symptomatic at the time for the effect to be significant
- Severe lipemia in some patients can interfere with measurements. Interference can be reduced by washing red cells and making an offline dilution to report out the A1C value
- Taking medications such as salicylates can have an effect, though rarely

Despite these limitations, the use of the glycohemoglobin measurement is still a powerful tool! Many studies have correlated the A1C level with the risk of developing complications. Many such complications may even result from the glycosylation of various tissues of the body in a manner similar to the glycosylation of hemoglobin. Thus, the glycosylation of hemoglobin may represent a surrogate of what is occurring to other tissues, and the measurement of glycohemoglobin may actually measure one of the processes that leads to the complications of diabetes.

Self-Monitoring of Blood Glucose (SMBG)

As noted above, the initial development of the means for patients to routinely monitor their glucose levels during their normal daily routine was one of the major milestones in the history of diabetes treatment. Previously, the only way to get serial readings, or a profile of daily blood glucose patterns, was by hospitalization. This intervention altered the daily routine so much that many of the changes that were made in insulin treatment programs failed to maintain control when the patient was discharged.

By using SMBG, a more accurate picture of the patient's glucose patterns can be obtained when he or she is involved in a usual daily routine. Whether or not an initial intervention to regulate glucose control occurs as an inpatient or outpatient, it can now be thought of as "the beginning" of the control process, not "the end." The goals of these interventions are to determine the best treatment program, provide relevant educational interventions, and initiate the insulinization regimen in a controlled setting. Then the next stage of "fine tuning" the program, with the patient living a normal lifestyle, leads to more effective treatment programs.

In addition, the development of self-monitoring techniques has been the cornerstone of the physiologic insulin replacement programs. Obviously, without SMBG, adjusting insulin doses based on glucose levels would be impractical. As an extension of this concept, the landmark study, the Diabetes Control and Complications Trial (DCCT), which proved once and for all that "tight" (physiologic) control does reduce the risk of complications, would have been impossible without SMBG. Many of the commonplace components of current diabetes treatment would have been impossible without this significant treatment advance.

The Significance of Blood Glucose Measurements

Blood glucose levels are in constant flux. One must try to extrapolate from a series of individual measurements — snapshots, as it were, of the glucose level — what the day-long pattern of glucose levels might have been. Just like a weather forecast and knowledge of the phases of the moon would help one predict what ocean levels might have been between a series of photographs taken at the seashore, knowing about factors that influence glucose levels can be crucial if patterns are to be interpreted.

Monitoring Logs

In order to interpret the patterns of blood glucose levels, it is important for the patient to keep a record of the various factors that can influence glucose levels, such as variations in food consumption, activity level, and timing variations. For this reason, many patients who successfully interpret their glucose patterns utilize a well-formatted record log. While computerized meters with memories can be useful tools, those that cannot record variations in daily events that are crucial to interpreting the results of their monitoring, only provide part of the data needed. Some newer, electronically sophisticated meters such as those on a PDA platform can record this important data. Conversely, many patients still use the hand-written log successfully. Appendix 3-A is an example of such a log.

A log should have space to record monitoring results — often both pre- and postprandial values, as well as middle-of-the-night results and other times of significance. You should be able to read across a row and see a number of values for various times on a given day. You should also be able to scan down a column and see the values for a particular time of day for a number of days running. Graph sheet records should be avoided. Scanning is impossible, and the implications that the blood glucose level "went from point A directly to point B" or that "point A was the lowest glucose level that day," can be quite misleading. Also, this result section should not be encumbered by a listing of other data such as the exact time of monitoring or insulin or medication dose, as these other numbers will make it difficult to scan and get an impression of the glucose result averages and variations. A separate section should be used to record insulin doses or medication, particularly if a program is in use that allows daily variations in the doses. Medication doses, which typically aren't adjusted on a daily basis, are usually only noted if there is a change.

A "comment" section should be available to record significant variations in the crucial factors that affect control. However, one might also note items like "bowling night" or "stressful day at the office," as these factors might affect diabetes control as well. Brevity of these comments is important, although they should be written so that one can look back on them at a later time and really use them to interpret glucose patterns.

Some patients attempt to write everything that they eat for a given day in the small box allotted for comments. Besides needing a magnifying glass to read this information, it is nearly impossible to go back and make sense of it. Food records, if requested by a dietitian, should be kept on a separate sheet of paper. However, some notation — "over ate" or "light lunch" — might be sufficient on the SMBG log sheet to note a variation from normal. Some people use a simple scoring system for variations.

Using food consumption as an example, if a typical day gets a score of "0," then slightly more food would get "+1" and much more eating would get "+2," while slightly less eating would get "−1" and much less would get "−2." A more formalized method of quantifying food consumption and adjusting insulin doses, referred to as "carbohydrate counting," is discussed in Chapter 5.

Once one begins using this system, patterns and associations may be seen that can be useful in adjusting diabetes treatment. Details concerning how to use patterns in making treatment decisions can be found in specific treatment chapters.

While one can argue for the use of hand-written logs, there are computerized functions that are also helpful in analyzing the data. Probably the most important one would be to determine the average, and perhaps range, mean, and/or median, of the test results at a given time of day. Such information can help detect times when glucose levels are off-target, and this can help determine treatment changes. Averages of all tests for periods such as a week or month are somewhat useful in gauging trends over time. The number of test results that are above or below a target range at a given time can also be useful. Many of the other graphing functions can be confusing and should be used and interpreted with caution. Some of the newer glucose monitors on PDA platforms, mentioned above, allow more data entry and are opening the door to future equipment that can integrate more information about daily control parameters.

Self-Monitoring Equipment

As with all electronic equipment, rapid advancements are occurring in the technology for SMBG meters. Improvements have lead to faster reading times, smaller and more portable sizes, and easier-to-use test strips, while all the while purporting better accuracy. Certainly, the rudimentary visually-read strip methods of the past are no longer recommended unless no other metered alternative is available. Some of the meters have computerized memories that store and analyze data or feed it to a home computer; PDA input and capabilities further expand their functionality. However, as was discussed in the section on record-keeping, there still may be an argument for keeping paper records with respect to correlating glucose results with life events for those who are not facile with the electronics of these more sophisticated meters.

The overall cost of SMBG over the course of the year may be somewhat high, but with the growing appreciation of the importance of these monitoring methods, many health insurance policies cover all or some of the costs if the materials are prescribed by a physician. For many, the cost of self-monitoring is money well spent. In the long run, the improvements in diabetes control that can result from SMBG should reduce the costs of healthcare and lost earnings. It should be noted, in this context, that people treated with antidiabetes medications as well as those treated with insulin benefit from monitoring, as the glucose patterns detected can be a reflection of their underlying pathophysiology and help with treatment decisions. In addition, the feedback on lifestyle decisions can serve as an effective behavior modification tool.

Hopes for noninvasive glucose testing have buoyed people with diabetes for many years. However, promises that the technology was "just around the corner" have also been made for many years. We are still not at that corner, but we may be getting closer. Less invasive devices are now beginning to appear on the market. Many meters are capable of using blood sites other than the finger, and more improvements will undoubtedly be available shortly.

Also, real-time continuous monitoring devices are now available. Using an inserted transcutaneous sensor similar to the infusion catheters that deliver insulin as part of an insulin pump, these devices measure glucose levels throughout the day, and have a display showing real-time glucose values and patterns. These devices also have adjustable alarms that sound when the glucose level reaches preset high and low target levels. This new technology has been shown to reduce both hyper- and hypoglycyemic excursions, and can be quite useful for optimizing diabtes control and minizing hypoglycemia. These devices are less accurate than current fingerstick glucose monitors and are not substitutes for conventional monitoring; patients using continuous sensors need to perform fingerstick capillary glucose measurements at meal-time and also to calibrate the sensor.

Of concern to clinicians is what to do with all the data that will certainly be generated from more and more technologically sophisticated monitors. Additionally, what will patients do with it? Many patients who are not used to seeing fasting glucose levels, or perhaps premeal measurements, or certainly post-meal values, will now be overwhelmed with glucose values. Unless these patients understand the natural variations of glucose patterns throughout different parts of the day and, in particular, in response to meals, there will be a temptation for them to overtreat some of the elevated postprandial glucose values, with potential for harm. **Clearly, careful patient education must accompany the use of any of these monitoring devices so that appropriate clinical decisions can be made.**

SMBG Procedure

Most currently used techniques for SMBG require that a blood sample be obtained by pricking the finger with a lancet. Some people can prick themselves freehand, while most now prefer using one of various fingerpricking devices that hold the lancet and, via a spring-mechanism, pierce the skin. Many of the devices come equipped with various "guards" or "platforms," which can be used to adjust the depth to which the lancet enters the finger. These devices may be purchased without a prescription in some states, while in others a prescription is required.

The lancing device is used to obtain a drop of blood. The finger is the usual source — the skin is pierced to one side of the fingertip, which has fewer nerve endings and is thus not as painful as the center. The ear lobe may be an alternative but more difficult site from which to obtain blood. Also, as noted, glucose meters are now available that allow lancing of the forearm or the palm side at the base of the thumb, which may be less painful if accuracy concerns can be addressed.

The drop of blood is transferred to the test strip, which usually contains chemicals involved in the testing methodology. Depending on the meter and strip model, the meter senses the effect of the reaction of the glucose in the blood droplet with the chemicals on the test strip and produces a glucose reading.

Testing (Checking) vs. Monitoring

There is a distinct difference between "testing" or "checking" a glucose value, and "monitoring" diabetes. Monitoring is an overall plan for watching diabetes control. Testing or checking is the act of performing a specific measurement — an SMBG test or an A1C test. There is an important difference. Patients cannot monitor their diabetes without testing, but, unfortunately, patients often test without monitoring. Regardless of how often a patient performs tests, the results should be considered part of the monitoring plan. Whether or not a patient tests his or her blood once every 5 days or 5 times a day, he or she must understand what to do with the results, how to interpret them, what action they should imply, and when to call for help.

It is important that all patients who are taught to test should also be taught a monitoring plan. The discussions of blood testing schedules below all relate the frequency of testing to the interpretation and use of the result and actions that should ensue.

Some people prefer to use the term blood glucose "check" rather than "test," as the latter term has connotations of evaluation and results which can be "good" or "bad." To avoid people feeling that the results of this process have some judgmental impact on how they are viewed, the term "checking" is sometimes used. For the purpose of this book, we will usually refer to the process of testing. However, when talking with a patient who is feeling particularly down about not achieving results that they expect or feel that others expect of them, the term "checking" may be a kinder terminology.

Frequency of Testing

The goals of monitoring will usually dictate the frequency of testing that will be needed. Thus, the reason for monitoring — what one hopes to learn from it — must be decided first. If a patient accepts the rationale for the monitoring program, then he or she will be much more likely to perform the required tests. The design of the monitoring program, therefore, should occur with the patient's participation. The patient may be a passive participant, just listening to the reasons that a particular approach is being suggested, or an active participant, providing insight into his or her own lifestyle that affects the monitoring program design. Either way, by presenting and developing the program in this manner, the patient has a better understanding of the "why" of the monitoring program, and the "what to do" of result interpretation.

Key considerations in designing a monitoring program include:

- **the need to obtain information about the patients underlying pathophysiology through interpretation of daily glucose patterns**
- **the importance of gauging the efficacy of diabetes treatment**

- the role of feedback to the patient in impacting self-management decisions
- the degree of willingness or ability of a patient to perform tests, including physical limitations, cost considerations, personal schedule, or tolerance for discomfort
- safety while performing certain tasks such as driving

Glucose patterns during the course of the day can provide a window to the relative predominance of the various pathophysiologic abnormalities that can lead to diabetes. Particularly for people with type 2 diabetes, the etiology may fall anywhere in a spectrum between insulin resistance and insulin secretory deficiency. While not always fully reliable, glucose patterns do provide a hint as to which defects may be significant and, therefore, help with selection of specific pharmacologic agents for treatment.

For example, the characteristic fasting hyperglycemia of type 2 diabetes, caused by hepatic insulin resistance leading to increased hepatic glucose production in the fasting state, is suggestive of significant degrees of insulin resistance. Mild postprandial hyperglycemia is typical of early type 2 diabetes with blunted first-phase insulin response; significant postprandial hyperglycemia suggests a more significant insulin secretory defect typical of later stages of type 2 diabetes.

For patients of the Joslin Clinic, blood testing schedules are individualized; however, they tend to fall into broad schedule categories.

Sporadic Testing. People using this program usually check their blood less than once a day. This is not optimal. It is typically the default mode for many suboptimally adherent people with type 2 diabetes. While it gives a vague idea of typical glucose values, the patterns are often not evident. Frequently, people adopting this approach have significant obstacles to testing, and if these obstacles can be addressed, a more useful testing frequency can result. With the newer, easier, and more comfortable testing equipment, very few people should resort to this level of testing.

Nevertheless, sporadic testing is better than no testing, and it can give some insight into the underlying pathophysiology as well as the efficacy and selection of pharmacologic treatments if the patient varies the time of testing each day. Testing before each meal, and occasionally after a meal or during the night, when looked at in aggregate over a longer period of time, can give some sense of pathophysiology and medication selection. (See Chapter 8 for a more detailed discussion of how this monitoring pattern may be used in this regard.)

Systematic Testing. This is a program for people who are willing and able to test 1 or 2 times per day. Left to their own devices, such people tend to check their blood at the same time(s) each day, providing the same, repeated information day after day. Instead, they should be encouraged to vary the times that they test among those times that provide useful monitoring information. Usually, before meals and bedtime are the most commonly recommended times from which to choose testing times. However, occasionally such patients should be encouraged to perform their daily quotient of tests before and after a given meal to get a sense for the postprandial glucose excursion. Alternatively, occasional nocturnal or exercise-related testing might be useful.

The uses of systematic testing as a monitoring program are similar to those for the sporadic tester. However, the more frequent testing allows better interpretation of the results, and the daily monitoring can be more effective in providing feedback to the patient on the impact of lifestyle events on glucose control. It can also be combined with a more intensive block of testing, described below.

Block Testing. Blocks of blood tests consist of a minimum of 3 to 4 daily tests, and as many as 7-8 for a short number of days — often 3–4 in a row. These blocks give a useful sense of the inherent glucose patterns but allow time between the days during which the block of tests is performed for a less frequent schedule. Usually, patients will perform 1or 2 blocks of tests per month. Often, block testing can be inserted into a program of systematic testing to improve the quality of the monitoring data. The goal of the blocks is to gauge the efficacy of the treatment, while the goal of testing between blocks may be just to monitor for evidence of trouble.

Post-Prandial Testing. Obtaining readings 2 hours postprandially is useful, particularly during these stretches of intensive block testing days, as postprandial hyperglycemia has been implicated in increased macrovascular risk. This type of testing is particularly useful:

- for patients whose A1C is elevated but fasting glucose is on target.
- for patients who are using glucose lowering agents targeted at post-prandial glucose such as the short-acting secretagogues (repaglinide and nateglinide) or the incretin-mimetics (GLP-1 agonists or DPP-IV antigonists).
- and as an evaluation tool for patients who are making dietary and physical activity changes

Intensive Daily Monitoring. This approach to self-monitoring consists of testing the blood 4 or more times per day, every day. This approach is recommended for those with type 1 diabetes using either conventional-type therapies, one of the intensified conventional therapies, or physiologic insulin replacement programs (see Chapter 11). For these latter programs, daily insulin dose adjustments are made based on the results of the tests, using dosing algorithms and/or formulas for adjustment based on carbohydrate intake (see "Carbohydrate Counting," Chapter 5) and activity level.

Fructosamine Tests

In addition to the blood monitoring described above, a fructosamine test has been available through laboratories since the early 1980s. The main advantage of this test is that it can detect overall changes in blood glucose control over a shorter time-span than the A1c. Fructosamine levels indicate the level of blood glucose control over the past two or three weeks. So, when rapid changes are being made in a diabetes treatment plan, this test can indicate in a more timely fashion than an A1C test how well the changes are working and whether other changes should be considered. Home fructosamine testing kits are also available.

The fructosamine test can be potentially helpful for people making changes in their diabetes treatment plan. It can also be helpful to people with diabetes that do not closely monitor their blood glucose levels with multiple daily home tests. But a once-a-week fructosamine test should not be considered a substitute for daily monitoring, as a normal fructosamine test doesn't mean that blood glucose have been normal for the past 2 to 3 weeks. As with the A1C measurement, someone with wide swings in blood glucose levels might have a normal fructosamine test but would really have serious problems with his or her overall treatment plan that would require adjustment. This would be uncovered by frequent daily home blood glucose monitoring.

The fructosamine test offers information that augments that provided by home blood glucose monitoring and A1C tests. For people who are changing a treatment program, it may be particularly useful. For those who are not currently doing frequent blood glucose tests at home, it may provide a first step in getting oriented toward self-testing and toward taking action in their overall diabetes management.

The Office Blood Glucose Measurement

The measurement of blood glucose levels in a healthcare professional's office still may have some utility even though the patient may be engaged in regular SMBG. Obtaining such a test helps correlate and corroborate the self-monitoring results. If a patient reports values all between 80 to 120 mg/dl, and the lab reports back a value of 350 mg/dl, there is clearly something amiss. However, it might not be that the patient is either incorrectly performing the tests or misrepresenting the results. For example, if a patient always reports preprandial values, and the office test is postprandial, it may be a revelation of a time during the day when glucose levels are particularly high, resulting in higher A1C levels. Also, many patients perform fasting tests early in the morning before really moving about very much. They may have significantly higher values in the office due to the adrenaline surge resulting from fighting traffic during the drive in or the frantic search for a parking place just prior to having the blood drawn. Nevertheless, in most instances, the office test can gauge the precision of the self-monitoring that the individual has reported.

Many physicians now have an office laboratory that gives almost immediate results, allowing "on-the-spot" decisions. Some use meters similar to those used by patients to measure the glucose level on a capillary sample. Keep in mind that blood test results may vary according to the site from which the blood sample is taken. The fingertip or earlobe sample from capillaries is blood heading for tissues and thus contains more glucose. It is often 20 to 30 mg/dl higher than that from venous blood, which is returning to the heart and lungs after some of the glucose has been used. At fasting levels, the results are pretty much equal, but in samples drawn after eating, this difference may be seen. Table 2-5 in Chapter 2 lists the expected normal venous blood glucose levels, as well as suggested target levels.

Generally speaking, glucose levels in capillary whole blood is approximately 10% lower than those in plasma or serum. We normally multiply meter values (whole blood) by 1.1 to correlate with plasma values from commercial labs. This calculation is based on patients with an average hematocrit of 41%. Such calculations can verify meter accuracy unless the meter is a newer model that gives plasma-like readings directly.

Urine Testing for Glucose

With the predominance of SMBG, there is rarely a role for urine glucose testing. For many years prior to blood testing, urine testing was the only self-monitoring method available. One can test urine because when elevated glucose levels exceed the renal threshold, glucose is cleared in the urine via an osmotic diuresis. However, urine glucose measurements have two significant drawbacks. They reflect glucose levels over the recent past, but not the current moment, and they indicate when the glucose level is high, but negative urine glucose does not indicate whether the blood level is normal or too low.

The only advantages to urine testing are that it is easy to use, inexpensive, and painless. However, the significant disadvantages outweigh the advantages. It poorly correlates with actual blood glucose levels and its accuracy is dependent on renal threshold, which varies from person to person, and with a given person, from time to time.

With the ease of current self-blood glucose monitoring devices, the only setting in which urine glucose testing would be indicated is when a patient is absolutely unwilling or unable to do any SMBG tests, and there is no other person available to assist in such testing. In these situations, urine glucose testing would be somewhat better than nothing. Making an estimate of the renal threshold is also helpful in interpreting urine glucose results. Obtain urine and blood glucose levels at the same time on a number of occasions and compare values, looking for the highest blood glucose value for which there is a negative urine glucose reading. That is the renal threshold.

One additional reason that urine testing is still valid today is to determine the cause of increased urinary production. Excess urinary production or increased frequency without a significant urinary glucose content would suggest that the problem was the result of some other process.

When testing urinary glucose for monitoring purposes, it is recommended that a second voided specimen be tested. The patient should empty the bladder of urine that has collected over a long period of time, wait one-half hour, and then void again. Glucose testing should be performed on this second, freshly made specimen.

Twenty-Four-Hour Urine Glucose Test. Before the advent of the glycohemoglobin measurement, 24-hour urine collections were used to measure glucose loss, which reflected, to some degree, the average level of control over a 24-hour period. A person who does not have diabetes should have minimal urinary glucose loss, if any, over a 24-hour period. Ideally, a person with diabetes should not lose much either, but practically speaking, good regulation of diabetes in an adult should result in a loss no greater than 5% of the total carbohydrate intake for the day. Now, with A1C measurements, 24-hour urine collections are rarely used.

Urine Or Blood Fingerstick Testing For Ketones

Measurement of urinary or blood ketones remains an important part of a diabetes monitoring program. Ketone production and resulting ketonuria or ketonemia occur when fat is metabolized for use as an energy source that, depending on the setting, may or may not be desirable.

Settings when ketone production may occur include:

- extreme or rapid weight loss
- insulin deficiency
- pregnancy if there are insufficient calories to meet increased energy needs
- extreme exercise

With regard to weight loss, a person intentionally may undereat, which leads to a decrease in insulin production. Decreased levels of insulin allow fat mobilization and metabolism. Similarly, if someone is undernourished and engages in physical activity, ketone production may occur. However, the ketone production accompanying hyperglycemia in a person with type 1 diabetes may reflect a significant insulin deficiency. Glucose levels rise due to this insulin lack, which also allows fat metabolism to occur.

Urine testing for ketones. Urine acetone or blood beta-hydroxybutyrate ketone testing should usually be performed whenever there is significant elevation in blood glucose levels, usually above about 250 mg/dl, particularly in the setting of some other physiologic stress such as an illness that can increase insulin requirements. It can be quite useful in differentiating hyperglycemia due to such a stress from the hyperglycemic rebound seen after a hypoglycemic reaction. *Rebound hyperglycemia is usually accompanied by a urinary acetone level of "zero" or "trace," while hyperglycemia due to a significant stress or absolute insulin deficiency is often accompanied by urinary acetone readings of "small" to "large" or elevated blood ketone readings.*

Blood Ketone Testing. Ketone testing is recommended for patients with reduced or no insulin production who are ill. The presence of ketones in the urine or blood can alert the patient and provider to impending diabetic ketoacidiosis. The ketone body that is detected in capillary blood is beta-hydroxybutyrate (B-OHB). It is produced from fat breakdown used if glucose is unavailable. For people with type 1 diabetes, information about the presence of ketones in the blood and the level of ketone is important in treating mild ketonemia at home and avoiding emergency room or hospital visits.

Checklist for Initiation, Design, and Revision of a Diabetes Self-Monitoring Program

The following issues should be addressed in the initiation, design, and revision of a self-monitoring program for a patient. The key is individualization of the program to the patient's abilities and needs. Also, there should be periodic reassessment of the success of this program, adjusting its intensity based on actual experience from its use.

1. *What information is really needed?*
    a. for the healthcare providers to design and modify the treatment program
    b. for the patient to use as feedback on his/her self-care routine
    c. as an alert of potential acute problems
2. *Does the patient have any physical or mental limitations that may affect testing ability or methods?*
    a. visual limitations
    b. dexterity
    c. vascular or neuropathic, or concerns regarding infections
    d. mental limitations affecting technique, understanding, or ability to interpret results
3. *Are there any economic, social, scheduling, or work/school-related obstacles to the monitoring recommendations?*
4. *What is the patient's professed willingness to do the testing?*
5. *If already on a testing program, how successful has the patient been at following the regimen?*
6. *Based on the above assessment, have you designed an individualized monitoring program and schedule that the patient or a significant other can self-manage, that will get reasonable and useful information, and that can prompt appropriate action when needed?*
7. *Has the patient or will the patient receive proper teaching?*
    a. techniques and equipment use
    b. record-keeping (for both glucose values and other key information)
    c. use and interpretation of result
8. *Does the patient know his/her specific targeted values or ranges?*
9. *Does the patient understand what to do when values do not fall in those ranges?*
10. *Does the patient understand the difference between values reflecting acute concern vs. those reflecting longer-term control concerns?*
11. *Does the patient know when and how to self-manage certain off-target values, and does he or she know when values warrant a call to a medical professional for help?*
12. *Does the patient know how to manage "sick days"?*
13. *Does the patient need to know how to test for ketones, and if so, in what setting, using what methodology? Does he or she know how to interpret the results, and when to call for help?*

Key to Successful Monitoring

Self-monitoring of blood glucose is an important component of all diabetes treatment programs. It is the key to achieving excellent control of blood glucose levels in a safe and effective manner, allowing careful tailoring of dosages of insulin or antidiabetes medications to the needs of each person.

While it plays somewhat different roles for insulin-using and non-insulin-using patients, it is important for both. For non-insulin-using patients, it can help delineate daily glucose patterns that can reflect underlying pathophysiologic abnormalities, helping in medication selection. For patients using insulin, a self-monitoring program combined with a thoughtfully designed treatment plan can eliminate the frequent, severe hypoglycemia of years past while achieving excellent control. The old fear that "tight control means lots of hypoglycemic reactions" is no longer valid if self-monitoring and a physiologic insulin replacement program are utilized.

The success of a self-monitoring program is dependent upon the motivation of the patient to undertake an appropriate testing schedule. **Patients are more likely to monitor if they are involved in the selection or design of the self-monitoring program, and if they have specific guidelines as to what to do with the results of their tests.** Whether they adjust their insulin, get feedback on lifestyle, or know when to call the healthcare provider, a monitoring program must involve performing tests, correlating the test results with other components of the diabetes treatment program, and a resulting action plan. Looking ahead, newer monitoring methods will make this task easier in the years to come. For all these efforts, the reward is improved, safe diabetes control, which can positively impact the patient's quality of life. This benefit, in and of itself, should be a significant reward for the effort of monitoring.

Appendix 3-A

Joslin Diabetes Center

DIABETES MONITORING RECORD

MR# _____

Name: _____

Phone #: (_____)_____

_____
Street Address

_____
City   State   Zip

	GLUCOSE MONITORING RESULTS					INSULIN DOSES										Comments
						Before Breakfast		Before Lunch		Before Supper		Bedtime				
Date 20__	Before Break-fast	Before Lunch	Before Supper	At Bed-time	Other	Rapid	Long/ Inter/ Mix	Rapid	Long/ Inter	Rapid	Long/ Inter/ Mix	Rapid	Long/ Inter			

KEY: *Rapid* = Regular, lispro, aspart, glulisine or inhaled insulin
Inter = Intermediate Insulin: NPH (N)
Long = Long-acting Insulin: glargine or detemir
Mix = 70/30, 75/25, 50/50

In "Comments" Section above record variations to Activity, Food Consumption, or Timing

For pre- and post-meals, use [⬚]

Prescribed Product Name(s) _____

_____

GENERAL COMMENTS:_____

_____

_____

Physician / NP / Diabetes Educator : _____ Date:_____

4

Adipose Tissue as an Endocrine Gland: A Possible Key in Understanding the Metabolic Mysteries

Osama Hamdy, MD, PhD, FACE

Today, we are looking at fat in a whole new light! Until recently, adipose tissue was regarded as a passive depot for lipids that somehow contributed to the metabolic and cardiovascular burden, but in and of itself was an inert bulk. How wrong we seem to have been! There is now increasing evidence which points to an important role of adipocytes as an active endocrine organ whose metabolic and secretory products (hormones, prohormones, cytokines and enzymes) play a major role in total-body metabolism.

This chapter, new to this edition, explores our evolving understanding of the role of adipose tissue as an active organ, producing substances that may play a central role in the development of type 2 diabetes and the vascular dysfunction that often accompanies it. As the concept that adipose tissue can function as an endocrine organ is a relatively new concept for clinicians, we have devoted this chapter to a more in-depth look at what is known in this area. The more practical treatment recommendations follow in Chapter 5, for those who are looking for more of the applicability of nutritional principles to diabetes management. However, the implications of adipose as an active metabolic organ will undoubtedly expand over the next few years, impacting treatments for the hyperglycemia of type 2 diabetes as well as therapies for other components of the metabolic syndrome. Thus, this material sheds an exciting new light on many of the existing treatments discussed elsewhere in this book. Certainly, it provides a rationale for many of the nutritional recommendations that you will find in the chapter that follows. Further, newer treatments are on the horizon which target adipose tissue and the endocrine secretions of this tissue. Thus, it is likely that during the useful lifetime of this book, clinicians will hear more about these potential new treatments. The background information provided by this chapter should be helpful in understanding the importance of such treatments and in putting them into a proper therapeutic and pharmacologic context.

Therefore, in this chapter, we indulge in a discussion of evolving physiologic perspectives — perspectives with a very practical implication which, increasingly, are being recognized as perhaps the etiologic keys to many of the treatments we have been using for decades, and some that are on the horizon.

Understanding the Endocrinologic Role of Adipose Tissue

It has been largely over the past decade that we have learned that the impact of obesity on both insulin resistance and endothelial dysfunction (the early stage of atherosclerosis) is mediated through the release of the cytokine hormones produced in the adipose tissue. Cytokines are proteins produced in hematopoetic and non-hematopoetic cell types, which play a role in immune responses. Their dysfunctional secretion often plays a role in immunological, inflammatory, and infectious diseases. The cytokine hormones produced by adipose are collectively called adipocytokines or adipokines.

It has been evident from studies in recent years that the components of the metabolic syndrome may be mediated through a common underlying metabolic process. The metabolic syndrome is the clustering of metabolic abnormalities, discussed in more detail in Chapters 7 and 15, but defined by the presence of at least 3 of the following: elevated triglycerides, low HDL, elevated fasting glucose, increased waist circumference, and/or elevated blood pressure. Insulin resistance has been thought to be the common thread in this syndrome, but the role of the inflammatory process has also been implicated in both its etiology and the mechanisms by which the syndrome leads to vascular dysfunction. Therefore, pathophysiologic interrelationships among these vascular risk factors are likely to be of importance, and from a clinical perspective, whatever can be determined to increase insulin resistance and/or the inflammatory response becomes a potential treatment target.

It is for this reason that the products of adipose tissue, the adipokines, have become the focus of a great deal of interest for their potential etiologic role in the metabolic syndrome and vascular disease, and are likely to become even more relevant clinically as treatments targeting them are developed. The adipokines are a group of pharmacologically active proteins which, like other cytokines, are related to inflammatory processes and stimulation of the immune system. They also play an important role in the adipose tissue physiology and in initiating several metabolic and cardiovascular abnormalities, not only in overweight and obese individuals, but also in some lean persons with higher visceral fat mass. These adipokines include adiponectin, leptin, tumor necrosis factor-alpha (TNF-α), interleukin-6 (IL-6), and plasminogen-activating inhibitor-I (PAI-1) among many others.

An increased amount of adipose tissue, with a disproportionate distribution between central and peripheral body regions, is related to altered serum levels of these cytokines, which can have significant clinical consequences. Except for leptin and adiponectin, other cytokines are produced not only from fat cells but also from the macrophages that infiltrate the adipose-tissue. It has been seen that when people get older or fatter, more macrophages infiltrate the adipose tissue and consequently produce more proinflammatory cytokines.

In contrast to the harmful effect of most cytokines, adiponectin, a cytokine also produced by adipose tissue, has beneficial effects, and protects against the later development of type 2 diabetes. Adiponectin is relatively abundant in plasma and at generally higher levels among women than men. Low plasma adiponectin is found in obese individuals and in patients with coronary artery disease. A ten percent weight reduction in obese people leads to a significant increase in the adiponectin level (40–60%) in both obese diabetic and non-diabetic individuals.

Therefore, one way to look at the pharmacology of the various treatments of type 2 diabetes is to think of how those treatments impact adipokines. For example, it has been reported that treatment with thiazolidinediones (e.g. pioglitazone and rosiglitazone, see Chapter 8) may normalize or even increase adiponectin gene expression. In one study, the administration of thiazolidinediones for 3 months resulted in increased adiponectin levels in both lean, obese non-diabetic and obese diabetic subjects. Adiponectin is also involved in the modulation of inflammatory responses, as it seems to attenuate the pro-inflammatory effect of TNF-α. It has also been shown that adiponectin inhibits many functions of mature macrophage, such as the cytokine production discussed above, as well as phagocytosis. Adiponectin also modulates endothelial function and has an inhibitory effect on proliferation of vascular smooth muscles. Therefore, in trying to understand how the various treatments for type 2 diabetes may work to reduce not only hyperglycemia, but the risk of vascular disease, the impact on adiponectin may hold the key.

Leptin is another adipocyte-derived hormone that circulates in the serum. The physiologic effects of leptin, mediated either through direct stimulation or through activation of specific centers in the hypothalamus, are to decrease food intake, increase energy expenditure, influence glucose and fat metabolism and alter neuroendocrine function. Interestingly, serum levels of leptin increase with increased fat mass. Leptin does not seem to suppress the appetite of obese individuals, which raises the possibility of leptin resistance in obese individuals, similar to insulin resistance.

What is very interesting about leptin is that it is expressed predominantly by subcutaneous rather than visceral fat cells. Women also seem to have higher leptin levels than men, which could be either related to the increased percentage of peripheral body fat in women, or a result of stimulation of leptin production by estrogen/progesterone. Studies have demonstrated that fat mass and gender are the main independent predictors of leptin concentration in people with type 2 diabetes, and that insulin secretion and the degree of insulin resistance contribute significantly to leptin levels. Leptin therapy in lipodystrophic patients was shown to improve hepatic and peripheral glucose metabolism and reduce hepatic and muscle triglyceride content, suggesting that leptin acts as a signal that contributes to regulation of total body sensitivity to insulin. It was also found that leptin was independently associated with cardiovascular mortality.

Although both adiponectin and leptin are integrally related to the metabolic or "insulin resistance" syndrome, adiponectin is more strongly related to the presence of visceral abdominal fat, while leptin is more closely related to the presence of subcutaneous fat content. The implications of that association are still not fully understood, and in the coming years, further research will undoubtedly shed additional light on the relationships between these two adipokines, as well as their relationships to adiposity and disease. This work may also lead to the prospect of their clinical use as targets or mediators in the treatment of overweight and obese subjects with insulin resistance or the metabolic syndrome.

Harmful Effects of Some Adipokines

Many of the adipokines have harmful physiologic effects that are now being recognized as being of clinical importance in the etiology of vascular disease. As we consider the many treatments discussed later in this book, which seek to reduce the risk of vascular disease, the targeting of the inflammatory process may be a key underlying pharmacologic mechanism. With this in mind, it has become clear that adipose tissue is a major source of such pro-inflammatory cytokines such as TNF-α. Obesity in humans is associated with increased production of TNF-α and also increased gene expression of its receptors. TNF-α is known to be directly linked to cardiovascular disease. Plasma levels of TNF-α have been shown to be increased in individuals with premature cardiovascular disease independent of insulin sensitivity. Table 4-1 below outlines many of the roles in the pathogenesis of the vascular lesion that have been postulated for TNF-α.

PAI-1 is another important bioactive substance produced by adipose tissue. While PAI-1 gene expression has been detected in both subcutaneous and visceral fat, it correlates better with visceral adiposity. High level of PAI-1 is a strong indicator of increased cardiovascular risk. In humans, it has been shown that improvement in insulin sensitivity, either through weight reduction or medications, will lower circulating levels of PAI-1. Such decrease was found to correlate with the amount of weight lost and also with the degree of decline in serum triglycerides.

TABLE 4-1.   Roles of TNF-α in the pathogenesis of the vascular lesion

- Stimulates the production of adhesion molecules on the surface of the vascular endothelium, which work like a glue that traps the circulating monocytes from the blood stream.
- It then stimulates the migration of these trapped monocytes through the endothelial barrier to the subendothelial area where they are transformed into macrophages, which engulf the oxidized LDL and are themselves transformed into the foam cells that form the core of the atheromatous plaque.
- Stimulates the migration and proliferation of the vascular smooth muscle cells.
- Stimulates the production of the proteolytic enzymes that facilitate the rupture of the fibrous cap that would otherwise protect and separate the atheromatous plaque from the vascular lumen. Once exposed to the flowing blood, platelet aggregation and clot formation is likely to occur.
- Increases with obesity; has also been noted to decrease significantly with weight reduction.

Body Fat Distribution and Cardiovascular Risk

Over the last few years, it has become evident that central fat distribution (the so-called "apple-shaped" body) is more strongly associated with several metabolic and cardiovascular problems than total adiposity. This relationship between increased visceral adiposity and the risk of developing type 2 diabetes and CAD seems to also be related to the increased presence of the recognized coronary heart disease risk factors such as hyperglycemia, hypertension and dyslipidemia. It is, in fact, the waist circumference that is the key measure relating to risk profiling. For people with the same BMI, those with a larger waist circumference are at a significantly increased risk for coronary artery disease. In clinical practice, the waist circumference and waist to hip ratio (WHR) are the commonly used anthropometric measures to diagnose abdominal obesity. These measures correlate with the total amount of visceral fat measured by abdominal CT scanning.

As a result of the recognition of these relationships, the Adult-Treatment Panel III (ATP-III) of the National Cholesterol Education Program has adopted the increased waist circumference as a major criterion for clinical diagnosis of the metabolic syndrome. A waist circumference of equal to or greater than 102 cm. (> 40″) in men or 88 cm. (> 35″) in women is a cut off for increased risk. More importantly, accumulation of visceral fat remains also the major independent cardiovascular risk factor, even within the normal range of body mass index (BMI), and even at lower waist circumference than the above mentioned figures in certain ethic populations such as Asian, Indian and Chinese. This observation leads researchers and clinicians alike to believe that clinical diagnosis of visceral adiposity may be more important than the current diagnosis of obesity using body mass index (BMI), body weight or even percentage of total body fat.

Accumulating evidence also points to a major difference between the intraabdominal visceral fat and the peripheral or subcutaneous fat in the pathogenesis of these medical problems, both in lean and obese individuals. In contrast to the accumulation of fat in the gluteo-femoral regions, the accumulated fat in the intra-abdominal or visceral depots is strongly associated with all obesity-related complications. The relationship between visceral fat, as quantified by abdominal CT scanning, and CAD seems to be independent of age, BMI and the amount of subcutaneous fat in men with familial hypercholesterolemia. Moreover, abdominal obesity was also found to be associated with accelerated atherosclerosis independent of overall obesity and other risk factors in middle-aged men with no prior atherosclerotic disease.

Visceral Adiposity (Metabolic Obesity)

Visceral adiposity is defined as fat accumulation around the viscera and inside the intra-abdominal solid organs. Although this phenomenon is more common in overweight and obese individuals, as noted above, it can also occur in lean individuals with a normal BMI and, independent of the overall adiposity, this particular type of fat seems to play an important role in the development of type 2 diabetes and atherosclerosis. The progressive accumulation of intraabdominal fat increases hepatic and adipose-tissue insulin resistance and its consequent metabolic abnormalities like glucose intolerance, low HDL-cholesterol, elevated triglycerides and hypertension. This package of metabolic abnormalities is called the *metabolic syndrome,* and is discussed in other contexts throughout this book, particularly in discussions of type 2 diabetes and cardiovascular complications. Some also refer to this syndrome as the *insulin resistance syndrome* considering insulin resistance as its fundamental etiology. It is worth mentioning that the definition of metabolic syndrome and its phenotype characteristics is far from firmly established and academic debate is ongoing over which criteria should be included, and their relative etiologic, diagnostic, and prognostic significance.

The most appealing hypothesis to explain the relationship between visceral fat accumulation and insulin resistance is that visceral adipocytes are more lipolytically active, which results in an influx of a large amount of free fatty acids into the portal circulation and to the liver. This hypothesis is called the *liptoxicity theory.* The other theory that has recently gained a lot of acceptance is that visceral adipose tissue and its resident macrophages produce more proinflammatory cytokines like TNF-α and IL-6 that induce insulin resistance.

There are major ethnic and gender differences in the rate of accumulation of visceral fat. For example, African American women have a lower amount of abdominal visceral fat in comparison to white women, but much higher than African American men. Meanwhile, Japanese men and women have a significantly greater amount of abdominal visceral fat compared to Caucasians. Genetic factors like β3-adrenergic receptor polymorphism are another determinant factor of abdominal visceral fat accumulation. Many other factors also play a role in determining the volume of visceral fat, including

- environmental factors
- imbalance of sex hormones (in particular low serum-free testosterone in men)
- growth hormone
- IGF-1
- insulin
- excessive intake of sucrose and/or saturated fat
- lack of physical activity.

Age is also a major defining factor. At any given waist circumference, older people have a larger amount of visceral fat than younger individuals.

Visceral adiposity is associated with significant lipid abnormalities that include:

- elevated serum levels of small-dense LDL-cholesterol particles
- high apo-B
- hypertriglyceridemia
- reduced HDL-cholesterol

Although central adiposity is associated with impaired insulin sensitivity and blood glucose abnormalities, isolated peripheral adiposity does not have any apparent effect on glucose homeostasis. As excessive accumulation of visceral fat also occurs in lean individuals, the term "metabolic obesity" may be a better new definition of obesity when metabolic and cardiovascular risks are considered. It may identify, more accurately, those individuals at high risk for diabetes and CAD based on their anatomical fat distribution irrespective of their corresponding BMI.

Measurement of Visceral Fat

Current knowledge makes it also possible to subdivide body fat into at least three separate and measurable compartments: subcutaneous, intramuscular and visceral fat. The current gold standard techniques for measuring visceral fat volume are the abdominal CT (at L4-L5) and the MRI. These methods are not widely used because of their cost. Commercial software is currently available for calculating visceral fat volume. Using these techniques has confirmed the original assumption that body fat is mostly localized in the subcutaneous space and only partially in the visceral area. Interestingly, they also showed that fat in the central line (around the waist) is predominately subcutaneous and not visceral. This may explain the difference in clinical value between measuring the volume of visceral fat directly and measuring it indirectly through measuring waist circumference.

Dual-energy X-ray absorptiometry (DEXA) can be used to accurately measure total body fat and regional fat distribution. DEXA is more accurate than anthropometric measures and more practical and cost effective than CT or MRI scans. However, DEXA cannot distinguish between subcutaneous and visceral abdominal fat depots, or between subcutaneous and intramuscular peripheral fat depots.

Abdominal ultrasonography is another suitable technique for measuring visceral fat. A good correlation has been found between measuring visceral fat volume using abdominal ultrasound and abdominal CT scanning. Measurements should be performed at the end of quiet inspiration and by compressing the transducer against the abdomen to limit distortion of the abdominal cavity during scanning. The distance between the peritoneum and the lumbar spine is used as a measure of visceral fat. This distance should be measured at 3 positions along the horizontal line between the highest point of iliac crest and the lower costal margin, and each measure should be repeated three times. The reproducibility of this technique is excellent with a coefficient of variability around 4–5%. Using this protocol, it may be possible to easily measure visceral fat volume in clinical practice, which may yield more reliable information than simple anthropometric measurements. Its accuracy is closer to abdominal CT or MRI while being less costly.

However for the time being, these methods are not usually performed to assess visceral adiposity; waist circumference seems to be the easiest anthropometric measurement that can be used by healthcare professionals in order to diagnose visceral adiposity, or at least to get a rough impression of the visceral fat volume.

The Paradoxical Effect of Peripheral Fat Accumulation

There is much less data on the physiologic and clinical role of the peripheral fat mass. Interestingly, large hip circumference has been found to be an independent predictor of lower cardiovascular and diabetes-related mortality. It also seems that fat depots exhibit different influences on lipid metabolism, with central fat mass promoting and peripheral fat mass counteracting atherogenicity. Peripheral fat mass has been found to negatively correlate with both atherogenic metabolic risk factors and aortic calcification in women. Hip circumference and leg fat also showed a strong negative association with atherogenic lipid and glucose metabolites. It is interesting that a relative lack of peripheral fat leads to significantly poorer insulin sensitivity.

It is postulated that increased leg fat may reflect underlying hormonal factors (e.g. estrogen) that regulate preferential deposition of fat in the hip and thigh area. The protective effect of a large hip circumference may be due to the high lipoprotein lipase activity and low fatty acid turnover of gluteo-femoral adipose tissue. There is also evidence to suggest that peripheral fat accumulation plays an important role in modulating insulin resistance through regulating visceral fat accumulation and visceral fat production of TNF-α. In an experiment with animals, reduction of peripheral fat resulted in excessive accumulation of visceral fat and more production of TNF-α. Thus, from a clinical and endocrinologic perspective, all fat is not alike!

Biological and Genetic Differences between Visceral and Subcutaneous Body Fat

It has recently been shown that the functional differences between visceral and the subcutaneous adipocytes are related to their anatomical location. The severity of atherosclerosis is significantly lower in generally obese people compared with those with predominantly central obesity. Adipocytes from the visceral abdominal region are more sensitive to lipolytic stimuli and are more resistant to suppression of lipolysis by insulin than the adipocytes from gluteo-femoral subcutaneous region. The metabolic characteristics of the adipocytes from the subcutaneous abdominal region tend to be intermediate. Consequently, the systemic flux of free fatty acids is higher in individuals with a preponderance of abdominal fat. An overexposure of hepatic and extra hepatic tissue to FFA promotes abnormal insulin dynamics and action. Moreover, abdominal fat may directly impact hepatic free fatty acid flux due to its proximity to the portal circulation, and consequently increases triglyceride synthesis and decreases hepatic insulin clearance. Other contributing mechanisms include abnormal expression and secretion of fat-derived cytokines including resistin, leptin, adiponectin, TNF-α and IL-6.

Recent evidence also indicates that there are several gene loci which determine the propensity to store fat in the abdominal region. Differences in several gene expressions in visceral fat in comparison to subcutaneous fat may account for the differences in the metabolic risks between the two fat depots. Many of those genes that are involved in glucose homeostasis, insulin action, or in lipid metabolism are expressed more in visceral fat than in subcutaneous fat.

Modification of Body Fat Distribution

Lifestyle modifications in the form of caloric restriction and increased physical activity, and medications such as metformin and PPARγ agonists like pioglitazone and rosiglitazone, are the most common modalities used for treating insulin resistance. Except for metformin, reduction of visceral adiposity is a common feature of these interventions. Caloric restriction and exercise result in weight loss, lower W/H ratio and improvement of insulin sensitivity through reducing visceral fat and total body fat volume. In contrast, treatment with the thiazolidinediones, pioglitazone or rosiglitazone, results in weight gain but also lowers W/H ratio and improves insulin sensitivity through selective increase of lower body fat with possible reduction in visceral fat volume. PPARγ agonists selectively stimulate adipocyte proliferation, but mostly in peripheral adipose tissue so consequently the result is body fat redistribution. This observation also confirms a site-specific responsiveness of these compounds and suggests that the improvement in insulin sensitivity with PPARγ agonists may be a result of favorable fat redistribution in association with reduction in both intrahepatic and intramuscular fat. Treatment with these medications is discussed in more detail in Chapter 8.

Visceral fat is also sensitive to exercise. Regular exercise that is balanced between cardiovascular and resistance exercise has been shown to reduce visceral fat volume. Interestingly, most of the fat loss during the first 2 weeks of caloric restriction and exercise is from the visceral fat. But if one compares a given level of caloric deficit brought on either by caloric restriction or increased energy expenditure by exercise, the deficit brought on by the increased exercise more effectively reduces the volume of visceral fat.

Recent evidence has also shown that reducing the caloric intake from carbohydrates from 55–60% down to around 40% is associated with significant reduction of visceral fat and improvement of insulin sensitivity. If this change is associated with caloric reduction and increased protein intake from 15% to around 20–30% in patients with no microalbuminuria or impaired kidney function, it results in more weight reduction, a decrease in triglycerides and an increase in HDL.

So far, it is unclear how much reduction in visceral adipose tissue is required to induce favorable metabolic changes. It seems that even moderate reduction of visceral fat, as seen with short-term weight reduction programs, yields metabolic benefits with regard to lipid profile, insulin sensitivity and blood pressure similar to that observed after major weight reduction.

Effects of Selective Removal of Visceral or Subcutaneous Fat

Surgical removal of visceral fat in experimental animals reversed hepatic insulin resistance. It also prevented age-related deterioration in peripheral and hepatic insulin action. Meanwhile it decreased gene expression of TNF-α and leptin in subcutaneous adipose tissue. Furthermore, removal of visceral fat delayed the onset of diabetes in the Zucker fatty rats, the model of obesity and diabetes.

In contrast, surgical removal of subcutaneous adipose tissue of similar amount did not have any noticeable effect on any of the metabolic parameters. Similarly, surgical removal of large amount of abdominal subcutaneous fat by liposuction in a group of diabetic and non-diabetic individuals did not improve insulin sensitivity in muscles, liver or adipose tissues, and did not change plasma concentrations of circulating mediators of inflammation, including C-reactive protein, IL-6, and TNF-a. It also did not change blood pressure, plasma glucose, and serum insulin or lipid profile. Interestingly, the weight loss observed in this liposuction study was equal or even far more than weight loss observed in many lifestyle modification studies, yet the weight loss brought on by lifestyle changes resulted in significant improvement in insulin sensitivity and improvement of cardiovascular risk factors. The only explanation for this observation is that liposuction only reduces subcutaneous fat mass without changing visceral, intramuscular, or hepatic fat mass, which is only reduced by weight reduction brought about by diet and exercise.

Future Directions

So how will this growing knowledge base impact the efficacy of the clinician in his or her efforts to blunt the impact of the metabolic syndrome and its related conditions? In the past, clinicians, faced with patients who had diabetes, dyslipidemia, or other stigmata of this syndrome would tell people to "lose weight" knowing fully that the likelihood of success was small. Fad diets abounded, with their fast-off, and then faster-back-on patterns! Yet, now we are on the brink of an era where many of the concepts described above, included for the first time in this edition at the risk of being more theoretical than most chapters, may very shortly be taking that final leap into daily clinical care in a very relevant way.

The understandings described above help us better appreciate how existing treatments work, both at reducing a targeted metabolic parameter for which they have a specific indication, as well as for pleiotropic effects on other metabolic manifestations mediated through underlying mechanisms which are only now beginning to be understood. New treatments are currently being developed to target these specific factors, the adipokines, and their target tissues. Dietary modifications, which address these issues more precisely, are being designed and initiated, and pharmacologic agents that target abdominal adiposity, at this writing, are undergoing FDA review. These treatments may lead to more successful weight loss programs, and more effectively blunt the impact of the endocrine effects of adipose. And, certainly, understanding the issues mechanistically helps put the treatment principles discussed in the next few chapters into a perspective that is more understandable and logical. The principles of medical nutrition therapy, exercise, and pharmacologic treatment for type 2 diabetes and its macrovascular complications take on a new light in the context of the mechanisms discussed above, and a new relevance as we better understand the etiologic targets and downstream implications of our therapeutic interventions.

5

Medical Nutrition Therapy

Amy P. Campbell, MS, RD, CDE and Richard S. Beaser, MD

The Challenge

One of Dr. Elliott P. Joslin's greatest contributions to the treatment of people with diabetes was his belief in empowering patients to manage their own care and his advocacy of comprehensive patient education that makes such self-care possible. Of course, when viewed from today's world, what those "empowered" patients of Dr. Joslin's time could actually do appears minimal. As in the early days of the modern diabetes management era, however, self-management of nutrition is one area in which patient empowerment is central. Perhaps too much so, many a healthcare provider has lamented, frustrated over seeming lack of adherence by patients! It is the skill to mold a medical nutrition treatment plan to a patient's medical needs and lifestyle patterns that can be the most challenging component of the treatment of diabetes.

The challenge, of course, is to translate scientifically based nutritional recommendations into practical daily eating guidelines. To insist on the ideal would be foolish, as few could follow such recommendations and many would quit in frustration. However, to forget the ideal would forsake the rigor of our treatment goals that patients deserve. The construction of an individualized medical nutrition plan is the science of metabolism blended with the art of perceiving what is realistic for a particular patient, tempered with patience and understanding. It is in this mixed recipe that the optimal balance may be established.

So what is that science? And how do we translate that science into practical education for patients so they can successfully establish and follow a healthy nutritional program? What kind of meal planning approach will work with which patients, and how is that approach determined?

The physiology of adipose tissue and its impact on metabolism is outlined in the previous chapter. This information provides the platform on which those who work with patients approach the nutritional recommendations and support that are important in reaching the therapeutic goals.

For a dietitian, knowledge of the role of adipose and the pull-through to clinical practice is important and probably has been part of his or her training already. However, for other medical professionals caring for people with diabetes, a level of knowledge in the area of medical nutrition therapy is essential. So intertwined are modern treatment modalities that an understanding of how nutrition prescriptions are designed and how self-care is instructed is essential if any medical professional hopes to optimally utilize current pharmacotherapies of diabetes, dyslipidemia, and hypertension.

Initiation of medical nutrition therapy begins with a realization — by both the patient and the medical professional — that the therapy is needed in the first place. Too many patients, once diagnosed, report that they were advised to "avoid sugar." Whether or not many medical professionals actually are making this simplistic and erroneous suggestion, many patients have the *impression* that this is the approach their practitioner has advised. *Knowing* what the ideal nutritional approach may be is insufficient if the nature of such treatment cannot be adequately communicated to the patient.

And the process of emphasizing the importance of medical nutritional therapy is not solely the responsibility of the dietitian or nutritionist. All medical professionals must support the need for a carefully devised nutritional component of treatment. Though this might seem trite or pedantic, it carries even more importance today in this era of polypharmacy.

With all of the newer pharmacologic tools now available, medical nutrition therapy has seemingly been pushed into the background. In truth, new antidiabetes medications *can* produce near normoglycemia, whereas years ago, sulfonylureas alone might not have succeeded. Further, the adjustable insulin programs offer variations in premeal, rapid-acting insulins to allow variations in food types and quantities.

Nevertheless, a proper medical nutrition program is still quite important from a number of perspectives. Proper adherence to a nutrition program for a person with type 2 diabetes can help reduce the number of medications and the dosage needed to control glucose levels, as well as help ameliorate other related problems such as dyslipidemia and hypertension. In addition, a nutrition program geared toward calorie reduction can help with weight loss, along with improved glycemic control. For those with type 1 diabetes or insulin-treated type 2 diabetes, these issues also apply, but also a proper sense as to the baseline nutritional program allows more systematic — and thus more accurate — insulin dose adjustments for variations. Keep in mind, as well, that with excessive food consumption driving excessive insulin doses for coverage, a person with type 1 diabetes can gain considerable weight.

A Clinician's Approach to Medical Nutrition Therapy

A registered dietitian is uniquely qualified to provide medical nutrition therapy (MNT), and is an invaluable member of the patient's healthcare team. The initiation of a medical nutrition therapy program for a patient begins with a thorough patient assessment (addressed later in this chapter). This assessment should allow the provider to:

- focus on a patient's metabolic needs
- gauge lifestyle patterns
- help set goals
- guide professional intervention and evaluation

From the information gleaned in the assessment process, specific nutrition recommendations can be developed. The current design of medical nutrition therapy for diabetes stems from the recommendations, reviewed below, of a 1994 ADA expert panel. It is the challenge to healthcare providers to translate, initiate, and support these recommendations so that they become practical, individualized nutrition recommendations that are also integrated components of an overall treatment strategy.

Nutrition Therapy Is Not New

Long before insulin was discovered and used as a treatment, diabetes mellitus, which means "the production of great quantities of sweet urine," was described as being a disorder in which one's body was unable to use carbohydrate as fuel. Thus, the logical treatment was to eliminate carbohydrate from the diet. However, as carbohydrate is the body's major energy source, its elimination resulted in the body's utilization of alternative energy sources — fat and protein. Functionally, the original pre-insulin-era treatment for diabetes was marked diet restriction bordering on starvation.

Of course, for those with type 2 diabetes, this approach may not have been so bad, but it did not provide adequate glucose control for many and was not ideal from the perspective of metabolic needs. Carbohydrate is an important stimulus of insulin production by the β-cells. For people with type 2 diabetes who had developed significant insufficiency of insulin secretory capacity, these early low-carbohydrate diets may have been counterproductive, as they may have understimulated insulin secretion.

As nutrition counseling evolved into the insulin era, the guidelines for carbohydrate intake, then one-third of the daily caloric total, were still insufficient by today's standards. With one-third of the intake as carbohydrate, the remaining intake was about 15% to 20% protein and the remainder was fat. Now, it is known that high saturated-fat diets contribute to dyslipidemias. Over time, we have come to realize that people with diabetes can, and should, handle more carbohydrate. Current recommendations for the percentage of total daily calories that should come from carbohydrate vary, depending on the individual's type of diabetes, metabolic goals and personal lifestyle. For example, an overweight person with type 2 diabetes should aim for approximately 40% of total calories from carbohydrate, whereas, for a lean person with type 1 diabetes 50% to 60% of the total daily calories coming from carbohydrate may be appropriate. Fat content should also be reduced. (Unfortunately, the actual diet of the average American today consists of almost 40% of the daily calories coming from fat!) It has been known for some time now that high-fiber diets are useful, as they provide more bulk, which gives a feeling of "fullness," allowing people to feel satisfied more easily. Fiber also may slow carbohydrate absorption from the bowel. And one type of fiber, called soluble fiber, can help lower blood cholesterol levels.

The Body's Fuel

We have often been told that "we are what we eat." There is considerable truth to this old adage, and it is central to the role of nutrition in the treatment of diabetes and related metabolic disorders. Food consists of three key macronutrients: carbohydrate, protein, and fat.

Carbohydrate is the primary source of fuel for the body. The body can utilize this fuel for immediate needs, or it can store it in the liver and muscle tissue in the form of glycogen for future use. Stored energy provides for varying energy requirements throughout the day and from day to day. Protein can provide an alternative source of energy if it is needed. However, the major alternative energy source after utilization of stored glycogen is fat, which is also an efficient storage form of energy.

From both the functional standpoint as well as from the nutritional perspective, diabetes can be thought of as being a condition in which there is impairment in the body's ability to use, store, and retrieve these food fuels. The treatment of diabetes focuses on an attempt to correct this impairment.

There are three factors to consider when approaching analysis of a medical nutrition program:

- food quantity
- food types
- timing of food intake

To maintain glucose homeostasis, each of these three components of nutritional therapy must be considered. The proper type of food must get into the body in the proper amount and at the proper time. Doing so allows the available insulin, whether endogenous or exogenous, to be matched in terms of both quantity and time of availability in order to insure proper utilization of the incoming nutrients for immediate energy needs or storage for later use.

Quantity of Food

The measure of food-energy is the calorie (technically, a "kilocalorie," abbreviated "kcal"). The three types of nutrients — carbohydrate, protein, and fat — all provide calories, but carbohydrate is the primary source, providing 4 calories per gram. Protein provides a slower, more sustained energy supply, also contributing 4 calories per gram. Protein, however, is better used for functions other than providing energy. Fat, a concentrated energy source, serves as a long-term storage depot for energy. It provides 9 calories per gram.

Basal energy needs differ from person to person, depending on factors such as age, sex, activity level, and body weight.

The preferred method for determining a patient's caloric requirements is to calculate it based on the patient's usual eating style. By conducting a thorough 24-hour recall and food history assessment, a close approximation of the typical intake of calories and grams of carbohydrate, protein and fat can be determined. This level can then be adjusted based on the mutually determined goals of blood glucose control, weight change, and lifestyle.

Alternatively, formulas can be used to approximate the number of calories needed to maintain weight. Once maintenance calories are set, the calories can be adjusted up or down to gain or lose weight.

Another simple method for estimating daily caloric requirements for an average (although somewhat inactive) adult of normal weight would be:

- 25 calories per kilogram (2.2 lbs.) of desirable body weight per day (or 11 calories/lb. of ideal body weight per day) for weight maintenance.
  - Add 20% to this total if moderately active
  - Add 40% to this total if very active
  - Add calories if weight gain is desired, or for pregnant (300 calories) or lactating women (500 calories)

The energy needs for children range between 36 and 45 kcal/lb. As children age they need fewer calories. Adolescent boys need 20 to 36 kcal/lb and girls need 15 to 20 kcal/lb, depending on their physical activity.

Adjustments in caloric intake above or below the estimated basal caloric needs can result in weight changes. A caloric intake below basal requirements will lead to the use of noncarbohydrate fuels, hopefully fat, leading to weight loss. To gain weight, of course, we must do the opposite. A change of 3500 kcal up or down will result in change in body weight of approximately 1 lb. So, if 25 kcal/kg (11 kcal/lb) body weight represents the caloric level needed to maintain present weight for a person of average activity, then a reduction in that caloric intake by approximately 500 kcal/day can result in weight reduction of about 2 to 4 lbs/

month. Losses of slightly more than this — 4 to 8 lbs/month — might be appropriate for the most highly motivated individuals, but may not be for an overweight or obese person with type 2 diabetes unless this weight reduction is medically supervised.

Other factors also affect daily caloric needs:

- Women usually require fewer calories than men because they are smaller in size and frame and have less muscle mass.
- Smaller people usually require fewer calories to maintain their weight.
- Younger, more active people need more calories than older people, especially during periods of growth.
- Caloric needs increase with some types of physical stress, such as after severe injury or illness or during pregnancy and lactation.

The additional fuel needed to power physical activity increases caloric needs. While an active lifestyle requires more calories, it does not require more insulin than that which would be required to maintain glucose control if less activity were performed. Though active people with diabetes, in order to maintain current body weight, could eat additional food to fuel increased activity and continue to take the same insulin doses as if they were less active, the better course would be to adjust their insulin.

Food Types

Food types or nutrients can be divided into two categories, macronutrients and micronutrients. To understand how to utilize these nutrients in a medical nutritional treatment plan requires a basic understanding of the nutritional roles of each. Macronutrients — carbohydrate, protein and fat — will be covered in detail here; the micronutrients, vitamins and minerals, will be discussed later.

As noted above, in 1994, the ADA revised its nutritional recommendations, stating that there is no standard ADA or diabetic diet! A meal plan must be individualized to each person's personal eating style and metabolic needs. In fact, for many people with diabetes, the dietary guidelines are in essence the same as those that would be recommended as a healthy nutritional plan for most adults.

Carbohydrate

Carbohydrate is the major source of energy for the body's needs. It is the major constituent of the "starchy" foods such as breads, cereals, grains, and pasta. These polysaccharide carbohydrates are referred to as complex carbohydrates, as compared with the refined or simple mono- and di-saccharide carbohydrates like sugar. Carbohydrate is also the main component of "sugary" foods, such as cake, cookies, candy, table sugar, milk, fruits and vegetables.

In the past, the recommendation for people with diabetes was to consume primarily complex, or starchy, carbohydrates. The assumption was that these sources of carbohydrate were more slowly absorbed, and thus were present at a time that was more closely coordinated with either the second-phase insulin secretion of a patient with type 2 diabetes or the regular insulin action pattern for someone treated with exogenous insulin therapy.

Today, however, much more is known about carbohydrate. Research shows that eating 50 grams of carbohydrate from a sugar, such as maple syrup, has the same effect on blood glucose as eating an equivalent amount of carbohydrate from a starch, such as bread. In fact, more than twenty research studies show that when individuals choose a variety of foods containing either starches or sugars in meals, if the total amount of carbohydrate is the same, the glucose response will be essentially the same. A key education point for patients is that because foods containing either starches or sugars are digested into glucose at approximately the same rate, it is important to control the total amount (and not the type) of carbohydrate consumed. Of course, good nutrition principles prevail, and the message regarding sweet foods should still be one of moderation, as these foods are often high in fat and calories and provide little nutritional value.

Glycemic Index

The concept of the "glycemic index" was developed by staff at the University of Toronto and shows how certain food affects blood glucose levels. A more precise definition of glycemic index (GI) is: a system of ranking foods containing equal amounts of carbohydrate according to how much they raise blood glucose in comparison with a reference food (50 grams of glucose or 50 grams of bread).

The glycemic index of a carbohydrate food is determined by assigning that food a number from 0 to 100, where 100 means that 1 gm of carbohydrate from this food raises the blood glucose to the same level as 1 gm of carbohydrates from bread. In other words, foods with lower GI have less of an effect on blood glucose than do foods with higher GI. Low GI foods are ranked between 0 and 50; intermediate GI foods are ranked from 56 and 69, and high GI foods are ranked 70 or higher. Some foods are surprisingly fairly low on the glycemic index: the glycemic response of sucrose, for example, resembles more closely that of rice or potatoes. Fruits and milk (sugars) produce a much lower glycemic response than starches. Even M&Ms, the chocolate-coated candy, have a lower glycemic index than other, more healthful foods, including pasta.

To further complicate matters, many factors can affect the glycemic index of a food, including how it is prepared and in what form it is eaten. Furthermore, the glycemic index can be challenging for patients to apply to their daily food choices because foods are compared with one another not in usual portions but in equivalent amounts of carbohydrate. For example, a pound and a half of carrots and one cup of pasta each contain 50 grams of carbohydrate, and this amount is used to determine their GI even though it is very unlikely that anyone would consume one and a half pounds of carrots at one time.

Because of the difficulty of relating GI with portions sizes, some researchers suggest using another approach, called the glycemic load (GL). The GL combines the GI value and the carbohydrate content of an average serving of a food or meal, and is calculated by multiplying the GI number of a food by the number of grams of carbohydrate in a serving and then dividing by 100. A GL of 10 or less is low; 11–19 is medium; and 20 or more is high.

The American Diabetes Association concludes in its evidence-based nutrition recommendations that research does not support the glycemic index as a primary method of meal planning for people with diabetes. Recent research also casts some doubt on the effectiveness of this approach as an effective meal-planning tool. The current trend is to focus more on total carbohydrate intake than the specific breakdown among the starchy and sugary foods. Research has shed new light on the methods used by our bodies to get needed nutrition. Not all carbohydrates have the same effects on blood glucose levels. Thus, while it is not necessary to eliminate potatoes, it is important for people with diabetes to choose a variety of starches from day to day and to understand the differences among the various choices. The glycemic index and glycemic load may be beneficial for people with diabetes, and this view is in accord with Joslin's Nutrition Guideline, but these tools should be used only as adjuncts to other meal planning methods, such as carbohydrate counting. People adjusting their rapid-acting insulin based on carbohydrate intake can actually develop their own glycemic index by carefully counting carbohydrate grams and monitoring blood glucose levels before and after meals.

Carbohydrate Content

How much carbohydrate do we really need? Before insulin was discovered in 1921, the diets recommended by Joslin physicians and others treating people with diabetes were high in fat, high in protein, and low in carbohydrate. This made sense to those physicians — diabetes is a condition in which patients cannot metabolize carbohydrate, so remove carbohydrate from the diet! These diets were not unlike those advocated today in some commercial diet plans for weight reduction like "South Beach" or the "Atkins" program.

Our understanding of the nutritional needs of people with diabetes has come a long way since those early days. We know that about 100% of consumed carbohydrates are converted to glucose and serve as the main source of energy in our diet. Carbohydrate sources are bread, pasta, rice, cereals, fruit, milk, table sugar and sweets.

An analysis of the current low-carbohydrate/high-protein diets advocated by some reveals that the caloric range for weight loss is from 1000 to 1600 kcals. There is also a recommended calorie level for weight maintenance of 1800 kcals. Of course these diets work, they contain fewer calories! What is not discussed in these diet plans is their ability to fit it into a healthy lifestyle. Are they practical? Are there food limitations? Are they providing enough vitamins and minerals that are known to aid in keeping good health? What impact do these diets have on increasing the risk of coronary artery disease?

The fact is that low-carbohydrate/high-protein diets cause ketosis, electrolyte loss and dehydration. They may exacerbate kidney disease and gout, and may cause calcium depletion. Because some of these commercial plans promote the eating of highly saturated fat foods, they also may contribute to coronary heart disease. While these diets may be a short-term fix, they are not ideal for long-term health. In addition, people with diabetes who also have kidney, liver or heart disease, or who are pregnant or lactating should not follow a very low-carbohydrate/high-protein diet.

The ADA no longer recommends that a specific percentage of calories come from carbohydrate; however, it does advise against restricting total carbohydrate to less than 130 grams per day. The source and distribution of carbohydrate calories among foods with differing glycemic indices is secondary in concern to the total carbohydrate content. Nevertheless, unrefined, unprocessed carbohydrate foods should be used whenever possible. Joslin Diabetes Center's *Clinical Nutrition Guideline for Overweight and Obese Adults with Type 2 Diabetes, Prediabetes or at High Risk for Developing Type 2 Diabetes* recommends approximately 40% of calories from carbohydrate, the total not to be less than 130 grams per day, in accordance with the Recommended Dietary Allowance. This modest decrease in carbohydrate may improve postprandial blood glucose levels and enhance weight loss by utilizing stored fat for energy without causing ketosis or dehydration.

Carbohydrate Metabolism

After digestion and absorption into the bloodstream, carbohydrate has three key destinations, and insulin is important for all three to be reached. Carbohydrate can be:

- used to provide for immediate energy needs
- stored as glycogen, primarily in liver and muscle, to serve as a rapidly accessible energy supply (e.g., source of glucose for rebound hyperglycemia or fuel for muscle undertaking sudden activity)
- converted to fat, an almost unlimited potential storage space that can be used when glycogen stores are filled

Insulin must be present for glucose to take any of the three pathways described above, including the storage of fat in adipose cells. As a result, many patients think that insulin makes you fat. Of course, this is not true! Insulin is non-caloric! However, insulin, when given to a person with previously uncontrolled glucose levels, reduces calorie loss through glycosuria, can temporarily promote edema, and, when not balanced properly with food intake, can cause hypoglycemia, necessitating excess food consumption. Proper insulin use, balanced in a physiologic manner with carbohydrate intake, should not lead to excessive weight gain, although in the short run some increase in weight may occur.

Fiber

Fiber refers to a group of carbohydrate foods of plant origin (fruits, vegetables, grains, nuts and legumes) that the human gastrointestinal system cannot digest or absorb. Fiber has no caloric value and may be insoluble or soluble. Typical foods that are high in insoluble fiber are wheat bran, as found in bran flakes, bran muffins, or whole wheat bread. Insoluble fiber absorbs, but does not dissolve in, water, increasing gastrointestinal transit time. This fiber is not digested and contributes to stool bulk, occasionally acting as a laxative.

Foods high in soluble fiber include apples, citrus fruits, oat bran, oatmeal, dried beans and peas, and many vegetables. Soluble fiber slows gastric emptying, which can affect glycemic response if large enough quantities are eaten, and thus can be useful for people with diabetes. Soluble fibers are also known as "gel-forming" or "gummy" fibers because when dissolved in water, they form a gummy gel, which slows down glucose absorption and blunts postprandial glucose elevations. They likely accomplish this by disbursing the incoming food into various parts of this gel structure, retarding movement of nutrients toward the gut wall for absorption. Digestive enzymes may also become caught in the gel, slowing their interaction with foodstuffs.

The current recommendation for fiber intake is to aim for a minimum of 20–35 grams of fiber per day. Research shows that people with type 2 diabetes can lower their blood glucose significantly by increasing the amount of fiber in their diet to approximately 50 grams per day. *Joslin's Nutrition Guideline* promotes this amount, as well, if the patient can tolerate it. The average fiber intake in the United States ranges from 10 to 13 grams per day; most people will find meeting the goal of 50 grams per day to be challenging, and perhaps not realistic unless they take additional fiber supplements. When educating patients on increasing fiber intake, it is important that they be advised to increase fiber *gradually* (by 3–5 grams/day) to prevent bloating. Also, at least 8 cups of beverages need to be consumed each day, as a high-fiber diet without enough fluid can lead to constipation. People with gastroparesis may need a low fiber diet due to the slower emptying of stomach contents during digestion.

Soluble fibers have the advantage of being useful in treating dyslipidemia as compared to insoluble fibers. Oat bran (in oat bran cereal and oatmeal), pectin (in citrus fruits and apple peel), and legumes (dried beans and peas) all contain an ample amount of soluble fiber that help to lower the level of cholesterol in the blood.

Protein

Just as carbohydrates are constructed from building blocks of glucose, so are proteins made from amino acids constituents. Amino acids are also important components of hormones, antibodies, and bodily structural components. They provide energy to the body in the setting of carbohydrate insufficiency.

The recommended daily allowance (RDA) for protein is 0.8 g/kg of body weight. According to the Institute of Medicine, protein should constitute about 10% to 35% of the total calories for the day, although the ADA suggests aiming for 15% to 20% of calories from protein. Appropriate dietary protein sources include skinless poultry, fish and seafood, lean meat and tofu.

With regard to type 2 diabetes, protein may aid in creating a sensation of fullness; maintaining muscle mass during weight reduction; and improving glucose uptake by muscles without increasing postprandial blood glucose. Thus, *Joslin's Nutrition Guideline* suggests aiming for approximately 20 to 30% of total calories from protein, as long as signs of diabetic kidney disease (microalbuminuria, increased serum creatinine or decreased creatinine clearance) are absent.

Fat

Fat (primarily triglycerides) is a dense energy source, providing 9 calories/gram in comparison to carbohydrate or protein, which provide 4 calories/gram.) However, because fat is metabolized via different pathways than carbohydrate and protein, it has less immediate effect on blood glucose levels. Yet, fat delays the emptying of food into the intestines, and thus may slow down the rise in the blood glucose if included as part of a mixed meal. A high-fat meal may result in a high blood glucose many hours later than expected due to delayed gastric emptying of carbohydrate and protein.

Fat is also a component of certain molecules and structures in the body, though not all of these fats are manufactured by the body. Some of these essential fats (linoleic and linolenic acids) must therefore be included as part of a normal diet.

People with diabetes often have elevated plasma cholesterol and triglyceride levels and lower levels of high-density lipoproteins (HDL) than nondiabetic individuals. Evidence suggests that lowering plasma lipid levels can reduce the occurrence of cardiovascular disease either through dietary adjustments or, if needed, with medications.

Dietary fat is digested into fatty acids, which are then absorbed into the bloodstream or stored. When the level of insulin is low, such as during weight loss or ketoacidosis, the opposite occurs — fat comes out of storage and is an alternative source of energy. The by-products of the use of fat as an energy source are known as ketones. **If ketones are seen during weight loss in a person with type 2 diabetes, despite well-controlled blood glucose levels, they indicate that the meal plan is successful.** *However,* **the presence of ketones in a person with type 1 diabetes with high blood glucose levels due to sickness or missed insulin injections shows a dangerous insulin insufficiency and indicates that more insulin is needed immediately.**

Cholesterol and triglycerides travel in the bloodstream as part of lipoprotein particles. Lipoproteins are classified by density and size. Low-density lipoproteins (LDL), or "bad cholesterol", usually carry cholesterol. High levels of LDL are dangerous because they deposit the cholesterol in the vascular epithelium. However, high-density lipoproteins (HDL), the so-called "good cholesterol" carry cholesterol away from blood vessel walls, back to the liver, where it is disposed of.

Triglycerides are made up of three fatty acid molecules. Fatty acids can be saturated or unsaturated. The choice of fats is important. In general, most saturated fats can increase cholesterol levels and are more harmful than unsaturated fats. Stearic acid and the medium-chain triglycerides are exceptions to this rule. Animal fats, which are usually solid at room temperature, are saturated fats. Palm and coconut oil are also saturated. Saturated fats raise blood cholesterol levels by interfering with the entry of cholesterol into cells. This causes cholesterol to remain in the blood stream longer and to become part of the plaque that builds up in the blood vessels.

Cholesterol intake should be limited to less than 300 mg/day. However, for patients with high LDL (>100 mg/dL), it should be lowered to less than 200 mg/day. By comparison, the average American consumes between 200 and 300 mg of cholesterol per day.

Trans fat is a type of fat formed from partial hydrogenation of oil, a chemical process that changes a liquid oil into a solid fat. The process involves adding hydrogen to liquid oil and turning it into solid or semisolid fat. *Trans* fats are found in many processed foods, including snack foods, cookies, some margarines and fast foods. *Trans* fats raise LDL-cholesterol level and significantly increase the risk for coronary artery disease more than any type of fat. For this reason, it should be limited as much as possible. As of January 1, 2006, the FDA has required that all food manufacturers list *trans* fat on the nutrition label, along with saturated fat and dietary cholesterol. *Joslin's Nutrition Guideline* recommends complete elimination of trans fat from the diabetes meal plan.

Monounsaturated fats such as olive, peanut, and canola oils may help reduce cholesterol levels and raise HDL levels. Therefore, these are usually recommended as best sources of fat. Keep in mind, however, that all fats are dense in calories.

Polyunsaturated fats are also preferred over saturated fats. The primary sources of polyunsaturated fats are the vegetable oils such as corn, soy, safflower, and sunflower oils. These fats are liquid at room temperature. While polyunsaturated fats are considered to be "heart healthy," the use of monounsaturated fats is preferred, as monounsaturated fats may help raise HDL cholesterol levels in addition to lowering LDL cholesterol. Polyunsaturated fats contain just as many calories as all other fats. Remember, too, that if these "good" oils are hydrogenated (as may be indicated on the ingredient label) they can raise the LDL (the "bad" cholesterol).

Fish is a source of two types of omega-3 fatty acids: eicosapentanoic acid (EPA) and docosahexanoic acid (DHA). Omega-3 fatty acids may help lower the risk of cardiovascular disease by in reducing triglyceride and blood pressure levels, and decreasing the risk of arrhythmias. Good sources of omega-3 fatty acids include fatty fish, such as salmon, herring, mackerel, trout and sardines. The American Heart Association recommends eating at least two servings of fatty fish per week. Supplements may be recommended for people who are not able to consume adequate omega-3 fatty acids by food alone. The use of such supplements should be discussed with and monitored by a healthcare provider, and this is especially important for people who are taking blood-thinning medications.

Another type of omega-3 fatty acid, called alpha-linolenic acid and found in walnuts, canola oil, flaxseed and olive oil, is another essential fatty acid and is thought to help decrease blood clotting and decrease inflammatory processes in the body. Patients should be encouraged to obtain alpha-linolenic acid from food sources rather than from supplements.

The current ADA recommendation is to base the percentage of calories that may be derived from fat on the patient's specific nutritional assessment, treatment goals, and lipid levels. A general guideline, based on the USDA Dietary Guidelines for Americans 2005, for those who are at a healthy weight and whose lipid levels are not a concern would be to limit fat intake to 20% to 35% of total calories; of this, less than 10% should be saturated (although the ADA does recommend that less than 7% of calories come from saturated fat).

Joslin's Nutrition Guideline for overweight or obese patients with type 2 diabetes recommends aiming for 30 to 35% of calories from fat, and limiting saturated fat to less than 10% of total calories or to less than 7% of total calories if LDL cholesterol is greater than 100 mg/dl. Polyunsaturated fat should comprise no more than 10% of calories, and the remaining 15 to 20% of total calories should come from monounsaturated fats

Two dietary substances that have recently attracted attention, called plant stanols and plant sterols, have the ability to lower blood cholesterol levels, and their daily consumption is recommended as part of a "heart-healthy" diet. It has been known for more than 50 years that these substances can lower blood cholesterol levels. Plant stanols and sterols are found naturally in many fruits, vegetables, nuts, seeds, legumes and vegetable oils, although the amounts in these foods are not high enough to significantly impact cholesterol levels. Some food manufacturers have developed products that contain appreciable amounts of either of these ingredients. Two margarines on the market, Benecol and Take Control, contain plant stanol esters and plant sterol esters, respectively. These substances block dietary cholesterol absorption, resulting in a significant lowering of total serum and LDL cholesterol levels averaging 10%. The National Cholesterol Education Program's ATP III Guidelines recommend

2 grams plant stanols as part of a daily diet that is low in saturated fat and cholesterol to help reduce heart disease.

Sweeteners

Sweeteners are categorized as nutritive (containing calories) and non-nutritive (non-caloric). Different sweeteners can have different effects on blood glucose levels.

Nutritive Sweeteners

For many years, the common nutritive sweetener, sugar (sucrose), was excluded from diabetes meal plans in order to avoid the significant postprandial excursions in glucose levels that it might cause, as well as to reduce the caloric intake of those hoping to lose weight. Other nutritive sweeteners that did not cause such postprandial excursions, as well as non-nutritive sweeteners, replaced this sugar. However, as more was learned about the true glycemic indices of various foods, both alone and in combinations, the concerns over the hyperglycemic effects of sucrose lessened. Further, people who selected alternative nutritive sweeteners, thinking that the "sugar-free" designation would allow unlimited consumption soon learned that "sugar-free" does not mean "carbohydrate free!"

All nutritive sweeteners must be included in daily carbohydrate allotments. Commonly used nutritive sweeteners in addition to sucrose include the sugars fructose and dextrose, as well as honey, corn syrup and molasses. All of these substances contain the same number of calories per gram (4), and, in significant amounts, all can elevate the blood glucose level.

The sugars in common usage consist of six carbon atoms or hexoses. One of these sugar molecules is called a "monosaccharide," while two bonded together are a "disaccharide." Glucose and fructose are monosaccharide hexose sugars. Sucrose, a disaccharide made up of glucose and fructose, is the most common sweetener used by manufacturers to sweeten their products and the one that those with diabetes have tried hardest to avoid.

Recently, as a result of improved understanding and better treatment tools, more sucrose has been included as part of the medical nutrition therapy prescription. Properties such as the bulking effect of sugar, which is lacking in non-nutritive sweeteners, make it difficult to eliminate entirely in some recipes. Also, sucrose when combined with other ingredients high in fat, such as in ice cream, may not cause an overwhelming glucose elevation in the immediate postprandial period. In addition, with very rapid-acting insulins, as well as antidiabetes mediations that specifically stimulate postprandial insulin release, insulin effect can now be more focused during the postprandial period. Some sucrose may be allowed as part of the carbohydrate content of a full meal (or as dessert). Calories still count, however, and for those on weight-loss diets, extra calories such as those in dessert-type foods are not advisable. If such foods are eaten, the usual recommendation is to have the patient carefully monitor postprandial glucose excursions and, with the help of a dietitian or other provider, develop his or her own medication adjustment scale for such foods.

Fructose (or "fruit sugar" or "levulose") is found in fruits and honey, and is 1.0 to 1.8 times as sweet as sucrose. Fructose plus glucose make up sucrose. Fructose is absorbed into the bloodstream more slowly than sucrose and appears to cause a slower rise of the blood glucose level for a given concentration of calories in persons with well-controlled diabetes. However, it is still a sugar and requires insulin for proper utilization. People who have high blood glucose levels due to insufficient insulin convert fructose to glucose, which results in a further rise in blood glucose level. Fructose may also worsen pre-existing problems with hypertriglyceridemia. The routine use of fructose as a substitute for sucrose in small quantities such as in cooking and baking is reasonable.

The *sugar alcohols* are basically sugar molecules converted to their alcohol form. Commonly used sugar alcohols include sorbitol, xylitol, mannitol, and hydrogenated starch hydrolysates. These substances contain approximately 2 calories per gram. Compared with glucose and sucrose, they are not completely absorbed and thus cause less postprandial hyperglycemia. But herein lies the problem, as well. Poor absorption can result in an osmotic diarrhea when these substances are consumed in large quantities (over 30 grams daily), although some patients will experience diarrhea, cramps and gas with smaller amounts. Sorbitol, for example, is found in many products such as ice cream, chewing gum, and "sugar-free" candy and baked goods. A key education point concerning foods containing sugar alcohols is that these "sugar-free" foods still contain carbohydrate — sometimes as much as the regular version, as well as calories and fat, and thus need to be counted in the diabetes meal plan.

Non-nutritive Sweeteners

Non-nutritive sweeteners provide almost no calories and do not affect blood glucose levels. These include:

- Aspartame: Nutrasweet, Equal, Sweet Mate
- Saccharin: Sucaryl, Sugar Twin, Sweet Magic, Sweet 'n Low
- Acesulfame-K: Sunette, Sweet One
- Sucralose: Splenda

Artificial sweeteners have improved the quality of life for many people with diabetes and those who are trying to lose weight. All of the non-nutritive sweeteners have undergone the FDA's rigorous safety testing.

Saccharin is 375 times sweeter than sucrose by weight. It has been available for some time, as it was first developed in the late 19th century. Until the advent of aspartame, saccharin was the leading non-nutritive sweetener, used in many soft drinks and as a tabletop sweetener, although many people complain that it has a displeasing aftertaste. A study suggesting a higher incidence of bladder cancer in animals given saccharin lead to a reduction in saccharin use several years ago. However, these animals were fed very large and unrealistic doses of it, and there is no evidence of a cancer risk in humans. In 2000, saccharin was dropped from the FDA's cancer-causing chemical list.

Aspartame is considered a non-nutritive sweetener. Although it does contain 4 calories per gram, it is 180 times as sweet as sucrose, and it is effective in such tiny doses that it essentially has no real caloric value. Aspartame is made synthetically from the two naturally occurring amino acids aspartic acid and phenlyalanine. As it is made from phenylalanine, people with phenylketonuria (PKU) who cannot metabolize phenylalanine should avoid aspartame.

The Food and Drug Administration approved the use of aspartame in 1981. It is found in numerous products from cereals to soft drinks to chewing gum and does not have the same aftertaste as saccharin. It is added to products under the brand name Nutrasweet, while the tabletop form is marketed as Equal. Equal contains some added dextrose and dried corn syrup to allow its granular form to flow. Each packet is as sweet as 2 teaspoons of sugar, and provides 4 calories (compared with 32 calories for 2 teaspoons of table sugar). Aspartame is unstable at high temperatures and loses its sugar-like sweetness, so it is usually not used during the cooking process.

Aspartame has also faced some controversy. While extensive studies have not shown aspartame to be toxic, there have been a few reports that in some persons it may trigger migraine headaches or diarrhea. Some people are "sensitive" to aspartame, and even small quantities make them feel uncomfortable; thus they must be cautious in selecting commercially prepared foods to avoid aspartame. Fortunately, these complications appear to be relatively rare. Nevertheless, recommendations by both the ADA and the FDA suggest limiting the daily intake of aspartame to 23 mg per pound of body weight (50 mg/kg). For a person weighing 150 pounds, this would be about 3400 mg daily, a difficult amount to consume when you consider that one can of diet soda contains 170 to 200 mg of aspartame and that a packet of Equal contains 35 mg of aspartame. It should be noted that several health groups, including the American Medical Association, the American Diabetes Association, and the American Academy of Pediatrics Committee on Nutrition, have issued statements in support of the use of aspartame.

Acesulfame K. (acesulfame potassium) is a sweetener approved by the FDA in 1988 that is approximately 200 times sweeter than sucrose. It is derived from acetoacetic acid and chemically resembles saccharin. Acesulfame K is stable both in liquid form and for cooking and has no major health warnings. Some people do complain that it has a bitter taste when used in high concentrations, which is why this sweetener may be combined with other low-calorie sweeteners to improve the taste profile.

Sucralose, approved for use by the FDA in 1998, is a non-caloric sweetener made from sugar. It is 600 times sweeter than sucrose. Its stability enables it to retain sweetness over a wide range of temperatures, which allows it to be used in a variety of foods. It is found as a low-calorie sweetener (Splenda) in fruits, juices, baked goods, sauces and syrups. More than 100 studies conducted over 20 years demonstrate the safety of this sweetener. Sucralose is safe for use during pregnancy.

Neotame, approved for use by the FDA in 2002, is the fifth non-nutritive sweetener available in the United States. This sweetener, which is approximately 8000 times sweeter than sucrose, is expected to be used in a wide variety of foods, including beverages, frozen desserts, dairy products, baked goods and chewing gum. Neotame is not yet widely used in products, although there are a few beverages and candies available that contain it.

Stevia. Some people use stevia as a sweetening agent. Stevia is a South American shrub whose leaves have been used for centuries in South American cultures to sweeten a beverage called yerba mate. Stevioside, the main ingredient in stevia, is three hundred times sweeter than sucrose and is calorie-free. The FDA has not approved stevia to be used as a sweetener, but because it is an herb and is thus considered a dietary supplement, it can be purchased in health food stores. While other countries use stevia as a sweetener, the United States, Canada and the European Union cite lack of safety evidence as reasons for non-approval. Large amounts of stevia given to animals have led to problems with the reproductive system, problems with carbohydrate absorption, and the formation of a mutagenic compound that could be carcinogenic.

Vitamins, Minerals and Supplements

If the diet is adequate, there may be no need for additional vitamins. It is important to determine whether your patients are taking any dietary supplements. Though you need to offer advice if any supplements they may be taking are harmful, be mindful not to be judgmental, as it is important for patients to be involved in their self-treatment. In addition, many people take supplements based on their cultural beliefs about nutrition and medicine.

Patients who are at risk for nutritional deficiencies and for whom you might want to suggest a vitamin supplement are vegetarians, the elderly, pregnant or lactating women, those with poor metabolic control, those who experience malabsorption, who have had myocardial infarctions or congestive heart failure, or people who are following very-low-calorie diets. Women with diabetes may need a calcium and vitamin D supplement to optimize bone health and prevent osteoporosis. Some younger women may need an iron supplement if they have or are at risk for iron-deficiency anemia.

A study by researchers at the Beetham Eye Institute at Joslin Diabetes Center showed high doses of **vitamin E** supplements to be effective in improving blood flow in the retina of the eye and the kidneys in patients with type 1 diabetes. Caution is recommended, however, in suggesting vitamin E supplements to diabetes patients, as further studies are needed to confirm these findings. Furthermore, a recent study indicates that high doses of vitamin E may actually be harmful to older people.

When treating people with diabetes, keep in mind that both deficiencies and overdoses of the B vitamins can cause symptoms similar to diabetic neuropathies.

Those studying **chromium** have found that, in the Chinese population, supplements up to 200 mcg improved blood glucose levels, which makes sense, given that chromium is a trace mineral that helps insulin do its job. However, another, more recent study has shown that chromium given in doses of either 500 or 1000 mcg did not improve blood glucose control in obese patients with poorly-controlled type 2 diabetes. The chromium did not produce any greater reduction in A1C levels than a placebo. Furthermore, true chromium deficiencies are rare, and there is some doubt that chromium will have any benefit unless a deficiency is present. The faddists' suggestions to use chromium as an antidiabetic agent may also carry some risk — chromium excess has been shown to be harmful in lab animals.

Cinnamon is a popular spice used extensively to season many different foods. Over the past several years, cinnamon has been used as a dietary supplement by many people with diabetes to help lower blood glucose levels. Phenols, antioxidants found in this spice, are involved with glucose transport and curbing inflammation in the body. In addition, polyphenol, another antioxidant found in cinnamon, has insulin-like properties which help to lower glucose levels. One study involving people with type 2 diabetes who were given various doses of cinnamon (1, 3 or 6 grams) showed beneficial effects: All doses of cinnamon lowered fasting glucose, LDL cholesterol, total cholesterol and triglyceride levels. Cinnamon is considered to be quite safe, with no significant harmful side effects, other than possibly causing an allergic reaction in certain individuals. However, the use of cinnamon oil should be avoided due to its toxic properties. At this time, there is no standard recommendation for dosing for cinnamon, but research indicates that one gram (1/5ᵗʰ of a teaspoon) of cinnamon is a reasonable starting dose. Type 2 diabetes patients interested in trying cinnamon should be encouraged to monitor glucose levels carefully, noting any episodes of hypoglycemia that might warrant a medication adjustment.

Also, people who are magnesium-deficient may see an improvement in their blood glucose once they begin taking magnesium as a supplement. Magnesium is known to increase insulin sensitivity. Poor metabolic control can lead to losses of magnesium in the urine. The daily value (DV) for magnesium is 400 mg.

Because it is rare that people will obtain all of their vitamins and minerals from food sources, it's good practice to recommend a multivitamin/mineral supplement to adult patients with diabetes. Men and postmenopausal women should aim to choose a supplement without iron.

Sodium

Both the American Diabetes Association and the American Heart Association recommend keeping sodium intake to no more than approximately 2300 mg per day, which amounts to a teaspoon of salt. Because many people with type 2 diabetes have either high blood pressure or are salt sensitive (i.e., more likely to develop high blood pressure), it's recommended that these people be educated on ways to reduce sodium intake in the diet. Sodium intake may need to be adjusted based on other medical conditions that might be present such as hypertension or congestive heart failure. Salt restriction may not be advisable for patients with orthostatic hypotension.

Timing of Eating

Though the timing of food consumption is important, newer pharmacologic treatment agents have made the need for precision of meal timing less crucial.

For people whose diabetes is not insulin-treated, the total daily caloric intake should be modified based upon the person's individual goals. For those people who tend to skip meals, distribution of calories throughout the day may need to be addressed.

For people treated with insulin, food intake should coincide with the peak action times of the insulin. Typically, traditional diabetic meal plans often included several snacks consumed at insulin peak times. However, newer insulins and insulin treatment designs allow more flexibility. The rapid-acting insulins that peak sooner and mimic the timing of natural insulins, such as lispro, aspart, and glulisine, are being combined with effectively designed basal insulin programs using repeated injections of intermediate insulin (NPH), or more commonly the long-acting insulins glargine or detemir (see Chapter 9). These basal programs recreate the smoother, peakless, natural basal effects more precisely and avoid having large quantities of intermediate or long-acting insulin peaking at once. Therefore, meal timing can now be more flexible, as it is not as crucial to match a meal with the time that a large insulin dose may be having significant action.

Obesity

Obesity is epidemic in today's society among people with and without diabetes. While medical conditions may be the cause of obesity in a small minority, the basic reason that most are obese is that they consume more calories than they burn for energy. Obesity is becoming more of a problem in children, as well, and the result is that the incidence of type 2 diabetes in this young population has increased markedly in recent years. Contributing to this epidemic may be factors such as cutbacks in funding for school physical education, too much television, or the popularity of computer and video games. The 12 year old of a previous generation spent a weekend afternoon playing outside with friends, while 12 year olds now are more likely to spend that afternoon sitting at the computer, online with friends. To make matters worse, many eat out of habit and nibble while sitting by the computer, by the television or when doing homework.

Body mass index (BMI), which evaluates weight in relation to height, is the traditional gauge to measure obesity. It is defined as the body weight in kilograms divided by the square of the height in meters, or the weight in lbs multiplied by 703 and divided by the square of the height in inches.

$$BMI = \frac{\text{Body weight(lbs.)} \times 703}{\text{Height (inches)}^2} \quad \text{or} \quad BMI = \frac{\text{Body weight (kg)}}{\text{Height (meters)}^2}$$

As BMI levels increase over 25, so, too, does the health risk (see Table 5-1). According to the National Heart, Blood and Lung Institute (NHBLI), "overweight" is defined as a BMI of 25 to 29.9 kg/m², "obesity" is defined as a BMI $\geq$30 kg/m² and severe obesity as a BMI>40 kg/m²

Another key measure in weight and body-fat assessment is waist circumference. It is now known that waist circumference is a stronger predictor of cardiovascular disease (CVD) outcomes than BMI. Measuring the waist circumference gives an indication of the extent of abdominal fat, or central adiposity, which is fat that is more "metabolically active." A high amount of abdominal fat predisposes a person, not only for heart disease, but also for type 2 diabetes, high blood pressure and dyslipidemia as well. American men with a waist circumference of 40 inches or greater, and American women with a waist circumference of 35 inches or greater are at increased risk for CVD. In other ethnic groups such as Asians, the risk starts to increase at much lower waist circumference.

Waist circumference, along with BMI, blood pressure, blood glucose and blood lipid levels, should be measured in a primary care setting to identify those patients who are at cardiovascular risk.

Unfortunately, in many cultures obesity is confused with prosperity and good health. Obesity can also run in families, both through inherited tendency and also by learned eating habits and ethnic diet preference. Psychological issues can also contribute. Loneliness, depression, and anxiety can lead people to seek gratification by eating. Specific considerations for developing a weight loss program will be discussed later in this chapter.

Weight Loss

To lose weight, people must either take in fewer calories or burn up more calories — or both. Exercise alone does not usually result in significant weight loss; it is effective when accompanied by a lower caloric intake and behavioral modification. With weight loss, insulin works more effectively and less insulin is needed. Triglyceride levels also decrease, and glucose tolerance improves, signifying improved diabetes control. The

Table 5-1. Body Mass Index (BMI)

BMI	19	20	21	22	23	24	25	26	27	28	29	30	31	32	33	34	35
Height (inches)							Body Weight (pounds)										
58	91	96	100	105	110	115	119	124	129	134	138	143	148	153	158	162	167
59	94	99	104	109	114	119	124	128	133	138	143	148	153	158	163	168	173
60	97	102	107	112	118	123	128	133	138	143	148	153	158	163	168	174	179
61	100	106	111	116	122	127	132	137	143	148	153	158	164	169	174	180	185
62	104	109	115	120	126	131	136	142	147	153	158	164	169	175	180	186	191
63	107	113	118	124	130	135	141	146	152	158	163	169	175	180	186	191	197
64	110	116	122	128	134	140	145	151	157	163	169	174	180	186	192	197	204
65	114	120	126	132	138	144	150	156	162	168	174	180	186	192	198	204	210
66	118	124	130	136	142	148	155	161	167	173	179	186	192	198	204	210	216
67	121	127	134	140	146	153	159	166	172	178	185	191	198	204	211	217	223
68	125	131	138	144	151	158	164	171	177	184	190	197	203	210	216	223	230
69	128	135	142	149	155	162	169	176	182	189	196	203	209	216	223	230	236
70	132	139	146	153	160	167	174	181	188	195	202	209	216	222	229	236	243
71	136	143	150	157	165	172	179	186	193	200	208	215	222	229	236	243	250
72	140	147	154	162	169	177	184	191	199	206	213	221	228	235	242	250	258

Source: National Heart and Lung Institute. (http://www.nhlbi.nih.gov/guidelines/obesity/bmi_tbl.htm)

amount of energy used and the basal metabolic rate decrease with weight loss as a result of a low-calorie diet alone; this can slow down metabolism and may cause a "plateau" in weight loss. Adding exercise, especially with a relatively higher protein intake usually makes the difference by maintaining lean muscle mass. To summarize this dual pronged approach to weight loss, Dr. Joslin, in a humorous vein, has been quoted in many past publications musing that one of the best exercises is pushing oneself away from the table before one is full!

Other forces can affect the ability to achieve a desired weight:

- age
- ethnic customs and beliefs
- family habits
- lifestyle factors
- psychological issues

Setting a realistic weight-loss goal is an important part of any weight-loss program. Rapid-weight-loss programs rarely work in the long-run and should be avoided or only used in extreme situations. In addition, telling a person who is 50 pounds overweight that his or her goal is to lose those 50 pounds is of little use, as the person will invariably fail because such a goal is overwhelming. Once the initial weight loss plateaus, frustration often leads people to abandon their efforts.

Goals should be short- to medium-term, and realistic. The 1994 nutrition recommendations developed by the ADA changed the way we send messages to our patients about setting unrealistic goals for weight loss.

Moderate weight loss can result in a significant improvement in blood glucose in people with type 2 diabetes who are overweight or obese. It may not even be necessary to achieve "desirable" body weight — in many instances, a 10 to 20 pound weight loss (7 to 10% of body weight) is sufficient to significantly improve insulin sensitivity and glycemic control. Therefore, achieving a "reasonable" weight (the weight that a patient and provider agree can be achieved and maintained) may be a more realistic goal.

In addition, targets should be designed in steps or increments. For example, a person who is 50 pounds overweight might be given a goal of losing 10 pounds over a 3–6 month period. This goal is realistic and not so overwhelming. In addition, someone 50 pounds above ideal body weight may only need to lose 10 to 20 pounds to have a significant impact on metabolic parameters.

Providing a weight-loss goal is often ineffective if it is not accompanied by recommendations for specific behavior changes. Determine caloric intake levels as previously discussed and then use those levels along with information obtained from the nutritional assessment to design a specific medical nutrition therapy plan.

Initiating Medical Nutrition Therapy

From the initial diagnosis of diabetes, it is important that all healthcare professionals emphasize the central role that medical nutrition therapy has in the overall treatment strategy. While the availability of newer medications lightens the burden on dietary adherence in achieving glucose control goals, reaching such goals is not nearly as likely to occur without a proper medical nutrition program. *Patients need to hear this message from the beginning, and repeatedly throughout the course of treatment.*

A medical nutrition therapy program for a person with diabetes should be designed and prescribed just as any other medical treatment would be. In designing this program, the theories discussed above are translated into practical guidelines for individuals to follow. The ADA, the American Dietetic Association and Joslin Diabetes Center have developed guidelines and curricula for nutrition education.

Nutrition education is not a one-time event. It is an ongoing process. The first time patients are presented with the nutrition prescription, they tend to be overwhelmed, and reinforcement after they have tried to follow that prescription can increase the efficacy of the process. Behavioral change takes time and needs to be approached in small steps rather than by attempting to make one large lifestyle adjustment. For that reason, follow-up visits with a dietitian are most important.

The Role of the Dietitian

The registered dietitian (RD) is an important part of the diabetes healthcare delivery team. An RD is a medical professional with a postgraduate degree in the field of nutrition and has passed a national qualifying exam. The RD may be certified by the National Certification Board for Diabetes Educators, indicated by the initials "CDE" or "Certified Diabetes Educator" used after his or her name.

The role of the dietitian in the prescription and implementation of the medically prescribed nutrition recommendations can be the crucial link to successful lifestyle changes. Healthcare providers should identify dietitians in their area with interest and expertise in the design of meal plans for people with diabetes and use their consultative services regularly. The local American Diabetes Association chapter, other diabetes groups, or local hospitals can be resources for identifying such dietitians.

The Nutrition Prescription

The nutrition prescription, which, optimally, is designed by a registered dietitian, involves calculating caloric levels and determining appropriate combinations of nutrients while taking into account the weight, clinical goals, activities level, and health status of the patient. Goals for healthy eating should include the following:

- individualized calorie levels for growth/maintenance or weight loss
- blood glucose control
- normalization of blood lipid levels
- blood pressure control

Patient Assessment

The first step in implementing a nutrition prescription is to perform a careful patient assessment. This assessment should cover the patient's current habits, issues and needs with respect to the nutritional recommendations. Identifying the patient's readiness to learn will affect the ultimate treatment plan with respect to time, course of initiation, degree of changes to be anticipated, and prospects for ultimate success. The issues and questions included in the following checklist may be included in a nutritional assessment:

Patient Nutrition Assessment

1. Is the patient performing self-monitoring of blood glucose?
2. Is the patient keeping, or has he ever kept, a food record?
3. What type and how much physical activity does she presently do? Is she planning to change (increase) her activity level?

4. Does he have any concerns relating to finances or psychosocial issues that would impede his success at lifestyle changes?
5. What cultural factors and beliefs might be influencing her food choices and eating style?
6. What are his present medications and nutritional supplements?
7. What is the patient's weight history? Weight goals?
8. What are his recent laboratory values for A1C, fasting lipid profile, microalbumin/creatinine ratio?
9. What is the patient's current eating style?
10. Does the patient currently follow any meal plan?
    - How much effort is made to change to a healthier meal plan?
    - How close is the patient's actual intake to that prescribed by the meal plan?
11. How skilled is the patient at assessing food choices?
12. What foods does the patient avoid?
    - What foods does the patient eat excessively? (Based on the answers to the two questions above, an initial focus on food choice instruction can be determined.)
    - Does the patient know how to read a food label accurately?
    - Is the patient able to describe how different foods affect his blood glucose levels?
12. How skilled is the patient at assessing portion sizes?
    - Are portion sizes reasonable and controlled?
    - Are portions estimated or measured?
    - Does the patient need help estimating portion size?
13. Does the patient time meals and other food consumption appropriately?
    - Does he eat three balanced meals daily?
    - Does she skip meals?
    - Does he "graze"?
    - Are the intervals between meals optimal?
    - Have the diabetes medications and/or insulin been accurately based on the patient's usual eating style?
    - If the patient is adjusting his insulin intake based on the amount of carbohydrate he eats, is he doing this correctly?
14. Are the patient's eating habits consistent? How important it is to eat at regular intervals and to eat about the same amount of carbohydrate may vary, depending on treatment. For those not adjusting insulin, it

is crucial to be consistent about eating times. For those who do make compensatory adjustments, more flexibility may be allowed. Nevertheless, the degree of variability must be determined:

– Does your patient eat about the same time each day?
– Is the amount of carbohydrate eaten fairly consistent from day to day?

Planning Meals

Once the patient has been assessed and overall treatment goals have been determined with the patient, a meal plan is designed based on lifestyle and dietary preferences. Individualized degrees of consistency and nutritional balance are incorporated into this plan.

The meal planning approaches are categorized from basic to advanced:

- following healthy eating guidelines
- use of preplanned menus
- use of exchange or food choice lists
- use of counting methods

Healthy Eating Guidelines

Patients who are new to diabetes can make immediate improvements in their eating habits until they have the opportunity to meet with an RD. They can be given guidance in choosing healthy foods using a picture of a plate divided into suggested servings (see Figure 5-1). It is not expected that calories would be calculated at this point in the process; this is just a starting point.

The key changes targeted by healthy eating guidelines include:

- emphasizing limiting saturated and trans fats and added sugars
  - selecting substitute foods
  - food grouping and portion size
  - timing of meals
- eating a consistent amount of carbohydrate day-to-day
- increasing intake of fresh fruits and vegetables and whole-grain carbohydrates

Figure 5-1. Plate Method

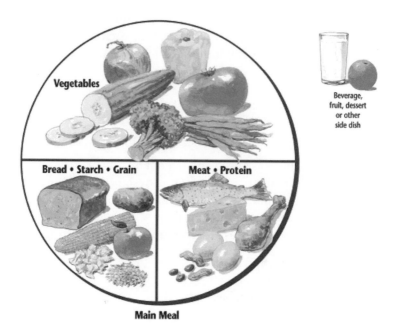

Preplanned Menus

Following preplanned, written menus can be helpful for patients who would benefit from having specific, written instructions with less flexibility. While this approach lacks variety, it emphasizes structure for those who need it.

Food Choice Lists

Food choice list, also known as exchange list, programs are useful for patients who are willing to follow a more structured system to control blood glucose or weight but want some flexibility to create their own menus.

The food choice lists categorize foods based on composition and by grouping foods that have similar calories, carbohydrate, protein and fat. Within each food group, foods may be substituted or exchanged for one another in the designated amounts. The nutrient distribution of these choices are summarized in Table 5-2.

If your patient is able to see a dietitian, the dietitian will work with the patient to create a meal plan — that is, the dietitian will determine the number of calories the patient needs per day and the proper number and ratio of carbohydrate, protein, and fat, and will then distribute these among the day's meals and snacks. Then the dietitian will write the number of choices (a choice is a certain amount of food, e.g., ½ cup, 1 oz.) allowed from each food group for each meal on a form similar to the one shown in Appendix 5-A. Thus, for breakfast a person who needs 60 grams of carbohydrate, 1 oz. of protein and 0 to 1 servings of fat will be allowed 1 fruit, 1 milk, 2 starch choices, 1 meat choice and 1 fat choice. By looking at a food choice list (see Appendix 5-B), the patient can select among appropriate and varied choices for the meal.

Carbohydrate Counting

Carbohydrate counting, a method of keeping track of the grams of carbohydrate one eats at meals and snacks, is a form of meal planning that has become increasingly popular. It can be used by anyone with diabetes, but is particularly useful for those who have an insulin treatment program that utilizes variable doses of rapid-acting insulin. **Carbohydrate counting is based on the premise that carbohydrate foods have the greatest impact on blood glucose, since almost all of it is converted to glucose, and all forms of carbohydrate have about the *same* effect on the blood glucose; therefore, carbohydrate foods can be easily exchanged for each other.** (An interesting perspective for your patients: while one might think that a teaspoon of sugar would make blood glucose rise faster than ½ cup of potatoes, in fact the potatoes will contribute about 15 grams of carbohydrate, while a level teaspoon of sugar will only give 4 grams of carbohydrate. Therefore the potatoes will have about three times the effect on blood glucose as the table sugar. Of course, though the blood glucose responds in the same way if two foods have equal amounts of carbohydrate, not all carbohydrates are equally healthy, and this fact needs to be emphasized to patients as well.)

There are two methods of carbohydrate counting. One method is referred to as a *consistent carbohydrate plan*, or *basic carbohydrate counting*. Patients using this method, and who know how many carbohydrate, protein

Table 5-2. Exchanges at a Glance

Food Group	Carbohydrate	Protein	Fat	Calories
Starch	15	3	trace	80
Fruit	15	0	0	60
Milk				
Skim	12	8	0	80
Low-fat (1%)	12	8	3	107
Low-fat (2%)	12	8	5	125
Whole	12	8	8	150
Other				
carbohydrates	15	0		varies
Vegetables	5	2	0	28
Protein				
non-fat	0	7	0	40–45
low-fat	0	7	3	55
medium-fat	0	7	5	75
high-fat	0	7	8	100
Fat	0	0	5	45

and fat choices they should have at each meal, are allowed to swap foods of equal carbohydrate content. Thus, a fruit or a starch or a milk choice are all approximately 15 grams of carbohydrate and can be interchanged with each other. As an example, a patient may be given a goal of 60 grams of carbohydrate at a particular meal. The patient can then decide how he or she will "spend" those 60 grams of carbohydrate. Patients treated with antidiabetes medications or who are on a fixed insulin dose program may choose to use this method.

The second approach to carbohydrate counting is referred to as a *flexible carbohydrate plan,* or *advanced carbohydrate counting.* This method can be used by patients who are competent in adjusting their doses of rapid-acting insulin in response to the type and amount of carbohydrate desired at meals and snacks. Thus, most of these patients tend to be using programs consisting of multiple daily insulin injections or an insulin pump (see Chapter 11).

Rather than retrospectively considering the past glucose patterns to determine the current insulin dose, the flexible carbohydrate counting method focuses attention on the planned, current food intake. The more carbohydrate that one plans to consume, the more insulin that is taken. In addition, further dose adjustments can be made to accommodate for the actual blood glucose level before the food is eaten. So, for example, if the patient's pre-meal blood glucose level is above target, the patient would take a "correction" dose of insulin along with the insulin needed to cover the carbohydrate at the meal. This method works well with people who are willing to do pre-and post-prandial blood glucose monitoring and keep detailed food and blood glucose records.

Patients must have a working knowledge of food and carbohydrate content from labels, food count books, or food lists in order to estimate the grams of carbohydrate in the meals and snacks that they eat.

Necessity of Carbohydrate Counting for Patients Using an Insulin Pump

Patients who are using a pump (see Chapter 11) rely on carbohydrate counting to ensure that they have programmed their pump to deliver the proper bolus dose of insulin. While the basal insulin controls blood glucose in the patient's fasting state and typically provides 50% of one's insulin needs, the bolus is a larger amount of insulin delivered by the pump to "cover" the food the patient eats. (A bolus can also quickly reduce a high blood glucose.) Bolus doses are matched to the carbohydrate content of each meal or snack eaten.

In order to determine what the bolus dose should be, one must first determine his insulin to carbohydrate ratio (I:Carb), which tells how much carbohydrate (thus the need for carbohydrate counting) 1 unit of insulin (rapid-acting or regular) will "cover." There are several ways to determine the I:Carb. One such method involves using what is call the 450 Rule. Here's how this works:

- Determine the patient's total daily dose (TDD) of insulin. This includes both rapid-acting and long-acting, or basal, insulin.
- Divide 450 by the TDD to derive the ratio. For example, if the TDD is

50 units, 450 divided by 50 equals 9. Therefore, the starting I:Carb is 1:9. This means that one unit of rapid-acting insulin "covers" 9 grams of carbohydrate.

- To use the ratio, the patient would then calculate the number of grams of carbohydrate he plans to consume at his meal. For example, if the patient will be eating 45 grams of carbohydrate, he would divide the 45 grams of carb by 9, which equals 5. This means that the patient would need to take 5 units of insulin to cover the 45 grams of carbohydrate.

Some endocrinologists advocate using the 500 Rule, rather than the 450 Rule. There is not much evidence supporting the benefits of one rule over the other, and since most I:Carb ratios need fine-tuning anyway, the initial calculation of such a ratio is merely a starting point, and the use of 450 or 500 is based upon personal preference.

The I:Carb, in general, is related to how insulin-sensitive a person is, and will vary from person to person. (The same person may have slightly different I:Carb ratios that they use for different times of the day, as well.) All patients choosing to use this advanced form of carbohydrate counting must, at least initially, be willing to check postprandial blood glucose levels in order to determine if the ratio is correct. If, for example, the 3-hour postprandial blood glucose is 40 points higher than target range (usually 100–120 mg/dl), and the patient is certain that the carbohydrate grams were accurately counted and the ratio used correctly, the ratio is probably incorrect and will need to be fine-tuned. The ratio used for each meal must be evaluated.

Once the I:Carb ratio is established, the patient's bolus dose can be calculated by taking into account the following factors:

- the amount of carbohydrate the patient plans to eat
- the I:Carb ratio
- the patient's blood glucose at the time the bolus is being calculated
- how much 1 unit of insulin will reduce the patient's blood glucose when it is above her target range (the patient's sensitivity factor)
- the length of time since the last bolus

One other important component of advanced carbohydrate counting involves the use of the sensitivity, or correction, factor. The Insulin:Carb ratio covers carbohydrate consumed at a meal. But if the pre-meal blood glucose level is above target, additional insulin is required to lower the glucose level back to target range. This is where use of the sensitivity factor comes in. The sensitivity factor is defined as the amount of blood glucose (mg/dl) that is lowered by 1 unit of rapid-acting insulin. Joslin Diabetes Center uses the 1500 Rule to calculate the sensitivity factor, although other institutions may prefer to use the 1800 Rule. Again, the point is that these formulas are merely starting points, and, just as with the I:Carb, the sensitivity factor needs to be evaluated and fine-tuned, if necessary.

The steps for calculating the sensitivity factor are as follows:

- Determine the total daily dose (TDD) of insulin, which includes both rapid-acting insulin and long-acting insulin.
- Divide 1500 by the TDD to determine the sensitivity factor. For example, if the TDD is 50, divide 1500 by 50 and the result is 30. This means that a unit of rapid-acting insulin will lower the blood glucose level by approximately 30 points.

Most people have a sensitivity factor between 30 and 50, although patients who are extremely insulin resistant may have a sensitivity factor of 10, for example, and those who are very insulin sensitive may have a sensitivity factor of 80.

Here is an example as to how the sensitivity factor is used:

- The patient's pre-meal blood glucose level is 250, and his target blood glucose is 100. Therefore, the blood glucose is 150 points higher than target.
- Divide 150 by the sensitivity factor of 30, which equals 5.
- The patient would need to add 5 units of rapid-acting insulin to his mealtime dose (calculated using his I:Carb ratio) to bring his blood glucose level back to target range postprandially.

The sensitivity factor is most commonly used when pre-meal blood glucose levels are high, as in the example above. It may also be used to correct a high blood glucose level apart from meals. Patients using pump therapy may need to correct apart from meals, for example. However, patients should be instructed not to randomly correct for high blood glucose levels, and should receive appropriate instruction from their healthcare team before doing so, in order to limit episodes of potentially severe hypoglycemia.

Most likely, patients interested in pump therapy will have been referred to specialists in diabetes care and management, and this specialist or, more likely, a diabetes team, will have helped the patient determine his or her I:Carb ratio, sensitivity factor, and the appropriate basal and bolus dose — and will have taught him or her how and when adjustments are necessary. As a member of the patient's overall healthcare team, however, it is important for the primary care provider to understand these basics of intensive therapy (see Chapter 10).

Evaluation of the Success of a Nutrition Plan

Whatever meal planning approach is selected, it is important that it be an integrated part of an overall diabetes treatment program initiated to reach specific goals of therapy. These goals must be measured, and if they are not being reached, adjustments in the treatment are needed.

For a person with type 2 diabetes whose diabetes is being controlled by diet alone, specific metabolic goals have been defined by Joslin and by the ADA: achieve an A1C level that is below 7%. If this goal is not met within a defined time period — 6–8 weeks — then more aggressive treatment is warranted.

The meal plan may need to be adjusted and/or the patient may need to start pharmacologic therapy. Antidiabetes medication therapies are usually the next step. Similarly, if medical nutrition therapy and medications fail to achieve targeted glycemic goals, progression to insulin must be considered. Monitoring progress towards reaching goals and helping evaluate the overall effectiveness of the meal plan can be done using a number of parameters:

- **Glucose control:** Are the glucose monitoring (SMBG) results approaching target levels? Is there improvement in the fasting, premeal and postprandial levels? Is hypoglycemia or hyperglycemia a problem? Is the A1C level below 7%?
- **Lipid Levels:** Are the lipid levels improving: total cholesterol, HDL, LDL and triglycerides?
- **Weight:** Is the patient losing or gaining weight (if that is the desired goal)?

- **Patient Satisfaction:** Is the patient satisfied with the approach chosen? Is he or she meeting overall nutritional needs? What difficulties is he or she having?

Food Labels

People have become more conscious of what they eat and the ingredients of the foods that they purchase. In 1994, the US government mandated that specific nutritional information be provided on food labels, making it easier for everyone, including people with diabetes, to determine more precisely what they are consuming. Ingredients are listed, as well as calories per serving and amounts of protein, carbohydrate, and fat.

There are still many pitfalls in understanding labels. Some are difficult to read and hard to understand. Words do not always mean what they say, particularly with regard to the so-called "dietetic" foods.

Patients should be advised to pay particular attention to the serving size, as the other nutritional measures, such as calories, fat and carbohydrate, are based on this parameter. The serving size may or may not relate to the serving size on exchange lists, but can be used for comparison. In advising patients about labels, ask them what serving size they would usually have. Remind them that if they usually eat one cup and the portion on the label is for 1/2 cup, they are getting twice as many nutrients and calories.

An example of a healthy food product is defined as the following and can be used in comparing items:

- saturated fat <1 gm/serving
- low-fat <3 gms/serving
- fiber >3 gms/serving
- sodium
  - snack item: <400 mg/serving
  - entree <800 mg/serving

As of January 1, 2006, the FDA requires all food manufacturers to list the trans fat content on the Nutrition Facts label. Trans fat, just like saturated fat, can raise LDL cholesterol levels, increasing the risk for heart disease. At this time, there is no Daily Value for trans fat, but the overall goal is to educate patients to choose foods with as little trans fat as possible.

"Dietetic" Foods

Many people mistake "dietetic" for "diabetic." Another common error is to assume that all "dietetic" and "sugar-free" foods are low in calories or have no carbohydrate. This is not true, and can be misleading to many patients.

In the past, patients were advised to strictly avoid sucrose, but this is not felt to be such a concern today. The total carbohydrate and caloric contents are important, however. Thus, patients need to be informed consumers and read past the packaging designations and consult the actual nutrition labeling. Some "dietetic" foods may be useful for people with diabetes. These include sugar-free soft drinks, sugar-free gelatin, artificial sweeteners, dietetic jellies and syrups, and reduced-calorie dressings. The most important point is to read the label. Even if the product is lower in calories than the "real" product, such foods still may contain more calories than the consumer bargained for. Also, patients should look out for the nutritive sweeteners (sucrose, fructose, sorbitol) that can still increase blood glucose levels.

The labeling laws allow manufacturers to declare an item "sugar-free" in bright, bold print. The "sugar" that they are referring to is sucrose, and often the print is less bold when they state that they have replaced the sucrose with another carbohydrate (such as fructose, sorbitol, or others). These may have as many calories and carbohydrates, and may cause an elevation of blood glucose level equal to the sucrose they replaced.

The "dietetic" designation only indicates that the product has fewer calories than the standard version. For example, "diet candy" may have only 80 calories per piece, where the "regular" version has 150! Also, beware of what might have been used to replace the missing calories. For example, in the candy in question, the fat content might have been increased so as to maintain the expected consistency. Thus, the "healthier" *sounding* product might not be as healthy as the regular counterpart!

Alcohol

Alcohol may be used in moderation by patients who have good glucose control and for whom there is no other contraindication. Alcohol blocks hepatic glucose production, which can functionally increase the clinical efficacy of insulin and make recovery from hypoglycemia more difficult. Also, the effects of alcohol consumption can have detrimental effects on a patient's ability to follow self-care procedures or to recognize early hypoglycemic symptoms so as to prevent more severe consequences.

Keep in mind also that alcohol contains calories, so that even without other specific reasons to restrict drinking, those patients following a calorie-restricted meal plan must include the caloric content of such beverages in the daily intake calculation. In addition, calories from alcohol lack nutritional benefit, and should not be substituted for more important components of the nutrition prescription. Often, reduction of the calories in alcohol consumption can be a successful component of a weight-loss strategy.

Nevertheless, in recent years, the evolution of more responsible attitudes toward alcohol consumption and the availability of products such as light and alcohol-free beers have made the social aspects of moderate drinking more compatible with adherence to nutritional plans for people with diabetes. When incorporating alcohol into a nutrition program, a compensatory reduction in fat intake should occur based on the quantity of alcohol consumed at 7 kcal/gram. The carbohydrate content of sweetened drinks must also be taken into consideration.

Alcohol recommendations for adults with diabetes are similar to those for the general public: men should limit alcoholic drinks to two or less per day, and women one or less per day. One "drink" contains about 15 grams of alcohol and is defined as:

- 12 oz. of beer (preferably light)
- 5 oz. wine
- 1 ½ oz. distilled spirits (scotch, whiskey, rum, vodka)

People with diabetes who take insulin or diabetes pills that can lower blood glucose levels should be instructed to drink alcohol with food to reduce the risk of hypoglycemia. No food should be omitted in exchange for an alcoholic beverage.

Certain people should not drink alcohol, including pregnant and lactating women, and those people with medical problems such as pancreatitis, advanced neuropathy, and alcohol abuse. Patients with extremely elevated triglyceride levels should be encouraged to avoid alcohol. Excessive amounts of alcohol may increase blood pressure and may worsen diabetic retinopathy. Finally, patients who take metformin should avoid drinking large amounts of alcohol due to the increased risk of lactic acidosis.

Vegetarian Diets

A properly designed vegetarian meal plan can be very healthy. Vegetarians often have a lower morbidity and mortality from macrovascular diseases (which are worsened by dietary fats found in animal meat) than do nonvegetarians. Vegetarian diets are inherently higher in carbohydrate, but planned carefully, they can be well tolerated. It is important that patients and patients' families be well educated when adopting this type of nutrition plan, especially if the diet is for a child with diabetes, as deficiencies may develop, particularly of iron, calcium and/or vitamin B12.

Legumes (dried beans and peas) have a very low glycemic index and their high fiber content can help lower cholesterol levels. However, people who follow a strict vegetarian ("vegan") diet (eliminating all animal protein including dairy and eggs) must ensure that they derive their protein sources from cereals and grains in order to maintain an adequate intake of protein. Patients who are interested in following a vegetarian meal plan should be referred to a registered dietitian.

Fasting

Fasting is not recommended for people with diabetes, particularly those treated with insulin. For those with type 2 diabetes, consumed food is important to stimulate endogenous insulin, and thus is important in metabolic homeostasis. Fasting for the purpose of losing weight can be dangerous for anyone and should not be undertaken except under strict supervision by a physician.

For some, there are religious reasons to fast. Some people fast for periods of about a day, such as for the Jewish holiday of Yom Kippur. Over the years, rabbis have been confronted with the question of how people with diabetes should handle this situation. Many have suggested that an individual's health takes precedence over religious observance and have therefore condoned the decision not to fast. Some live the "spirit" if not the letter of the law by consuming a drink of sugar-containing liquid (juice or soda) every hour or two, to equal 1 ounce for every hour of fasting. Some choose small amounts of food. In response to this approach, some rabbis have commented that while a full meal would be a big sin, many small snacks would be just tiny sins and in total would not be very much of a sin at all!

The fast of Ramadan, observed by Muslims, represents a one-month period in which only 2 meals are eaten, an early breakfast and a later dinner with no lunch. The duration of fasting extends for 8–16 hours between sunrise and sunset and depends on the season of the year. Insulin-sensitizing medications do not cause hypoglycemia and are usually safe in comparison to insulin-stimulating medications, which should be limited to use with the evening meal if needed. Insulin regimens usually need some adjustment. Avoidance of NPH insulin (due to peaking during fasting), and use of longer-acting insulin and rapid-acting insulin are preferable. Using SMBG may help in appropriate adjustments of diabetes treatment to compensate for this time change. As for diet, it is advisable to delay the first meal as long as possible toward sunrise. It is also advisable that this meal contain a higher percentage of calories from protein and carbohydrate that are high in fiber content to last for a longer period during the fast. The morning dose of rapid or short-acting insulin must be lowered by 20–30%. The second meal should be a balanced meal with a modest amount of carbohydrate to avoid a sudden rise in blood glucose levels. Many people prefer to eat a smaller snack, like soup or dates, followed within a few hours by a larger meal. In such instances, insulin should be injected with the larger meal to avoid insulin overlap. Dates are very high in carbohydrates and should be limited to 1–2 pieces for breaking the fast. Sweets that are high in sugar should be avoided and sweeteners should be used when applicable.

Food Records

People with diabetes are often asked to keep records of their food and/or carbohydrate intake, as well as activity level and blood glucose results. A completed food record is an invaluable tool to determine if the current diabetes treatment plan is successful or not. Encourage patients to keep at least a three-day food record prior to seeing a dietitian for the first time. Thereafter, a dietitian may ask the patient to continue to keep food records, especially if the patient is experiencing fluctuating blood glucose levels, is trying to lose weight, or is in the process of evaluating an insulin-to-carbohydrate ratio, for example.

Appendix 5-A

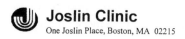 **Joslin Clinic**
One Joslin Place, Boston, MA 02215

MEAL PLAN

JC#_____

NAME: _____

VISIT DATE:_____

REFERRING MD:_____

Dietitian:_____   Phone:_____
Date:_____

CHO_____ g   PRO_____ g   FAT_____ g   CALORIES_____
Other Diet Modifications:_____

MEAL	SAMPLE MENU AND/OR SPECIAL INSTRUCTIONS	
BREAKFAST Time_____		
_____ g CARBOHYDRATES		
_____ Starch		
_____ Fruit		
_____ Milk		
_____ OZ. PROTEIN		
_____ FAT		
MORNING SNACK Time_____ g carb_____		
LUNCH Time_____		
_____ g CARBOHYDRATES		
_____ Starch		
_____ Fruit		
_____ Milk		
_____ Vegetable		
_____ OZ. PROTEIN		
_____ FAT		
AFTERNOON SNACK Time_____ g carb _____		
DINNER Time_____		
_____ g CARBOHYDRATES		
_____ Starch		
_____ Fruit		
_____ Milk		
_____ Vegetable		
_____ OZ. PROTEIN		
_____ FAT		
EVENING SNACK Time _____ g carb _____		

Appendix 5-B

 Joslin Diabetes Center
FOOD CHOICE LIST

CARBOHYDRATE FOODS

Grains / Breads / Starchy Vegetables (15 grams carb)

1 slice bread (1 oz)	1/3 cup cooked rice or pasta	1 small potato (3 oz)
1/4 large bagel (1 oz)	4-6 crackers*	½ cup corn or peas
½ hamburger or hot dog roll	½ cup cooked cereal	½ cup lentils or beans
½ English muffin	¾ cup dry cereal	1 cup winter squash
1 6-inch tortilla or pita bread	2 pancakes, 4" across*	1 cup broth based soup

Fruit (15 grams carb)

1 small fresh fruit	½ cup canned fruit or juice	¼ cup dried fruit
About 15 grapes	About 1 cup fresh berries	2 Tbsp raisins

Milk (15 grams carb)

1 cup fat free or low fat milk	¾ cup light-style yogurt	1 cup 2% fat milk*

Vegetables ("free" if 1 – 2 servings are eaten; 15 grams carb if 3 servings are eaten)

1 cup raw vegetables	½ cup cooked vegetables	½ cup vegetable or tomato juice

Other Carbohydrates (15 grams carb)

½ cup low fat frozen yogurt	¾ oz. pretzels/snack crackers	1 Tbsp jam, sugar or syrup
2 small cookies*	15 potato chips*	2-inch square brownie*

* starred items also have one additional fat serving (5 grams of fat)

MEATS / PROTEIN FOODS (5 grams fat, 0 grams carb)

1 ounce cooked lean meat, fish or poultry	¼ cup tuna	2 Tbsp peanut butter**
	¼ cup low fat cottage cheese	2 ounces tofu
1 ounce low fat cheese	2 Tbsp grated parmesan	1 egg or ¼ cup egg substitute

FAT FOODS (5 grams fat, 0 grams carb)

1 tsp butter° or margarine	1 Tbsp salad dressing	1 ½ Tbsp flax seed
1 tsp oil or mayonnaise	2 Tbsp reduced fat salad dressing	2 Tbsp cream or half & half°
2 tsp peanut butter	10 peanuts	1 Tbsp cream cheese°
2 Tbsp (1 oz) avocado	4 walnut halves	1 strip bacon°

° these items are sources of saturated fat

FREE FOODS (A free food has less than 20 calories per serving. Limit foods with serving sizes to 3 per day)

1 Tbsp fat-free cream cheese	1 Tbsp catsup	Diet/sugar-free soft drinks
1 Tbsp liquid non-dairy creamer	2 tsp low sugar/light jam or jelly	Sugar-free gelatin
¼ cup salsa	1 cup raw vegetables	Herbs, spices, seasonings

6

Physical Activity for Fitness

Richard S. Beaser, MD,
Edward S. Horton, MD and
Catherine A. Mullooly, MS,
RCEP, CDE

Introduction

Exercise is probably one of the earliest treatments for diabetes. It was noted in writings of ancient physicians and it has remained, along with diet, weight management and the use of insulin, an important part of the treatment troika. In recent years, the benefits of fitness derived from a physically active lifestyle have been extolled for everyone, not just those with diabetes. The result has been a renewed interest in this component of diabetes management as a primary focus of treatment, rather than merely as an action in the daily routine for which compensatory adjustments in food, insulin and other antidiabetic medications are necessary.

A physically active lifestyle has multiple fitness and health benefits for people with and without diabetes, including:

- reduction of cardiovascular risk
- improved lipid profile
  - decreased triglycerides
  - increased high-density cholesterol

- improvements in mild to moderate hypertension
- increased energy expenditure, promoting
  - weight reduction and weight management
  - preservation of lean body mass
- increased strength and flexibility
  - enhanced bone density
  - improved posture and balance
  - decreased risk of falls and injuries
- increased ease of daily activities
- improved sense of well-being

For people who *do* have diabetes, the impact of a physically active lifestyle can extend beyond the usual issues of fitness, because it may:

- lower blood glucose concentrations
- reduce glycohemoglobin levels (A1C)
- reduce the dose of oral diabetes medications and/or insulin needed
- increase the chance that the diabetes can be managed without any pharmacologic intervention
- increase insulin sensitivity
- reduce hyperinsulinemia

People with diabetes have a two to four times greater incidence of cardiovascular disease (CVD) compared to age and gender matched people without diabetes, and CVD is responsible for approximately 75% of diabetes-related deaths. A fitness regimen is an important tool in reducing these statistics. Its effects in improving insulin sensitivity and glucose control, combined with the benefits of cardiovascular training and resulting reductions in lipids and hypertension, clearly have significant implications for macrovascular health. For the person with diabetes or prediabetes, a program of regular physical activity impacts glucose metabolism not only by directly lowering the blood glucose levels, but also by improving the body's sensitivity to the effects of insulin. Indeed, it has recently been suggested that a fitness regimen, including weight reduction, can reduce the occurrence of type 2 diabetes. Two major studies, The Finnish Diabetes Prevention Study and The Diabetes Prevention Program (DPP) found that people at high risk for developing type 2 diabetes can lower their chances of getting the disease by as much as 58% by modest, sustained weight loss (10–15 pounds) and about 30 minutes of moderate intensity physical activity each day.

Effects of Physical Activity on People without Diabetes

When people are at rest, circulating free fatty acids provide up to 90% of the needed fuel for the skeletal muscle. Physical exertion, however, significantly increases energy requirements, which can come from a number of sources. Fat stored in muscle and free fatty acids released into the circulation from adipose tissue are two major sources. In addition, normal exercising muscle rapidly increases glucose utilization, which is obtained through the breakdown of glycogen stores in muscle and liver and the uptake of glucose from the circulation. During physical exertion insulin levels drop, while levels of counterregulatory hormone such as epinephrine, glucagon, and cortisol will rise. These hormone shifts result in further increases in blood levels of glucose and free fatty acids that can be used for energy, and reduce the risk of hypoglycemia.

The fuel for short bursts of physical exertion is primarily glucose. Muscle glycogen is used initially, followed after about two to three minutes by glucose from the circulating blood. After about 15 minutes of activity, however, the glucose used for fuel and maintaining adequate blood glucose levels comes increasingly from glucose newly made in the liver from glycogen breakdown or through gluconeogenesis. Blood glucose levels may actually rise in this circumstance, as glucose production may be greater than glucose utilization. Some energy can also be provided by the breakdown of protein into amino acids and their direct metabolism, or conversion, into glucose in the liver (especially alanine).

After about 30 minutes of physical exertion, as glycogen stores in liver and muscle start to become depleted, new production of glucose (gluconeogenesis) increasingly begins to supply glucose needs. However, such glucose production often cannot keep up with needs. To provide for these needs, and also to prevent overutilization of glucose and resulting hypoglycemia, the body turns to the free fatty acids for more of its energy supply.

Exercise results in increased insulin sensitivity, leading to increased glucose uptake by muscle cells during the post-exercise period. This effect may be seen for as long as twelve hours, and in some cases as long as twenty-four hours, after the physical activity has been completed, and is related to the rebuilding of the glycogen stores in the muscle and liver. This phenomenon is commonly referred to as the "lag effect." Insulin must be available for this process to occur, but there also must be enough glucose in the blood from which to make the glycogen. In people with diabetes, if the blood glucose levels are too low after physical exertion or there is too much insulin, the rebuilding of the glycogen stores can result in hypoglycemic reactions over the next several hours.

Effect of Physical Activity on People with Diabetes

Type 1 Diabetes

The ability of someone with type 1 diabetes to compensate for physical exertion is determined by the amount of available insulin, the degree of diabetes control, and the state of hydration. In theory, and often in reality, the person with well-controlled diabetes with insulin and food/fuel in proper balance can handle activity just as well as someone without diabetes. However, if the control is poor and the balance of these components is not well established, physical exertion can trigger significant metabolic aberrations.

In a person with poorly controlled diabetes, there is increased glucose production by the liver, as well as increased release of fat from adipose cells. This occurs as the deficient levels of insulin result in even higher blood glucose levels during physical exertion, with excessive hepatic glucose production adding to the problem.

The metabolism of free fatty acids results in the increased production of ketones. Thus, exercise by a person with poorly controlled type 1 diabetes results in elevated levels of glucose, as well as rising levels of ketones from the utilization of free fatty acids as an alternative fuel.

There is another interesting change that occurs with physical exertion in people with diabetes. As long as the diabetes is well-controlled and sufficient insulin is present, the additional glucose needed to fuel increased activity does not require an incremental amount of insulin. Muscle contraction itself increases glucose uptake by muscle fibers. As a result, more glucose utilization can occur per unit of insulin by working muscle than by resting muscle. For these reasons, physical activity is one of the three major factors affecting blood glucose levels, along with food and insulin.

Type 2 Diabetes

Exercise or physical exertion by a person with type 2 diabetes usually leads to a reduction in blood glucose levels. This is particularly so for people with type 2 diabetes who are in the hyperinsulinemic phase of the disease, as physical exertion does not induce as much of an insulin reduction as it would in someone without diabetes. Physical exertion increases insulin sensitivity, and as insulin resistance is a hallmark of type 2 diabetes, physical exertion directly works counter to the pathophysiologic abnormality causing this condition to occur. In fact, if those with type 2 diabetes are treated with oral antidiabetic medications or insulin, symptomatic hypoglycemia may develop. They may also demonstrate a significant lag effect, with the hypoglycemic effect persisting or occurring a number of hours after the activity has occurred.

The most striking benefit of an improved fitness level for the patient with type 2 diabetes is the increase in insulin sensitivity that can result. It is well known that lack of physical exertion can lead to some impairment in glucose tolerance, even in a person who does not have diabetes. Many people with type 2 diabetes are sedentary and this certainly contributes to their insulin resistance. By contrast, when such people participate in some form of endurance training or physical fitness program, they can experience improvements in insulin sensitivity. Even very obese individuals will improve glucose metabolism in response to a regular physical activity program. People with type 2 diabetes undergoing physical fitness training can demonstrate reductions in both fasting and postprandial glucose values, benefits not generally seen in people with type 1 diabetes.

The Physical Fitness Program

There are three components of a physical fitness program: cardiopulmonary endurance, flexibility and strength training. Cardiopulmonary endurance training is exercise carried out over an extended period of time and requiring sustained energy expenditure. It stimulates the heart and lungs and uses most of the body muscles for at least 30 or more minutes each session. Strength training is physical exertion such as weight lifting that applies heavy resistance to specific muscle groups. Flexibility involves stretching of specific muscle groups and increasing range of motion. It is important in the "warm up" and "cool down" phases of an exercise session. Most physicians and exercise physiologists recommend endurance training or a combination of endurance and strength training as the most useful activity for adults because of the beneficial stress effect on the cardiovascular and metabolic systems. Although all types of exercise are recommended for most people with diabetes, more time should be spent on endurance exercises.

Evaluation before Starting

Before starting a fitness program, your patients with diabetes should first be carefully evaluated. This evaluation is important at any age. It is assumed that older individuals have increased risk of heart, lung, or circulatory disease, particularly if they have multiple macrovascular risk factors. Medical clearance prior to starting the fitness program is assumed to be most important in this age group. Yet younger people with long-term diabetes still have a potential for underlying circulatory or cardiac disease as well, and should also undergo evaluation prior to starting a physical exertion program.

People can still engage in a physically active lifestyle in spite of the presence of diabetes complications, but an evaluation of these complications is important before starting the physical fitness regimen. These findings will be useful to identify any necessary modifications to the fitness program. A poorly designed program can exacerbate complications. Specific complications to focus on during an evaluation include:

- Proliferative retinopathy
  - vitreous hemorrhage
  - retinal detachment
- Nephropathy
  - increased proteinuria

- Peripheral neuropathy
  - soft-tissue and joint injuries
  - falls
- Autonomic neuropathy
  - decreased cardiovascular response to physical exertion
  - decreased maximum aerobic capacity
  - impaired response to dehydration
  - postural hypotension

As noted above, each- evaluation must be individualized. However, for people with diabetes, the evaluation should focus on areas in which complications are likely to be present:

1. *Cardiovascular system* — Take a detailed history, focusing on cardiovascular risk factors in addition to the diabetes, including:

   - dyslipidemia
   - hypertension
   - smoking history
   - gender
   - age
   - family history
   - weight
   - active vs. sedentary lifestyle
   - duration of diabetes
   - any history of cardiac or vascular disease

   Look for symptoms suggestive of coronary artery disease. An exercise tolerance test, or perhaps a stress echo or stress thallium, should be considered, particularly if the patient is over 35 years of age or has had type 1 diabetes or type 2 diabetes for over 10 years *or* type 2 diabetes and at least one of the following:
   - microalbuminuria
   - overweight/obesity: BMI > 28km/m2
   - dyslipidemia: LDL-C $\geq$ 100mg/dl, HDL- C , 40 mg.dl, TG > 200 mg/dl
   - known macrovascular disease (PVD)
   - family h/o CAD: under 55 y/o
   - hypertension; > 140/90 mmHg on 3 occasions

- smoker
- start of a new physical activity program
- autonomic neuropathy evidenced by
  ♦ cardiac autonomic function abnormalities
  ♦ orthostatic hypotension
  ♦ erectile dysfunction
  ♦ gastroparesis

Be aware that people with diabetes may have atypical symptoms of coronary disease. Significant occlusion of coronary arteries may be present with either no anginal symptoms at all ("silent ischemia") or with angina pain being manifest in an atypical manner such as jaw or shoulder pain ("anginal equivalents"). If there is any suggestion of cardiovascular disease, it is recommended that the patient participate in a supervised cardiovascular fitness program.

Screening for autonomic neuropathy affecting cardiac function can consist of listening for decreased respiratory rhythm variation, as well as measurement of postural blood pressures, watching for an excessive (20mmHg. with standing) drop in systolic blood pressure. A resting tachycardia of 100 beats/minute is also a good screen. Certainly, a history of postural symptoms such as dizziness or lightheadedness should be a warning of possible problems. People with significant autonomic dysfunction, particularly postural hypotension, might consider armchair exercise routines rather than activities involving walking or standing. Patients with autonomic dysfunction affecting cardiac function may not be able to achieve increases in heart rate comparable to those with no dysfunction. Therefore, caution should be taken not to push these people to exert themselves to the usual predicted maximum heart-rate levels. They might not be able to increase their pumping frequency as much and could, with significant exertion, experience cardiac insufficiency.

2. *Eyes* — All patients starting a physical fitness program should have a thorough dilated (or equivalent) evaluation by an ophthalmologist. Patients with severe or progressive diabetic retinopathy should not perform certain physical activities, as changes in blood pressure induced by these activities can increase the risk of blood vessel leakage or hemorrhage. Low to moderate intensity options are usually better for these

people. For people who do have active proliferative retinopathy, vigorous activity may precipitate a vitreous hemorrhage or retinal detachment. Such individuals should be advised not to participate in anaerobic activities or physical movements that include jarring, straining, or Valsalva-like maneuvers. The degree of retinopathy often dictates the risk associated with physical exertion.

3. *Renal Function* — The sudden or significant increases in blood pressure that can occur during physical exertion can increase renal pressure and, with preexisting diabetic renal disease, further worsen renal function. This concern is particularly acute with physical movements that cause a Valsalva maneuver such as lifting and straining. Systolic blood pressure response should not exceed 180 mmHg. Also, exercise will often result in increased microalbuminuria, which is usually transient and is not harmful. However, if a patient is found to have microalbuminura on a routine screening examination, be sure to obtain an exercise history and, if the patient has participated in strenuous exercise within the previous 24–48 hours, repeat the test after at least 48 hours without strenuous exercise.

4. *Lower Extremities* — Patients should undergo a careful examination of their lower extremities, with particular attention to detection of:

   - neuropathies
   - peripheral vascular disease orthopedic or podiatric abnormalities and/or histories

   Low-impact activities such as swimming that minimize trauma to the lower extremities should be considered. Any evidence of injury, particularly to the skin integrity, should be monitored closely. Proper footwear for different physical activities is also very important.

In addition, **for everyone with diabetes, the quality of diabetes control needs to be assessed prior to initiating a physical fitness program. If poor, control should be improved before the physical fitness program begins.** In general, for people with type 1 diabetes, physical exertion should not be performed unless the blood glucose level is below 250–300 mg/dl, except in the immediate post-prandial state. There should also be no evidence of ketosis in such individuals (see Table 6-2).

TABLE 6-1.　Considerations for Activity Limitation in Patients with Diabetic Retinopathy (DR)

Severity of DR	Acceptable Activities	Discouraged Activities	Reevaluation
No DR	Dictated by medical status	Dictated by medical status	12 months
Mild NPDR*	Dictated by medical status	Dictated by medical status	6–12 months
Moderate NPDR*	Dictated by medical status	Activities that dramatically elevate blood pressure: • power lifting • heavy Valsalva	4–6 months
Severe NPDR*	Dictated by medical status	Activities that substantially increase systolic blood pressure: • Valsalva maneuvers • active jarring: – boxing – heavy competitive sports	2–4 months (may require laser surgery)
PDR*	Low-impact cardiovascular conditioning: • swimming • walking • low-impact aerobics • stationary cycling • endurance exercises	Strenuous activities: • Valsalva maneuvers • pounding or jarring: – weight lifting – jogging – high-impact aerobics – racquet sports – strenuous trumpet playing	1–2 months (may require laser surgery)

* NPDR = nonproliferative diabetic retinopathy; PDR = proliferative diabetic retinopathy.

TABLE 6-2. When Patients with Diabetes May Exercise

Type 1	If blood glucose is 250 mg/dl or higher, check for ketones; – if **positive** for ketones—DO NOT exercise. If blood glucose is between 251 and 300 mg/dl: – if negative for ketones, it is okay to engage in physical activity. If blood glucose is over 300 mg/dl: – if negative for ketones, exercise with *extreme caution*
Children with type 1	Follow the guidelines above — **except** that it is okay to engage in physical activity with blood glucose of up to 400 mg/dl.
Type 2	Can engage in physical activity with blood glucose levels of up to 400 mg/dl (regardless of whether or not using insulin)

Diabetes control should be maximized through careful attention to glucose patterns, insulin doses and adjustments, and dietary guidelines. The patient should be educated on the adjustments for his or her program to compensate for physical exertion in order to avoid hyper-or hypoglycemia. Frequently adjustments of medications are needed, both for insulin and oral treatments. Usually, if an oral medication needs adjustment, it is an insulin secretagogue. These medication doses may be reduced if the individual engages in intermittent, acute increases in daily physical activity.

Prescribing the Fitness Program

A prescription for a fitness program should take into account four things:

1) type of activity
2) intensity
3) duration of each session
4) frequency of the sessions

TABLE 6-3. **Physical Activities Beneficial to People with Diabetes**

Individual Activities	
Brisk walking	Running or jogging
Swimming	Bicycling (including stationary)
Dancing	Skiing (downhill and cross-country)
Rowing	Skating (ice and roller)
Badminton	Golf (with brisk walking only!)
Wrestling	Stair climbing
Fencing	Tennis
Handball	Squash
Racquetball	Inline skating
Aquaerobics	Aerobic dance
Team Activities	
Soccer	Volleyball (vigorous only!)
Basketball	Hockey (ice and field)
Lacrosse	

Type

Aerobic activities are usually the preferred form of physical activity, and walking is the most commonly chosen of the types of aerobic activities. If this weight-bearing activity is not well tolerated, then other options can be utilized. Non-weight-bearing alternatives include armchair exercise, aqua aerobics, arm ergometry, rowing and stationery cycling.

Strength training may also be included in a physical fitness program if no contraindications exist. These types of movements improve muscle mass as well as contribute to improved posture, balance, gait and ease of daily activities. People with significant physical limitations can benefit from gentle strengthening exercises, such as walking, stair climbing and specific leg muscle strengthening exercises and the use of elastic exercise bands, to improve activities of daily living.

Physical movements to improve flexibility may also be recommended. These activities may be particularly useful for people who, with aging, have diminished flexibility. Yoga, tai chi and range-of-motion exercises are some examples.

Table 6-3 lists some appropriate activities for people with diabetes.

Choices will vary depending on ability, personal interest, climate, and available facilities. All fitness program recommendations should be individualized based on physical condition, medical conditions, and personal interest and goals.

Intensity

The intensity of physical exertion is determined by monitoring the heart rate and other signs of stress. Heart rate is measured by taking the pulse at the carotid artery, the temple, or the radial artery or by placing the hand on the chest. The heart rate should be measured within 5 seconds of stopping activity. People who are just starting an fitness program should also monitor their pulse rate four or five times during an physical activity session. Suggest to patients that that they can estimate their pulse rate by measuring it for 10 seconds and multiplying by 6, which will give them the heart rate per minute. Alternatively, affordable and accurate heart monitors are now available for use during physical activity.

Remind patients who use medications such as beta-blockers that these drugs may affect the heart rate. Also, the cardiac effects of diabetic autonomic neuropathy may affect the heart rate. In circumstances such as these, the pulse rate may underestimate the actual stress on the body, and caution must be taken. In these instances, the "Ratings of Perceived Exertion Scales" described below can be used.

Other signs of stress include labored breathing, light-headedness, angina, or a very pale face.

It is important that the person performing the fitness program be advised to work to the correct intensity in order to insure safety, as well as to maximize enjoyment. Increasing the heart rate as little as twenty to thirty beats per minute above the resting rate can provide significant health benefits.

There are several methods one can use when determining the appropriate level of intensity with physical exertion or of the physical fitness program:

1. *Heart Rate Reserve Method*

   If the desired goal is to improve fitness levels using aerobic activities, heart rates during physical exertion of between the intensity levels of 60% and 85% of the increment to maximal heart rate can be calculated

TABLE 6-4.   Exercise Heart Rate Calculation

TO CALCULATE EXERCISE HEART RATE (HR):

Formula: HRmax. = Max HR achieved on a Graded Exercise Test (GXT) or an Exercise Tolerance Test (ETT).
[Note: For a person with diabetes under the age of 35 who is otherwise healthy, an estimated Exercise Heart Rate may be calculated by using the formula: 220 − age.]

> HRrest = Pulse at rest
> Exercise Heart Rate =
> > [(HRmax - HRrest) x 60% and 85%] + HRrest

Example: Age = 70 and HRrest = 60 beats/minute (bpm)
HRmax = 150 bpm
Exercise HR = [(150 bpm - 60 bpm) x 60% and 85%]
+ 60 bpm = 114 - 137 bpm

---

using the **heart rate reserve** method (Karvonen formula — see Table 6-4). Remember that this formula is a guideline and the target heart rate can be adjusted based on the individual's response to physical exertion.

2. *Alternative Methods*
   - *Rate of Perceived Exertion Scale* — Another method of measuring the intensity of physical exertion is to have people monitor how they *feel* during physical activity. If they are short of breath, dizzy, fatigued or experience pain, they should reduce the intensity or rest. These subjective methods can be used if monitoring the heart rate is too cumbersome.

     A common method used for ratings of perceived exertion is the Borg RPE scale (also called the "Borg Scale" or the "RPE Scale"). It was developed by Gunner Borg (see *Resources* at the end of this chapter) and is constructed so that given ratings grow linearly with heart rate during physical exertion. It can be used in the same way as heart rate to estimate working capacity and to prescribe intensity during the physical activity. Patients may, for example, target their physical exertion to a particular level that is described by such terms as "somewhat hard" or "hard," and may be advised to stop exercising if they would describe the level of intensity as "very hard." Cardiac rehabilitation programs and patients taking certain medications are often advised to utilize this method for determining individualized workload intensities. An exercise physiologist can be helpful in explaining and implementing the use of this method to the appropriate patients.

- Intensity can also be monitored by instructing the patient to follow the "Talk Test" rule. If at any time they cannot breathe comfortably — or talk — they should slow down the pace of physical exertion or stop and rest.

Duration

The duration of physical activity depends on goals and objectives. The physical activity session should last:

- 20 to 40 minutes for blood glucose control
- 45 to 60 minutes for weight loss/weight maintenance

For those patients who are severely deconditioned, several short bouts of physical activity may be necessary to get started, such as four sessions a day lasting 5 minutes each. As the patient becomes better conditioned over time, the duration of the physical activity can increase. If the individual is limited by his fitness level, alternating intervals of physical activity with rest periods may be helpful in developing the needed stamina to eventually lengthen the duration of the session. For example, a person might alternate 3 to 5 minutes of cycling with 1-to 2-minute rest periods, allowing a sufficient amount of physical activity to be performed even if the individual is poorly conditioned.

The duration and frequency of activity sessions is often dependant on age, time available for physical activity and level of endurance fitness. For sedentary individuals, any increase in regular physical activity should improve cardiovascular fitness.

Frequency

As with duration, the frequency of physical activity also depends on goals and objectives. In general, physical activity sessions should occur:

- 3 to 4 times weekly for blood glucose control
- 5 to 7 times weekly for weight loss

People participating in strength training may want to perform these type of workouts 2 days a week. Those doing strength training to improve activities of daily living may want to do up to 3–4 sessions a week.

General Recommendation

It is often recommended that patients consult with an exercise physiologist or physical therapist to assist in determining the best fitness program. In general, for people seeking to initiate a fitness program, a recommendation of exercising three sessions per week, performed on nonconsecutive days, is the minimum ideal activity level. Each physical activity session should last between 20 and 30 minutes. Activity should reach 50% to 55% of maximal aerobic capacity, or approximately 70% of an age-adjusted maximal heart rate (220 minus age in years).

Patients should start with that level of physical exertion with the intention of slowly increasing it. People who have been physically inactive should increase the activity slowly. A gradual increase will also allow time to determine appropriate adaptations in the insulin or oral agent doses and in the meal plan in order to compensate. Table 6-5 gives estimates of various activity levels as part of an exercise prescription. Unless the patient is above the "sedentary" level at the start, he or she should begin at that level and work upward in activity level from there. The activities used for this estimation are those listed in Table 6-3.

An ultimate goal of the physical fitness program for most people should be exercising at 70% to 85% of maximal heart rate for 30 to 60 minutes, at least three to five times weekly. However, the elderly, or those with limitations due to other medical conditions, will still get some benefit from more limited physical exertion. Taking brisk walks of 30 minutes or more three times weekly can be beneficial to almost anyone.

The Physical Fitness Routine

The physical activity session consists of 1) the warm-up phase, 2) the workout or exercise phase, and 3) the "cool-down" phase.

The warm-up should include a period of 5 to 10 minutes of light activity preceding the workout or exercise session. For example, begin with a leisurely walking pace before increasing to a power walk or jogging tempo. Or use a stationary cycle for 5–10 minutes before performing a more strenuous lifting routine. This approach will gradually increase blood flow to the working muscles to prepare them for the more vigorous workout phase and possibly reduce the chance of injury. The workout phase should be followed by a gradual cool-down over the remaining 5 to 10 minutes of the activity session. The final phase may include light aerobic activity and stretching movements. This helps restore the energy expenditures and the blood flow to the resting state.

Motivation

Once patients decide to start a fitness program, it takes motivation to continue after the first enthusiasm wanes. The program works better if it is designed specifically for the individual, with his or her input. It should be written down. Goals should be short-term, focusing on an interval such as two weeks. They should also be realistic. Patients should let family or friends know of their fitness plans, so they can encourage the patient to stick with the workout program, perhaps joining them to provide the added motivation of knowing that "someone is watching!" Activities should be selected that the patient enjoys. Alternate activities should also be included in the plan so that bad weather, equipment failure, etc., will not provide an excuse to skip a workout session. The intensity and duration of the activity must be realistic so that the patient does not overexert herself. A bad experience can turn someone off to the fitness program altogether. Written schedules also help, especially in integrating physical exertion with eating and insulin. Small rewards for reaching goals are helpful too, but often the best reward is the feeling of accomplishment, or merely just feeling good!

Physical Activity for People with Disabilities

When disabilities affect a person's ability to be independent, or when medical conditions limit an individual's ability to get out and move, some

TABLE 6-5.   The Exercise Prescription

This table lists the various levels of activity by frequency, duration, time, and intensity. Unless a patient is currently more active than the "sedentary" level, he or she should start at that level and increase sequentially.

Activity Level	Frequency (sessions/ week)	Duration (minutes/ session)	Total time/ week (minutes)	Intensity (heart rate based on Karvonen Formula)
Sedentary	4–6	10–20	40–80	40–60%
Somewhat active	4–6	15–30	90–120	50–75%
Moderately active	3–5	30–45	120–180	60–80%
Very active	3–5	30–60	180–300	60–85%
Athlete	5–7	60–120	300–840	70–85%

form of activity may still be possible, and, in fact, often quite valuable. Such physical fitness programs must be individualized to the person's particular abilities and disabilities, and consultation with an exercise physiologist may be recommended. There are also videos that are available that are geared for people with disabilities or lesser levels of fitness, showing armchair exercises, or even bed exercises that can help maintain muscle strength and cardiovascular health. Similarly, television broadcasts of fitness programs for those with some limitations might be available. So-called senior fitness programs often include activities such as Tai Chi, stretching, aerobic dance, or weight lifting. Home exercise equipment such as stationary bicycles or treadmills might also be considered.

Adjusting Diabetes Treatment to Meet the Demands of Physical Exertion

While the glucose lowering effect of physical activity may be beneficial, it is also important that it be balanced with the two other major components of glucose control — food and insulin. Successfully achieving this balance requires many of the skills that are basic to diabetes self-care, though the application of these skills does differ somewhat between the two major types of diabetes.

Self-Care Skills Applied to Physical Exertion

Self-monitoring of blood glucose (SMBG) is central to developing a self-care routine that maintains metabolic balance. Monitoring before and after — even during — physical exertion allows the patient to observe the impact of physical activity on blood glucose levels and to chart the course of glucose variations as affected by the activity performed. In addition, monitoring helps document the presence of hypoglycemia, even if symptoms are not obvious, and also helps guide the development of hypoglycemic avoidance strategies.

No matter how much care is taken, hypoglycemia is still a possibility during and after physical exertion. Patients should always have hypoglycemia treatment items (see Chapter 12) readily available during physical activity. As hypoglycemic symptoms may not always be present or obvious during physical exertion, blood glucose values, rather than symptoms, should be the determinant of a hypoglycemic event.

Physical Activity and Type 2 Diabetes

As noted previously, endurance training for people with type 2 diabetes can be quite beneficial, as it lowers insulin resistance and improves glucose tolerance. Over time, the right endurance program may allow the dose of insulin or oral antidiabetic medication to be reduced. However, as physical exertion can be detrimental in the presence of an absolute deficiency, it is important to identify those people with type 2 diabetes who have progressed to this point of β-cell dysfunction. It is a good rule that those with type 2 diabetes who do not use insulin should not begin physical exertion if the blood glucose level is above, or close to, 400 mg/dl.

For those patients who have type 2 diabetes adequately controlled using oral antidiabetic medications, and who are engaged in a physical fitness program, monitoring blood glucose levels can help determine appropriate medication adjustments. The goal for these people may include weight loss and/or reduced medication dose. As some antidiabetes medications can cause hypoglycemia, particularly those medications that increase insulin secretory capacity, careful self-monitoring is important. If hypoglycemia is detected either through testing or by recognition of symptoms during or after physical exertion and it is confirmed by testing, the medication dosage may be reduced. Medication dose reduction is certainly preferable to extra snacking if weight loss is a goal. Improvements in physical fitness can also increase insulin sensitivity, so dose reduction for all days, not just the physically active days, can often be achieved.

When occasional physical exertion results in hypoglycemia, however, it is often ineffective to reduce the oral agent dose, particularly if the increased activity is not predictable. Instead, small snacks before or after physical exertion on those occasional active days may be needed to prevent hypoglycemia despite any efforts at weight reduction.

For people with type 2 diabetes who use insulin, the approach is similar to that taken by people with type 1 diabetes using insulin, and the guidelines listed in the sections below apply.

Physical Activity and Type 1 Diabetes

While promoting physical fitness is an important part of therapy for people with type 1 diabetes, proper adjustment of the insulin dose and food consumption is essential to maintain proper diabetes control. With such adjustments, these individuals have the potential to perform as well in sports or other activities as those who do not have diabetes.

Through proper diabetes management training, patients can develop the skills to more effectively self-manage a fitness program. Often there can be great benefit from consultation with an exercise physiologist experienced in advising people with diabetes. With input from these specialists, patients can develop proper fitness routines, and become skilled in adjusting food and insulin to maintain smooth glucose control. It is not only the stereotypic young, athletic individual who should consult with an exercise physiologist. Physical activity, tailored to individual abilities and medical conditions, is of great benefit to all people, including those in the later years of life.

Even if an exercise physiologist is not consulted, a person with type 1 diabetes can begin a fitness program. However, there are a few key points for him or her to keep in mind when exercising. Like people with type 2 diabetes, those with type 1 diabetes must avoid physical exertion if their diabetes is out of control. For people with type 1, even more than those with type 2, elevated glucose levels, particularly if not due to a hypoglycemic event and rebound hyperglycemia, can reflect an insulin insufficiency. Exercising with hyperglycemia and with the presence of ketones may lead to increases in blood glucose levels or a worsening of the ketosis. **A blood glucose level over 250–300 mg/dl, especially with the presence of ketones, should be a warning not to be physically active until the abnormality is corrected.**

The insulin dose and food consumption may need adjustment to prevent hypoglycemia during or after a workout session. By keeping careful records of all parameters, including the differing types of physical activity, a patient can estimate a dose adjustment that works for him or her based on the duration, intensity, and frequency of exertion (see Table 6-6). Subsequently, through a sequential process of applying problem-solving skills, fine-tuning adjustments can be made to hone in on the proper balance of insulin, food, and activity that can be quite effective in maintaining glucose control. It should be emphasized that the development of this routine requires active patient participation in the process. Members of the healthcare team should recommend methods to estimate adjustments; but through actually trying various adjustments, many patients can self-train themselves to be quite skilled in management of the fitness program.

The importance of record-keeping cannot be emphasized enough. Detailed records of the blood glucose levels help patients determine for themselves which changes in the insulin dose and/or food consumption compensate properly for a given amount of physical exertion. Blood testing before and after physical exertion is a minimum requirement. It is also helpful to check blood glucose during an workout session to look for hypoglycemia, the symptoms of which may be masked by the sweating caused by the activity. Testing a few hours after the workout session can also be useful in gauging the strength of potential lag-effect, the post-exertion hypoglycemic tendency as glucose stores in muscle and liver are being replenished.

Physical exertion can have differing effects on glucose control depending on the time of day that it is performed. Specifically, at different times of day, various insulin doses may be at differing percentages of their peak activity (see Table 6-6). Temporal proximity to food consumption also plays a role.

For example, physical exertion should be done with caution just after

TABLE 6-6.   Insulin Adjustment Guidelines for Exercise

% To Decrease Peaking Insulin	Intensity of Physical Exertion	Duration of Physical Exertion
0%	Low, moderate or high intensity	Short duration
5%	Low intensity	Intermediate to long duration
10%	Moderate intensity	Intermediate duration
20%	Moderate intensity	Long duration
20%	High intensity	Intermediate duration
30%	High intensity	Long duration

Duration of Physical Exertion:
Short = less than 30 minutes (not necessary to adjust insulin)
Intermediate = 30–60 minutes
Long = 60 minutes or more

Intensity of Physical Exertion:
High intensity = high end of target heart rate
Moderate intensity = low end of target heart rate
Low intensity = not in target zone

Adjust the insulin with peak acting time concurrent with the exercise time:

Insulin	Peak range for adjustment
Rapid acting insulin analog (aspart, glulisine, lispro)	*0.5-3 hours*
Regular insulin	*1-5 hours*
Intermediate (NPH) insulin	*4-12 hours*
Peakless basal insulins (Detemir, Glargine) (It is generally recommended not to adjust peakless basal insulins)	*no peak action*

insulin injections are given. This would be particularly true for the rapid-acting insulins (aspart, glulisine, or lispro). Many people find that the best time to perform the fitness workout is at least an hour after a meal. Having reviewed all of these suggestions for optimal timing, however, many pragmatic healthcare professionals suggest that the best time to do the fitness workout is the time that the patient will actually be able to DO that activity! Insulin or snack adjustments to compensate for the diabetes can be worked out for almost any timing.

As physical movement is fueled by increased muscular glucose metabolism, hypoglycemia can occur if there is insufficient glucose available to these muscles, as when there is an excess of insulin or if the amount of stored glucose is already too low due to insufficient carbohydrate intake. **If diabetes is well-controlled, insulin doses should be decreased or food increased in anticipation of activity, and perhaps, for some, after activity as well. The preferred method for most people is to reduce the insulin dose.** Insulin reduction is less likely to result in hypoglycemia, and minimizing additional food consumption helps avoid weight gain. However, in some cases, both additional food consumption and decreased insulin dosages may be needed.

Low-Level Physical Exertion

Some reduction of the insulin dose that covers the period of physical exertion may be necessary when a person starts a fitness program. However, once the program has become part of the routine, occurring at least 3 to 4 times per week, people with ideal body weight who are not trying to lose weight often do not need to adjust their insulin for occasional, moderate physical exertion of short duration (under 30 minutes). For more intense or prolonged periods of exertion, however, insulin dose reduction or a snack may be needed, especially if the activity is performed more than 1 or 2 hours after a meal. Fifteen grams of carbohydrate, for example, should be enough for 30 to 60 minutes of moderate physical exertion such as "friendly" tennis, leisurely biking, or walking. People should get into the habit of checking their glucose level prior to each workout session and adjusting the snack based on the result of that glucose test. The lower the blood glucose level at the start of activity, the more food may be needed. In a relatively short time, most can become quite skillful in snack titration.

Vigorous Physical Exertion

For more vigorous activity, the preferred accommodation would also be to reduce the insulin doses. More food, perhaps half a sandwich (15 grams of carbohydrate and 7 to 8 grams of protein) can also be used to cover the first hour of activity. Table 6-7 lists some snack food options. Some of these are higher in fat than those commonly recommended for usual snacks. Fat slows intestinal absorption of food, leading to more prolonged and even availability of the food-supplied energy during the activity.

When the physical activity is unexpected and adjustments of insulin or calculated consumption of foods to provide even energy has not occurred, it is certainly acceptable, indeed recommended, to consume concentrated carbohydrates such as sugar-containing tonic or juices in anticipation of sudden bursts of activity. However, since these are short-lasting, a carbohydrate and protein-containing snack may still be required in order to maintain the blood glucose throughout the activity.

Longer Physical Exertion Sessions

When longer periods of activity are anticipated, insulin dose reductions are the primary means of compensatory adjustment. Initial estimates of the dose reduction may be off-target, but careful record-keeping, with notations as to the dose adjustments and the reasons for them, will allow later review of a number of such events to gauge accuracy and hone in on a more accurate dose adjustment estimate.

Supplemental snacks may also be used. However if relied upon to excess, the benefits of activity for weight management may be ameliorated. Snacks may be used, however, if the decision to undertake the activity occurs after the insulin dose has been taken. In such instances, snacks at 60-minute intervals may be required. These snacks can consist of 15 grams of carbohydrate plus 7 to 8 grams of protein. Snacking in this manner may be utilized, if needed, for all-day activities such as cross-country skiing or hiking, and patients should be told to take appropriate types and quantities of food along. Snack quantities may vary depending on the time of day and the amount of insulin that may be having its peak activity. Again, a problem-solving approach combined with good record-keeping will help determine the optimal quantities. For some very vigorous all-day ac-

TABLE 6-7. Snack Foods For Exercise

Dried fruit and nuts

Plain cookies

Granola bars

Yogurt (plain or fruit-flavored)

Pretzels

Various sandwiches

Nuts

Low-fat milk and muffins (corn or bran)

Junior baby foods

Low-fat cheese and crackers (e.g., rye wafers, Low-fat Triscuits, Rye Krisp Trail mix)

Low-fat cheese or peanut butter crackers

Sports Nutrition Bars

Sports Drinks

Diabetes Snack Bars

tivities, significantly more calories may be needed if sufficient reductions of insulin dose have not been made. For example, backpacking may require 5000 to 6000 calories per day, and the increase should be spread over the meals as well as the snacks.

Fluids are also quite important! A great deal of fluid may be lost as sweat, so sufficient intake prior to starting physical exertion is recommended. Water is recommended because it is most easily absorbed. Fluids are especially important for prolonged activity on a warm day or for activities that cause much sweating. Dehydration can worsen diabetes control.

An overweight person with type 1 diabetes may undertake an fitness program to lose weight. When weight loss is the goal, it is important to reduce the insulin doses so that extra snacking can be avoided. Again, trial and error, with frequent checking of blood glucose levels, will help determine the quantity of insulin reduction for a given amount of activity. Remember, too, that the "lag effect" can result in post-exertion hypoglycemia, so that more than one insulin dose may need to be reduced.

Conclusion

With careful attention to parameter adjustment, people with diabetes can enjoy the benefits of an fitness program without any deterioration of glucose control. It is important that people not become discouraged if the adjustment solutions are not evident early-on in the development of their activity routine. Encouragement, support from skilled educators, and patience will often bear fruit. However, when control cannot be maintained in concert with a fitness program, it may be an indication of the need to redesign the insulin program so that it more closely mimics normal insulin patterns. Chapters 9 and 10 detail methods to make such changes.

Suggested Reading

American College of Sports Medicine. *Exercise Management for Persons with Chronic Diseases and Disabilities*. Champaign, Il: Human Kinetics; 2003.

Borg, G. *Borg's Perceived Exertion and Pain Scales*. Human Kinetics: Champaign, IL, 1998.

Steppel JH, Horton, ES. Exercise in patients with diabetes mellitus. In Kahn CR, Weir GC, King GL, et al, eds. *Joslin's diabetes mellitus*. 14th ed. Philadelphia: Lippincott Williams & Wilkins, 2005 [649–657]

7

Type 2 Diabetes: Multiple Treatments for a Multicomponent Condition

Richard S. Beaser, MD

Introduction

The current term "type 2 diabetes" represents an evolution in terminology reflecting a progression in the understanding of this condition. The change to the Arabic numeral "2" from the Roman numeral "II" is only the latest in the evolution of descriptive terminology. This type of diabetes was previously known as non-insulin-dependent diabetes; maturity-onset diabetes, and adult-onset diabetes. Unfortunately, some people even called it "borderline" diabetes when insulin was not needed as therapy.

The change in terminology, while intended to eliminate confusion implied by the previous names, also reflects the varied pathophysiology, patient demographics, and treatment for this condition. Patients with type 2 diabetes may be both insulin treated and non-adult. And it is far from the trivial abnormality that the term "borderline" implies. Even when the glucose abnormalities are seemingly minimal, the potential impact on health can be significant.

Type 2 diabetes is by far the most common type of diabetes, representing close to 95% of all people with this condition. Unfortunately, too, it is probably more common than people realize. Its onset is often minimally symptomatic, and thus the insidious development of this condition often goes unrecognized for many years. Estimates have suggested that one-third of all people who actually have this condition do not yet know it! Yet, ignorance is not bliss. The hyperglycemia, as well as the other components of the insulin resistance syndrome, of which type 2 diabetes is a part, are silently impacting the vasculature, with significant long-term implications for morbidity and mortality.

Insulin Resistance

Type 2 diabetes is usually part of a spectrum of abnormalities often referred to as the "metabolic syndrome." The pathophysiologic hallmark of this condition is insulin resistance, manifest in liver and peripheral (primarily muscle and adipose) tissue. When insulin resistance is present, more insulin is required to produce a given degree of glucose-lowering effect. However, **for type 2 diabetes to be present, there needs to be dual defects: the insulin resistance and a relative or absolute insulin secretory insufficiency so that there is not enough insulin produced to overcome the insulin resistance.**

Insulin resistance is not always accompanied by type 2 diabetes. In fact, insulin resistance may be present, but with other clinical manifestations such as dyslipidemia and/or hypertension. If the pancreas is capable of making enough additional insulin to overcome the insulin resistance and maintain normal glucose tolerance, there is no hyperglycemia or clinical manifestation of diabetes. This is usually the case in early stages of type 2 diabetes. However, as the insulin resistance causes the body to need increased amounts of insulin, when the pancreas is able to respond by producing this additional insulin output, the patient is said to have become hyperinsulinemic. Hyperinsulinemia is *associated* with many of the other macrovascular risk factors that make up the metabolic syndrome, including dyslipidemia and hypertension. The exact etiologic relationship between the hyperinsulinemia and the development of these other conditions is not fully understood. However, many people believe that the hyperinsulinemia represents a marker for the syndrome rather than a cause of the risk factors in question.

Insulin resistance can be found in both the liver and peripheral tissues. With insulin resistance and insufficient compensatory hyperinsulinemia, increased hepatic glucose production occurs. This production is most often reflected clinically in elevations of fasting glucose levels. **When the fasting glucose level rises to above 100 mg/dl, it is classified as impaired fasting glucose, and when it rises to 126 mg/dl or above, diabetes is diagnosed.**

Peripheral insulin resistance is usually due to a number of defects, including post-insulin receptor binding defects, leading to decreased glucose transport and metabolism.

The Pathophysiology and Natural History of Type 2 Diabetes

For a number of years prior to the clinical manifestation of hyperglycemia, many people who will develop type 2 diabetes have an insidious increase in insulin resistance. During this time, the pancreas will increase insulin output, and normoglycemia is maintained.

However, for many people destined to develop type 2 diabetes, the ability of the pancreas to secrete enough additional insulin may decline. This decline may actually begin as many as 10 years prior to diagnosis of diabetes. It is usually a decrease in the early, or first phase, insulin secretion that occurs while second phase insulin secretion is increased. Concurrently, there is also a reduced suppression of glucagon in the postprandial state, which leads to increases in endogenous glucose production, further contributing to postprandial hyperglycemia.

When the insulin secretory capacity is significant enough to overcome the insulin resistance, normoglycemia is maintained. However, if that excess secretory capacity begins to wane, mild hyperglycemia may develop. If one compared this person's level of insulin secretion to that of someone without diabetes and with normal glucose levels, the insulin level would be elevated. However, in spite of this elevated insulin level, β-cell function is insufficient to overcome the insulin resistance. Thus, we say that this individual has a relative insufficiency of insulin secretory capacity and is unable to overcome insulin resistance.

It is at this time, when mild hyperglycemia develops, that diabetes *should* be diagnosed, but the lack of symptoms often leads to delays in disease discovery. Making the diagnosis earlier — at this stage in the progression — may be the best time to intervene with lifestyle changes that will prevent type 2 diabetes, as well as vascular disease, from progressing. In the Diabetes Prevention Program, intervening at the stage of impaired glucose tolerance with lifestyle changes resulted in a 58% reduction in diabetes progression as well as a 9% reduction in the number of persons with metabolic syndrome.

At the time that diabetes is diagnosed, there are a number of abnormalities in physiology that are likely to be present. Initially, the insulin resistance is more peripheral — muscle and adipose — reflecting decreases in postprandial glucose uptake. In addition, at the level of the beta-cell, there is a loss of first-phase insulin release. Normally, insulin is released in two phases. The first phase represents pre-made insulin within the beta-cell, and is released in the first 15 minutes after carbohydrate intake commences. It prevents a sharp rise in glucose levels in the immediate postprandial period. The second phase of insulin release represents newly manufactured insulin and begins as the first phase is subsiding. It lasts longer and provides sustained carbohydrate coverage for the remainder of the incoming nutrients.

With the loss of the first phase of insulin release, the postprandial glucose level often rises significantly. Also contributing to this is the lack of glucagon suppression, which further promotes production of endogenous glucose. However, as these patients retain their second-phase release, the higher postprandial glucose level leads to a greater amount of insulin produced during this period. For some patients at this stage, a pattern of reactive hypoglycemia may be seen. This happens because muscle is the main source of glucose uptake after meals and more insulin is needed to drive glucose into muscle cells than fat cells or to suppress the liver output of glucose. The higher insulin levels can lead to a drop in blood glucose 3 to 5 hours after a meal and symptoms of hypoglycemia may occur.

In addition, as the glucose level begins to rise, glucose toxicity can develop. Glucose toxicity is the paradoxical effect of hyperglycemia on insulin production and insulin action. Rather than driving the pancreas to make more insulin and the cells to be more insulin responsive, just the opposite occurs. Insulin secretory capacity is blunted, glucagon levels are elevated, and insulin resistance increases. Thus, there can be a vicious-cycle effect: the initial mild hyperglycemia can worsen beta-cell function and insulin sensitivity, leading to more hyperglycemia and more decreases in beta-cell function and insulin sensitivity. With time, more significant hyperglycemia can develop. Even fasting hyperglycemia that is minimally above normal levels can contribute to glucose toxicity and blunt first phase insulin response.

Once hyperglycemia begins to develop, the degree of insulin resistance plateaus. From that point on, most people maintain a static degree of insulin resistance, only varying as a result of external forces such as significant changes in food intake and activity level, physiologic stress, glucose toxicity, or glucose-sensitizing medications. The further progression of the disease is, from this point on, driven primarily by the decline in β-cell function.

During this period of time, glucose patterns, assessed from reviewing the patients' self-monitoring of blood glucose (SMBG) records, can reflect the progressive deterioration in insulin secretory capacity. From the initial abnormalities in postprandial glucose levels seen with the early stages of β-cell dysfunction, more significant pre-and postprandial glucose elevations can result. Fasting glucose levels can be more significantly elevated than those before lunch and supper, resulting from multiple factors such as the hyperglycemia of the dawn phenomenon, the lack of eating to stimulate insulin secretion increasing hepatic insulin resistance and decreasing insulin secretion. Fasting insulin levels are often elevated, yet still insufficient to normalize glucose levels. **When preprandial, and particularly fasting, glucose levels remain under 200 mg/dl and A1C values under about 9%, non-insulin antidiabetes treatments (oral and/or injectable exenatide) can often provide adequate glucose control early in the course of the disease, targeting pre- and post-prandial hyperglycemia.**

With progressive decrease of insulin capacity, glucose levels rise further and often herald the approaching need for exogenous insulin. **Fasting glucose levels at or over 200 mg/dl in a patient aggressively treated with pharmacologic and lifestyle modalities are usually a sign that endogenous insulin production is dropping below that which will sustain control without exogenous supplementation.** Longer duration of diabetes also suggests that exogenous insulin therapy will be needed. This elevated fasting glucose is often treated with bedtime insulin, while treatment with daytime antidiabetes medication is often still adequate for the remainder of the coverage needs (see Chapter 10).

With further decreases in insulin secretory capacity, progressive changes in glucose patterns beyond elevated fasting and immediate postprandial levels can be seen:

- *Rising glucose levels during the day* — In early stages of type 2 diabetes, the prebreakfast glucose levels are typically higher than values before lunch and supper. As insulin secretory deficiency progresses, the prelunch and presupper values rise, so that the fasting glucose is not notably higher than these later premeal values. This is one reflection of declining insulin secretory capacity.
- *Marked postprandial hyperglycemia* — Another reflection of a decline in insulin secretory capacity — the decline of second phase secretion — is a more marked difference between pre-and postprandial glucose levels. Loss of first-phase insulin response can cause postprandial hyperglycemia early-on in the natural history of this condition, but a more pronounced postprandial rise reflects more significant second-phase insufficiency.
- *Marked hyperglycemia throughout the day* — reflects further insulin secretory deficiency. Fasting glucose is elevated, and there are further elevations in values before lunch and supper. At this point, prandial coverage is insufficient and basal insulin also cannot return glucose values to baseline. Exogenous insulin therapy is almost certainly needed when glucose patterns reach this stage.
- *General lability in response to daily activities* — reflects even further deterioration in insulin secretory capacity and glucose homeostatic mechanisms. In all likelihood, when such instability in patterns is seen, insulin production levels have dropped to an absolute deficiency. Physiologic insulin replacement programs similar to those used to treat people with type 1 diabetes *are* recommended at this stage.

Treatment Goals

The goal of treating any type of diabetes can be summarized as being *the prevention of its acute and chronic complications.* As this applies to type 2 diabetes, the objectives really represent a more comprehensive approach to reducing macrovascular risk and include:

- **Glucose control.** Achieving this objective prevents acute complications of hypo-and hyperglycemia and, based on recent study data, reduces the risk of microvascular and neuropathic complications and contributes to reducing the risk of macrovascular complications. The EDIC study which was a follow up of the DCCT Study recently showed the importance of physiologic early glycemic control. Patients in the intensive treatment group whose control deteriorated after the main study, still had less progression in their microvascular disease compared to the standard treatment patients who had the higher A1C during the trial and whose control was now improved. Thus early tight glycemic control in these people with type 1 diabetes had a legacy effect on the vascular tissues. In addition, the physiologic glucose control also reduced the risk of macrovascular disease for the first time.

- **Reduction of cardiovascular risk factors and cardiovascular complications.** These include clinically targeting dyslipidemia, hypertension, hypercoagulability, obesity, vascular dysfunction, inactivity, and cigarette smoking.
- **Prevention of other complications,** including microvascular and neuropathic effects, by addressing issues such as treatment of microalbuminuria, regular ophthalmologic evaluations, and proper foot care. Interventions to achieve these goals are discussed in detail in other chapters devoted to the specific topics. However, specific considerations as these issues apply to people with type 2 diabetes are outlined below.

Developing a Medical Care Plan

Before initiating any specific therapeutic interventions for a patient with type 2 diabetes, a careful assessment of the patient's general condition, related issues such as socioeconomic, cultural and lifestyle considerations are important. Preparing such an inventory in one place as part of the initial diabetes evaluation record can be most helpful in visualizing the scope of interventions that will be necessary.

Development of this initial assessment begins with a careful and comprehensive patient history and physical examination. While many of the components of this assessment are similar to those that might be used for patients with type 1 diabetes, the focus should be on issues related to treatment concerns for type 2.

Medical History

The **history** should detail, in particular, the following information:

1. **History of diagnosis and treatment of diabetes**
   - *When was diagnosis made?*
   - *Estimate of how long the patient might have had diabetes prior to diagnosis, suggested by:*
     - suggestive symptoms
     - presence of complications at presentation
     - history of gestational diabetes or large babies
     - past impairment of glucose tolerance or fasting glucose
     - abnormal glucose levels in old records that may not have been acted upon
   - *How the diagnosis was made?*
     - acute presentation/presentation due to symptoms
     - discovery by accident
     - discovery concurrent with another illness
     - gestational diabetes
   - *Treatment history*
     - initiation of lifestyle changes (when, what, and how successful)
     - initiation of pharmacologic intervention (when, what medications, degree of control achieved and for how long, medication changes / combinations, insulin initiation and dosing pattern history)
     - initiation of treatments to reduce macrovascular risk factors and/ or provide direct vascular protection
     - weight changes before and since treatment initiation
     - treatment complications (hypoglycemia, hyperosmolar coma or diabetic ketoacidosis (DKA), adverse events relating to medication use)

2. **Diabetes educational history**
   - *Instruction on medical nutritional therapy (MNT)*
     - when (initial and refresher visits)
     - with whom (dietitian/nutritionist, nurse educator, physician, written or electronic, other)
     - details of calorie recommendations or other parameters

- adherence to program
- weight changes resulting from MNT
- *Basic diabetes education*
  - when (initial and refresher visits)
  - with whom (certified diabetes educator [CDE], other educator, physician, written or electronic, other)
  - subjects covered and current educational deficits. Of particular importance to those patients with type 2 diabetes would be:
    - self-blood glucose monitoring (SBGM) (what method/equipment taught, frequency of testing recommendation and adherence to recommendation, method and frequency of record-keeping and adherence to recommendation, interpretation and use of results)
    - foot care
    - eye care
    - recognition of signs and symptoms of macrovascular disease
    - effects, impact, and treatment adjustments for activity
- *Instruction on exercise or physical activity*
  - when (initial and refresher visits)
  - with whom (diabetes nurse educator, exercise physiologist, trainer, written or electronic, other)
  - factors limiting activity (other medical conditions, etc.)
  - initial activity recommendations
  - current type and frequency of activity
- *Current potential for further education*
  - level of patient interest or readiness to make lifestyle changes
  - financial obstacles
  - logistical obstacles (time constraints, difficulty with access to educational resources, etc.)
3. **History of conditions related to diabetes, the time of their diagnosis, and treatment history**
   - *Cardiovascular risk factors*
     - dyslipidemia
     - hypertension
     - microalbuminuria
     - hypercoagulability with prophylactic treatment
     - smoking

- – family history of premature cardiovascular disease
- – lifestyle (obesity, activity)
- *Cardiovascular end-organ effects (when, extent of impact, treatment initiated and its success, recurrences/chronic impact, current functional status)*
  - – coronary artery disease
  - – peripheral vascular disease
  - – cerebrovascular disease
  - – other (renovascular, etc.)
- *Microvascular status*
  - – frequency and most recent eye examination by qualified diabetes eye care professional, with results
  - – hypertension treatment
  - – microalbuminuria — presence, treatment, results of treatment
  - – renal function status (microalbuminuria history, creatinine/creatinine clearance)
- *Neuropathic complication assessment and treatment history*
  - – history suggestive of peripheral neuropathic changes (pain/hypesthesia, anesthesia, neuropathic ulcers, Charcot changes)
  - – mononeuropathies
  - – sexual function/reproductive problems
  - – bladder dysfunction
  - – GI symptoms suggestive of gastropathy (early satiety, etc.) or diabetic diarrhea (diarrhea alternating with constipation)
  - – orthostatic hypotension
  - – cardiac neuropathy (absence of respiratory rhythm variations)
- *Other foot issues*
  - – podiatry consultations (if ever, frequency, most recent, issues such as toe care, calluses, deformities)
  - – shoe use (types, frequency of shoe rotation/change)
  - – foot pain or discomfort (onset, duration, severity, precipitating factors and time of day most likely to occur)
  - – past foot injury/surgery
  - – foot deformities

4. **Current medications in use**
   - *Treating existing conditions*
   - *Preventing macrovascular disease or protecting vascular health*
   - *Birth control*

- *Prophylaxis (aspirin, vitamins, osteoporosis/menopausal, etc.)*
- *"Over-the-counter" medication habits*

5. **Family medical history**
   - *Of diabetes*
   - *Of macrovascular risk factors (especially dyslipidemia, hypertension)*
   - *Of macrovascular end organ disease*
   - *Of obesity*
   - *Of early non-accidental death*
   - *Of other genetic/endocrine disorders (thyroid disorders, etc.)*
   - *General family medical history*

6. **Personal/social history**
   - *Marital status*
   - *Family issues/stresses (ill relatives, marital discord, etc.)*
   - *Domestic violence*
   - *Living arrangement status (with whom, type of dwelling, who does cooking, etc.)*
   - *Occupational history*
     - type of work
     - activity level at work
     - work schedule (hours, meal times, variability of schedule/swing shifts, predictability of schedule, overnight travel requirements, dining out and entertainment requirements)
   - *Daily schedule for arising, meals, activity, bedtime*
   - *Substance use/abuse, current and past, with status of efforts to control (tobacco, alcohol, recreational drugs)*

7. **Other issues as part of a general medical history**

Physical Examination

The **physical examination** should include the basics of a comprehensive medical examination. For patients with type 2 diabetes, focus should be, in particular, on:

1. **Height/weight/waist circumference and/or BMI**
2. **Blood pressure lying/standing (checking for orthostatic changes)**
3. **Ophthalmologic examination (fundoscopy)**
4. **Examine for bruits (carotid, femoral)**

5. **Feet**
   - *General appearance of feet*
     - color (dusky look or dependent rubor? — suggestive of ischemia)
     - presence of hair (presence of hair suggests adequate circulation, however, absence does not necessarily suggest ischemia)
     - deformities
     - ulcers or other signs of infection
     - presence of calluses or potential pressure points
   - *Peripheral pulses*
   - *Signs of peripheral neuropathy*
     - light touch (monofilament)
     - vibration (tuning fork)
     - pin prick (pin or pin wheel)
   - *Shoes*
     - unusual or uneven wear
     - support
     - are they custom made or have special features?
6. **Cardiopulmonary examination**
   - *General examination*
   - *Cardiac rhythm abnormalities*
   - *Congestion or congestive heart failure*
   - *Presence or absence of respiratory variations of cardiac rhythm*
7. **Abdominal examination**
   - *General examination*
   - *Hepatic status*
   - *Signs suggestive of abdominal aneurysms*
   - *GI sounds*
8. **Male genitalia (if history of sexual or reproductive dysfunction)**
   - *General examination (normal anatomy?)*
   - *Presence of signs of past injury, Peyronie's disease, etc.*
9. **Female**
   - *Loss of lubrication for sexual activity*

Laboratory Assessments

Among the routine **laboratory assessments** performed, the following should be measured for people with type 2 diabetes:

- **Glucose**
- **A1C**
- **Renal and hepatic function** *(especially estimation of creatinine clearance or GFR, and transaminase levels)*
- **Lipid profile** *(total cholesterol, fasting triglycerides, HDL, LDL)*
- **Urinalysis** *(particularly to rule out infection, gross proteinuria, abnormal sediment)*
- **Microalbuminuria** *(microalbumin/creatinine ratio is usually sufficient)*
- **EKG**
- **CBC** *(rule out infections, or abnormalities that might render A1C less reliable)*

Outlining the Treatment Approach

Based on the initial assessment, clear treatment goals should be set and shared with the patient. These goals should be defined as specific parameters. A list of goal parameters to consider might include:

- **Glucose levels** *(fasting, before other meals, 1 to 2 hours postprandial)*
- **A1C**
- **Weight change**
- **Lipid levels**
- **Blood pressure levels**

The goals must be realistic. This might seem obvious, but it is often overlooked in the zeal of trying to achieve ideal results. Telling a person who is 50 pounds overweight that the weight-loss goal is 50 pounds might seem to him or her like an insurmountable task. However, a goal of losing 10 pounds might be more achievable, and probably would have a significant impact on key metabolic parameters. Similarly, while glucose and A1C goals should reflect Joslin or ADA guidelines, *initial* goals may be modified some, taking into consideration patient safety, abilities/willingness for self-care, and other medical conditions. Eventually, as the patient makes some progress, the goals may be changed to reflect Joslin or ADA targets.

As these goals should be set in conjunction with the patient, it is also important to them in terms of specific tasks, educational goals, or behavioral changes (See Chapter 23). Such goals might include:

- **Lifestyle adjustments**
  - Adoption of a new medical nutrition plan
  - Initiation of an activity (exercise) program (commensurate with cardiac and general medical status)
  - Changes in schedule or daily activities
- **Monitoring**
- *Starting a program of self-monitoring* of blood glucose, record-keeping, and/or adjustments of treatment parameters based on monitoring results
- *Monitoring blood pressure*
- *Getting blood drawn on a schedule* to check metabolic parameters
- **Taking medication or insulin for diabetes**
- **Taking medication for other conditions** (dyslipidemia, hypertension, microalbuminuria, hypercoagulability, vascular protection, etc.)
- **Identifying specific members of the healthcare team** (educators, dietitians, exercise physiologists, etc.)
- **Seeking care from other specialists** (ophthalmologists, podiatrists, vascular specialists, mental health professionals, cardiologists, etc.).

Finally, it is important to determine a regular schedule of medical care and follow-up with any of the healthcare professionals needed for comprehensive diabetes care, and for monitoring risk factors and/or early signs of complications.

Medical Nutrition Therapy

For decades it has been said that "diet is the cornerstone of treatment for type 2 diabetes." Of course, the common understanding of the word "diet" is that it is something that people undertake in order to lose weight — something that, by its nature, is temporary "until the weight is lost!" People with type 2 diabetes tend to be overweight (having, in particular, abdominal obesity or the so-called apple-shaped body habitus) — so the impression that weight loss is needed is partially right. People with type 2 diabetes generally *should* lose weight, but the effort to change eating habits must *not* be temporary. In addition, by implication, this focus on "diet" suggests that weight loss is the crucial component in achieving control of type 2 diabetes.

Being overweight — and overeating itself — both increase insulin resistance. However, as a result of the last few decades of experience treating type 2 diabetes, as well as recent advances and insights into effective treatment modalities, we now have a new perspective on the role of "diet" in the treatment of type 2 diabetes. First, we no longer refer to the eating plan as a "diet" because of the implication that it is just a temporary adjustment in eating to lose weight. What is needed for the treatment of type 2 diabetes is "medical nutrition therapy," which is a **treatment** that continues as long as the person has diabetes.

In addition, the primary focus is *not* weight loss. The goal is *metabolic control*, impacting glucose levels, lipid levels, and blood pressure. Weight loss may assist in reaching the desired goals or parameters. However, these parameters may be reached without significant weight loss, and even partial success with the recommended lifestyle changes may be beneficial in this era of expanded pharmaceutical treatment tools. The approach is not "all or nothing!"

Weight loss is still desired, recommended, and quite beneficial. In no way should it be implied that this is not an important goal and an integral part of the treatment program. However, it has long been recognized that many people have difficulty losing weight. There is tremendous anguish over the issue, causing much personal stress and interpersonal strife, particularly between spouses or other concerned family members or friends. The good news is that the pressure with regard to "diet" and weight loss is not as great as it used to be because of the new pharmacologic tools now available. Much research is underway to further understand the mechanisms leading to obesity — particularly abdominal obesity — and thus develop more effective treatments. There is now no excuse for waiting months and months for weight loss to occur; if a medical nutrition plan falls short in about 3 months, pharmacologic intervention is indicated.

Therefore, *it is important to individualize the medical nutrition therapy to the needs of each patient.* Treatment goals should be those set by the ADA or Joslin for glucose control, lipid status, and blood pressure control. Weight loss goals need to be individualized and realistic. To tell someone who has been fifty pounds overweight for much of his or her life to lose fifty pounds is almost certain to meet with discouraging failure. Telling that same person to lose five to ten pounds may be more likely to meet with success, and it may only take the loss of that amount of weight to approach or even reach the desired metabolic goals.

Consultation with a dietitian or nutritionist can be quite effective in assisting patients with integrating a medical nutrition therapy program into their lives. Details on medical nutrition therapy can be found in Chapter 5.

Physical Activity

For decades, it has also been said that, in addition to diet, exercise or physical activity is crucial to the control of type 2 diabetes. This statement, too, is correct. Exercise helps reduce blood glucose levels and insulin resistance. Details of the role of exercise in the treatment of diabetes can be found in Chapter 6.

However, like proper eating habits, exercise is often not undertaken by many people with type 2 diabetes as much as would be ideal. In addition, the word "exercise" is often frightening to people with type 2 diabetes, not just because they don't like doing it, but because for those with over-sedentary lifestyles, "exercise" often implies something a svelte, young person in tight clothing does at a gym for one to two hours a day. Indeed, the potential for silent coronary artery disease should make such exercise frightening for the medical professional as well until the patient with type 2 diabetes has had a cardiac evaluation!

The truth is that the term "exercise," as commonly used, may be ideal for those with type 2 diabetes, but is not the best *initial* approach. For people whose existence is primarily a sedentary one due to habit, age, or other medical conditions, just encouraging some moderate "activity" may be a sufficient increase in movement to have an impact on their metabolic status. Also, as with obesity, approaching activity gradually can often lead to greater success. Modest, periodic, stepwise increases in daily activity level can be more successful and medically safer than trying to push patients into a more aggressive activity program than they initially can tolerate.

Physical activity has a number of benefits for people with type 2 diabetes. It:

- improves glucose control
- assists with weight-loss efforts, particularly with regard to abdominal obesity

- increases energy expenditure
- increases lean body mass
- improves lipid profile.
- improves cardiovascular health
- improves psychological well-being, reducing stress and improving self-image

However, as explained in greater detail in Chapter 6, before a person with type 2 diabetes initiates an exercise program, there needs to be careful prescreening and medical clearance:

- **review glucose control** (although it might not be optimized until after the activity program has started) and make sure that the patient can adjust his or her treatment to reduce the risk of hypoglycemia and/or treat the hypoglycemia if it occurs
- **cardiovascular evaluation** (rule out occult coronary disease) and other measures of exercise tolerance and work capacity
- **ophthalmology evaluation** (rule out the presence of active proliferative retinopathy which could bleed as a result of exercise)
- **foot examination** to gauge the impact of peripheral vascular disease and neuropathy on exercise, and vice versa.

Indication for Antidiabetes Medications for Type 2 Diabetes

Antidiabetes medications are usually the first line therapy once lifestyle changes are no longer sufficient to achieve treatment goals for one with type 2 diabetes. The ADA has recommended that oral pharmacotherapy should be initiated for people with type 2 diabetes when:

- treatment goals are not met after 3 months of adhering to a medical nutrition therapy plan and exercise programs
- symptomatic hyperglycemia is present
- ketosis is present
- imminent surgery

In many cases, it doesn't take 3 months to determine that non-pharmacologic treatments will not work. The patient may be so clearly hyperglycemic, symptomatic, or have other serious conditions affecting, or affected by, the hyperglycemia that the need for intervention is more acute. The point that the ADA is making with the 3-month recommendation is that there should be a finite trial period of time to determine if lifestyle changes will be effective and can achieve control close to the therapeutic goal.

With the selection of medications now available to treat type 2 diabetes that specifically target the various pathophysiologic abnormalities, there is rarely a reason to delay treatment when goals are not met. In fact, the clinical trend is to start pharmacotherapy earlier in *both* the natural history of the type 2 diabetes and the progressive deterioration of glucose control. Monotherapy, combination therapy, and even therapy with medications *plus* insulin are being used to successfully control glucose levels in many of these patients. The various pharmacologic treatments for type 2 diabetes and how to use them are discussed in detail in Chapter 8, and designing insulin treatment programs is reviewed in Chapters 10 & 11.

Summary

The treatment of type 2 diabetes includes aggressive control of glucose. However, it also involves multiple lifestyle changes, including medical nutrition therapy and an activity program. Self-blood glucose monitoring (SMBG) is an important component of treatment, not just to provide "test results," but also to gauge glucose patterns reflective of the underlying pathologic spectrum of abnormalities causing the diabetes, as well as to involve the patient more effectively in his or her care.

As type 2 diabetes is so pathophysiologically tied to the metabolic syndrome and its array of cardiovascular risk factors, addressing these concerns is central to proper treatment for type 2 diabetes as well. Dyslipidemias, hypertension, vascular dysfunction, and hypercoagulability must be treated aggressively to maximize the potential for longevity and good health.

The outlook for those with type 2 diabetes is far better today than it was not too many years ago. With a renewed focus on lifestyle changes, new pharmacologic tools and a better understanding of risk factors and preventive strategies, there is a realistic hope of success in avoiding the many complications once thought to be inevitable. However, to do so requires effort by healthcare professionals as well as the patient and his or her family and others constituting the patient's personal support system. While the new treatment tools *do* make the management of this condition much easier, the lifestyle changes and the challenges of avoiding or treating the complications still remain, and are usually the most difficult part of this disease.

8

Pharmacotherapy of Type 2 Diabetes: Medications to Match the Pathophysiology

Richard S. Beaser, MD

Introduction

The development of oral medications to treat type 2 diabetes has been one of the major milestones in the modern era of diabetes treatment. Since the 1950s, it has been possible to treat type 2 diabetes with tablets. In recent years, newer medications have become available targeting specific components of the spectrum of pathophysiologic abnormalities, regulating glucose input, and also addressing glucose utilization and disposal through impacts on insulin resistance and insulin deficiency. This broadening of the reach of non-insulin medical therapies also now includes a non-insulin injectable medication. The power that these treatment tools bring to diabetes treatment has allowed more people with type 2 diabetes than ever before to approach a level of glucose control and near-normalization of glucose patterns that can significantly reduce their risk of complications.

The availability of oral medications for diabetes therapy was one of the significant milestones in the history of diabetes treatment. When these oral medications first became available, there were thousands of people who suspected or actually knew that they had diabetes, but, fearing insulin injections, did not seek medical attention. Physicians practicing at that time recall the many patients who suddenly appeared once oral treatments were available. Today, modern insulin administration is easier, provides better control, is more widely accepted by patients, and can be very appropriate for many with type 2 diabetes. Yet, the oral treatment boon has achieved widespread acceptance among people with diabetes and has contributed immensely to improved health and reduced disease impact. In fact, as is discussed in the chapter on macrovascular complications, comprehensive treatment of type 2 diabetes often involves the use of many medications to treat other metabolic abnormalities in an attempt to reduce macrovascular risk.

Using pills to treat diabetes was not a new concept even in the 1950s. German scientists found compounds with hypoglycemic effects as far back as 1920, although many of those early compounds were too toxic for human use. In many parts of the world, natural substances have been used for years as medications to lower glucose levels, and the search continues today for others that may be effective.

The comments at the end of the previous chapter on the treatment of type 2 diabetes provide the medical indications for pharmacotherapy for type 2 diabetes. Other than states of acute hyperglycemia, the primary indication for treatment with antidiabetes medications is the inability to achieve goals of therapy after no more than 3 months of nonpharmacologic intervention. The goals should be those of a diabetes organization such as the Joslin Diabetes Center (see Joslin's Clinical Guidelines, www.joslin.org) or the ADA, but such goals may otherwise be individualized for a particular patient.

The recent introduction of the many new pharmacologic agents to treat type 2 diabetes that can effectively approach individualized treatment goals has taken some of the pressure off nonpharmacologic treatments. Medical nutrition therapy and increased activity are still the primary therapies for type 2 diabetes, but many patients cannot alter these lifestyle parameters sufficiently to overcome metabolic abnormalities and optimize glucose control. In the past, this inability to make long-term lifestyle changes resulted in suboptimal control. Now, pharmacology can circumvent the inability to optimize the impact of lifestyle changes, and patients do not have to suffer the consequences of hyperglycemia resulting from inadequate pharmacology and the inability to change their habits. However, it does *not* mean that medical nutrition therapy and activity are any less important. This point must be emphasized to patients at the initiation of pharmacologic treatment, as well as throughout the course of their treatment. Pharmacologic management is not likely to be sufficiently effective — if effective at all — without some conscientious attention to lifestyle changes as well.

Options for Therapy

The medications available at this writing to treat type 2 diabetes can be grouped according to their chemical class and function:

- Medications that improve insulin action
  - Biguanides
  - Thiazolidinediones
- Medications that slow glucose absorption
  - α-Glucosidase inhibitors
- Medications that increase insulin secretion
  - Sulfonylureas
  - Meglitinides
  - D-phenylalanine derivatives
- Medications that restore or replicate incretin action on insulin secretion and glucagon suppression
  - GLP-1 agonists
  - DPP-IV inhibitors
- Medications that provide additional insulin
  - Exogenous pharmacologic insulin
  - Injected

It is important to note that insulin is included in this list. Insulin should not be thought of as a treatment of last resort when oral medications fail to work, or when the patient is perceived to be nonadherent. Insulin is an important part of this medication list with specific indications. It has typically been used when there is decreased endogenous insulin secretion or to decrease glucose toxicity. However, in recent years with the recognition that postprandial glycemia is a major contributor to elevated A1C levels on the lower end of the scale, and also may be a marker of increased macrovascular risk, the incentive to provide prandial insulin coverage has increased. Thus, it is possible that we will see the use of insulin not just reserved for the time when the absolute insulin secretory capacity has decreased, but also earlier in the natural history when it is the first phase insulin secretion that has diminished in capacity and it is needed to provide adequate prandial coverage. While this book has separate chapters on insulin use because of the administration and treatment design issues, functionally, it is just another tool in the treatment armamentarium.

General details about the use of insulin and treatment design can be found in Chapter 9. Comments relating to combination use of insulin and oral medications are included later in this chapter.

Medication Selection for Treatment of Type 2 Diabetes

There are a number of considerations in selecting a medication to treat type 2 diabetes:

- Underlying pathophysiology
  - severity of abnormalities
  - degree of insulin resistance vs. insulin deficiency
  - presence and severity of glucose toxicity
  - degree of postprandial hyperglycemia
- Overall patient condition
  - age
  - coexisting diseases, conditions, or abnormalities
  - patient lifestyle considerations
  - willingness and ability to use injected medication (exenatide, exogenous insulin)
- Characteristics and precautions of potential medications

Currently, there is no easy method in common clinical use to measure insulin resistance or insulin secretory capacity. Insulin clamp studies that are used in research protocols to measure insulin resistance are not practical in the outpatient office. Measurement of C-peptide can be used as a marker of endogenous insulin production. C-peptide is the connecting peptide that is severed from the proinsulin molecule in the final stage of insulin production. Unfortunately, patients for whom the clinical signs that reflect insulin secretory capacity are equivocal often have equivocal C-peptide levels, thus not helping clinical decisions. However, if future

trends lead to treatment of insulin resistance in the absence of hyperglycemia, and hyperinsulinemia is reflective of insulin resistance, then measuring C-peptide may become useful. At present, however, most clinicians do not feel it adds much to the medication selection decisions.

Clinical Markers

There are clinical markers that can reflect the predominance of the various
pathophysiologic components that contribute to type 2 diabetes. While
these markers cannot be relied on to provide completely accurate information about the underlying pathophysiology, they can help give the
healthcare professional enough of a clinical sense of the predominance of
the various defects to guide selection of treatments. They might also signal the need for additional attention to potential problems. These markers
include:

Body habitus: The so-called apple-shaped body (big belly) suggests
insulin resistance. Overweight in general suggests insulin resistance.

Age: Aging promotes insulin resistance. Therefore, the older
the person, the more likely he or she is to have insulin
resistance.

Weight change: Recent loss of weight, particularly concurrent with
poorly controlled diabetes, suggests insulin deficiency.
Weight gain tends to lead to insulin resistance. BMI
(Body Mass Index) greater than 27 is invariably associated with insulin resistance.

Duration of diabetes: The longer the patient has had type 2 diabetes, the
more likelihood that there is significant insulin defi-
ciency.

Gender: Women with type 2 diabetes lose the protection against
macrovascular disease that being female would normally bring. Attention to macrovascular risk factor reduction is important.

Ethnic group: Groups with an above-average incidence of type 2 diabetes and insulin resistance may benefit from treatment with a medication that reduces insulin resistance.

Coexisting diseases: The presence of other components of the insulin resistance syndrome suggest the presence of insulin resistance. These might include dyslipidemia, hypertension, or gout.

Side effect profile: The development of side effects from use of a medication might preclude its use. Similarly, the presence of another condition that might be exacerbated by a side effect might preclude use of the offending medication. (e.g., liver toxicity potential in someone with underlying hepatic disease)

Glucose patterns: Glucose patterns, can be suggestive of more specific underlying pathophysiology.

- Fasting hyperglycemia, with lower values before lunch and supper, is reflective of hepatic insulin resistance. The presence of other factors suggesting insulin resistance would support this conclusion. (Keep in mind that values that are generally elevated throughout the day may be more reflective of both insulin resistance as well as a more significant reduction in insulin secretory capacity.)

- Postprandial hyperglycemia is also a hallmark of type 2 diabetes, usually reflecting the loss of first-phase insulin release (insulin release in the first minutes after starting food consumption). Absent first-phase insulin release allows the postprandial glucose level to rise to higher levels, primarily in response to nutrients provided in the meal. However, first-phase insulin loss may also lead to a less effective suppression of hepatic glucose production as well.

- Glucose values that are unresponsive to oral therapy and lifestyle changes may suggest significant insulin deficiency. As insulin deficiency increases, patterns may progress through a number of stages that suggest declining insulin secretory capacity. Note that not all patients will demonstrate all stages and stages are often not as clear as described. These stages might include:

- Elevated fasting glucose (greater than those seen in earlier stages that may be responsive to oral therapy. Generally, fasting values >200 mg/dl suggest absolute insulin deficiency.)

- Rising glucose levels during the day (a general up-trend in glucose levels suggests that insulin secretion cannot keep up with needs)

- Marked postprandial hyperglycemia (suggests marked reductions in insulin secretory capabilities in response to meals, probably beyond loss of first-phase insulin release that is present early in the natural history of diabetes.)

- Marked hyperglycemia throughout the day (probably heralds generalized insulin deficiency)

- General lability in response to daily activities (the patterns typically seen with type 1 diabetes)

Using these markers to gauge the presence and predominance of the various pathophysiologic components of type 2 diabetes, the clinician can then select pharmacologic treatments to target these specific defects. A discussion of selecting medications based on this information will follow later in this chapter.

In a general sense, all non-insulin therapies used to treat type 2 diabetes require the presence of insulin or functional beta-cells in order to be effective. The source of that insulin may not necessarily be the pancreas (it could be exogenous), but significant differences exist among medications that reduce insulin resistance. Some exert their effect directly. All will have some effect on reducing insulin resistance by virtue of a reduction in glucose toxicity that accompanies reduced hyperglycemia.

How the Various Antidiabetes Medications Work

Listed below are general summaries of how the antidiabetes diabetes medications work with respect to the various pathophysiological states that constitute type 2 diabetes.

- **Medications that improve insulin action**
  - *Classes:* biguanides, thiazolidinediones
  - *Efficacy with respect to insulin resistance:* Reducing insulin resistance is the primary effect of these medications, whether that resistance is hepatic (primary action of the biguanide metformin) or peripheral (thiazolidinediones). Their clinical efficacy is dependent on the present degree of insulin resistance.
  - *Efficacy with respect to insulin level:* These medications can be effective as long as insulin is present, and that insulin may be of exogenous or endogenous origin. The key is just that insulin be present, and that there is some insulin resistance against which these medications can work. Therefore, in patients with type 2 diabetes and significant insulin resistance who also have significant loss of insulin secretory function, these medications could be effective along with either insulin secretagogues to stimulate endogenous insulin production, incretin mimetics, or replacement exogenous insulin therapy.

- **Medications that slow glucose absorption**
  - *Classes:* α-glucosidase inhibitors
  - *Efficacy with respect to insulin resistance:* Any medication that reduces glucose levels decreases glucose toxicity and thus decreases insulin resistance. They have little or no direct effect on insulin resistance.
  - *Efficacy with respect to insulin level:* An early defect of type 2 diabetes is loss of first-phase insulin secretion. Many people will initially have compensatory increases in second-phase insulin secretion. By delaying glucose absorption, these medications match the timing of incoming glucose to the insulin secretory patterns.

- **Medications that increase insulin secretion**
  - *Classes:* sulfonylureas, meglitinides, D-phenylalanine derivatives
  - *Efficacy with respect to insulin resistance:* Any medication that re-

duces glucose levels decreases glucose toxicity and thus decreases insulin resistance. They probably have little direct effect on insulin resistance, but their use often results in improvements in insulin sensitivity.

- *Efficacy with respect to insulin level:* Medications that increase insulin secretion exert their effect on β-cells. Therefore, functional β-cells must be present for these medications to have any effect. This does not preclude the use of exogenous insulin, however, particularly in the case of the sulfonylureas. When used with insulin therapy, these medications may be used to stimulate secretion of endogenous insulin in its more natural patterns, and allow a reduction in the amount of exogenous insulin being used.

  The direct secretagogues (sulfonylureas, meglitinide, D-Phenylalanine derivative) medications vary as to their binding to the SUR binding site, leading to differing insulin secretory responses. With more binding affinity such as is seen with glyburide, there is a more constant insulin secretory response. Lesser binding affinity, such as with glipizide and glimepiride, results in more meal-stimulation of insulin rather than tonic increases in insulin secretion. Nateglinide, with much less affinity, has predominantly meal-stimulated effects.

- **Medications that restore or replicate incretin action on insulin secretion and glucagon suppression**
  - *Classes:* GLP-1 Agonists, DPP-IV inhibitors
  - *Efficacy with respect to insulin resistance:* As with the direct secretagogues, medications that reduce hyperglycemia decrease glucose toxicity and insulin resistance.
  - *Efficacy with respect to insulin level:* The incretin replacement therapies work by increasing the level of GLP-1 activity, either by providing more of this enzyme, or inhibiting its degradation. A key effect of GLP-1 is to stimulate insulin secretion, so functional β-cells must be present for these medications to work. GLP-1 also suppresses glucagon, particularly in the postprandial state. Some treatments, particularly those that directly augment GLP-1 levels (GLP-1 Agonists), may also improve the feeling of satiety.

Side Effects and Contraindications

Side effects and contraindications vary among the available medications. In addition, the impact of side effects may vary from patient to patient. For example, the concern about potential hypoglycemia may be a minor concern for some, yet potentially life threatening for others. Patients may tolerate gastrointestintinal side effects differently. Some medications may have a potential for adverse hepatic effects, or cannot be used if hepatic or renal impairment are present. Therefore, screening renal or hepatic status prior to medication selection is important.

Also, keep in mind that many of these treatments for type 2 diabetes are contraindicated in women who are pregnant.

A more detailed listing of such concerns can be found in the *Medication Summaries* section at the end of this chapter.

The Classes of Antidiabetes Medications

Medication Comparisons

There are many studies of antidiabetes medications demonstrating their efficacy, safety, and utility for various indications, usually comparing the medication to a placebo, or perhaps to a sulfonylurea. However, making comparisons among the various medications used to treat type 2 diabetes is made more difficult by the fact that there are few head-to-head studies on comparable patient populations.

Many of the available studies that evaluate diabetes medications are designed and supported by pharmaceutical companies. Such studies are designed with specific objectives in mind: to obtain results that demonstrate the safety and efficacy of their medication for the purpose of FDA submission and specific usage indications, and to provide useful information about the medications for utilization by the pharmaceutical company's sales force. While these are not necessarily bad objectives and do provide useful data, they are not usually helpful in determining whether one medication vs. another is preferable in a given clinical situation.

The interpretation of data from these studies must be done carefully, particularly if one is tempted to compare one study to another. Baseline characteristics of the study populations often vary significantly with respect to key parameters that influence outcomes, such as degree of diabetes control (glucose levels and A1C), lipid levels, weight or BMI, age, gender, demographics, or duration of diabetes. Study design can be quite variable with respect to factors such as inclusion and exclusion criteria, study duration, treatment intervention and medication adjustment criteria. Studies initiated prior to the availability of results of studies such as the DCCT or UKPDS often have higher A1C starting points, because the impetus for achieving aggressive control in the general population was less and the medications to achieve it were fewer. Also, human studies committees allowed more control deterioration prior to the availability of conclusive proof that such levels of poor control were harmful. Drug naïve patients (patients with no previous exposure to oral diabetes therapy) usually have a greater hypoglycemic response to medications than do those who had previous therapy.

It is important to know the treatment history of study patients in order to properly interpret the data and compare it to data for other medications. Today, there is so much data suggesting the benefits of aggressive therapy of diabetes and all of the associated risk factors such as dyslipidemia and hypertension, that many study subjects are using, or have in the past used, some medications for macrovascular protection. Thus, studies seeking end-organ events as clinical endpoints often need large numbers of subjects, often difficult to recruit and expensive to treat, in order to show any statistically significant differences.

Therefore, in trying to compare medications within a class, or from class to class, using different studies, one *cannot* state with any certainty that slight differences in characteristics of medications are of any statistical or clinical significance. While markedly significant differences in outcome do suggest that differentiation among the medications may be real, one still cannot say so with absolute certainty. Further, lack of differences may be clouded by background blunting of study effect by other treatments. Therefore, studies or study data should be interpreted with caution. Use this information to determine an approximation of overall drug efficacy, comparative strength, accompanying effects, and side effects, rather than to draw any firm conclusions comparing one medication to another. Even end-organ impact can be difficult to gauge accurately.

Another area of caution when making comparisons among medications involves extrapolation of medication characteristics to others in the same class. Can you assume that the results of a study of a particular drug,

TABLE 8-1. Oral Medications Available in the United States to Treat Type 2 Diabetes

Class of Medication	Optimal Daily Dosing (mg)	Typical Daily Dosing Schedule
Insulin Secretagogues		
second generation sulfonylurea		
glyburide	1.25–20	Up to 20 mg as 1–2 daily doses
glyburide (micronized)	0.75–12	Up to 12 mg as 1–2 daily doses
glipizide	2.5–40	Up to 40 mg as 2 doses
glipizide GITS	2.5–20	Up to 20 mg as 1 dose
glimepiride	1–8	Up to 8 mg as 1 dose
meglitinides		
repaglinide	1.5–16	0.5–4 mg with each meal
D-phenylalanine derivative		
nateglinide	180–360 before each meal	60–120 mg with each meal
Incretin mimetic therapies		
GLP-1 agonists		
exenatide	5–10 mcg	5 mcg injected BID titrated to 10 mcg BID
DPP-4 inhibitors		
sitagliptin	100 mg	100 mg once daily (50 or 25 with renal dysfunction)
α-Glucosidase Inhibitors		
acarbose	25–300	25–100 mg with each meal
miglitol	25–300	25–100 mg with each meal
Biguanides		
metformin	500–2000	Up to 1000 mg BID (extended release: all presupper)
Thiazolidinediones		
rosiglitazone	4–8	Up to 8 mg as 1–2 doses
pioglitazone	15–45	Up to 45 mg as 1 dose

demonstrating an effect or indication, apply to others in the class? Should side effects or adverse events experienced with one medication be assumed to accompany others? These assumptions are risky, must be individualized carefully, and make drug-to-drug comparisons even more challenging.

With these concerns stated, listed below are descriptions of the various groups of antidiabetes medications available to treat type 2 diabetes. More details can be found at the end of this chapter in the *Medication Summaries*.

What do we call all these medications?

At this juncture, we probably should discuss nomenclature, which has gotten a bit convoluted of late! With the development of increasing numbers of medications used to treat diabetes came an interesting evolution in the way we refer to them. The term "oral hypoglycemic agents" or, shortened, "oral agents" was the term originally used to refer to the sulfonylureas, which were the first non-insulin, oral treatments for this condition. These medications increase insulin levels and lead to an increased *hypoglycemic* effect. As the mechanisms of action of these medications were not well understood when phenformin became available, this medication also was lumped under this original label, "oral agent."

In recent years, however, other medications with different mechanisms of action have become available, and, as well, we have learned more about how these medications work. It is clear, for example, that metformin reduces insulin resistance and is not likely to make people "hypoglycemic" as much as it reduces elevated glucose levels by reducing hepatic insulin resistance. It is really an oral "antihyperglycemic agent." Most recently, exenatide became available which is administered by injection, and thus is certainly not an "oral agent!"

Therefore, tracing the nomenclature forward can be an interesting exercise. Prior to the availability of the injected exenatide, many people referred to *all* of the oral diabetes medications as "oral agents" out of habit. However, those wishing to be precise (some might say "pharmacologically correct"!) would use this term *only* for sulfonylureas. The entire group of oral medications would be referred to by another name such as "oral antidiabetes medications" or "oral diabetes medications." Now, the enlarged group, including injectable and oral medications that are available to treat type 2 diabetes that are not insulin, are referred to by most as simply "antidiabetes medications."

Of course, injectable insulin is also considered by some to be an antidiabetes medication. Thus, at the risk of creating more confusion, for the purposes of discussions in this edition of this book, we will refer to non-insulin treatments as antidiabetes medications, and *all* available treatments for diabetes will be "antidiabetes medications plus insulin." Undoubtedly, this will all change again by the time we prepare the *next* edition!!

Medications that Improve Insulin Action

One could make the argument that all patients with type 2 diabetes could benefit from using a medication that reduces insulin resistance. Insulin resistance is felt to be the hallmark of type 2 diabetes and should be present in everyone who is properly diagnosed with this type of diabetes. In fact, it is present in people with type 2 diabetes before diabetes becomes clinically apparent.

Medications in this group of classes share the following characteristics:

- They require the presence of endogenous or exogenous insulin to have their effect.
- The patient must have insulin resistance for these medications to be effective.
- As these medications reduce insulin resistance rather than increase insulin quantity, they tend to be more effective at higher glucose levels. They are also not as likely to cause significant hypoglycemia as treatments that increase insulin levels.

Biguanides

- *General comments:* The one biguanide currently available in the United States is metformin, although in the past phenformin was available and others have been tried in various parts of the world. The primary mode of action of medications in this class is to decrease hepatic production of glucose. Therefore, the most predominant clinical manifestation is lowering of the fasting glucose level, which is the parameter most reflective of hepatic glucose production. To a lesser extent, these medications may also increase peripheral glucose utilization.

- *Anticipated efficacy:* Studies have suggested that treatment with metformin can result in a reduction of the A1C level by about 1.5% to 1.8%. In addition, data suggest that metformin may have some small beneficial effect on lipid profiles and can promote weight loss. The most common adverse events are gastrointestinal, especially diarrhea, affecting 30% of people starting metformin. However, it is usually mild, lasting about 2–3 weeks after initiation of therapy, and results in only a 4% to 5% drug discontinuation. The incidence of diarrhea may be reduced by taking the medication during or after meals and titrating the medication dose more slowly. This problem may also be reduced by use of the extended-release formulation. Subclinical reductions in vitamin B12 levels requiring no clinical intervention can also occur, affecting about 7% of people using metformin.

- *Clinical dosage:* Metformin is usually started as 500 mg orally BID, although 500 mg once daily can be used for a few weeks in patients in whom gastrointestinal disturbances occur. The use of the extended-release formulation would allow once-daily dosing and often cause less gastrointestinal side effects. Also, formulations with glyburide or glipizide provide for easier combination treatment. Dose response increases as the total daily dose is increased to 2000 mg daily. However, if the desired efficacy is not achieved at this dose level, adding a second agent to the therapeutic regimen should be considered. Doses higher than 2000 mg daily do not generally increase efficacy.

- *Adverse effects:* Lactic acidosis was a concern with a previous biguanide, phenformin, which is no longer on the market. Compared with phenformin, lactic acidosis associated with metformin therapy is extremely rare due to differences in metabolic pathways. The reported incidence of lactic acidosis in metformin-using patients is 0.03 cases/1000 patient-years. While the mortality rate for those people who do develop lactic acidosis can be quite high, the actual numbers of people dying from metformin-induced lactic acidosis is comparable to the mortality from sulfonylurea-induced hypoglycemic coma. Metformin-associated lactic acidosis occurs primarily in patients with specific contraindications to drug use. These include:

- renal disease (serum creatinine: >1.5 males, >1.4 females, or abnormal creatinine clearance)
- liver dysfunction
- congestive heart failure (CHF) under drug treatment
- history of alcohol abuse/binge drinking
- acute or chronic metabolic acidosis

Metformin should be withheld in conditions predisposing to renal insufficiency and/or hypoxia, including:

- cardiovascular collapse
- acute myocardial infarction
- acute CHF
- severe infections.

Metformin should be temporarily discontinued at the time of or prior to the use of iodinated contrast media or major surgical procedures and withheld for 48 hours subsequent to the procedure. It should be reinstituted only after renal function has been re-evaluated and found to be normal. An earlier requirement to stop metformin 48 hours prior to a contract study has been eliminated.

Thiazolidinediones

- *General comments:* The thiazolidinediones are a relatively new class of diabetes medications; the first member of this class, troglitazone, was introduced in the United States in 1997, but withdrawn in 2000 due to liver toxicity. The two remaining medications in this class, pioglitazone and rosiglitazone, don't seem to share this significant adverse characteristic. Thiazolidinediones are thought to work primarily by decreasing peripheral insulin resistance, affecting tissues such as muscle and adipose. Their effect is to increase basal and insulin-stimulated glucose transport.

  Many feel, however, that all of the efficacy of these medications cannot be explained solely on the basis of the peripheral effects, and there is evidence that they may also have some effect in reducing hepatic glucose output as well. Thiazolidinediones have no glucose-lowering effect in the absence of insulin, do not produce hypoglycemia when used alone, and have been shown to have some lipid-lowering and antihypertensive effects as well.

  All compounds contain the thiazolidinedione structure, with additional moieties added to affect bioavailability and potency. The apparent mechanism of action involves binding to nuclear receptors that regulate gene expression at the transcriptional level. Thiazolidinedione receptors include the peroxisome proliferator-activated receptors (PPAR family).

There has been some suggestion that this class of medications may have some effects beyond direct glucose control. Early studies suggest that use of these medications may lead to prolongation of the survival time of β-cells and could reduce the risk of endothelial damage. However, more data are needed before we can conclusively conclude that these beneficial effects can be ascribed to this medication class, or quantitate the impact. Other, more recent studies suggest some benefits by medications in this class in slowing the progression of the development of diabetes or blunting macrovascular events.

Medications of a different class that bind to multiple PPAR receptors ("Dual PPAR's") and may have significant effects on other related metabolic functions such as lipid metabolism were under development in the past, but development was stopped due to concern about adverse events. At this writing, there is no indication that work on these medications will resume.

- *Anticipated efficacy:* At this writing, there are no head-to-head studies. As studies of these medications individually vary according to inclusion/exclusion criteria, starting level of glucose control, and study design, comparisons are difficult. However, variations may be determined in the future if head-to-head studies are performed.
- *Clinical dosage:* There are differences in clinical doses that result from variations in binding affinity among the medications in this class. These doses result in similar clinical effect:
  - Pioglitazone doses: 15 to 45 mg/day
  - Rosiglitazone doses: 4 to 8 mg/day
- *Adverse experiences:* Other than the concern about liver toxicity noted above, the most significant side effect, which seems to be seen with both medications, is a tendency for edema, which can result in a dilutional anemia or exacerbated congestive heart failure (CHF). These medications should be used with caution in people with, or prone to, CHF, and ongoing monitoring is important. Also, a meta-analysis of studies of rosiglitazone suggests a greater risk of coronary artery events. These findings have stirred some controversy, and the

ongoing debate should be monitored for impact on usage of this medication. This concern does not seem to be shared by pioglitazone. Patients using these medications also tend to gain weight, often greater amounts than might be expected from the reduction in glycosuria and the fluid retention.

- *Drug interaction profiles:* Differences in drug interactions among these medications result from differences in cytochrome pathways for metabolism. (See *Medication Summaries* at the end of this chapter.)
- *Liver toxicity:* There has been considerable concern about the relationship between use of medications in this class, particularly troglitazone, and idiosyncratic hepatic injury. Small numbers of people treated with troglitazone were reported as having mild elevations of liver transaminase enzymes, but there were a few with more significant liver damage, and some deaths. With the availability of other thiazolidinediones, pioglitazone and rosiglitazone, which seemed to have much better safety profiles, Troglitazone was voluntarily removed from the market on Mach 21, 2000.

Nevertheless, persistent concerns over hepatotoxicity lead to recommendations for hepatic monitoring with the use of rosiglitazone and pioglitazone. Such recommendations were included in their initial package inserts upon release in 1999. As one might predict from statistical probabilities of occurrences, rare patients using these other medications have and will suffer some hepatic dysfunction and hepatic enzyme elevations (> 3 times the upper limit of normal). However, subsequently, and as of this writing, there seems to be enough experience to suggest that there is not likely to be a significant causal relationship between medication use and serious hepatic failure. Therefore, the liver function monitoring guidelines were reduced, and the current recommendation is to check the liver enzymes (ALT and AST) prior to the initiation of therapy, and then periodically thereafter, per the clinical judgment of the healthcare professional. However, as these types of recommendations are subject to further change, practitioners using these medications should watch for updated reports on hepatic function or precautions, should they be released, and for any changes in screening recommendations for all members of this medication class.

These are important medications in the control of diabetes. Their use, either alone or in combination with other treatments, has allowed considerable numbers of patients to achieve more effective glucose control than they ever had previously. Ironically, many of the elevations in liver enzymes seen are the result of fatty liver, rather than drug effects, and treatment to improve glucose control often leads to *improvements* in liver enzyme elevations, rather than worsening.

Initial doses and titration instructions are outlined in the *Medication Summaries*. As a general rule, it takes a minimum of two months to get a full sense of the efficacy of these medications in a given patient, and for some patients an even longer period of time may be needed. Thus, the titration is relatively slow, usually performed at intervals dictated by the timing of liver function monitoring.

If patients are using other diabetes medications and a thiazolidinedione is added, the dose of the other medication(s) should be continued at the same dose initially. However, as the dose of the thiazolidinedione is titrated, the dose of the other medication(s) may need to be reduced if glucose levels begin to fall, particularly below 120 mg/dl.

Patients utilizing thiazolidinediones often differ in their response to treatment. Some will show a substantial response to therapy, while others have a minimal response or no response at all. For those who respond, the efficacy can be impressive. Much of the data reported in the literature about thiazolidinedione efficacy is based on "intent-to-treat" studies in which patients are included in the drug treatment group based on random assignments. Thus, in an intent-to-treat analysis, responders and nonresponders are combined in the final efficacy analysis. While this is appropriate for clinical research and required for FDA submissions, in a clinical practice, patients who do not respond to a medication are usually not treated with that medication for a prolonged interval. Thus, over time, those patients who continue to use thiazolidinedione therapy are usually those with a clinically useful, and often quite impressive, response.

Weight gain has been seen as a side effect of thiazolidinedione therapy. This has been ascribed to both reduced glycosuria from the improvement in glucose control and the edema that can occur with treatment with these medications. However, many people think that the weight gain may be a result of other drug effects, such as increasing pre-adiposite differentiation. Most of the weight gain is felt to be subcutaneous fat rather than the more atherogenic and metabolically active intra-abdominal fat.

Studies of lipid effects have varied according to initial lipid and glucose levels of the study populations and therefore are difficult to compare. Most medications in this class lower free fatty acids and triglycerides, which may be part of the mechanism resulting in the drug's glucose lowering effect; these lipid changes lead to increased glucose uptake in muscle and decreased hepatic glucose production.

Summary

The medications that improve insulin action are effective as treatment for anyone who has diabetes and insulin resistance. As the medications reduce insulin resistance — allow the insulin that is present to work more effectively — they also require the presence of insulin in order to be effective. However, the source of that insulin may be either endogenous or exogenous. Patients who have become insulinopenic and who are receiving insulin injection therapy, but who have significant insulin resistance that impacts their diabetes control, might benefit from treatment with these medications.

Medications that Slow Glucose Absorption

The effect of this class of medications — slowing glucose absorption — is particularly helpful in improving glucose control for patients for whom the loss of first-phase insulin secretion is a predominant abnormality, often accompanied by a delay in second-phase and insulin resistance. The slowed glucose absorption and delayed rise in postprandial glucose absorption results in a better match between this glucose influx and the second — or later — phase of insulin release.

Normal insulin response occurs in two phases. The first phase is a rapid insulin release immediately following the ingestion of food. It is postulated that this phase is the result of release of pre-made insulin from β-cells and occurs after exposure of the cell to rising blood glucose levels. Loss of first-phase insulin release is a characteristic abnormality seen in people with type 2 diabetes. Subsequently, there is a more gradual, longer-lasting rise in insulin levels representing newly manufactured insulin, referred to as the second phase.

The loss of first-phase insulin release typically occurs early in the natural history of type 2 diabetes. The first-phase insulin response is also blunted by glucose toxicity, caused by the hyperglycemia present prior to food ingestion. When the first-phase insulin response is lost, the postprandial glucose levels rise unopposed and reach a higher-than-normal level. In the patient who still has otherwise adequate β-cell function and number, the second phase of insulin release, stimulated by this elevated postprandial glucose level, is often augmented. The result is the increased insulin secretion that leads to the hyperinsulinemia that has been noted previously.

Interestingly, some people who may not yet have diabetes, but have parts of the insulin resistance constellation, will begin to lose their first-phase insulin response. In fact, people with impaired glucose tolerance who demonstrate a loss of first-phase insulin secretion are more likely to develop frank diabetes, as compared with those who retain that first phase. With absent first-phase insulin release, a significant second-phase release can lead to reactive hypoglycemia hours after eating. This can be particularly significant if a rapidly absorbed glucose source is consumed, resulting in a sharp rise in postprandial glucose levels and marked second-phase insulin production.

Early phases of diabetes will be manifest by this pattern of insulin secretory abnormality and the resulting glucose pattern of postprandial hyperglycemia. In fact, about 50% of people destined to get type 2 diabetes, who have not yet met diagnostic criteria based on the fasting glucose level, will show some postprandial abnormality. In spite of the promulgation of the new diabetes diagnostic criteria based on a fasting glucose level, intended to make diagnosis easier, there is some evidence that the early clinical manifestation of an insulin secretory abnormality — postprandial hyperglycemia — might be an important marker of the insulin resistance syndrome and all of the inherent risks of earlier morbidity and mortality that it carries with it.

For patients who have diabetes and are at the stage at which this early insulin secretory defect is present, one can reduce the need for that missing or blunted first phase of insulin secretion if the incoming glucose load is absorbed more slowly. This is how the medications that slow glucose absorption work to improve glucose control. They blunt a sharp postprandial glucose rise that cannot be effectively held at appropriate levels by a first-phase insulin response, and then prolong the absorption of that glucose into the timeframe of the second-phase insulin release, when the presence of blood glucose more closely matches the presence of secreted insulin.

Thus, these medications have a specific niche in treatment for insulin resistant patients who have progressed to that phase in the natural history of the condition where first-phase insulin secretion is significantly de-creased, and often, also, there is a delay or reduction in the second phase.

Similarly, while reactive hypoglycemia is over-diagnosed and used as an explanation of many unrelated symptoms, for the patient with insulin resistance and a true reactive pattern, these medications are sometimes used to help ameliorate untoward symptoms.

α-Glucosidase Inhibitors

- *General comments:* α-Glucosidase inhibitors are the class of medica-tions that are currently used to slow glucose absorption. The mem-bers of this class that are currently available in the United States are acarbose and miglitol. These medications are competitive inhibitors of intestinal brush border a-glucosidases, which leads to the prolon-gation of carbohydrate absorption time from the gastrointestinal tract. The usual effect on lowering A1C levels is about 0.5 to 1%.
- *Anticipated efficacy:* As these medications are optimally effective in early stages of type 2 diabetes when glucose abnormalities are not as great as they may be later, the resulting impact on A1C-lowering is less than that seen with other classes of medications. However, there have been some suggestions that these medications may demon-strate greater A1C-lowering effect when used in patients with more advanced diabetes and higher initial A1C levels. In addition, not sur-prisingly, these medications are more effective in people who con-sume a diet higher in carbohydrates. Further, a study ("Stop NIDDM") suggests that the use of one of these medications, acar-bose, can reduce the progression from impaired glucose tolerance to type 2 diabetes and also can reduce the incidence of cardiovascular events.
- *Clinical dosage:* The usual starting dose of miglitol and acarbose is 25 mg TID. However, some physicians start with 12.5 mg before meals (although the tablet is not scored) and some elect to suggest 25 mg before just one or perhaps two meals initially.

  Usually, the medication is taken with the first bite of food at the 3 main daily meals. Doses are then gradually titrated upward, if neces-sary, based on the results of self-blood glucose testing and A1C,to 50 mg.TID, then 100 mg.TID.
- *Adverse effects:* Use may be limited by the typical side effects of flatulence, which is usually mild and self-limited, or diarrhea. These

occur in about 56% of people using acarbose, with 15% discontinuing use as a result; there are similar occurrences for miglitol. For most people, these symptoms subside after about three to four weeks of use. Mild elevations of liver enzymes (transaminases) are quite rarely seen with these medications, usually at higher doses.

Medications that Increase Insulin Secretion

Traditionally, the group of medications that increase insulin secretion were referred to as insulin secretagogues. The sulfonylureas, one class of medication in this grouping, were the first types of oral treatments for diabetes in common usage. Subsequently, the short-acting secretagogues became available with more immediate postprandial secretory effects.

There is now a new group of medications that work to increase insulin secretion, referred to by various names including the incretin mimetics or incretin replacement therapies. While technically also secretagogues, we will consider them in a separate grouping due to their differences in mode of action.

The traditional insulin secretagogues

As noted above, the "traditional" insulin secretagogues are divided into the longer-acting sulfonylureas, and the shorter-acting or prandial secretagogues, the meglitinides and D-phenylalanine derivatives. While the medications that decrease insulin resistance require the presence of insulin from any source in order to be effective, medications that increase insulin secretion require the presence of the functioning β-cells, as they act upon these cells to increase their insulin production.

These insulin secretagogues work by binding to the SUR binding site on the wall of he pancreatic β-cell. This triggers a closing of potassium channels, and a resulting depolarization leads to opening of the calcium channels. This, in turn, leads to an increase in intracellular Ca^{++}, which causes insulin release. The binding of these medications to the SUR binding sites can be tight or loose. Sulfonylureas tend to bind tightly, and thus there is a more tonic, longer acting insulin secretory response. Some of the other shorter-acting secretagogues bind more loosely, and thus have an immediate effect only, then come loose and the effect subsides. Thus, when taken before meals, their effect can be targeted to the postprandial period and also tend to be more dependent on glucose levels to modulate insulin secretion. Even within the sulfonylurea group, the binding affinity can vary, with glyburide binding the most tightly, thus leading to the most tonic, ongoing insulin secretory stimulation, with glimepiride and then glipizide binding somewhat less tightly.

While the primary impact of these medications is increased insulin secretion, the reduction of glucose levels can decrease glucose toxicity, and, indirectly, also reduce insulin resistance. This fact may explain the phenomenon that insulin levels do increase upon initiation of therapy with a sulfonylurea, one class of insulin secretagogues. However, after a number of months of therapy with improvement in glucose control, insulin levels often return to pretreatment levels. The reduction in glucose toxicity from the improvement in diabetes control may have the indirect effect of reducing insulin resistance, resulting in reduced insulin requirements. However, the direct effect of sulfonylureas to potentiate insulin action in liver and peripheral tissues (muscle and adipose) has also been proposed, and the actual clinical impact of these possible actions remains debatable.

Sulfonylureas

- *General comments:* As their primary mode of action, sulfonylureas increase insulin secretion in response to rising glucose levels. They also exhibit the indirect effects noted above, possibly increasing insulin action and decreasing hepatic insulin clearance.

  The sulfonylureas were the first class of oral medications for diabetes treatment that achieved widespread use throughout the world, and their availability is considered to be one of the significant milestones in the modern history of diabetes treatment.

  The first medication in this class, tolbutamide, became available for clinical use in 1955. Subsequently, three other medications, acetohexamide, tolazamide, and chlorporpamide became available. For two decades, these "first-generation" medications dominated the oral diabetes therapy market, shared, only briefly, but significantly, with the biguanide phenformin, which is no longer available. By the early 1980s, however, modifications of the basic sulfonylurea molecule led to the introduction of a second generation of sulfonylureas. These agents include **glyburide** (also known as glibenclamide), **glipizide,** and **gliclazide. Glimepiride** followed a few years later.

  The second-generation sulfonylureas (listed in Table 8-1) have essentially replaced the first generation agents in common usage due to numerous advantages:

- high level of potency relative to therapeutic dosage due to high affinity for the sulfonylurea receptor on the cell surface
- short half-life, yet 24-hour duration of action
- compared with many of the first-generation agents, these second generation agents can be given less frequently, increasing adherence
- theoretically fewer drug interactions and side effects

In addition, differing formulations of some of these agents (glipizide GITS, micronized glyburide, and combination tablets) can affect their pharmacologic action. (See *Medication Summaries*.)

Contraindications to the use of sulfonylureas include:

- type 1 diabetes or diabetes due to pancreatic resection
- pregnancy or gestational diabetes
- significant renal or hepatic disease
- a history of adverse reactions to sulfonylureas or related compounds
- treatment during acute stress such as infections, trauma, surgery
- acute hyperglycemia with ketosis or hyperosmolar states
- tendencies to develop severe hypoglycemia

- *Anticipated efficacy:* Generally, sulfonylureas can be expected to lower A1C levels by about 1–2 percentage points in a person with adequate β-cell function remaining.
- *Clinical dosage:* The dosing ranges for the various agents in this class are listed in Table 8-1 and in the *Medication Summaries*. Most of the therapeutic efficacy of sulfonylureas is seen in the first half of the usual dosing range. Dose titration is accomplished based on the results of SMBG and A1C levels.
- *Adverse effects:* There are relatively few adverse effects from sulfonylureas. The most common concerns are allergic reactions in people with sensitivity to sulfa drugs. Hypoglycemia is more likely to occur with the use of the sulfonylureas than with the use of medications from any other class due to the potential for generalized increases in insulin levels.

Meglitinides

- *General comments:* Meglitinides are a newer class of non-sulfonylurea insulin secretagogues. These medications are benzoic acid analogues, and the first drug introduced from this class is **repaglinide.** Repaglinide is a β-cell sensitizer that primes the cell for glucose-dependent release of insulin in the immediate postprandial period. Thus, from a clinical standpoint, the key difference is that the insulin release is more predominantly glucose-dependent, as opposed to the effect of sulfonylureas, in particular glyburide, which initiate insulin release more independent of the presence of glucose.

This medication can be effective in patients with the characteristic loss of first-phase insulin release. However, with a longer effect than nateglinide (see below), these medications probably can boost insulin response in the timeframe of the second phase of insulin release as well. Therefore, they would be useful for patients who are at the point in the natural history of their type 2 diabetes at which they are losing the glucose-stimulated insulin secretory function and are beginning to develop significant postprandial hyperglycemia. For patients needing an insulin secretagogue but who often eat meals on erratic schedules, of variable quantities, or who even skip meals, this medication can be adjusted based on these variables, with doses being omitted if a meal is missed.

- *Anticipated efficacy:* Generally, repaglinide, the meglitinide currently available, can be expected to lower A1C levels by about 1.6 to 1.9 A1C percentage points in a person with adequate β-cell function remaining.

- *Clinical dosing:* Repaglinide is indicated for use as monotherapy or in combination with metformin. It is given preprandially, titrated to doses between 0.5 and 4 mg prior to each meal, and can be used for up to four meals per day for a maximum dose of 16 mg/day. (See *Medication Summaries*).

- *Adverse effects:* Relatively few. As with sulfonylureas, hypersensitivity and hypoglycemia are adverse effects that might occur.

D-Phenylalanine Derivatives

- *General comments:* The representative medication of the class of D-phenylalanine is **nateglinide.** In spite of the similarity of the generic name to repaglinide, this medication is really in a separate structural class from repaglinide and, for that matter, from the sulfonylureas. The name similarity stems from the similarity of its clinical effects to those of repaglinide — the rapid, glucose-mediated stimulation of postprandial insulin release — and often people mistakenly include this in the meglitinide group, when technically it is not.

Nateglinide has an essentially flat dose-response curve, so the usual dose recommendation is 120 mg, with the 60-mg dose reserved for patients who are close to their therapeutic target. The glucose levels dictate the degree of response more than does the dose of medication. Nateglinide has a strong affinity for beta-cells. If it is taken before eating, its glucose-dependent effect in stimulating insulin release is extremely rapid, analogous to the first-phase insulin release that is lost in people with type 2 diabetes. Used as monotherapy in non-drug-naïve patients, data suggest an A1C drop of about 0.45%. As with other medications, drug-naïve patients, and those with higher pretreatment A1C levels, may have a greater response. For example, combined therapy with metformin may achieve an A1C drop of 1.5% or more. As with repaglinide, treatment can be tailored to meal schedules with respect to timing and the omission of the medication if a meal is skipped.

The key clinical difference between this medication and repaglinide is the time-course of action. Compared with repaglinide, nateglinide has a more rapid onset and results in a postprandial insulin secretory peak that comes even closer to the natural first-phase pattern than repaglinide would stimulate. Its shorter duration of action makes it less likely to cause hypoglycemia hours after the meal than is seen with repaglinide and considerably less likely than with sulfonylureas. However, the other side of this issue is that with less late efficacy, it might be less effective in patients who have developed significant defects in second-phase insulin secretion. Therefore, one would expect this medication to have clinically significant efficacy in patients with early type 2 diabetes, where the characteristic loss of first-phase insulin release has occurred, but before the condition has progressed further to include a significant second-phase insulin secretory deficiency or a reduction in β-cell mass as well.

Medications that Restore Incretin Function: The Incretin Mimetics

The existence of the incretin system has been known for a number of years, but it is not until recently that this knowledge has translated into a mode of treating diabetes. It had been observed for many years that when glucose was taken orally, the resulting insulin stimulatory response was greater than when glucose was given intravenously — over 50% greater in many instances. This effect was noted in the differences in expected response between an oral and intravenous glucose tolerance test. This difference in response is referred to as the *incretin effect*. It is primarily due to the effects of two hormones stimulated by the intestines and which stimulate insulin secretion and glucagon suppression, glucagon-like peptide-1 (GLP-1) and glucose-dependent insulinotropic polypeptide (GIP). These hormones, constituting the incretin effect and playing significant roles in mealtime insulin secretion, are major controlling influences on postprandial glycemia.

GLP-1 is secreted by the L-cells in the distal small intestine (jejunum and ileum) upon stimulation by the presence of incoming nutrients. GLP-1 is rapidly metabolized by the enzyme dipeptidyl-peptidase IV, or DPP-IV. GIP is also metabolized by this enzyme, but less efficiently. Thus, the half-life of GLP-1 is about 4–5 minutes.

People with type 2 diabetes have been found to have a reduced incretin effect, primarily due to reduced GLP-1 secretion, but decreased GIP effect as well. As the efficacy of GLP-1 remains, and it is the *secretion* that is effected, replacement of GLP-1 was targeted as a potential treatment intervention. GLP-1 has a number of actions that have been identified to date:

- stimulates insulin gene transcription and expression, and the resulting insulin synthesis
- increases β-cell mass by stimulating new cell formation and inhibition of apoptosis
- enhances glucose-dependent insulin secretion
- suppresses glucagon secretion
- slows gastric emptying (which blunts postprandial glucose excursions)
- improves insulin sensitivity
- reduces appetite and food intake

Thus, it seemed initially that with effects such as these, GLP-1 replacement would be a wonderful treatment option. However, as noted above, the rapid degradation by DPP-IV renders most of the GLP-1 inactive quite rapidly, and thus the natural form would not be a therapeutic option. To develop a pharmacologic means of replacing incretin function in people with type 2 diabetes, the options would be to find an alternative form of GLP-1 that was not degraded as rapidly as the natural form, or to inhibit the enzyme DPP-IV, so natural GLP-1 would remain active longer.

GLP-1 Agonists

- *General comments:* GLP-1 mimetic substances have been sought as a treatment to restore incretin function. The first one to reach the market was exenatide (brand name: Byetta). At this writing, others are under development.

  Exenatide was discovered when it was noted that a salivary protein from the Gila monster had properties similar to GLP-1! A synthetic version of this substance was produced and tested, and found to be effective. It has greater than 50% structural overlap with human GLP-1, binds to the human GLP-1 receptor on the β-cell, and is resistant to DPP-IV degradation, being measurable in plasma for as long as 10 hours after injection.

  Exenatide is indicated for use as adjunctive therapy to achieve targeted glycemic control in people with type 2 diabetes who are taking metformin, a sulfonylurea, or a combination of the two. It increases first phase and augments second phase insulin secretion. It also reduces glucagon secretion, particularly in the presence of hyperglycemia, but does not blunt glucagon response to hypoglycemia. It slows gastric emptying, resulting in slower entry of meal-derived glucose into the circulation. It has been shown to reduce appetite, leading to decreased food intake.

  Another long-acting GLP-1 agonist, liriglutide, is also under development.
- *Anticipated efficacy:* Generally, exenatide is used in combination with a sulfonylurea and/or metformin, and can achieve a reduction in A1C of up to 1%. It can also lead to a reduction in weight, most likely in combination with metformin alone where 3 kg reductions can be seen.
- *Clinical dosing:* Exenatide is initiated as injection therapy at a dose indicated for use as monotherapy or in combination with metformin. It is initiated at 5 mcg per dose, given with a prefilled pen device, twice daily within 60 minutes of the morning and evening meals.

After about a month, based on clinical response and absence or amelioration of side effects, it is increased to 10 mcg per dose, twice daily.
- *Adverse effects:* Other than hypoglycemia, the most common adverse
effect was nausea, usually mild to moderate. The nausea usually sub-
sided with continued therapy.

DPP-IV Inhibitors

- *General comments:* At this writing, one DPP-IV inhibitor, sitagliptin,
has received FDA approval and is on the market, and others are being developed. Normally, DPP-IV inactivates GLP-1, rapidly deplet-
ing the endogenous pool. DPP-IV inhibitors will block this degradation process, thus increasing the supply of endogenous GLP-1. Their
blocking of GLP-1 degradation will lead to improved glucose dependent insulin release, reduced hepatic glucose production, and
improved peripheral glucose utilization. Some of the other effects
of GLP-1 replacement are less clear, such as the effect on satiety and
β-cell preservation.

    Sitagliptin is indicated as an adjunct to diet and physical activity in
the treatment of type 2 diabetes as monotherapy, or in combination
with metformin or a thiazolidinedione.
- *Anticipated efficacy:* Improvements in A1C levels in initial studies
have shown improvements of about 0.5–1.0%, the greater improvements seen with higher initial A1C levels.
- *Clinical dosing:* DPP-IV inhibitors are oral medications, administered once daily. Sitagliptin is given as 100 mg tablets, although 50
mg tablets are used for people with moderate renal insufficiency, and
25 mg for those with severe renal dysfunction.
- *Adverse effects:* Studies with these medications showed no significant differences from placebo. Further details are available in the
package inserts for these medications.

Assembling a Treatment Program

A General Approach to Treatment

When nonpharmacologic interventions are deemed insufficient to achieve
treatment targets, treatment with antidiabetes medications would be

indicated. Initial medication selection can be made using the parameters to assess the predominance of the various pathophysiologic components of type 2 diabetes discussed earlier in this chapter. Selection of the initial medication, based on this assessment of pathophysiology, can then be made taking into consideration the characteristics of the various medications as outlined above and in the *Medication Summaries*.

With the array of new medications available, more precise treatments can be selected to target the predominant pathophysiologic defects and specific glucose pattern abnormalities. This evolution to a more precise targeting of pathophysiology with a carefully selected medication or medications has been occurring over the last decade. Keep in mind, also, that when hyperglycemia becomes manifest in someone with type 2 diabetes, there *must* be *two* significant defects present.

- By definition, people with type 2 diabetes have some degree of insulin resistance
- In order for glucose abnormalities to be present, there must be insulin secretory insufficiency. Even if there is hyperinsulinemia (excess insulin relative to normal), it is still insufficient to overcome that insulin resistance and normalize glycemia, and thus these patients have *relative* insulin secretory insufficiency.

The first key abnormality in insulin secretion usually seen is a blunting or loss of the first-phase insulin release. Early on, there may be a compensatory augmentation of the second-phase insulin release leading to hyperinsulinemia. Eventually, there may be a more complete loss of insulin secretory capacity.

Further, if there is significant hyperglycemia on presentation, one can anticipate that this hyperglycemia may also be causing glucose toxicity. Glucose toxicity, caused by significant hyperglycemia, paradoxically worsens insulin resistance and blunts insulin secretory capacity.

Therefore, one can and should assume that upon diagnosis of type 2 diabetes, there are multiple defects present and, thus, treatment with multiple pharmacologic agents with differing modes of action is not only reasonable, but in many instances may be recommended.

If the diagnosis of type 2 diabetes is truly made early in the natural history of the condition, the lifestyle changes of medical nutritional therapy and physical activity may be sufficient to achieve appropriate control. Improvements in nutrition and activity habits may reduce insulin resistance enough to restore insulin sensitivity to a level that corresponds to the insulin secretory capacity. If not, the combination of lifestyle changes and a single pharmacologic agent may be sufficient to achieve targeted levels of control.

However, in many cases, at the time of diagnosis, the condition has progressed significantly so that the impact of multiple defects can be considerable. Therefore, increasingly, clinicians have chosen to initiate combination therapy earlier in the natural history of this condition. Many are moving away from the traditional therapeutic approach of starting one medication and working it exclusively for a considerable period of time.

Now, with the recognition that multiple metabolic defects cause the glucose abnormalities, combination therapy is utilized sooner. While the selection of an initial medication may be made based on the usual clinical estimates of predominant metabolic defect, only a short time is allowed to pass during which clinical efficacy is measured and drug tolerance is assured. Shortly after initiation of this first medication, rather than increasing its dose, treatment with a second medication is initiated. Then, both are concurrently titrated to achieve optimal control, pharmacologically treating multiple defects concurrently. Third medications may also be added to the mix.

The advantages of this approach are:

- multiple defects are addressed, providing more effective treatment by more completely addressing the spectrum of underlying pathophysiologic components
- use of lower doses of each medication reduces the likelihood of adverse effects from any one of the medications

Taking this approach one step further, combination medications have now become available to simplify such therapy. These medications are discussed in detail in the *Medication Summaries* at the end of this chapter. Undoubtedly, as well, additional combinations may become available following publication of this book. Various ratios of the component medications found in these combination tablets allow concurrent initiation of dual therapy using one tablet to optimize convenience and compliance. For tablets such as the glyburide/metformin combination, there are differences in the pharmacodynamics of the glyburide, leading to earlier rises in drug levels.

The benefits of combination tablets should not be underappreciated. In this era of polypharmacy and of pharmaceutical plans doling out prescription refills in one-month aliquots, fewer pills to take not only reduces the chance for erroneous dosing and missed doses, but also may reduce the onerous timed trips to the pharmacy or the mailed-in request forms to refill a prescription at the precise time in a refill cycle.

How Much Treatment Is Needed?

To determine the answer to this question, there are a number of questions to be answered and steps to be taken:

- *What is the goal?* In general, the goal for the glucose control for people with type 2 diabetes is an A1C level that is at least < 7% (with normal 4%–6%), and ideally as low as can be safely and practically achieved. Aside from individualized situations where there might be contraindications to attempting to reach this goal, achieving an A1C level of <7% should be the target.

- *What is the starting point?* For a given patient, what is their starting A1C level? How far above a level of 7% is it? Anyone with an A1C >7% despite optimized medical nutrition therapy and exercise will probably need pharmacologic intervention, and the higher the starting A1C, the more likely monotherapy will not be sufficient.

- *What is the impact of nonpharmacologic therapy?* Have medical nutrition therapy and activity optimization been attempted? How long ago and with what impact? Would a "refresher" course be useful?

- *How acutely is intervention needed?* Is the patient markedly hyperglycemic with symptoms? Is there a complicating factor such as an acute or chronic infection or other physiologic stress? The presence of an infection might be leading to increased glucose levels, and thus infection treatment may be indicated. However, even with infection treatment, the resulting hyperglycemia may need more aggressive treatment.

Let's assume that nonpharmacologic interventions are optimized, that the hyperglycemia is not so excessive that it warrants acute aggressive intervention (usually insulin), and there are no complicating conditions such as infections. The key piece of information in determining the needed pharmacotherapy is the "distance" between the patient's current A1C and the 7% target. This information will give a sense as to how much therapy is needed — whether one medication is sufficient or multiple medications are required. Then, the next steps are to:

- Assess the predominance of the various pathophysiologic abnormalities as discussed earlier.
- Assess each of the appropriate medications to determine how much strength in A1C lowering they are likely to bring to that patient. Keep in mind when doing so that the data found in studies is based on differing A1C starting points. In clinical practice, most agents have more A1C-lowering effect when used in patients with higher initial A1C levels.
- Review the patient's overall medical condition in light of contraindications to the use of any medications.

Examples: We have provided a few examples below to give a sense as to how one might approach selecting therapy, and the various considerations that go into the decision-making process.

In an otherwise uncomplicated patient with optimized non-pharmacologic treatment parameters, if the A1C is 9%, the achievement of adequate control would require pharmacologic interventions that could lower the A1C by 2%. The assessment would therefore focus on what medications will address the predominant pathophysiologic components of his or her diabetes and can provide enough strength to lower the A1C to 7% or below.

In the example given above, with an A1C of 9%, there is likely to be multiple factors: insulin resistance, decreased insulin secretory reserve (both 1st phase leading to postprandial hyperglycemia and, to some degree, second phase, and also there is likely to be some glucose toxicity). Thus, the likelihood of *one* medication succeeding in lowering the A1C to 7% is relatively low, and this patient will likely need multiple medications. One might start with one medication but initiate the second fairly early in the treatment progression, or even initiate the combination together. Conversely, if this patient had shorter duration diabetes and was markedly overweight, suggesting more predominant insulin resistance, one could consider early initiation of a combination of metformin and a thiazolidinedione, provided the weight issues associated with the thiazolidinediones could be managed. If concern about insulin secretory reserve was present, but peripheral insulin resistance was also a concern, with more predominant hyperglycemia later in the day, a combination of a thiazolidinedione and sulfonylurea could be considered. In many of these situations, combination tablets are available, which would improve compliance and ease of administration.

If the patient's starting A1C is 8%, it is possible that the targeted A1C level could be achieved using only one medication, so single-drug therapy initially would be quite appropriate. Nevertheless, with the trend toward earlier combination therapy and the likely presence of dual or multiple defects, even this patient may benefit from combination therapy, probably at less than maximum doses. It can certainly be argued that using combination therapy earlier in the natural history of type 2 diabetes can establish targeted levels of glucose control in the early years when much of the potential damage of hyperglycemia goes on silently. In addition, many of the medications used often show better efficacy early on, before the pathophysiology of this condition progresses, allowing smaller doses of multiple medications to be effectively used.

Further, at this writing, we are just beginning to see the clinical impact of incretin replacement therapy. Exenatide, while it must be administered by injection, is easily dosed and the injections are relatively easy, and with its potential for weight loss, it is becoming a reasonable option as an add-on therapy to sulfonylureas and/or metformin. The DPP-IV inhibitors are also a good option, and may produce a more physiologic insulin and glucagon effect than a sulfonylurea, either alone or in a combination program. Their A1C lowering capacity may not be quite as much as for sulfonylureas, but they work in a glucose dependent manner which could have advantages in that they precisely target the insulin action when it is needed, and suppress glucagon. This may allow more physiologic restoration of insulin secretory patterns and could be effective, particularly in a combination treatment program.

Similarly, if the starting A1C were 9.7%, dual or even triple therapy might be needed, and the use of combination therapy quite early in the dosing progression would be strongly suggested.

Keep in mind that insulin may be needed as an initial treatment in a patient with:

- a markedly elevated A1C level
- significant symptoms of hyperglycemia, ketoacidosis, or hyperosmolar coma
- the need for rapid establishment of glucose control such as someone

with an infection, imminent surgery, or other extenuating medical conditions

- contraindications to use of enough of the oral medications such that it is unlikely that adequate control could be achieved without insulin therapy

Specific Medication Combinations

Although combination oral therapy has become much more popular in recent years, it is not a new idea. The first oral combination to achieve widespread use was treatment with the sulfonylurea chlorpropamide plus the biguanide phenformin (originally described by this author's father, Samuel Beaser, MD in 1958). This combination was in widespread use through the 1960s until phenformin was removed from the market for concerns that its use increased the risk of developing lactic acidosis. However, in spite of this safety concern, this early combination was quite successful, improving control and prolonging the duration of time people could achieve adequate control before needing insulin therapy.

Typically, people would titrate one medication to optimal dosage. If treatment goals were reached, the patient was continued on that dose until goals no longer were achievable. This was referred to as "secondary failure" — failure to achieve goals with a medication after initially succeeding.

With the introduction of the safer biguanide, metformin, early studies of its combination therapy with sulfonylureas also demonstrated efficacy. It was through these studies that the term "secondary failure" fell into disuse and was replaced with "treatment insufficiency" as people realized that the first therapy did not *fail* per se. Rather, it was no longer able to achieve targeted control. However, it did not necessarily *fail* to work at all. In the case of metformin added to glyburide, for example, the loss of the ability of glyburide to achieve targeted control, where it might have done so in the past, is not surprising. The progression of type 2 diabetes involves loss of β-cell mass resulting in reduced pancreatic insulin secretory capacity, and it makes sense that a medication that stimulates insulin production from β-cells would lose efficacy. Thus, with treatment insufficiency, the approach is not to substitute one new medication for the old, but rather to combine their effects.

From this initial classic combination, the list has grown to include many other combinations that have been tried and proven useful. Some are sanctioned by the FDA as having official usage indications; others are reported in the medical literature. Still a few others have less scientific basis for their use, but have been tried by practicing physicians and, because of therapeutic success and absence of adverse events, continue to be used. This list of combinations is in flux, as new indications or studies are being reported. Table 8-2 includes combinations with proven utility. This list will undoubtedly grow in the future.

Achieving a Proper Balance

When initiating and titrating combination therapy, it is important to strike a proper dosing balance between agents. For example, while medications that reduce insulin resistance usually do not cause significant hypoglycemia, when they are added to an insulin secretagogue, hypoglycemia is possible, particularly as the dose of medication that reduces insulin resistance is increased. In this instance, it is probably the insulin secretagogue that is precipitating the hypoglycemia, and it is the dose of this medication that should be reduced.

Triple Therapy

Triple therapy is not an unreasonable approach if dual therapy does not reach targeted treatment goals but the A1C is close enough to the treatment target for a 3rd medication to reasonably be expected to achieve. The disadvantages include program adherence, expense and the additive potential for adverse pharmacologic events and side effects. However, there is some logic to the "triple" approach. For example, extending the logic that patients with type 2 diabetes have multiple defects and, on diagnosis, need both reductions in insulin resistance and boosts in insulin levels, the insulin resistance component can itself benefit from multiple pharmacologic approaches. The use of metformin, with predominant impact on hepatic insulin resistance, in combination with a thiazolidinedione, which focuses its effect on peripheral insulin resistance, would aim a "double-barreled" treatment attack on the multiple sites of reduced insulin efficacy. Then, an insulin secretagogue can be added to provide more endogenous insulin to overcome insulin deficiencies. Similarly, with the incretin mimetic therapies now available, the spectrum of effects beyond insulin secretion — the impact of glucagon and appetite — would make these a useful adjunct to other therapies, per FDA approval guidelines.

TABLE 8-2.   **Possible Oral Therapy Combinations for Managing**
Type 2 Diabetes*

Sulfonylurea &	Biguanide
	Thiazolidinedione
	α-Glucosidase inhibitor
	GLP-1 agonist
Thiazolidinediones &	Sulfonylurea
	Biguanides
	GLP-1 agonist
	DPP-IV inhibitor
Biguanide &	Sulfonylurea
	α-Glucosidase inhibitor
	Thiazolidinediones
	Meglitinides
	GLP-1 agonist
	DPP-IV inhibitor
α-Glucosidase inhibitor &	Sulfonylurea
	Biguanide
Meglitinide &	Biguanide
D-Phenylalanine derivative &	Biguanide
GLP-1 Agonist &	Sulfonylurea
	Biguanide
	Thiazolidinedione
DPP-IV Inhibitor &	Biguanide
	Thiazolidinedione

*FDA-approved combinations, and multiple combination therapies, are subject to changes. Please check updated package inserts for the latest information.

Unfortunately, many clinicians and patients alike turn to triple therapy too late in the natural history of type 2 diabetes. They use it at a time when endogenous insulin secretory response is markedly reduced in hopes of preventing the inevitable, and probably appropriate, need for insulin. When they do so, the results are disappointing, leading to a negative impression of triple therapy as a concept, and/or the drugs used in particular. When the patient is becoming insulinopenic, insulin, not a third oral medication, is indicated.

When considering triple therapy, keep in mind that each oral medication can only lower an A1C a reasonably predictable and not overly great amount. Further, the effect of each "add-on" medication is probably less than that drug would have had if it were the first medication being used. Thus, a patient on double therapy with an A1C over 9% is not likely to get the needed 2% drop in A1C from a third medicine. A patient who is thin or losing weight and yet has markedly elevated glucose levels probably needs insulin. Therefore, before choosing the path of triple therapy, make sure that the pathophysiology warrants it, that the insulin secretory reserve is sufficient, and that glucose toxicity is not overwhelming. Frequently, at this clinical juncture, consultation, assessment, and support from a dedicated diabetes treatment team can provide valuable input on the most likely therapy to achieve treatment goals. (See *Joslin's Clinical Guidelines*, www.joslin.org.)

Conclusion

One of the most rapidly changing areas in diabetes treatment in recent years has been that of the non-insulin medications that are used to treat diabetes. From an approach of "one drug class tries to fit all" in the early 1960s, we have evolved to the current state in which a number of medications are available that seem to effectively treat most of the multiple defects that lead to the glucose abnormalities of type 2 diabetes.

But do they really?

As we develop the tools to more effectively correct the glucose abnormalities of type 2 diabetes, we grow to appreciate the complexity of this condition. While everyone agrees that treating glucose levels is crucial, the question remains: is doing so really enough to impact long-term cardiovascular risk?

Beyond bringing glucose levels down to normal, and perhaps lowering lipids and fixing the blood pressure, what may we be missing? What other components, or less obvious underlying abnormalities, may need aggressive treatment? Is insulin resistance the key to macrovascular risk, and therefore should we be treating it *regardless* of glucose levels? What about the finding that the inflammatory process is present, and may be impacting vascular function? What is the significance of the fact that, when people with impaired glucose tolerance show a loss of first-phase insulin release and resulting postprandial hyperglycemia, they have a *very* strong chance of developing future type 2 diabetes? And, do the newer tools to restore early postprandial insulin release and thus correct postprandial hyperglycemia, truly impact this key harbinger of long-term risk? Or are they just fixing a metabolic marker in the form of glucose levels without fixing some underlying pathophysiologic process as yet incompletely understood? What is the role of adipose, and the substances that it makes? What role are these playing in the clinical picture that is referred to as the *metabolic syndrome?* Are the components of this syndrome really the best constellation to reflect increased cardiovascular risk?

Clearly, we are closer to significantly impacting the metabolic abnormalities of type 2 diabetes than ever before. Yet, frustratingly, every time we take a step forward, the target doesn't necessarily become clearer, and, at times, seems further off than ever.

Yet, this *is* type 2 diabetes! Many thought of it as a "touch of sugar" for years — its connections with other risk factors and the impact on cardiovascular disease not yet recognized. Often, in assuming that the complications were inevitable, clinicians avoided "tormenting" patients with complex treatments. Now we realize that the inevitability is *not* so inevitable, but with these clinicians' fatalistic attitudes and treatment approaches, the resulting health impact *did* become a self-fulfilling prophecy.

Recognizing that there are many questions left to answer, and many more yet to be asked, one thing has become extremely clear. **People with type 2 diabetes require aggressive, multicomponent treatments if they are to reduce the risk of complications.** This leads to a conundrum that is really a microcosm of this modern era. Wouldn't it be better if people could just make the lifestyle changes — nutritional and increased physical activity — to "fix" or prevent these metabolic problems and prevent the need for all these expensive medications or the costly diseases that may result? Yet, the next question is, if they cannot make those changes, should we let people suffer the consequences of these metabolic abnormalities, or treat to block the impact. The economic cost of these treatments is growing in this era when many focus on reducing immediate costs. Yet, the belief is shared by many that costly as these treatments may be at present, they are reasonable expenditures precisely because they will reduce long-term complications and the attendant greater costs later on.

These are issues that healthcare providers, economists, sociologists, and politicians all have been arguing. Yet we are operating as if this theory is correct. While proceeding accordingly, as healthcare providers always wish to intercede and help, we must seek to prove this theory so that resources can be targeted to support these treatments more effectively. So too, proof would provide more impetus to the efforts to provide support for the lifestyle changes that we all, idealistically, feel would be a better solution.

At the same time, continued investigation into the complex entity known as the "metabolic syndrome" must continue unabated so we can more fully understand the pathophysiologic defects, their clinical manifestations, and their long-term impacts and thus develop more specific and targeted treatments to ameliorate them. Clinically, we have only scratched the surface.

The last edition of this book ended this chapter with the comment . . . *to be continued!!* — it's still an appropriate ending.

MEDICATION SUMMARIES

IMPORTANT NOTE: These Summaries are provided for the convenience of the reader, for general education purposes, and as a clinical guide only. They reflect the author's compilation of information and general usage patterns that were accurate at the time of manuscript preparation. They should not be a substitute for the latest package insert. All categories listed below, particularly indications, precautions, screening recommendations, side effects, and other usage recommendations are subject to change without notice. For expected effects on A1C levels based on published data, be aware that some studies may reflect change with respect to placebo or change with respect to baseline. A1C improvements are also usually greater in magnitude with a higher starting value, and studies often vary with respect to the initial A1C of the treatment groups. Drug interactions listed are only those with specific relationship to the medication(s) in question, and do not list the many medications that might generally increase or decrease glucose levels. Ultimately, clinicians should use these medications based on the latest available information in the package insert, and not the potentially dated information in these Summaries.

CONTENTS

MEDICATIONS THAT INCREASE
INSULIN SENSITIVITY

1. BIGUANIDES

Metformin Summary

Brand name: Glucophage, Glucophage XR

Action: Decreases hepatic glucose production through a reduction in hepatic insulin resistance. Insulin secretion is unchanged, but fasting and daytime insulin response may actually decrease due to improved insulin sensitivity.

Indications and combination usage: To improve glucose control in people with type 2 diabetes, used as monotherapy, and combination therapy with sulfonylureas, repaglinide, nateglinide, thiazolidine-diones, exenatide, and insulin

Required for efficacy: Insulin (exogenous or endogenous), insulin resistance

Manifestation on glucose patterns: Generalized improvement in glucose levels. Reduction in hepatic glucose production leads to reduced fasting glucose levels.

Metabolism and elimination: Excreted unchanged in the urine

Potential effect on A1C: A reduction of up to 1.8 % vs. placebo

Potential for hypoglycemia: Quite low in monotherapy. Increased in patients with marked reductions in caloric intake, undergoing strenuous exercise, using concomitant medications that increase insulin levels, and consuming excessive alcohol.

Significant adverse events/side effects:

- diarrhea
- flatulence
- lactic acidosis

Other side effects of note:

- subclinical reductions in vitamin B12 levels
- infrequent hypoglycemia in people not adequately nourished

Typical patient with optimal efficacy: Type 2 diabetes with significant signs of insulin resistance syndrome, especially obesity, dyslipidemia

Typical starting dose: 500 mg BID, taken with breakfast and supper (mealtime dosing helps reduce GI side effects. Start with 500 or 850 mg once daily if GI side effects are bothersome).

Tablet sizes:

- Glucophage (metformin)
  - 500 mg; 850 mg, 1000 mg
  - 500 mg/ml liquid
- Glucophage XR (metformin extended release)
  - 500 mg; 750 mg
  - (Note, extended release system requires intact tablet. DO NOT split or crush.)
- Combination Tablets (brand names in parentheses)
  - Metformin / glyburide (Glucovance)
    - metformin 250 mg and glyburide 1.25 mg
    - metformin 500 mg and glyburide 2.5 mg
    - metformin 500 mg and glyburide 5 mg
  - Metformin / glipizide (Metaglip)
    - metformin 250 mg and glipizide 2.5 mg
    - metformin 500 mg and glipizide 2.5 mg
    - metformin 500 mg and glipizide 5 mg
  - Metformin / rosiglitazone (Avandamet)
    - metformin 500 mg and rosiglitazone 1 mg
    - metformin 500 mg and rosiglitazone 2 mg
    - metformin 500 mg and rosiglitazone 4 mg
  - Metformin / pioglitazone (Actoplus Met)
  - Pioglitazone 15 mg and metformin 500 mg
  - Pioglitazone 15 mg and metformin 850 mg
  - Metformin / sitagliptin (Janumet)
    - metformin 500 mg and sitagliptin 50 mg
    - metformin 1000 mg and sitagliptin 50 mg

The utility of combination tablets includes:

- Improved adherence to treatment regime
- Addressing dual defects (for combinations with sulfonylureas,

insulin resistance and insulin secretory deficiency, for combination with thiazolidinedione, hepatic and peripheral insulin resistance) that are likely present as early as the time of diagnosis of type 2 diabetes

- For the lowest dose of the metformin/glyburide combination, the ability to utilize low doses of both medications concurrently

Typical dose titration pattern for metformin: Start with 500 mg BID; increase in 2 to 6 weeks as needed to 1000 mg every morning and 500 mg at suppertime, then in 2–6 weeks more, if needed, increase to 1000 mg BID. If extended release is used, full dose can be given once daily, usually at suppertime.

Optimal daily dose: 1000 mg BID

Maximal daily dose: 2550 mg (850 mg TID)

Other clinical effects:

- **Weight:** decreases
- **Lipids:** reduces: triglycerides, LDL, total cholesterol
- **Coagulation:** decreased plasminogen activator inhibitor

Drug interactions with potential for clinical significance:

- Most clinically significant interaction is cimetidine/metformin, leading to increased metformin levels
- Nifedipine enhances metformin absorption. Metformin has minimal effects on metformin
- Metformin has minimal effect on nifedipine
- Cationic drugs that are eliminated by the kidneys (including amiloride, digoxin, morphine, procainamide, quinidine, quinine, ranitidine, trimethoprin) have the potential for interaction with metformin by competing for common renal tubular transport systems. Theoretically, they may increase the metformin levels.

Contraindications and precautions:

- Known hypersensitivity to metformin
- To reduce risk of lactic acidosis, avoid use in contraindicated patients:
  - renal disease (serum creatinine : ≥1.5 mg/dl in males, ≥1.4 mg/dl in females, or abnormal creatinine clearance)
  - hepatic dysfunction has been associated with some cases of lactic

acidosis, so use of metformin should generally be avoided in patients with clinical or laboratory evidence of hepatic disease.
  - congestive heart failure (CHF) requiring pharmacologic treatment
  - history of alcohol abuse/binge drinking
  - acute or chronic metabolic acidosis, including diabetic ketoacidosis
- Metformin should be withheld in conditions predisposing to renal insufficiency and/or hypoxia, including:
  - cardiovascular collapse
  - acute myocardial infarction
  - acute CHF
  - severe infections
- Metformin should be temporarily discontinued in patients undergoing radiologic studies or surgical procedures involving intravascular administration of iodinated contrast materials at the time of the procedure. Metformin should be withheld for 48 hours subsequent to the procedure and reinstituted only after renal function has been reevaluated and found to be normal.
- May result in ovulation in anovulatory women
- Not indicated for use in pregnancy

Key advice to patients:

- Contact healthcare professional if deterioration of glucose control occurs.
- Contact healthcare professional for symptoms of hepatic disease: jaundice, anorexia, unexplained abdominal pain, nausea, vomiting, fatigue, or dark urine.
- Contact healthcare professional if anyone tells you that your kidneys are not working properly.
- Discuss potential for GI symptoms early in treatment (in particular, diarrhea), and the possibility of slower dose titration to reduce symptoms.
- Discuss symptoms of lactic acidosis (weakness, muscle pain, trouble breathing, stomach discomfort, dizziness or lightheadedness, irregular heart beat).
- Avoid excessive alcohol.
- Potential for resumed ovulation in anovulatory women.

2. THIAZOLIDINEDIONES

<u>CLASS SUMMARY:</u>

Action: Improves glucose control by improving insulin sensitivity. Works primarily to reduce peripheral insulin resistance (primarily muscle, adipose) but also can have hepatic effects. Thiazolidinediones are agonists for the peroxisome proliferators-activated receptor–gamma (PPARγ), which regulate transcription of insulin-responsive genes involved in glucose production, transport, and utilization, as well as fatty acid metabolism.

Required for efficacy: Insulin (exogenous or endogenous), insulin resistance

Manifestation on glucose patterns: general and postprandial glucose levels

Potential effect on A1C: ↓ 1%–2%

Titration: Because thiazolidinediones impact genes which are involved in glucose metabolism, their full clinical effect can take some time to be fully manifest. Upon treatment initiation or a change in dose, it may take as much as 2–4 months for the full clinical effect to be seen. Further, with this mode of action, if a patient has marked hyperglycemia requiring rapid reduction in glucose levels, thiazolidinediones should not be the primary mode of therapy, and a more rapid-acting treatment should be selected.

Significant adverse effects/side effects: Edema, anemia (probably dilutional), potential unmasking or exacerbation of congestive heart failure, weight gain. Based on meta-analyses, concerns have been raised about the relationship between rosiglitazone and coronary events.

Other potential adverse effects of note: rare hepatotoxicity (see below)

Typical patient with optimal efficacy: type 2 diabetes with significant signs of insulin resistance syndrome

Other effects:

- Weight: increases
- Lipids: variable among members of class, as studies have different

inclusion parameters and results are not consistent. Ultimately, many of the patients who would be candidates for thiazolidinedione treatment would also benefit from a statin, and one of these medications should be used in addition, if indicated.

- Procoagulant state: probable decrease

Class contraindications and precautions:

- Hepatic disease
- With the class tendency to produce edema and unmask/esacerbate congestive heart failure (CHF), use caution in the setting of current or potential CHF. Medications should be used with caution and careful monitoring in patients with mild to moderate heart failure (New York Heart Association (NYHA) Class 1 or 2) and not used in patients with more severe heart failure (NYHA Class 3 or 4).
- New onset or worsening macular edema has been noted very rarely with use of rosiglitazone. It is unclear if this is unique to rosiglitazone, or could be related to the class. Consider discontinuation of thiazolidinedione use, particularly rosiglitazone, if macular edema is diagnosed, and if a patient using a thiazolidinedione reports decreased visual acuity, consider the possibility of macular edema.

INDIVIDUAL MEDICATION SUMMARIES:

A. ROSIGLITAZONE (GENERIC)

Brand name: Avandia

Indications: Use as monotherapy, or in combination with sulfonylureas, metformin, or insulin.

Metabolism and elimination: Exclusively metabolized by cytochrome P450, CYP2C8 mostly, with CYP2C9 having a minor role. Excreted 64% in urine, 28% in feces.

Potential for hypoglycemia: Low when used as monotherapy. Increased when used in combination, particularly with an agent that increases insulin levels. Reduction of the dose of that other medication may be needed.

Possible adverse effects: Based on meta-analyses, concerns have been raised about the relationship between rosiglitazone and coronary events. See class effects for other possible issues.

Tablet sizes:

- 2 mg, 4mg, 8 mg
- Combination Tablets (brand names in parentheses):
  - Rosiglitazone/metformin (Avandamet)
    - rosiglitazone 1 mg and metformin 500 mg
    - rosiglitazone 2 mg and metformin 500 mg
    - rosiglitazone 4 mg and metformin 500 mg
  - Rosiglitazone/glimepiride (Avandaryl)
    - rosiglitazone 4 mg and glimepiride 1 mg
    - rosiglitazone 4 mg and glimepiride 2 mg
    - rosiglitazone 4 mg and glimepiride 4 mg

Typical starting dose of rosiglitazone: 4 mg per day, given at breakfast or in divided doses, 2 mg each at breakfast and suppertime

Typical dose titration pattern: increase every 4 to 8 weeks or more, as needed, to either 8 mg every morning, or 4 mg BID

Maximum daily dose: 8 mg daily, in single or divided dose; can be taken with or without food.

While initial recommendations were that better control could be achieved with BID dosing, long-term studies now suggest that this difference may not be significant, and once-daily dosing is probably adequate.

Drug interaction/metabolism: As rosiglitazone is primarily metabolized by CYP2C8, which is an uncommon pathway for drug metabolism, there are no clinically significant interactions with drugs metabolized by CYP3A4 such as nifedipine or oral contraceptives. Nevertheless, if changes in glucose control are noted with initiation or discontinuation of certain drugs which are metabolized by CYP3A4 (gembfibrozil inhibits, and may thus increase rosiglitazone effect, rifampin induces, and may decrease rosiglitazone effect), dose adjustments of diabetes treatments may be needed.

Contraindications and precautions:

- Can be used with renal impairment
- Contraindicated with hepatic dysfunction (ALT >2.5 ULN)
- As a precaution, it is recommended that liver enzymes be checked prior to initiation of therapy, and then periodically thereafter per the clinical judgment of the healthcare professional
- Rosiglitazone should not be initiated in people with elevated baseline liver enzyme levels (ALT > 2.5 X the upper limit of normal)
- Patients with mild elevations (ALT levels ≤ 2.5 X upper limit of normal) at baseline or during therapy should be evaluated to determine the cause of the liver enzyme elevation. Treatment can continue with caution and more frequent monitoring, per the judgment of the physician.
- If at any time, ALT levels increase to 3 X ULN, recheck enzyme levels a soon as possible. If ALT levels remain > 3 X ULN, therapy should be discontinued.
- Due to tendency for edema formation, rosiglitazone should not be used in people with New York Heart Association Class 3 or 4 cardiac status, unless the benefit is judged to outweigh the potential risk.
- Not indicated in pregnancy (Category C)
- May result in ovulation in an anovulatory female

Key advice to patients:

- Contact healthcare professional if deterioration of glucose control occurs.
- You need to have your liver function screened periodically when using rosiglitazone. Ask your healthcare provider about this screening.
- Contact healthcare professional for symptoms of liver disease: jaundice, anorexia, unexplained abdominal pain, nausea, vomiting, fatigue, or dark urine.
- Use of this medication with oral contraceptives could decrease the efficacy of these birth control medications.
- This medication is not indicated in pregnancy — contact healthcare professional if you become pregnant.
- This medication should not be used with severe heart failure, referred to as New York Heart Association Class 3 and 4 cardiac status, unless the benefit is judged to outweigh the potential risk. If heart

failure develops, carefully consider the risks of continuing this medication vs. its benefits. Consult a healthcare professional to discuss
this issue.
• Use of this medication may result in ovulation in anovulatory
women.

B. Pioglitazone (Generic)

Brand name: Actos

Indications: Monotherapy and combination therapy with sulfonylureas, metformin, and insulin

Metabolism and elimination: Hepatic metabolism via cytochrome
P450 (CYP2C8, CYP3A4). Most goes to bile and is excreted. A remaining 15 to 30% is eliminated in the urine.

Potential for hypoglycemia: Low when used as monotherapy. Increased when used in combination, particularly with an agent that increases insulin levels. Reduction of the dose of that other medication
may be needed.

Possible adverse effects: See class effects.

Tablet sizes:

• 15 mg, 30mg, 45 mg
• Combination Tablets (brand names in parentheses):
  – Pioglitazone/metformin (Actoplus Met)
    ♦ pioglitazone 15 mg and metformin 500 mg
    ♦ pioglitazone 15 mg and metformin 850 mg
  – Pioglitazone/glimepiride (Duetact)
    ♦ pioglitazone 30 mg and glimepiride 2 mg
    ♦ pioglitazone 30 mg and glimepiride 4 mg

Typical starting dose: 15 mg/day, given once daily before breakfast,
for monotherapy or combination therapy. Can be given with or without
food.

Typical dose titration pattern: Increase every 4 to 8 weeks or more, as
needed, to 30 mg, and then 45 mg daily. Full doses can be given at once
before breakfast.

Maximal daily dose: 45 mg

Drug interaction/metabolism: Three active metabolites via CYP3A4 and CYP2C8. In vitro, ketoconazole inhibits the metabolism of pioglitazone by 85%; with unknown clinical significance, but more frequent evaluation of glycemic control is recommended. Further drug interaction studies with drugs metabolized by the CYP3A4 pathway are not available at this writing.

Contraindications and precautions:

- Known hypersensitivity to thiazolidinediones
- Contraindicated in patients with impaired hepatic function as reflected by ALT > 2.5 X the upper limit of normal (ULN)
- Measurement of liver enzymes:
  - Determine baseline ALT, and then periodically thereafter, per the judgment of the physician.
  - People with mildly elevated liver enzymes (ALT 1 to 2.5 X ULN) at baseline or at any time during therapy should be evaluated to determine the cause.
  - Initiation of, or continuation of, therapy with pioglitazone should proceed with caution and should include appropriate follow-up and more frequent liver monitoring.
  - If ALT > 2.5 X ULN liver function tests should be evaluated more frequently until the levels return to normal or pretreatment values.
  - If ALT > 3 X ULN during pioglitazone therapy, retest promptly and discontinue if ALT remains >3 X ULN or if patient shows signs of liver disease such as jaundice.
- Can be used to treat patients with renal insufficiency. No dose adjustment is usually needed.
- Not indicated in pregnancy (Category C)
- Due to tendency for edema formation, rosiglitazone should not be used in people with New York Heart Association Class 3 or 4 cardiac status, unless the benefit is judged to outweigh the potential risk.
- May result in ovulation in anovulatory women

Key advice to patients:

- Contact healthcare professional if deterioration of glucose control occurs.

- You need to have your liver function screened with a blood test every 2 months for the first month of the use of this medication and periodically thereafter. Be sure you have made these arrangements with your healthcare provider.
- Contact healthcare professional for symptoms of hepatic disease: jaundice, anorexia, unexplained abdominal pain, nausea, vomiting, fatigue, or dark urine.
- Use of this medication with oral contraceptives could decrease the efficacy of these birth control medications.
- This medication is not indicated in pregnancy — contact healthcare professional if you become pregnant.
- This medication should not be used with severe heart failure, referred to as New York Heart Association Class 3 and 4 cardiac status, unless the benefit is judged to outweigh the potential risk. If heart failure develops, carefully consider the risks of continuing this medication vs. its benefits. Consult a healthcare professional to discuss this issue.
- Use of this medication may result in ovulation in anovulatory women.

MEDICATIONS THAT BLOCK GLUCOSE ABSORPTION

3. α-GLUCOSIDASE INHIBITORS

CLASS SUMMARY:

Action: competitive, reversible inhibitors of intestinal brush border α-glucosidase enzymes, which leads to delayed glucose absorption from the gastrointestinal tract and a lowering of postprandial hyperglycemia.

Required for efficacy: some remaining insulin secretory capacity by the pancreas

Manifestation on glucose patterns: reduces elevations of postprandial glucose levels

Potential effect on A1C: ↓0.5%–1%

Significant side effects: flatulence, which is usually mild and self-limited, or diarrhea

Other side effects of note: rare elevations of liver transaminases

Typical patient with optimal efficacy: early type 2 diabetes with significant postprandial hyperglycemia

Contraindications: inflammatory bowel disease, colon ulceration, intestinal obstruction, significant renal disease (creatinine > 2.0 mg/dl)

Other Effects:

- **Weight:** minimal increase
- **Lipids:** negligible

Contraindications: inflammatory bowel disease, colon ulceration, intestinal obstruction, significant renal disease (creatinine > 2.0 mg/dl)

INDIVIDUAL MEDICATION SUMMARIES

A. ACARBOSE (GENERIC)

Brand name: Precose

Indications: Monotherapy or in combination with a sulfonylurea, metformin, or insulin

Pharmacology:

- Less than 2% absorbed
- Most excreted in the feces. A few metabolites are absorbed and are excreted in the urine.
- Metabolized in the GI tract by intestinal bacteria

Typical starting dose:

- 25 mg orally given TID with the first bite of each meal
- Can titrate more slowly based on clinical need or side effects, starting with 25 mg once daily, and then increasing to 25 mg TID

Typical dose titration pattern:

- 25 mg TID, adjusted upward every 4 to 8 weeks to a maximum of 100 mg TID
- Can start with lower dose and/or frequency for milder effect or to reduce likelihood of adverse symptoms

Optimal dose:

- Depends on clinical effect and side effects, but usually 50–100 mg TID
- Maximum dose:
    - Weight $\leq$ 60 kg: 50 mg TID
    - Weight $>$ 60 kg: 100 mg TID

Tablet size:

- 25 mg, 50 mg, 100 mg

Drug interactions:

- May affect bioavailabiity of digoxin and require a dose adjustment of digoxin
- Intestinal adsorbents (charcoal) and digestive preparations may reduce the effect
- Drugs that potentiate hyperglycemia: thiazides, other diuretics, corticosteroids, phenothiazines, thyroid products, estrogens, oral contraceptives, phenytoin, nicotinic acid, sympathomimetics, calcium channel blockers, and isoniazid

Contraindications and precautions:

- Contraindications with known hypersensitivity to the drug and in the treatment of diabetic ketoacidosis
- Contraindicated in patients with inflammatory bowel disease or other significant bowel, intestinal, or digestive conditions
- Doesn't usually cause hypoglycemia
- Can cause transient elevations of serum transaminase levels
- Pregnancy: category B — use only if clearly needed

Key advice to patients:

- Take only 3 times daily.
- Discuss side effects and the possibility of adjusting titration schedule if side effects are excessive.
- Hypoglycemia treatment: Hypoglycemia may occur with use of these medications, particularly in combination with a medication that increases insulin levels. Keep in mind that these medications will delay the absorption of glucose that is consumed in the form of complex carbohydrates. Hypoglycemia must therefore be treated with a form of glucose (e.g., glucose tablets) rather than a complex form of carbohydrate.

B. MIGLITOL (GENERIC)

Brand name: Glyset

Indications: Monotherapy or in combination with a sulfonylurea

Pharmacology:

- Absorption depends on dose: 25-mg dose: 100% absorbed; 100-mg dose: 50%–75% absorbed. Absorption is not involved in therapeutic effect
- Metabolism: not metabolized
- Excretion: mostly renal as unchanged drug

Typical starting dose:

- 25 mg orally given TID with the first bite of each meal
- Can titrate more slowly based on clinical need or side effects, starting with 25 mg once daily, and then increasing to 25 mg TID

Typical dose titration pattern:

- 25 mg TID, adjusted upward every 4 to 8 weeks to a maximum of 100 mg TID
- Can start with lower dose and/or frequency for milder effect or to reduce the likelihood of adverse symptoms

Optimal dose:

- Depends on clinical effect and side effects, but usually 50–100 mg TID
- Maximum dose: 100 mg TID

Tablet size:

- Tablet size: 25 mg, 50 mg, 100 mg

Drug interactions:

- Drugs that potentiate hyperglycemia: thiazides, other diuretics, corticosteroids, phenothiazines, thyroid products, estrogens, oral contraceptives, phenytoin, nicotinic acid, sympathomimetics, calcium channel blockers, and isoniazid
- Intestinal adsorbents (charcoal) and digestive preparations may reduce the effect

Contraindications and precautions:

- Contraindications with known hypersensitivity to the drug
- Treatment of diabetic ketoacidosis
- Contraindicated in patients with inflammatory bowel disease or other significant bowel, intestinal, or digestive conditions
- Doesn't usually cause hypoglycemia
- Can cause transient elevations of serum transaminase levels
- Do not use in patients with a creatinine level > 2.0 mg/dl
- Pregnancy: category B — use only if clearly needed

Key advice to patients:

- Take only TID.
- Discuss side effects and the possibility of adjusting titration schedule if side effects are excessive.
- Hypoglycemia Treatment: Hypoglycemia may occur with use of these medications, particularly in combination with a medication that increases insulin levels. Keep in mind that these medications will delay the absorption of glucose that is consumed in the form of complex carbohydrates. Hypoglycemia must therefore be treated with a form of glucose (e.g., glucose tablets), rather than a complex form of carbohydrate.

MEDICATIONS THAT INCREASE INSULIN SECRETION

4. SULFONYLUREAS

CLASS SUMMARY:

Action: Insulin secretagogues. Initial effects are to increase insulin secretory capacity. With establishment of long-term glucose control, this increase may not persist and other extrapancreatic effects, either direct or indirect, may also occur.

Required for efficacy: Some remaining endogenous pancreatic insulin secretory capacity

Manifestation on glucose patterns: General reductions in elevated glucose levels throughout the day

Potential effect on A1C: ↓ 1%–2 %

Significant adverse effects/side effects: weight gain, hypoglycemia (particularly in older individuals who may undereat or miss meals)

Other potential adverse effects of note: Past concerns about increased risk of coronary events (stemming from the University Group Diabetes Project study) seem to have diminished with the findings of the United Kingdom Prospective Diabetes Study (UKPDS) showing no increased cardiac risk with sulfonylurea use. However, some suggestion that use of these medications in the acute post-infarct period worsens outcomes has led many to avoid their use in these situations, often switching to insulin therapy.

Typical patient with optimal efficacy: Type 2 diabetes with insufficient insulin secretory capacity (relative or absolute), yet enough beta-cell function remaining for some stimulation of further insulin secretion to be possible.

Other effects:

- Weight: increases
- Lipids: no significant effect

INDIVIDUAL MEDICATION SUMMARIES:

Capsule Information on First-Generation Agents Still in Occasional Use:

- **Tolbutamide (Orinase)**
  - Short-acting sulfonylurea
  - Half-life 4.5–6.5 hours
  - Duration of action 6–10 hours
  - Metabolized in the liver to inactive metabolites, which are excreted via the kidney. This medication may be used in mild renal impairment.
  - Dose range 500–3000 mg daily, usually given 2–3 times daily
  - Comment: short duration and frequent dosing requirement make compliance an issue
- **Tolazamide (Tolinase)**
  - Intermediate duration of action
  - Half-life 7 hours
  - Duration 16–24 hours
  - Metabolized in the liver to mildly active metabolites, which are excreted via the kidney
  - Dosing range 100–1000 mg daily, taken 1–2 times daily
- **Chlorpropamide (Diabinese)**
  - Very long duration of action
  - Half-life 36 hours
  - Duration can extend for 2–3 days
  - Metabolized incompletely in the liver to metabolites with hypoglycemic activity, excreted via the kidney. Contraindicated with renal impairment.
  - Dosing range 100–500 mg/day, usually in a single dose
  - Adverse effect is the chlorporpamide-alcohol flush (Antabuse-like reaction)
  - Long duration of action makes it potent but hypoglycemia can persist for a long time

Second-Generation Agents:

A. GLYBURIDE (GENERIC)

ALTERNATE GENERIC NAME: GLYBENCLAMIDE

Brand Names: Diabeta, Micronase

Pharmacology:
- Half-life biphasic: 4 and 10 hours
- Duration of action 16–24 hours
- Metabolized in the liver to weakly active and inactive metabolites, which are excreted in liver (50%) and bile (50%). This is different from other sulfonylureas, which have primarily a renal excretion.

Typical starting dose:
- 2.5 to 5 mg daily, in single dose. Can start with 1.25 mg if there is concern about possible hypoglycemia or decreased drug clearance.

Typical dose titration pattern:
- Range 1.25–20 mg daily

Optimal dose:
- 10 mg/daily. Usually given once or twice daily

Tablet size:

- Glyburide: 1.25 mg, 2.5 mg, 5 mg, 10 mg
- Combination Tablets:
  – Metformin / glyburide (Glucovance)
    ♦ glyburide 1.25 mg and metformin 250 mg
    ♦ glyburide 2.5 mg and metformin 500 mg
    ♦ glyburide 5 mg and metformin 500 mg

The utility of this combination tablet includes:

- The ability to utilize low doses of both medications concurrently (some not otherwise available)
- Improved adherence to treatment regimen and ease of use
- Ability to "dual defect" of insulin resistance and insulin secretory deficiency, particularly early in the natural history in a conveniently dosed single tablet

Potential drug interactions:

- *Hypoglycemic* effects may be potentiated by the following medications: NSAIDS, salicylates, sulfonamides, alcohol, fibrates, chloramphenicol, probenecid, allopurinol, coumarins, trimethoprim, mono-amine oxidase inhibitors, ß-blockers. Interactions with cipro-floxacin causing a potentiation of hypoglycemic effect have been described.

- *Hyperglycemia* may potentiated by the following medications: cort-icosteriods, thiazides, other diuretics, barbiturates, rifampin, pheno-thiazines, thyroid products, estrogens, oral contraceptives, pheny-toin, nicotinic acid, sympathomimetics, calcium channel blocking drugs, and isoniazid. Interactions with miconazone and fluconazone causing hypoglycemia have been described.

Contraindications and precautions:

- Known sensitivity to glyburide and in the treatment of diabetic ketoacidosis, with or without coma
- Hypoglycemia
- Pregnancy: category B — use only if clearly needed

Information for patients:

- Discuss risks of hypoglycemia.

ALTERNATE FORMULATION OF GLYBURIDE: MICRONIZED FORMULATION OF GLYBURIDE

Brand name: Glynase PresTab

Differences in action/pharmacology from glyburide: The micronized glyburide provides somewhat greater bioavailability per milligram than standard glyburide, with peak drug levels occurring at 2–3 hours (4 hours for gyburide)

Differences in dosing: Dosing: while 3 mg of micronized glyburide has a somewhat similar efficacy to 5 mg of glyburide, the actual peak drug availability curves differ slightly and some retitration is often nec-essary when a switch is made

Typical starting dose:

- Usual starting dose 1.5 to 3 mg daily, in a single dose

Typical dose titration pattern:

- Dosing range 1.5 to 12 mg daily

Optimal dose:

- Optimal dose 6 mg daily, in single or divided dose

Tablet size: 1.5 mg, 3 mg, 6 mg

Other categories: Same as for glyburide — see above

B. Glipizide (Generic)

Brand name: Glucotrol

Pharmacology:

- Half-life of 2–4 hours
- Duration of action 12–24 hours
- Metabolized in liver to inactive metabolites with excretion primarily via kidney and small amounts in bile

Typical starting dose:

- 5 mg daily, in single dose. Can start with 2.5 if there is concern about possible hypoglycemia or decreased drug clearance.

Typical dose titration pattern:

- Dosing range 2.5–40 mg daily

Optimal dose:

- 20 mg/daily. Usually given once or twice daily.

Tablet size:

- Glipizide: 5 mg, 10 mg
- Combination Tablets (brand name in parentheses):
  - Metformin/glipizide (Metaglip)
    - glipizide 2.5 mg and metformin 250 mg
    - glipizide 2.5 mg and metformin 500 mg
    - glipizide 5 mg and metformin 500 mg

The utility of this combination tablet includes:

- Improved adherence to treatment regimen and ease of use
- Ability to "dual defect" of insulin resistance and insulin secretory deficiency,

Potential drug interactions:

- *Hypoglycemic* effects may be potentiated by the following medications: NSAIDS, salicylates, sulfonamides, alcohol, fibrates, chloramphenicol, probenecid, allopurinol, coumarins, trimethoprim, monoamine oxidase inhibitors, ß-blockers. Interactions with cipro-floxacin causing a potentiation of hypoglycemic effect have been described.

- *Hyperglycemia* may potentiated by the following medications: corticosteriods, thiazides, other diuretics, barbiturates, rifampin, phenothiazines, thyroid products, estrogens, oral contraceptives, phenytoin, nicotinic acid, sympathomimetics, calcium channel blocking drugs, and isoniazid. Interactions with miconazone and fluconazone causing hypoglycemia have been described.

Contraindications and precautions:

- Contraindications with known hypersensitivity to the drug and in the treatment of diabetic ketoacidosis, with or without coma
- Precautions: metabolism and excretion slowed with renal or hepatic disease; can cause hypoglycemia
- Pregnancy: category C — not indicated for use

Information for patients:

- Discuss risks of hypoglycemia.

ALTERNATE FORMULATION OF GLIPIZIDE: THE GLIPIZIDE "GITS"
(GASTROINTESTINAL THERAPEUTIC SYSTEM), OR GLIPIZIDE XL

Brand name: Glucotrol XL

Differences in action/pharmacology from glipizide: These tablets consist of an osmotically active drug core surrounded by a semipermeable membrane. Drug is released into the gastro-intestinal tract through an orifice in the membrane at a controlled rate during the transit of the tablet. This formulation produces a constant drug release, resulting in even drug availability over the 24-hour duration of action period.

Typical starting dose:

- Usual starting dose 5 mg daily, in a single dose

Typical dose titration pattern:

- Dosing range 5 to 20 mg daily, usually in single dose
- Start with 5 mg daily, and titrate up to 10 mg daily
- As the added advantage of going to 20 mg daily is not great, once the 10 mg dose is reached, usually another medication is added rather than increasing to glipizide XL 20 mg daily as the next step

Optimal dose:

- Optimal dose 10 mg daily, in single dose
- Maximum dose 20 mg daily in a single dose

Tablet information for patients size: 2.5 mg, 5 mg, 10 mg

Information for patients

- Discuss risks of hypoglycemia.
- Tell patients that they must swallow this pill whole. They might see pill casing pass out in the stool — this is normal.
- Do not cut pill in half or crush.

Other categories: Same as for glipizide — see above.

C. GLIMEPIRIDE (GENERIC)

Brand names: Amaryl

Pharmacology:

- Half-life: 3–7 hours
- Duration of action 24 hours
- Metabolized in liver to weakly active metabolites. Excreted by kidney (60%) and bile (40%).

Typical starting dose:

- 1–2 mg daily, in single dose at breakfast or the main meal. People who are potentially sensitive to these medications should start with 1 mg.

Typical dose titration pattern:

• Dosing range 1–4 mg given once daily

Optimal dose:

• 2 mg/daily. Usually given as a single dose.
• Maximum dose 4 mg/daily, given as a single dose.

Tablet size: 1 mg, 2 mg, 4 mg

• Combination Tablets (brand names in parentheses):
  – pioglitazone/glimepiride (Duetact)
  – pioglitazone 30 mg and glimepiride 2 mg
  – pioglitazone 30 mg and glimepiride 4 mg
  – rosiglitazone / glimepiride (Avandaryl)
  – rosiglitazone 4 mg and glimepiride 1 mg
  – rosiglitazone 4 mg and glimepiride 2 mg
  – rosiglitazone 4 mg and glimepiride 4 mg

Potential drug interactions:

• *Hypoglycemic* effects may be potentiated by the following medications: NSAIDS, salicylates, sulfonamides, alcohol, fibrates, chloramphenicol, probenecid, allopurinol, coumarins, trimethoprim, monoamine oxidase inhibitors, ß-blockers. Interactions with cipro-floxacin causing a potentiation of hypoglycemic effect have been described.

• *Hyperglycemia* may potentiated by the following medications: corticosteriods, thiazides, other diuretics, barbiturates, rifampin, phenothiazines, thyroid produc\ts, estrogens, oral contraceptives, phenytoin, nicotinic acid, sympathomimetics, calcium channel blocking drugs, and isoniazid. Interactions with miconazone and fluconazone causing hypoglycemia have been described.

Contraindications and precautions:

• Known sensitivity to glimepiride, and in the treatment of diabetic ketoacidosis, with or without coma
• Hypoglycemia
• Pregnancy: category C — not indicated

Information for patients:

- Discuss risks of hypoglycemia.

D. GLICLAZIDE (GENERIC) — NOT AVAILABLE IN THE UNITED STATES

Brand name: Diamicron

Summary:

- Half-life 6–12 hours
- Duration of action 16–24 hours
- Metabolized in liver to metabolites that are probably inactive, and excreted by kidney (70%) and bile (30%)
- Dosage 80–160 mg given 1–2 times daily

5. MEGLITINIDES

REPAGLINIDE SUMMARY

Brand name: Prandin

Action: stimulates the glucose-dependent postprandial insulin release from functioning β-cells

Pharmacology:

- Completely absorbed from GI tract
- Peak serum level at about 1 hour, dissipation in 3–4 hours
- Peak insulin response is seen 10 minutes after administration
- Metabolism: Cytochrome P-450 system, specifically 3A4. Metabolites are not active. Most eliminated by GI route.

Required for efficacy: Functioning β-cells

Manifestation on glucose patterns: Primarily reduces postprandial glucose excursions. However, impact on overall control can also lead to reductions in fasting and preprandial glucose levels as well.

Potential effect on A1c: ↓ 1.6%–1.9% vs. placebo; somewhat greater in drug naïve patients

Significant averse effects/side effects:

- Hypoglycemia

Other side effects of note:

- Weight: increase
- Lipids: no significant effects

Typical patient with optimal efficacy: Type 2 diabetes with loss of postprandial, particularly first-phase, insulin release, manifest by significant elevations in glucose levels between the pre-and postprandial period. Useful for patients with erratic meal schedules or who skip meals, particularly if they have been having difficulty with hypoglycemia using sulfonylureas.

Tablet Sizes: 0.5 mg, 1 mg, 2 mg

Dosing: Starting dose:

- Drug-naïve (no prior oral medication): 0.5 mg, 0–30 minutes before each meal (15 minutes is ideal)
- Prior oral therapy: 1–2 mg 0–30 minutes before each meal (15 minutes is ideal)

Dose Titration:

- Maximum efficacy at each dosing level seen in 1–2 weeks
- Titrate upward to maximum of 4 mg before each meal
- Can be given for up to 4 meals per day. Doses may vary before specific meals, adjusted for food quantity and differing response. If meal is omitted, medication is omitted.
- Indicated also for use with metformin

Optimal dose:

- Most of the therapeutic efficacy is seen in the first half of the dosing range, i.e., up through 2 mg preprandially

Other clinical effects:

- Weight: decrease
- Lipids: reduces: triglycerides, LDL, total cholesterol
- Coagulation: decreased plasminogen activator inhibitor

Drug interactions:

- Increases repaglinide metabolism: rafampin, barbiturates, carbamazepine
- Decreases repaglinide metabolism: angifungals, erythromycin
- Increases repaglinide effect: NASIDs, ß-blockers, sulfonamides, salicylates, chloramphenicol, coumadin, MAOIs, probenecid
- Decreases repaglinide action: corticosteroids, calcium channel blockers, oral contraceptives, thiazide diuretics, thyroid preparations, estrogens, pheonthiazines, phentoyn, rifampin, isoniazid, phenobargital, sympathomimetics

Contraindications and precautions:

- Known hypersensitivity to repaglinide
- Type 1 diabetes and ketoacidosis
- Hepatic insufficiency can cause elevated repaglinide blood levels as well as decrease gluconeogenesis, leading to hypoglycemia. Use cautiously, and have longer intervals between dose adjustments to allow full assessment of response.
- Renal insufficiency: initial doses do not need to be adjusted, but subsequent increases should be made with caution. Repaglinide not tested in people with creatinine clearance < 20 mg/ml or on hemodialysis.
- Pregnancy category C

Key advice to patients:

- Contact healthcare professional if deterioration of glucose control occurs.
- Explain risk of hypoglycemia.
- Explain premeal dosing instructions (0–30 minutes premeal, 15 minutes being ideal), adjustments for missed meals (skip dose) or meals of various sizes (may adjust per individualized needs).

6. D-PHENYLALANINE DERIVATIVES

NATEGLINIDE SUMMARY

Brand name: Starlix

Indications: Monotherapy or in combination with metformin.

Action: Stimulates the rapid, glucose-dependent postprandial insulin release from functioning β-cells.

Pharmacokinetics: Stimulates pancreatic insulin secretion within 20 minutes of oral administration. Peak levels at 1 hour after dosing, and return to baseline at 4 hours after dosing.

Required for efficacy: Functioning β-cells

Metabolism: In the liver, primarily by CYP2C9 (70%) with some contribution by CYP3A4 (30%), to 3 major and several minor metabolites, none active. There is no significant interaction with other medications metabolized through similar mechanisms.

Elimination: 83% urinary excretion, of which 84% is metabolized drug, 16% is intact drug.

Manifestation on glucose patterns: Primarily reduces postprandial glucose excursions. Significantly lesser effect of fasting glucose levels.

Potential effect on A1C: ↓0.45% vs. baseline in non-drug naïve patients, with initial study A1C level 8.3%. Additional efficacy when used in combination with metformin.

Significant side effects:

• Mild hypoglycemia

Other side effects of note:

• Weight: slight increase
• Lipids: no significant effects on fasting lipids. Can decrease postprandial triglycerides

Typical patient with optimal efficacy: Type 2 diabetes with a predominant defect of loss of first-phase insulin release, as manifest by significant elevations in glucose levels between the pre-and postprandial period. This might be the thinner patient with type 2 diabetes, with fasting glucose levels above 125 mg/dl, but not close to 200 mg/dl or above. Also, for patients on biguanide or thiazolidinedione with suboptimal control, but who need insulin stimulatory effect to be meal-targeted to avoid hypoglycemia.

Dosing:

- 120 mg 1–30 minutes before meals. If no meal is eaten, no dose is taken. This is the usual dose for most patients, and no titration needed. Response is glucose dependent, not dose dependent.
- Taking medication after meals results in reduced drug levels
- For patients with A1C values close to target and for whom only minimal additional drug effect is desired, the 60-mg tablet is available
- Indicated also for use with metformin
- Same doses for patients with renal impairment and mild hepatic dysfunction

Additional precaution: Response to drug is dependent on glucose load. Therefore, if inadvertent overdose is taken without food, minimal hypoglycemia is likely to occur. However, if one attempts to "treat" such an overdose with glucose, the glucose load will stimulate a brisk insulin secretory response and the resultant hypoglycemia is likely to be *worse!*

MEDICATIONS THAT RESTORE INCRETIN FUNCTION

7. GLP-1 AGONISTS

Exenatide Summary

Brand name: Byetta

Indications: Monotherapy or in combination with a sulfonylurea and/or metformin

Action: Enhances glucose-dependent insulin secretion by the β-cell, suppresses inappropriately elevated glucagon secretion, and slows gastric emptying

Pharmacology: Injected drug reaches peak plasma concentration in 2.1 hours. Elimination by glomerular filtration with subsequent proteolytic degradation. Concentrations measurably present for 10 hours post-administration.

Required for efficacy: β-cells with some functional capacity remaining

Manifestation on glucose patterns: Generalized improvement in glucose levels, particularly postprandially. Reduction in hepatic glucose production leads to reduced fasting glucose levels.

Metabolism and elimination: Excreted unchanged in the urine

Potential effect on A1C: ↓ 0.4–0.9%, depending on starting A1C and use of combination therapeutic agents

Potential for hypoglycemia:

- Hypoglycemia: primarily when used in combination with a sulfonylurea. Not increased over placebo in combination with metformin alone.

Significant adverse events/side effects:

- Nausea: usually moderate and dose dependent. Decreased over time with continued therapy. Lead to withdrawal of therapy in 3% of patients.
- Pancreatitis: The use of exenatide has been very rarely associated with the development of pancreatitis. As a more common side effect of exenatide use is nausea unassociated with pancreatitis, clinicians should be cognizant of the need to differentiate GI symptoms that are and are not caused by pancreatitis. Clinicians are encouraged to discuss possible GI symptoms with their patients, and tell them to watch in particular for any persistent, unexplained abdominal pain, which could be quite severe and possibly accompanied by vomiting. The discomfort may or may not be accompanied by vomiting. In instances of such severe pain, the use of exenatide should be stopped if pancreatitis is suspected and the diagnosis of pancreatitis should be confirmed, including by the performance of enzyme testing. If pancreatitis is confirmed, exenatide should not be restarted unless an alternate cause of the pancreatitis is identified.

Typical patient with optimal efficacy: Type 2 diabetes, overweight, with postprandial hyperglycemia

Typical starting dose: 5 mcg per dose administered twice daily at any time within the 60-minute period before the morning and evening meals. Do not administer after a meal. Injection by prefill pen SC into the thigh, abdomen, or upper arm.

Prefilled pen dosage sizes:

- 5 mcg per dose, 60 doses, 1.2 ml
- 10 mcg per dose, 60 doses 2.4 ml

Titration and optimal daily dose: After 1 month of therapy at 5 mcg/dose level, if patient is without significant problems with nausea or hypoglycemia, increase to 10 mcg/dose with is the usual maintenance dose. When given with metformin, the dose of metformin usually does not need to be reduced. When given with sulfonylurea, a reduction in dose is often warranted initially to reduce the risk of hypoglycemia.

Maximal daily dose: 10 mcg/dose, given BID

Other clinical effects:

- Reduces appetite
- Slows gastric emptying

Drug interactions with potential for clinical significance:

- The effect of exenatide to slow gastric emptying may reduce the absorption of other orally administered medications. Use with caution in combination with medications which require rapid gastrointestinal absorption. Medications that are dependent on threshold concentrations for efficacy such as contraceptives and antibiotics should be taken at least 1 hour before an injection of exenatide. If such medications are to be taken with food, have the person take them with a snack at which exenatide is not administered.

Contraindications and precautions:

- Persons with hypersensitivity to exenatide or one of its components
- In patients with mild to moderate renal impairment (creatinine clearance 30–80 ml/min) clearance was only mildly reduced, and no dose reduction is needed. However, exenatide is not recommended in people with end-stage renal disease/dialysis (creatinine clearance < 30 ml/min).

- Not recommended for use in people with severe gastrointestinal disease
- Pregnancy Category C

Key advice to patients:

- Explain use of prefill pen devices, injection technique, and titration plan.
- Explain use of detachable needles and equipment disposal techniques.
- Explain potential for adverse events, including nausea and hypoglycemia.
- Advise regarding potential reduction in appetite.
- Advise that they should inform their physician if they become pregnant or plan pregnancy.

8. DPP-IV INHIBITORS

SITAGLIPTIN SUMMARY

Brand name: Januvia

Indications: Monotherapy or in combination with a metformin or a thiazolidinedione

Action: Enhances glucose-dependent insulin secretion by the β-cell, suppresses inappropriately elevated glucagon secretion

Pharmacology: Sitagliptin reaches it peak plasma concentration in 1–4 hours post administration. The absolute bioavailability is 87%. It may be administered with or without food. Approximately 79% of the drug is excreted unchanged in the urine, with metabolism being a minor pathway of elimination.

Required for efficacy: β-cells with some functional capacity remaining

Manifestation on glucose patterns: Generalized improvement in glucose levels, particularly postprandially.

Potential effect on A1C: ↓ 0.5–1.0%, depending on starting A1C and use of combination therapeutic agents

Potential for hypoglycemia:

- Hypoglycemia is not a significant problem with normal usage

Significant adverse events/side effects:

- Not significantly different from placebo. Details in package insert.

Typical patient with optimal efficacy: Type 2 diabetes, particularly those with postprandial hyperglycemia

Typical dose: 100 mg once daily. Use 50 mg daily for patients with moderate renal insufficiency, and 25 mg daily for patients with severe renal insufficiency or end stage renal disease. No dose titration.

Also available as a combination tablet with metformin:

- Sitagliptin/metformin (Janumet)
  - sitagliptin 50 mg and metformin 500
  - sitagliptin 50 mg and metformin 1000 mg

Other suggested clinical effects:

- May reduce appetite and promote weight loss
- Slows gastric emptying

Drug interactions with potential for clinical significance:

- None significant

Contraindications and precautions:

- No contraindications
- Precaution, with dose adjustment, in patients with mild to moderate renal impairment

VILAGLIPTIN

Brand name: Galvus

- Under FDA review at the time of this writing

9

Using Insulin To Treat Diabetes — General Principles

Richard S. Beaser, MD

Introduction

The year insulin was discovered by Drs. Frederick Banting and Charles Best of Toronto — 1921 — is the year that is commonly thought of as being the beginning of the modern era of treatment of type 1 diabetes. That landmark discovery allowed people with type 1 diabetes to survive beyond a few months of diagnosis and, over the ensuing decades with newer insulins and insulin delivery systems, strive to come closer and closer to a "normal" lifestyle.

However, in the early years insulin therapy was quite rudimentary. The earliest insulin available, known as "regular" insulin, was relatively short acting. Regular insulin's effect dissipated after a few hours, so truly insulinopenic patients needed to repeat injections frequently. It became clear that insulin worked most effectively and safely when given in conjunction with food, which provided the best chance to establish a balance between hyper- and hypoglycemic glucose levels. Thus, the premeal dosing schedules were developed.

Longer-acting insulins succeeded in freeing patients from frequent injections. In 1946, isophane insulin, which we now know as NPH, for

"Neutral Protamine Hagedorn" was developed, and in the 1950s, lente, another insulin with similar action, was developed. Modern forms of these two intermediate insulins evolved into general usage and were the mainstay of insulin therapy for many years. Only now, with the evolution to the use of insulin analogs, has the use of these insulins dropped off, and for the most part only NPH remains as the intermediate-acting insulin currently available.

Due to the relatively short duration of action of the intermediate insulins relative to the 24-hour day — particularly at lower doses — there were numerous attempts to make a longer-acting insulin. This led to the development of ultralente, the first long-acting insulin with effects that cover most of the day. With these advances, patients quickly moved from multiple daily injections to treatment regimens using one or, at most, two daily injections. A feeling of liberation permeated the ranks of people with diabetes.

It was at this time that physicians such as Elliott P. Joslin began to think that more aggressive treatment of diabetes might just be the key to reducing the risk of developing long-term complications. (Many argued that complications were inevitable, that the life of a person with diabetes was hard enough, and that keeping the insulin schedule simple — such as taking only one injection of NPH each morning — would make what years of life they had more comfortable and convenient.) Joslin, and those with similar views on control, focused on what was called "tight control." In reality, this usually consisted of an insulin regimen referred to as a "split-mix" — regular and NPH or lente mixed and given before breakfast and before supper, along with strict attention to diet and exercise. What was happening, in reality, was a recognition that insulin replacement is more effective and safer if it resembles, to some degree, natural insulin secretory patterns.

This era, with polarized camps of clinicians and researchers advocating either loose or tight glucose control, ran through to the early 1980s. During this time, insulin manufacturing techniques improved, including the one for extracting insulin from animal pancreases, and the commercially available insulins became purer. Purer insulins reduced the likelihood of insulin allergies, lipohypertrophy and lipoatrophy. It also had action times that were more and more predictable.

The early 1980s saw the dawn of the modern insulin era, with a focus on replacement of endogenous insulin with exogenous injections in a manner that was able even more precisely to mimic normal physiologic insulin action patterns. This era was heralded by a number of significant advances that, in sum, improved the ability of exogenous insulin to mimic natural physiologic insulin secretion. These were:

- The development of human insulin, guaranteeing sufficient insulin supplies to all in need, with minimal impurities and human-like amino acid structure to minimize insulin antibody production. The precision of the action of injected insulin was thus improved, allowing the design of more precise insulin treatment schedules.
- The development of methods for self-monitoring blood glucose (SMBG). Previously, urine testing, which was dependent on renal thresholds and indicated only glucose excess, led to treatments that sought to "shoot the top off" of high glucose levels with no regard to lows and patterns. Now, blood testing allows glucose patterns to be more clearly traced. These patterns assist in insulin treatment design. Also, with essentially instantaneous glucose measurements, patients can self-adjust insulin doses based on actual, current glucose levels.
- The development of methods to measure glycosylated hemoglobin (A1C), thus reflecting the average glucose level over a 2- to 3-month period. This technique gave us a much more accurate measure of glucose control. It provided a valid yardstick to measure success of therapy. It was speculated that hemoglobin glycosylation might also be a model of the process that leads to the development of long-term complications — the glycosylation of other tissues. Subsequent studies confirmed the correlation between the A1C level and the risk for the development of long-term complications.

The availability of these three tools allowed for the development of treatments that more accurately mimicked normal insulin action patterns. They also allowed the design of key studies that were performed over the next two decades that proved, once and for all, that aggressive control — but control that is based on replacing normal physiologic patterns — did, indeed, reduce the risk of complications. The key study among these was the Diabetes Control and Complications Trial (DCCT), and the follow-up study, Epidemiology of Diabetes Interventions and Complications (EDIC), which clearly showed that physiologic insulin replacement reduces microvascular and neuropathic complications of diabetes, and the impact of early intervention with physiologic insulin replacement was seen for many years.

Today, the key to insulin treatment is to design treatments that replace insulin in a manner that resembles normal physiologic patterns. For those with type 1 diabetes, this means focusing on careful monitoring of glucose levels and adjusting doses accordingly, as well as accommodating variations in food consumption and activity.

Endogenous Insulin

Insulin is a peptide hormone manufactured by the β-cells within the islets of Langerhans in the pancreas. A precursor molecule, proinsulin, is manufactured first. Then a section of that molecule, "C-peptide" (connecting peptide), is cleaved off, leaving the insulin molecule, which consists of two amino acid chains, the "A" chain and the "B" chain. Insulin is secreted in two phases in response to stimulation by rising glucose levels. The first phase represents pre-made insulin stored within secretory granules in the β-cell. It occurs over about 15 minutes after stimulation by rising glucose levels. The second phase represents release of newly manufactured insulin and occurs over a more prolonged period of time. The normal fasting or "basal" blood level of insulin in humans varies from 1 to 30 micro-units (1/1,000,000 of a unit) per ml of blood. In nondiabetic individuals, the postprandial blood level increases from insulin released in both phases, with the highest levels 0.5 to 1.5 hours postprandially. It returns to basal levels in about three hours.

Insulin for Exogenous Therapy

Commercially available insulin for treatment of diabetes has a number of characteristics that impact clinical utility. These characteristics are listed and discussed individually below.

- Biologic activity
- Species
- Concentration
- Purity
- Type, brand, and mode of delivery

Biologic Activity — The Unit

Insulin is measured in units, which measures a specific amount of biologic activity. The unit is an international measure and is consistent throughout the world. It always represents the same amount of clinical activity for every type of insulin. Keep in mind that the time course of insulins may differ, making some insulins *seem* to be more potent on a unit for unit basis. In reality, the more rapid-acting insulins produce an earlier, sharper rise in insulin levels than the longer-acting insulins. In describing unit-based potency, insulin action may be illustrated by an upward curve in which the time of most effect on glucose levels is indicated by the top or peak of the curve. The "area under the curve" should, theoretically, be constant for a unit of insulin — it is just shaped differently from insulin type to insulin type.

Species

Differences exist among species in some of the amino acids that make up the structure of the A and B chains of insulin. Until the development of the human-like insulins that came to market in the early 1980s, the most commonly used insulins were extracted from beef and pork pancreases. Porcine insulin is the insulin most like human insulin; the amino acid chains differ in only one amino acid substitution. Bovine insulin has three amino acids that differ from human insulin. Insulin from almost any animal can be effective in humans, and availability and local dietary practices have often dictated the selection. Insulin has been prepared from the pancreases of sheep, from tuna in Japan, and during World War II from whales in some countries. However, the differences in amino acid structure and sequence can produce antigenicity that can impact insulin action. This issue is discussed later in this chapter.

The human insulins developed in the 1980's have resulted in reduced antigenicity. However, the importance of the development of these insulins goes beyond mere insulin efficacy. The increases in the number of people with diabetes is proportionately just a bit greater than the increases in world population and much faster than the supply of animal pancreas! Estimates were made that by the dawn of the millennium there would have been a shortage of animal-source insulin if an alternative were not found. Indeed, economic and distribution issues still limit the availability of insulin in some parts of the world. However, with the development of synthetic and other genetically programmed insulins, supply should be sufficient to prevent a significant shortage.

Concentration

Most insulin used today is "U-100" which designates the concentration of 100 units of insulin per ml of volume. In the past there have been other concentrations such as U-40 or U-80. Today, these different concentrations are primarily used in veterinary care. The designation "U" with a number following indicates the concentration as measured by the number of units per ml of fluid volume. The differences between these insulins is concentration, not *strength* of the unit — a unit is always a unit! The U-100 is now used in much of the world.

It is important that patients match their insulin concentration to the proper syringe — U-100 insulin should be used with U-100 syringes. While most insulins — and thus most syringes — are U-100, occasionally outside the U.S. patients will encounter insulins and/or syringes of different concentrations. For patients comfortable with arithmetic, such conversions are not difficult, but they present potential for error.

For example, U-40 insulin would be 2.5 times less concentrated than U-100 insulin. Thus, to draw up a specified number of units, you would need to draw 2.5 times the volume of U-40 insulin. 20 units of U-40 insulin in a U-100 syringe are equal to 50 units on the volume marker of the syringe. Conversely, 25 units of U-100 insulin in a U-40 syringe are equal to 10 units on the volume marker.

The most commonly used U-100 syringes in use in the United States are 100 units, 50 units, and 30 units. Larger syringes containing 200 units are also available.

Other concentrations: U-500 insulin is also available for patients with extreme insulin resistance. U-500 insulin can be obtained by prescription and special order. On the other end of the spectrum, some children may require very small amounts of insulin. As it can be difficult to draw such small amounts in standard syringes, insulin can be diluted to U-10, U-25, or U-50 using diluting fluid obtained directly from the insulin manufacturer.

TABLE 9-1. Use of Syringes that Do Not Match the Insulin Being Used

If your insulin is	And your syringe is	Then if you draw up one unit of liquid in the syringe, it actually contains (units) of insulin
U-100	U-40	2.5
U-100	U-80	1.25
U-500	U-100	5
U-40	U-100	.4
U-80	U-100	.8
U-40	U-80	.5

Insulin Purity

The purity of insulin has improved markedly in the past few decades. During the many years of dependence on animal-source insulins, the challenge was extraction and purification from animal pancreatic tissue. The human insulins, however, are essentially impurity-free. Like differences in species, impurities can stimulate antibody formation, the consequences of which are discussed below.

Insulin Type, Brand and Mode of Delivery

We have evolved a number of modern insulins in common usage today. These insulins are listed in Table 9-2. Current insulins are used in combination to mimic the basal/bolus effect of natural insulin action as closely as is deemed necessary for a given patient.

Short-Acting Insulins

Short-acting insulins are termed **"regular"** insulins. The peak of regular insulin occurs at 3 hours, somewhat after the 0.5 to 1.5 hour timeframe during which most of the postprandial glucose rise is seen. Until recently, however, it was the most practical insulin for mealtime coverage. Its use has been either in combination with longer-acting insulins as part of

TABLE 9-2. Pharmacodynamics Of Current Insulin Preparations

Insulin Type	Product	Onset	Peak	Duration
Rapid-Acting				
Insulin aspart analog Insulin glulisine analog Insulin lispro analog	NovoLog Apidra Humalog	10–30 minutes	0.5–3 hours	3–5 hours
Short-Acting				
Regular insulin	Humulin R Novolin R	30 minutes	1–5 hours	8 hours
Intermediate-Acting				
NPH insulin	Humulin N Novolin N	1–4 hours	4–12 hours	14–26 hours
Long-Acting ("Basal"–like)				
Insulin detemir Insulin glargine	Levemir Lantus	1–2 hours	Minimal peak	Up to 24 hours
Premixed Insulin Combinations				
50% Human Insulin Isophane Suspension (NPH); 50% Regular				Humulin 50/50
70% Human Insulin Isophane Suspension (NPH); 30% Regular				Humulin 70/30
70% Human Insulin Isophane Suspension (NPH); 30% Regular				Novolin 70/30
50% lispro protamine suspension (NPL); 50% lispro				Humalog Mix 50/50
75% lispro protamine suspension (NPL); 25% lispro				Humalog Mix 75/25
70% insulin aspart protamine suspension (intermediate); 30% aspart				NovoLog Mix 70/30

conventional insulin therapy programs or given preprandially to provide postprandial coverage as part of physiologic insulin replacement programs. With the delay in onset and 3-hour peak, regular insulin has often been administered well before the meal in hopes of increasing its efficacy at countering the postprandial glucose rise. Typical intervals between injection and meals are 20 to 30 minutes. Some people wait even longer. Attempts at prolonging this interval to help lower higher preprandial glucose levels have also been tried.

The "tail" of regular insulin's action often lasts longer than 6 hours, primarily in people with long-standing diabetes, particularly those with significant antibody levels. In reality, regular insulin's effect probably adds ("piggy-backs") onto the action of the insulin working in the next timeframe. This effect makes it more difficult to determine which insulin is acting at what times and how to adjust insulins to maintain smooth glucose patterns. Regular insulin given at suppertime probably has significant action tailing off into the overnight period as well.

Rapid-Acting Insulin

The newer rapid-acting insulin includes insulin **aspart** (or just aspart, brand name NovoLog), insulin **glulisine** (or just glulisine, brand name Apidra), and insulin **lispro** (or just lispro, brand name Humalog). These insulins have an action pattern that more closely matches the postprandial glucose excursions than does the action pattern of regular insulin. They are clear insulins, and are often substituted for, and used similarly to, regular insulin. Their action characteristics are significantly different from regular, however, and must be understood in order to effectively and safely use these products.

Rapid-acting insulins have the advantage of their very rapid onset and short duration of action, which more closely mimics the action pattern of endogenously secreted insulin. This benefit is probably best seen when the insulin is given before meals to provide coverage of postprandial glucose. An added benefit is that the use of these insulins with a good long-acting basal insulin (discussed below) provides increased flexibility of meal times. Further, it is not necessary to wait 20 or 30 minutes for the insulin to begin to act, as one should with regular insulin. These insulins can be used as part of a conventionally designed insulin replacement program (see Chapter 10) as well as a physiologic insulin replacement program (Chapter 11). As the action of these insulins begins to run out at

about 3 hours, and meals — and thus subsequent insulin doses — are usually more than 3 hours apart, it is important that these insulins be used
with some form of basal insulin, particularly for patients with type 1 diabetes. In those patients who are truly insulinopenic, if only rapid-acting
insulin were used, there would be a significant nadir in the insulin level
between doses if the preprandial rapid-acting insulin were given without
some background of basal insulin. This would result in rising glucose levels in the late hours after meals from glycogenolosis and gluconeogenesis,
which would not be sufficiently suppressed due to the waning insulin
levels.

Similarly, when foods take longer than average to be absorbed, extending insulin action beyond that of the rapid-acting insulin may be needed.
Situations when this may be an issue occur when a patient eats foods with
high fat content or with patients who experience delayed food absorption
due to gastroparesis. Basal insulin or the use of regular insulin may be
needed. Also, use caution when rapid-acting insulins are given to lower
hyperglycemia at a time when food is not to be given subsequently. In
spite of significant hyperglycemia, hypoglycemia is more likely to result
with rapid-acting insulin than with the use of regular insulin. This does
not mean that these insulins should not be used for this purpose, just that
they should be used with caution.

The rapid-acting insulins work as rapidly as they do because the
changes that have been made in the amino acid structure makes them
quite unstable when in the crystalline state in the insulin bottle. With minimal dilution by subcutaneous fluid upon injection, the hexameric crystals begin to dissociate rapidly into monomers, which are the size most
readily absorbed.

This crystal dissociation also occurs when these insulins are exposed to
other insulins such as NPH. Therefore, once one of these insulins is mixed
with NPH, it needs to be administered within 5 minutes. It cannot be cus-
tom-mixed in advance — a practice common for those who wish to minimize the equipment they carry out to a restaurant or elsewhere or for
those needing assistance from others to draw up their insulin. However,
the use of commercially manufactured fixed mixtures of lispro and intermediate insulins may make such advance preparation possible if the
ratios of rapid-acting insulin to intermediate insulin fit the patient's
needs.

In addition, because of the rapid onset, rapid-acting insulin should be given no more than 15 minutes before eating. For many patients, it may be safer to take these insulins with the first bite of food. Certainly, when first starting to use this type of insulin, taking it with the first bite of food is safer until the patient's response to this insulin is determined. Patients should be particularly cautious when eating away from home, when the exact time that food will be available can be out of their control. In such circumstances, taking the injection as the food appears is probably safest. If episodes of hypoglycemia occur immediately before a meal, lispro may be injected at the completion of the meal as well.

Many people starting insulin therapy initially use rapid-acting insulins because of the advantages discussed above. Many people also switch to rapid-acting insulins for similar reasons, which might include, but are not limited to:

- problems with hypoglycemia 3 to 6 hours after a dose of regular insulin is used
- significant postprandial hyperglycemia not safely amenable to any other insulin dose adjustments
- change to a program using insulin coverage before each meal plus a long-acting basal insulin

Switching from regular to rapid-acting insulins

- Switching insulins using the same treatment regimen:
  For many patients, the rapid-acting insulin dose may be equivalent to the dose of regular. However, it may be safer to decrease the dose initially and titrate upward as needed. Fewer units of rapid-acting insulin may be needed to cover the same amount of food or to lower a high glucose level.

- Switching insulins using a different treatment regimen:
  Estimate the insulin dose for the new program the same way you would with regular insulin. Start with a slightly lower rapid-acting insulin dose than you would with regular insulin. If the patient is generally hyperglycemic, you might want to concurrently increase the intermediate, long-acting, or basal insulin. (See Chapter 10 for details of specific programs.)

- Check blood glucose often; particularly check before and 1 to 1.5 hours after meals. The dose is too much if:
  - blood glucose after a meal has not risen approximately 40 mg/dl above the premeal value
  - hypoglycemia is experienced 1 to 3 hours after a meal.

- Keep in mind that regular insulin typically peaks in 3 to 4 hours but can have a prolonged action of 4 to 8 hours. This prolonged action is not usually seen with rapid-acting insulin. As a result, the morning and evening intermediate, long-acting, or basal insulin may need to be increased due to the shorter duration of insulin lispro.

Intermediate Insulin

The intermediate insulin, **NPH,** was used for years, given 2 or even 3 times daily, to provide the basal insulin supply. Some tried to use larger doses of NPH, and another intermediate insulin recently retired from the market, lente, given once daily, to cover 24 hours. However, this approach was not ideal, as it did not replace the insulin in a manner very close to the natural insulin action patterns. Today, NPH is still used in conventional insulin programs, given 1–3 times daily, to provide background insulin, given at bedtime to target fasting glucose levels, occasionally given as part of a program using long-acting basal insulin with rapid-acting insulin to boost the basal insulin level during a specific part of the day, or given as part of a fixed mixture in a split-mix type program. NPH insulin contains protamine, which can potentially act as an antigen and stimulate an immunologic response. However, this rarely has any noticeable clinical effect.

Long-Acting Insulin

Long-acting "Basal" Insulins

For many years, ultralente was the long-acting insulin that was in common usage to provide prolonged basal insulin coverage. Its peak was quite blunt and, when given twice daily before breakfast and before supper, produced a fairly even basal effect. It was used along with some form of mealtime insulin coverage using regular or rapid-acting insulin. With the development of the newer long-acting basal analogs, with smoother and more reliable action patterns, the use of ultralente dropped dramatically.

The recent development of insulin analogues that more smoothly and reliably provide long-acting basal insulin effects has relegated ultralente to the realm of diabetes history. The first such product to reach the market was insulin **glargine** (or just glargine, brand name Lantus), followed more recently by the second, insulin **detemir** (or just detemir, brand name Levemir).

These long-acting insulins represent molecules that are modifications of the human insulin chain. Glargine has a substitution of glycine at position 21 of the chain and adding two arginines at position 30 of the chain. Detemir reflects the omission of threonine in position B30 and the attachment of a C14 fatty acid chain to amino acid B29. These molecular adjustments alters the release pattern of these insulins from the injection site so as to be smooth and continuous, lasting up to 24 hours. Thus, they have a flat action profile that effectively mimics a natural basal effect. One advantage of these insulins is that they can effectively lower fasting glucose levels with minimal nocturnal hypoglycemia.

Insulins glargine and detemir can be used to treat patients with either type 1 or type 2 diabetes as part of a treatment program aimed at mimicking normal insulin action patterns. Studies suggest that detemir may have a bit more of a peaking action and a duration which may be a little shorter, and may have a more consistent action pattern from one day to the next. This has led to its use as a twice-daily insulin, possibly in uneven doses so as to alter the basal insulin levels during the day vs. the night. Yet, doing this requires an additional daily injection. For some people it does last the full 24 hours, and can be given once daily.

Fixed Mixtures of Insulin

Insulin is also available in premixed solutions of short- or rapid-acting insulin and NPH or NPH-like insulins. The available products are listed in Table 9-2. Over the last few years, these insulin combinations have come and gone from the market, so it is likely that further changes to this list may occur.

The most common use of the premixed insulins is in treating patients with type 2 diabetes who would have difficulty mixing insulin. However, as these mixtures have a fixed ratio of the two insulins, the treatment is limited to the available ratios, without the ability for adjustments of one insulin without adjusting the other as well. For patients who can custom-mix and for whom such flexibility is important, fixed mixtures should not be used. These would include:

- children and adolescents
- anyone with type 1 diabetes
- thin (and thus more insulin-sensitive) people with type 2 diabetes
- pregnant women

Exceptions to this list would be those who have low visual acuity and would thus be prone to errors preparing the doses.

Inhaled Insulin

Having available an insulin that does not have to be injected has been considered by many to be a major milestone in the long history of insulin treatment. The first such insulin was marketed from 2006 to 2007, but, in spite of the feeling by many that non-injected insulin is the holy grail of insulin development, it was not commercially successful and had limitations on its medical utility. The inhaler was cumbersome and dose adjustments could not be made in small enough increments to make it practical for many. Yet, while this early inhaled insulin was a small, faltering step in the history of exogenous insulins, it is a giant conceptual leap in the evolution of insulin delivery that will be followed by further efforts. Other insulins that can be delivered either by inhalation or other non-injected delivery methods are in various stages of development at this writing, and will likely come to market in the near future, though details of pharmacology and usage parameters of these insulins are yet to be made public.

Given this first experience with non-injected insulin, it is difficult to gauge how it might have changed the indication for insulin therapy and potential insulin replacement program design. Theoretically, its availability could help target early postprandial hyperglycemia due to first phase insulin loss, whereas now using injection therapy for this early pathophysiologic defect is rarely accepted by patients. It might also improve patient acceptance of true physiologic insulin replacement, with "basal bolus" insulin administration requiring insulin dosing before each meal, and possibly snacks (see Chapter 11).

Once other, more refined non-injected insulin products are available in the future, the full clinical implication of this mode of administration will be determined, making clearer whether non-injected insulins reflect a true milestone in the development of exogenous insulins, or merely a footnote in the history of diabetes treatments.

Insulin Antibodies

Insulin antibodies can affect the efficacy of a treatment program and have significant clinical impact. With the development of newer insulins with improved purity that are identical to human insulin in structure, the effects of the less pure animal insulins used previously are more clearly appreciated.

People who had been exposed to these less pure animal insulins developed significant titers of insulin antibodies. These antibodies bind to the foreign substance to inactivate it, or even destroy it. Although the differences between human insulin and some animal insulins are minimal, they are still recognized as being a foreign protein, stimulating antibody production. Patients who used animal insulins for many years may have significant antibody titers and significant levels of antibody-bound insulin.

While the antibody-bound insulin is not liberated all at once, there can be an ongoing exchange between free and bound insulin. This effect results in blunting of the insulin peak, some delay in the time that the peak occurs, and a longer duration of action than is listed for that insulin. This explains why an intermediate insulin, supposedly acting for only 12 to 16 hours, actually can be effective for 18 to 30 hours, as was seen years ago when people were treated with one morning injection of intermediate insulin only. Many of the original studies determining peak times and the duration of action were undertaken with people without diabetes or with newly discovered diabetes without significant levels of insulin antibodies.

Antibodies to animal insulins as well as to impurities have also been implicated in the etiology of the lipodystrophies: the fatty buildup (lipohypertrophy) or wasting (lipoatrophy) at injection sites. They also may be the cause of insulin allergies and occasionally of insulin resistance.

Insulin Allergy

With the use of the purer, human insulins, the incidence of insulin allergy is declining. Nevertheless, some patients still develop localized or systemic reactions to the insulin or its components such as the protamine in

NPH. Sensitivity to any substance used to make a particular syringe (e.g., latex) should be ruled out when evaluating local allergic response.

Localized reactions may include itching, burning, erythema, or hive formation at the site of needle insertion. As such symptoms may also be caused by improper injection technique such as intradermal injection, the patient's technique should be reviewed. However, a true allergic response could be the cause. Systemic reactions are even more rare, but do occur. Systemic allergy can manifest itself as urticaria, bronchospasm, or even anaphylaxis. For true systemic allergic responses in a person who must use insulin, desensitization may be necessary.

Insulin Storage

It is important that insulin be stored in a manner that maximizes its efficacy. In addition, it is recommended that patients keep one or two vials or adequate cartridges/penfills available as back-up in the refrigerator.

Insulin storage recommendations often change, and may also vary from product to product. Listed below are some general guidelines. However, it is important to keep up with changing storage recommendations. Information supplied with the insulin or the manufacturer's website can often guide you on the specifics for each insulin, and for vials vs. cartridges/pens.

General rules for storage of insulin vials:

- Insulin vials in use can be stored in the refrigerator or at room temperature.
- Insulin should never be frozen.
- Insulin in use can be kept at room temperature (59–86° F) for up to 1 month. The potency of the insulin may be altered after that.
- The storage recommendations for insulin vials are similar for the major companies that produce them.

  - Unopened vials, refrigerated, can be kept until their expiration dates.
  - For opened vials, the recommendation is to discard after about 28 days for most insulins, regardless of whether they have been stored at room temperature or not. While glargine stored at room

temperature should be discarded after 28 days, detemir may be kept, once used, at room temperature for 42 days

- Keep insulin bottle(s) away from direct sunlight or heat and in a cool, dry place.
- Avoid exposing the bottles to temperature extremes (< 36° F or > 86° F).

General rules for storage of insulin cartridges and premixed insulins:

- Cartridges (pen-filled) of regular and lispro may be stored for 4 weeks at room temperature.
- Many of the pens/cartridges should be kept at room temperature and not refrigerated once usage has started.
- 70/30 cartridges and pens can be stored at room temperature for a maximum of 10–14 days
- Manually prefilled syringes containing NPH insulin should be stored in the refrigerator. Patients must adequately resuspend this mixture when they are ready to inject it by rolling the syringe in their hand before injecting. These prefilled syringes should be used within 21 days of preparation.

Insulin should also be discarded if there is any suggestion of reduced potency, contamination, or if white crystals appear in the insulin or the inside of the bottle. Any bottle of insulin that is normally clear (regular or rapid-acting) that is noted to be cloudy or discolored should also be discarded. It is a good rule that if there is any question, the safest step is to discard an insulin bottle and replace it. Patients should be told to always keep at least one or two extra bottles of each insulin on hand, refrigerated.

Also, keep in mind that there is a large margin of safety with the expiration date on the insulin bottle. This date is the earliest time before which there is absolutely no doubt about full insulin potency. After the expiration date, the insulin may slowly start losing some strength. Unlike a bottle of milk which sours past the expiration date, the issue with insulin is usually potency, and not that it has spoiled.

Insulin Injection — The Syringe

Insulin syringes are manufactured to match the concentration of the insulin being used and also come in various sizes and gradations, making it easier for some patients to use smaller quantities of insulin per injection. In the United States, the insulin use is primarily U-100, and therefore so are the syringes. Total capacity of syringes available for common usage are 30, 50 and 100 units total capacity.

Most people now use disposable syringes and needles. Rarely does anyone still use the reusable glass syringes and reusable needles. The disposable plastic syringes cannot be boiled to sterilize and usually come with pre-attached needles. The needles typically range in gauge from 29 to 31 gauge.

Syringe Preparation Techniques

Insulin injection techniques are relatively simple. Nevertheless, some people with poor eyesight, limited dexterity, or reduced intellect may have difficulty. Poor technique can be a major source of dosing errors, leading to potentially dangerous inaccuracies. The ability to prepare one's own insulin syringes avoids the dependence on others that can have a significant psychological and logistical impact on people with diabetes and their families.

Self-mixing also promotes independence and flexibility. Premixed insulins can reduce the likelihood of mixing errors, however they limit dosing flexibility. Pens can make injection techniques simpler, but until a pen is developed that can custom mix insulin, their use is limited to fixed, premixed insulin or single insulin types. The ability to custom-mix insulins can be an important skill.

Educators skilled in teaching self-injection and mixing techniques should be utilized to help patients develop the skills and accuracy needed for injecting insulin. Figure 9-1 and Figure 9-2 provide descriptions and diagrams of insulin syringe preparation techniques. Practitioners prescribing insulin treatment programs should use these descriptions to determine whether a given patient is likely to succeed in learning self-injection techniques. Educators can use them as a guide to their own teaching techniques.

Injection Techniques

Proper technique is important, and a patient who is learning insulin injection for the first time is often best taught by a Certified Diabetes Educator (CDE) who is skilled at such instruction. However, for practices located a distance from the nearest CDE, it is often useful to have someone from the office staff learn to teach insulin injection and management techniques. Support materials to assist in doing so are available from Joslin Diabetes Center and other diabetes organizations. Insulin injection techniques are included in the description of insulin dose preparation in Figures 9-1 and 9-2. These figures may be helpful in explaining such techniques to your patients.

The following points should be emphasized to patients learning to self-inject insulin:

- Prepare the skin by cleansing with an alcohol wipe. Cleansing technique is *very* important so as to avoid infection at or around the site of injection
- Grasp some tissue firmly, but not too tightly, between the thumb and one finger of one hand, holding the syringe in the other hand. A good amount of skin and tissue beneath the skin should be included in this grasp so that the injection will be well beneath the surface of the skin.
- If using an arm, the "grasp" can be simulated by pushing the arm against a solid object to push up the skin.
- Do not be concerned if a small amount of blood appears after the needle is withdrawn. Simply press the spot gently and briefly with cotton soaked with alcohol or an alcohol pad.
- Air bubbles can be avoided if the patient does not shake the insulin bottle but rather rolls it gently between the palms of the hands for mixing. The biggest worry about small amounts of air bubbles is reduced quantity of insulin, not air embolus (which would take over 100 ml).
- Insulin should be injected into subcutaneous fatty tissues. The published data on onset, peak and duration of insulin action are based upon insulin injected into subcutaneous tissue. If insulin is absorbed too deeply and into muscle, it is absorbed more rapidly. If it is injected too superficially (subdermal injection), absorption will be slower and less predictable, resulting in hyperglycemia.

FIGURE 9-1.   How To Draw Up and Inject Insulin

Single Dose

1. Wipe off top of bottle with alcohol swab (cotton and alcohol).

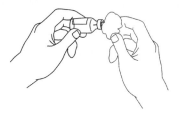

2. Roll bottle upside down and sideways between hands. Clear insulins do not need to be rolled.

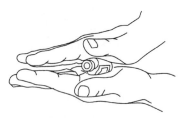

3. Pull plunger of syringe to number of units of insulin you should inject.

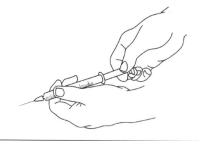

4. Put needle through top of insulin bottle and push plunger down. This puts air into the bottle of insulin.

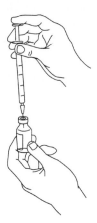

5. With needle still in bottle, turn bottle upside down.

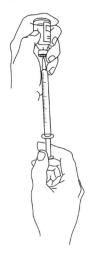

6. Pull plunger halfway down to fill the syringe with insulin. Check syringe for bubbles. If you do not see bubbles, push plunger to number of units of insulin you should inject. Remove needle from bottle.

If you see air bubbles, push all of the insulin back into the bottle. Then do Step 5 and Step 6 again.

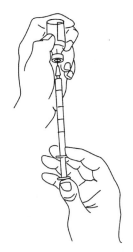

7. Wash the area with soap and water.

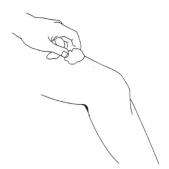

8. Pinch skin, pick up syringe like a pencil and push needle straight into skin. Push plunger down.

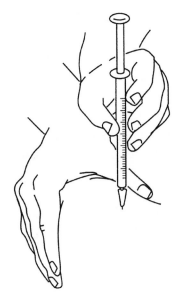

9. Let go of skin and pull needle from skin.

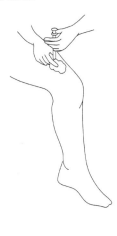

FIGURE 9-2.   Mixed Dose

1. Wipe off top of bottles with alcohol swab (cotton and alcohol).

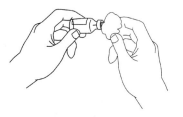

2. Roll cloudy bottle upside down and sideways between hands.

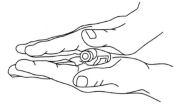

3. Pull plunger of syringe to number of units of cloudy insulin you should inject.

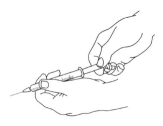

4. Put needle through top of cloudy insulin bottle. Keeping bottle upright on table, push plunger down, putting air into bottle. Take needle out. Syringe should be empty.

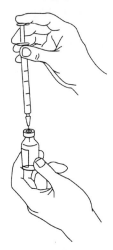

5. Pull plunger of syringe to number of units of clear insulin you should inject.

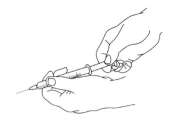

6. Put needle through top of clear insulin bottle. Keep bottle upright on table. Push plunger down.

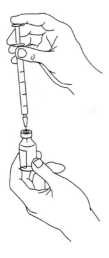

7. Leave needle in clear bottle and turn bottle upside down.

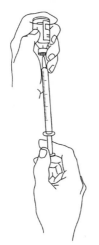

8. Pull plunger out about 10 units past the number of units of clear insulin you should inject. Check insulin in syringe for bubbles. If you do not see bubbles, push plunger to number of units of clear insulin you should inject. Remove needle from bottle.

If you see bubbles, push all of the insulin back into the bottle. Then do Steps 5–8 again.

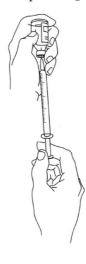

(Continued)

9. Turn cloudy bottle upside down. Put needle through top of bottle.

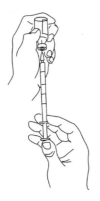

10. Pull plunger slowly to the number of total units of clear and cloudy insulins you should inject. Remove needle from bottle.

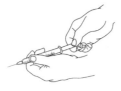

11. Wash the area with soap and water.

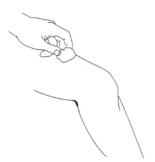

12. Pinch skin, pick up syringe like a pencil and push needle straight into skin. Push plunger down.

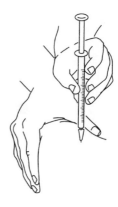

13. Let go of skin and pull needle from skin.

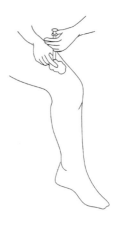

Additional Guidelines for Mixing Insulin:

- Do not mix insulin that differs in purity or source.
- Draw the clear insulin into the syringe first.
- Be sure to eliminate all air bubbles in the syringe before injecting.
- Refrigerated premixtures of regular and NPH are stable for up to 21 days.
- Store syringes with needles pointing up, so suspended particles do not clog the needles.
- It is important to inject a mixture within 5 minutes or after 24 hours to ensure consistency of insulin action.

  - Insulin lispro starts to bind to the longer-acting insulin after it has been mixed in a syringe for 5 minutes. This insulin should not be held in a mixed form for longer than 5 minutes.
  - Regular insulin starts to bind to the longer-acting insulin after it has been mixed for five minutes. Binding is usually complete in 24 hours. During the period of binding, the effects of insulin are unpredictable.

- DO NOT mix any of the long-acting basal insulins with any other insulin in the same syringe.

It is ideal to standardize the interval between mixing and injecting insulin, so the amount of binding is equal with each injection.

Common Mixtures

Regular and NPH

- Prefilled insulin is stable for 3 weeks when stored in the refrigerator.
- Refrigerate prefilled syringes until day of use.

Rapid-acting insulin and NPH

- Inject within 5 minutes of mixing.
- Rapid-acting insulins lose their potency when mixed with other insulin for more than five minutes.
- Should not be premixed and then refrigerated for later use.

Insulin Pens

The newer pen devices allow simpler injection techniques with more portable injection equipment. Many people using premeal insulin doses like to use these devices because of their convenience. However, the pens currently available can inject from only one cartridge of insulin. Therefore, they can be used to inject only a single type or premixed insulin. For patients needing two types injected in custom or variable amounts, use of the pen would necessitate two injections. Some patients so prefer the convenience of these devices that they do not mind the second injection. Many use these, in spite of the need for two injections, for just the injection times that they are away from home, typically lunch or dinner times.

Needles for the insulin pens can often be of finer gauge than those for standard syringes because they do not need to puncture the top of an insulin vial. For this reason, many people feel that these needles are more comfortable to use than the thicker syringe needles.

The techniques for use of the pens vary from product to product. They are relatively simple to use, however, and the technique can be taught to most patients quite easily. In general, these devices include a means to select the number of units to be given and then a simple injection mechanism for pushing the insulin out through the needle. Some pens are reusable and take cartridges for insulin refills, but most manufacturers are moving toward totally disposable pens, which are discarded once empty.

Automatic Injection Aids and Jet Injectors

Some people with diabetes may be squeamish about self-injecting, and over the years, various devices have been marketed in hopes of overcoming such problems.

The simplest such device is a small automatic injector that helps insert the needle beneath the skin. The syringe is filled with insulin as usual and placed into the injector. Then the injector is spring-cocked. The injection site is cleansed, and the injector is set against the skin. A small trigger is touched which forces the needle through the skin. The individual then pushes the plunger down, injecting the insulin.

"Jet injectors" have been available for many years as an aid to those who have difficulty with needle injections. While these do not use needles, they force the insulin through the skin with pressurized air. Unfortunately, these devices are not usually a significant improvement over syringes and needles. They are expensive, cumbersome, and the pain, while not as sharp as with a needle, is a dull thud that many also find objectionable. These devices do serve as an alternative for people who are completely unable to bear the trauma of injections. However, there has been a question as to the consistency of delivered insulin dose. The rate of absorption of the insulin is often increased when one of these devices is used, so the insulin dose(s) may need to be changed.

Assuming newer, non-injectable insulins are developed in the future, the need for these types of automatic and jet injectors will likely decline.

Insulin infusion pumps and other mechanical insulin delivery devices are other ways to deliver insulin to the body, and will be discussed in Chapter 11.

Injection Aids for People with Low Vision

For people with low vision, self-injecting insulin can be a challenge that threatens what remaining independence they may have. Using devices to assist them with self-injecting can make a significant difference for such individuals. Syringe magnifiers can be used to assist in reading syringe gradations. Insulin gauges and click-count syringes that click-count the number of units are available to help draw up the proper amount of insulin if reading the scale is difficult. Keep in mind that the use of pens may be easier for people with reduced vision than the standard syringes.

Injection Sites

Rotation of injection sites has been part of the insulin self-management curriculum since the beginning of insulin therapy. Early on, medical practitioners recognized that localized irritation can occur from frequent injections, and in frequently injected areas the skin can become thickened and scarred, delaying absorption. Rotating injection sites allows the trauma from previous injections to resolve, and reduces focal fatty deposits (lipohypertrophy) or fatty wasting (lipoatrophy), known collectively as lipodystrophies. Insulin injected into areas of lipohypertrophy may not be absorbed uniformly or predictably, possibly leading to erratic glucose control. There is also a greater tendency for insulin leakage from injection sites over hypertrophied tissue, further impacting the quality of control.

With the newer, less antigenic insulins and sharper, finer needles, many people become less concerned with strict site rotation. For example, the most common site for insulin injection has traditionally been, and still is, the thigh. Most people have enough flesh in this area, and it is easy to reach. Many like this area and, because they do, they tend not to rotate sites. Yet, site rotation is still important to optimize absorption and preserve sites, particularly if people are using treatment programs consisting of three or four daily injections. What they save from less antigenic insulins and less traumatic needles, they lose in the frequency of injections. Site preservation is still important.

Other possible injection sites are the upper arms and across the front of the abdomen as well as toward the sides (see Figure 9-3). Use of the abdomen should be encouraged, as it is easy to reach, is a vast area, many patients have extra fat tissue there, and abdominal tissue is easy to grasp. However, patients should avoid the 2-inch radius around the navel. The upper buttocks may be hard to reach, but other members of the family might help. An individual could inject his or her buttocks by leaning back against a piece of furniture such as a dresser or table edge so that the tissue is compressed firmly. Areas to avoid include the area close to or below the knee or into the very inside of the thigh. Ideally, enough rotation can occur so that a given area is not used more often than once per month.

Suggested options for a rotation schedule might include:

- Inject in a particular region of the body such as the entire abdomen for 1 to 4 weeks. Be sure to rotate injections within that area. Then move on to another area.
- Match the site of injection to the same time of day to allow for consistency in absorption from day to day. For example, inject the prebreakfast insulin dose into the abdomen every day; inject presupper insulin dose into the thigh and the nighttime insulin dose into the buttocks. Within each area, injection sites should also be rotated.

FIGURE 9-3.   Injection Sites

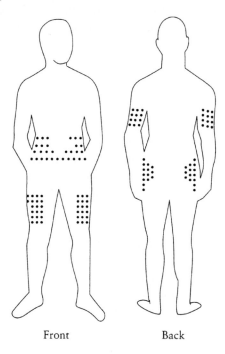

Front   Back

Rates of insulin absorption can vary from site to site. Below are listed sites from fastest absorption (abdomen) to slowest (buttocks):

- abdomen
- arm
- thigh
- buttocks

The clinical implications of differences in absorption go beyond being merely an explanation for variable control. Some people vary sites to change the insulin action timing, based on glucose levels. For example:

- If the blood glucose level is high, one might inject into the abdomen to lower the glucose level more rapidly.
- For elevated fasting glucose levels due to insufficient duration of action of supper intermediate insulin, injecting that insulin into a site

with slower absorption such as the hip may prolong its action some-what, though the effect of this maneuver would probably be mini-mal. Moving the nighttime intermediate insulin to bedtime might be a better solution.

Syringe Reuse

For reasons of economics, syringe availability, or disposal restrictions, some people may reuse disposable syringes. The ADA conducted studies that suggested that it is probably safe and practical for syringes to be re-used if a patient wishes to. Following are guidelines for reusing insulin syringes:

- Flush the syringe with air after use to prevent the needle from clog-ging with insulin sticking to the sides of a syringe.
- Do not wipe the needle with alcohol.
- Recap needle when not being used.
- Store the syringe to be reused at room temperature.
- Keep the outside of the syringe clean and dry; handle only when nec-essary.
- Do not reuse a needle that is bent or dull.
- Throw the syringe away if the needle touches anything other than the skin at the injection site or the top of the insulin bottle.
- Clean the top of the insulin bottle with alcohol before drawing up in-sulin.
- Observe injection sites for signs of infection.
  NOTE: With repeated use, needles may become dull and unit mark-ings on the syringe may wear off. It is therefore recommended that syringes only be reused within a 24-hour period.

People who should not reuse insulin syringes would include those with:

- poor personal hygiene
- open hand wounds
- known susceptibility to infection
- immunosuppression or who are immunocompromised

Disposal of Syringes

It is a good safety practice, and good for the environment as well, to dispose of syringes and lancets properly. Guidelines for proper disposal of these devices are listed below:

- Place syringe or lancet directly into a puncture resistant container with a tight cap or lid (a plastic bleach jug, liquid detergent bottle, or paint can, for example). Avoid using breakable glass containers or recyclable containers. A container with a small opening is preferable in order to prevent spills.
- Keep the container out of reach of small children and in the same room where injections and blood glucose tests are done.
- When the container is full, seal and tape securely.
- Certain states or towns may have special requirements for disposal of used syringes and lancets. Patients should check with the local Board of Health regarding disposal regulations before disposing of needles and lancets.

10

Designing a Conventional Insulin Treatment Program

Richard S. Beaser, MD

Introduction

The availability of insulin therapy is a life-sustaining miracle for many people, and a means to a much healthier life for many more. It is unfortunate, therefore, that insulin therapy has traditionally suffered from the unfortunate necessity of having to be delivered by injection. Many people have had difficulty getting past this fact, and this has lead to all sorts of interesting behavior! Physicians even use the possibility of insulin injections to threaten their patients: "If you don't *(fill in the blank with whatever adherence issue is being neglected)*, we will have to start insulin." It is thought of as a last resort: "We have tried *everything* that is available to control your diabetes. There is nothing else left. We *have* to start insulin."

Often patients will use their dread of injections to motivate themselves to follow their meal or physical activity plans. Some patients who are already using maximum oral therapies but achieving suboptimal control have been known to tape a picture of an insulin syringe onto the refrigerator to remind themselves of the consequences of eating too much!

Yet, when initiated under the proper circumstances, insulin is a physiologically appropriate and very effective therapy for diabetes. Those with type 1 diabetes need it to survive. Those with type 2 diabetes have traditionally started insulin when their condition has progressed to the point at which their endogenous insulin production is insufficient to maintain their good health. And for medical professionals, our attitudes about insulin often impact patients' acceptance of this therapy more than we might imagine. Patients will sense it if we adopt the attitude that insulin is a therapy to be dreaded. But they will also sense it if we feel that, when indicated, insulin is a therapy that can maintain or even improve health considerably. *"The good news is that we have insulin available to control your diabetes!"*

As discussed in the previous chapter, the future development of clinically useful, non-injected insulin may make insulin administration easier, and could lead to initiation of insulin therapy to cover prandial insulin needs earlier in the natural history of type 2 diabetes. Even now, the injection of insulin, using pens and finer needles, is easier and without significant discomfort. Also, other treatments for insulin, such as exenatide, are injected medications, making insulin not quite as unique. Thus, we really do need to change our thinking about insulin. It is one of the available treatments for diabetes and should be used as needed. The concern about injections really should not be considered a major obstacle.

Indications for Insulin Therapy

Type 1 Diabetes

For the person with type 1 diabetes, the indication for insulin therapy is the establishment of the diagnosis. By definition, people with type 1 diabetes must be treated with insulin. On first pass, this statement seems self-evident. However, from a clinical standpoint, it is sometimes less obvious than one might think.

For those with the classic onset of type 1 diabetes, presenting with marked hyperglycemia, weight loss, dehydration, and perhaps some ketonemia, insulin therapy is obviously needed immediately. There is no question; patients feel poorly and rarely argue. Such is the case for most children or adolescents who are diagnosed with diabetes. It is usually assumed that they have type 1 diabetes, and insulin therapy is initiated. Traditionally, this assumption is correct. However, with the growing incidence of obesity in childhood, as playing baseball is being forsaken for playing computer games, we are seeing more kids with type 2 diabetes. A detailed discussion of the diagnosis and differentiation of diabetes types in children can be found in Chapter 21. The key point, however, is that all diabetes in young people is not necessarily type 1.

Nor is all diabetes in older people type 2. For many adults, the more gradual onset that is typical of type 1 diabetes in older individuals may not make it readily apparent which type is present. It is not uncommon to achieve reasonable control for these patients in the early stages of their disease using oral medications, often sulfonylureas. Nevertheless, the slowly declining β-cell mass gradually leads to deterioration of control and eventually to the need for exogenous insulin therapy.

A thinner person may have some insulin resistance, less obvious without obesity to further worsen the condition. When this person gets diabetes, he or she is probably further along the spectrum of insulin secretory deficiency, probably has insulin resistance, and is well on the way to developing an absolute insulin secretory deficiency. The clinical picture can be mixed.

Thus, type 1 and type 2 diabetes are not always clinically distinct entities resulting from distinctly different pathophysiologic deficits, sharing only glucose elevations and complications. Indeed, while classic type 1 and type 2 diabetes differ in etiology and clinical presentations, in some individuals, clear clinical distinctions may blur. Does it matter?

Not if the clinician monitors the progress of therapy and the overall clinical scenario! That non-obese adult who presents with mild to moderate hyperglycemia that is initially manageable with oral therapies may have less insulin resistance than his more obese counterparts. His lack of obesity probably delayed the time in life that the glucose abnormalities became manifest. When they finally do, there is less hyperinsulinemia and more advanced deterioration in insulin production capacity. While initially, oral medications might work, before long, β-cell mass will decline further, and the clinical picture will more and more resemble type 1 diabetes. The vigilant clinician will recognize this progression and initiate insulin therapy in time.

The Honeymoon Phase

The honeymoon phase of type 1 diabetes can lead some to believe that either the diagnosis of diabetes was incorrect in the first place or at least that the determination that the diagnosis was type 1 diabetes was erroneous and the initiation of insulin therapy unnecessary. Of course, for those who understand the natural history of type 1 diabetes, this assumption is clearly incorrect.

The honeymoon phase of type 1 diabetes classically occurs a few weeks after diagnosis and initiation of insulin therapy. It is less common in younger children and most common in people diagnosed with type 1 diabetes in their late teens or early adulthood. With the onset of classic, auto-immune type 1 diabetes, at the time of diagnosis there is considerable inflammation of the islets of Langerhans from the immune assault. When exogenous insulin therapy is initiated, the need for pancreatic insulin production decreases, and with decreased metabolic activity in the β-cells, the inflammation subsides. Some β-cell function returns as cells that were inflamed but not yet destroyed resume insulin production. The honeymoon phase thus represents the recovery of some β-cell function.

As this recovery occurs, it is accompanied clinically by an increasing frequency of hypoglycemic reactions. Insulin doses are usually lowered in response, and may drop to as low as 0.1 unit/kg body weight.

Many good reasons have been advanced for not stopping insulin therapy during a honeymoon period. Many argue that stopping insulin may lead to patients thinking that their diabetes has been cured. With this impression, they might be very reluctant to face the need to restart insulin subsequently.

However, there are physiologic arguments for not stopping insulin as well. In the past when more antigenic insulins were in use, the argument was that stopping and restarting insulin was more likely to stimulate allergic responses. While this is less of an issue now, it has been replaced by another, similar concern. Recently, there have been suggestions that aggressive, physiologic glucose control with exogenous insulin therapy decreases the metabolic demands on the β-cells, and with decreased metabolic activity they are less likely to stimulate the autoimmune assault that is thought to lead to β-cell destruction. Some theorize that this approach may prolong the honeymoon phase or perhaps ultimately lead to a decrease in the degree of β-cell destruction when the autoimmune process eventually becomes quiescent, leading to more stable glucose patterns.

While both of these theories are not conclusively proven, many feel that they are suggestive enough to argue for early initiation of insulin therapy in an aggressive, physiologic manner.

Type 2 Diabetes

As suggested at the beginning of this chapter, the temptation to use insulin therapy as a threat, a punishment for non-adherence, or a treatment of last resort for people with type 2 diabetes should be avoided. In truth, insulin is indicated as an appropriate treatment when dictated by the underlying pathophysiology of a given patient's diabetes, which falls into four categories:

1. Glucose toxicity (decreased insulin sensitivity resulting from marked hyperglycemia)
2. Needed to adequately treat postprandial hyperglycemia
3. Insufficient endogenous insulin production (sufficient decline in β-cell mass)
4. Contraindications to the use of oral medications

Clinical scenarios that reflect these four categories include those listed below. As you can see, there is some overlap:

1. Glucose toxicity
   – marked hyperglycemia at presentation with diabetes
   – severe hyperglycemia with ketonemia and/or ketonuria
   – prolonged hyperglycemia despite maximal doses of antidiabetes medications
   – hyperglycemia in patients using antidiabetes medication therapy due to inadequate adherence to nutrition and/or exercise plan
2. Needed to adequately treat postprandial hyperglycemia
   – traditional non-insulin treatments can often cover postprandial glucose levels; however, with the concern that marked postprandial hyperglycemia may increase cardiovascular risk, and with the availability of newer medications that more efficiently and safely target this glucose pattern (incretin mimetics and non-injected insulin which now makes pre-meal dosing easier), we are likely to see more targeted treatments being initiated for postprandial hyperglycemia. Many experts argue that treatments targeting postprandial hyperglycemia earlier in the natural history of type 2 diabetes — not waiting for more significant insulin secretory

deficiency — may reduce cardiovascular risk and insulin resistance.

3. Insufficient endogenous insulin production
   - significant hyperglycemia at presentation with diabetes due to decreased β-cell mass or function; hyperglycemia despite maximal doses of antidiabetes medications may be due to decreased β-cell mass or function
   - increased insulin requirements due to acute injury, stress, infection or surgery (effectively, this represents increased insulin requirements in the setting of β-cells that cannot keep up with this increased insulin requirement)
4. Contraindications to the use of antidiabetes medications
   - renal disease
   - hepatic disease
   - pregnancy
   - allergy or serious reaction to antidiabetes medications
   - excessive side effects from antidiabetes medications

Past concerns about the effect of hyperinsulinemia due to injected insulin are no longer thought to be an issue. While hyperinsulinemia is a hallmark of type 2 diabetes, there is little evidence to suggest that exogenous insulin therapy increases atherogenic risk for patients with type 2 diabetes. If insulin is indicated for someone with type 2 diabetes, it should be used.

Conversely, if there are clinical indications that the endogenous insulin secretory reserve is still sufficient and none of the listed indications for insulin therapy is present, then non-insulin therapies, either alone or in combination, may be considered. Such patients usually:

- are overweight and not losing weight
- are non-adherent to lifestyle recommendations
- are mildly to moderately hyperglycemic, but often less so with episodic reductions in food intake or increases in activity.
- have no marked postprandial hyperglycemia, or postprandial glycemia is adequately controllable without insulin

Non-insulin therapies for type 2 diabetes, including oral treatments and non-insulin injectable treatments, are discussed in Chapter 8.

Insulinopenia

From the clinical perspective, an important determination as to whether or not insulin therapy is needed would be whether the patient is, in fact, insulinopenic. Measuring insulin or C-peptide levels is not a practical way to make this determination. For those for whom insulin secretory capacity if measured by laboratory methods would appear clearly elevated or depressed, the corresponding clinical picture is rarely ambiguous. When there is doubt based on clinical parameters, the chemical measures are usually equivocal as well. Therefore, in such circumstances, treatment decisions should be based on clinical need — the degree of hyperglycemia or key glucose patterns such as postprandial hyperglycemia, the presence or absence of other metabolic abnormalities, or other concomitant medical conditions. If a patient is closely monitored, any error in choosing this initial therapy can be quickly remedied as the clinical need becomes obvious.

Nevertheless, if one can detect the presence or absence of clinical signs of insulinopenia, one can more accurately choose the initial therapy. The following signs are suggestive of insulinopenia:

- longer duration of diabetes
- thinner patient or declining weight
- ketonuria
- glucose patterns, unresponsive to non-insulin antidiabetes medications, showing:
  - elevated fasting glucose
  - rising glucose levels during the day
  - marked postprandial hyperglycemia
  - marked hyperglycemia throughout the day
  - general lability in response to daily activities

Goals of Insulin Treatment

The objective of an insulin treatment program is to provide sufficient insulin for the utilization of glucose as energy or its storage as glycogen for later use. It is therefore important to establish a proper balance among the insulin that is administered and the other two major factors that patients can control, which contribute to determining the glucose level: food and activity.

It is important to remember that there are many other influences on glucose levels that can vary from day to day, even hour to hour. These can be difficult to identify and, even when they can be identified, it is often difficult to quantitate their actual impact on glucose control. Among such factors for injected insulin are:

- emotional stress
- timing of injections, activity, food
- insulin species (human insulin is more rapidly absorbed than animal insulin, which binds to proteins upon injection. Most insulin in use in the United States is human insulin.)
- contamination of the insulin vial by another type of insulin due to improper mixing technique
- injection site quality (presence of lipodistrophy or scarring)
- injection depth (see Chapter 8)
- excess air in the injected insulin (reduces actual amount of insulin delivered)
- quantity of insulin (larger amounts of insulin injected into one spot take longer to be absorbed than smaller amounts similarly injected)
- deterioration of the quality of insulin (proximity to expiration date, duration in use and at room temperature, exposure to extremes of temperature)
- ambient temperature (in warmer environments, there is more cutaneous circulation to dissipate body heat, resulting in more rapid insulin absorption)
- proximity of injected insulin to microvasculature (close proximity increases speed of absorption)
- speed and efficiency of gastrointestinal absorption of food

And there are undoubtedly more!

People needing insulin therapy vary with respect to the degree of instability in their glucose patterns. People with type 2 diabetes with a predominance of insulin resistance tend to have more stable patterns. They are more likely to have some endogenous insulin secretory capacity remaining, which covers the extreme excursions of glucose levels. Conversely, those with negligible endogenous secretory capacity, particularly if counterregulatory function is compromised, may have more erratic patterns, and thus more difficulty maintaining control. Therefore, the design of the insulin treatment program — its complexity, how closely it must mimic normal patterns, and how much dose variability it incorporates — is dictated by the degree of inherent stability a given patient may have.

Patients with absolute deficiencies of insulin secretory capacity need replacement programs that come close to mimicking normal insulin patterns. Such programs often use multiple insulin injections. They also may provide guidelines for adjusting insulin doses based on the variations in actual glucose levels and/or in compensation for other parameters that can impact glucose control, such as eating. By using such a program, one tries to compensate for the variability inherent in one's glucose patterns due to *all* factors, those we can identify and those that are beyond our control.

For those people with some remaining insulin secretory capacity and/or insulin resistance, endogenous insulin can stabilize glucose patterns, and the design of the replacement program is often simpler. Fewer daily insulin injections may be required to provide the needed supplementation to maintain an adequate physiologic pattern, and, with some endogenous insulin secretory variability in response to actual blood glucose levels, the complexity of daily variations of exogenous insulin dosing variations may be less.

Nevertheless, rarely does one daily injection of one type of insulin provide the best possible insulin coverage, and most people would benefit from some variation of insulin dosage based on daily lifestyle variations or actual glucose levels. Further, the perspective that covering postprandial hyperglycemia in people with type 2 diabetes may reduce macrovascular risk often leads to recommendations for more physiologic replacement programs for these people as well. The closer one can come to an insulin replacement program that is designed to resemble normal physiologic insulin patterns in terms of both insulin levels as well as responsiveness to daily variables, the better the control and the more comfortable the insulin action that will result.

Glucose Monitoring Programs for Patients Using Insulin

Careful self-monitoring of blood glucose (SMBG) (see Chapter 3) is essential to maintain proper balance. The design of the treatment program often dictates the optimal monitoring schedule. For people using replacement programs seeking to closely mimic natural physiologic insulin patterns (see Chapter 11), checking at least four times daily is essential — and checking even more frequently is often needed. Those with more stable patterns and simpler treatment designs may not need to test as frequently. Unfortunately, in an era when provision of supplies is determined by insurance carriers rather than physicians, the number of daily test strips provided is often a fixed number for *everyone* using insulin — such as "three." If a larger supply is prescribed, physicians must provide insurers with detailed explanations.

Whatever the motivation for the development of monitoring and other procedures, it is important that healthcare providers not assume that insurance company policies reflect optimal care. Take the time to explain why a given patient needs more strips. The benefits of this effort to the patient's health, and the eventual savings of your time, will become apparent.

Some guidelines for monitoring frequency and patterns are outlined below. Keep in mind that any monitoring program must be individualized to each person's lifestyle, schedule, metabolic patterns, insulin regimen, and willingness to monitor. Combinations and hybrids of programs listed below may be appropriate as well.

Low monitoring level:
- Appropriate for patients with some residual insulin secretory capacity, using a fixed daily dose of insulin, particularly if there are reasons why more frequent glucose checking is not possible.
- Possible schedules for glucose checks:
  - once daily, varying times among premeal and bedtime
  - twice daily, fasting daily, and supper alternating with bedtime as the second checking time
  - block checking — one of the above patterns, but, in addition, 1 to 2 times per month, the patients checks 4 to 6 times daily, premeals, postmeals, nocturnal, for 3 to 4 days in a row.
- Use of results in monitoring program:
  - patterns used to adjust insulin schedule or doses
  - blocks allow closer look at patterns
  - once- or twice-daily checking will provide warning of longer-term trends in glucose levels

- if circumstances present higher likelihood of acute changes in glucose levels (sick-days, marked activity changes, holiday overeating), more frequent checking is indicated

Intermediate monitoring frequency
- Appropriate for patients with limited residual insulin secretory capacity or significant insulin resistance using a more complex insulin program of two to three daily injections, with some dose variation based on monitoring results and other parameters ("intensified conventional" therapy).
- Possible schedules for glucose checks:
  - three checks daily, at insulin injection times
  - twice daily at times when variable doses of rapid-acting insulin are given, plus an additional daily check at variable times to determine the efficacy of the injected insulin (e.g., prelunch, bedtime, nocturnal, postprandial)
  - block checking as above might also be performed at this level
- Use of results in monitoring program:
  - daily adjustment of rapid-acting insulin per an intensified conventional insulin treatment program
  - glucose patterns through routine checking and block checking can be used to adjust insulin schedules or doses, or to recognize the need for sick-day coverage

Intensive monitoring frequency
- Appropriate for patients with negligible residual insulin secretory capacity and/or significant variations in daily schedule, often comprising the majority of people using an intensified conventional or physiologic insulin replacement program (see Chapter 11).
- Possible schedules for glucose checks:
  - a minimum of four checks daily, premeal and at bedtime
  - above noted checks four times daily plus regular checking at other times: nocturnal, postprandial
- Use of results in monitoring program:
  - daily adjustment of rapid-acting insulin per an intensified conventional or physiologic insulin replacement program
  - patterns used to make adjustments of insulin schedule or doses, or initiate sick-day coverage

Initiation of Insulin Therapy for Type 1 Diabetes

The first objective in initiation of insulin therapy for someone with newly diagnosed type 1 diabetes is to correct any existing metabolic abnormalities and ameliorate symptoms. For patients presenting with diabetic ketoacidosis (DKA), a discussion of treatment will be found in Chapter 13. It is hoped, however, that DKA will not be the presenting event, and the diabetes will be discovered before the patient becomes so metabolically compromised.

The more common presentation of type 1 diabetes is moderate hyperglycemia, with symptoms such as polyuria, polydypsia, polyphagia, weight loss, and/or blurred vision. Assuming that there is no ketonemia present, the current trend is to treat such patients as outpatients. However, with this typical presentation of type 1 diabetes, it may be difficult to gauge how rapidly the patient's metabolic status is deteriorating. It is possible that ketosis could develop within a day or two. Therefore, the first objective is to start insulin immediately.

When a patient has only moderate hyperglycemia and no ketosis, a physician in a busy office at the end of a work day, may be tempted to tell a patient to return the next morning (or on Monday morning!) to start insulin. However, the speed of potential deterioration of control is not always evident. The safest approach in this circumstance would be to give a simple injection of a small amount of intermediate or long-acting basal insulin (0.1–0.2 units/kg of body weight) to provide overnight coverage and suppress ketogenesis. Doing so will likely prevent further metabolic deterioration until a proper insulin program can be initiated. However, for marked hyperglycemia, and certainly with ketonemia, a more aggressive approach is recommended, with hospitalization for those with the most severe metabolic compromise.

Ideally, in any circumstance, the initiation of insulin therapy should occur immediately upon diagnosis of type 1 diabetes. Doing so requires that a program be designed and that the patient's educational process begin immediately. Unlike patients diagnosed with type 2 diabetes who may begin insulin therapy with only bedtime insulin, those with type 1 diabetes should use a multidose insulin program as the initial regimen. Unless patient considerations intervene, it is rarely, if ever, appropriate for a patient with type 1 diabetes to begin an ongoing treatment program of one daily injection alone. Other than, perhaps, during a honeymoon period, such programs do not adequately mimic normal insulin action patterns, and it is important that patients accept the need for multiple injections from the start.

In the past, physicians would treat newly diagnosed and hospitalized patients with injections of regular insulin every 4 to 6 hours for a couple of days, based on a sliding scale of some sort. Then they added up the amount of insulin used in 24 hours and divided it into a two injection, regular and intermediate insulin program. *This method is no longer appropriate.* First, we no longer hospitalize non-metabolically compromised patients, making such "round-the-clock" insulin dosing impractical. Second, as noted above, by giving some insulin — almost any reasonable amount — ketosis is suppressed. Therefore, most physicians now determine the design of the insulin program (number and schedule of injections) and initiate it with relatively low doses of insulin and then titrate the insulin doses upward as needed. Ketone production is suppressed, and the patient can be gently eased into control, while getting used to self-administration on an outpatient basis.

Choosing the Appropriate Insulin Program

There is a spectrum in the complexity of insulin therapies that can be roughly grouped into three categories, although the dividing lines between them often to blur for some patients. A choice of the initial level of intensity should be based on metabolic needs, variability of lifestyle (particularly timing and activity), and patient willingness to perform glucose monitoring and give injections. As a rule, to achieve a given level of diabetes control, the more complex (i.e., physiologic) the program, the more flexibility in lifestyle is permissible.

1. *Conventional insulin therapy* utilizes two to three daily injections with the insulin doses essentially remaining the same from day-to-day. Doses are adjusted only for significant variations in food consumption, activity, or event timing.
2. *Intensified or "more physiologic" conventional therapy* usually utilizes two to three daily injections, but does not include an injection before every meal (lunchtime injections are usually omitted), which, by definition, is true physiologic therapy. Adjustment scales for rapid-acting insulin doses given prior to meals (breakfast and supper) are

developed. These programs may be easier to self-manage for some patients than true physiologic insulin replacement therapies and may be streamlined to involve SMBG. However, they can be more effective and flexible than conventional therapies, and by providing adjustments based on self-monitoring, they may also increase SMBG adherence.

3. ***Physiologic insulin replacement therapy*** utilizes rapid-acting insulin before each of the three daily meals. These insulin doses are adjusted based on glucose level, food consumption, activity, etc. Often, a program such as carbohydrate counting is used to assist in such dose adjustments In addition, some form of basal insulin is used such as glargine or detemir. In the past, multiple doses of intermediate insulin were used, but this alternative approach is rarely used today with the availability of the longer-acting basal insulins. Externally worn insulin pumps (continuous subcutaneous insulin infusion or CSII) fall into this category of intensive therapy as well. Pumps administer bolus doses of rapid-acting insulin before meals and provide a slow infusion of that same insulin to produce the basal effect. The goal of a physiologic insulin replacement program is to achieve normoglycemia and optimization of lifestyle flexibility. These types of programs, then called "intensive insulin therapy," were used in many landmark studies of the impact of aggressive diabetes control such as the DCCT and Kumamoto studies. They are discussed in detail in Chapter 11.

Recent improvements in insulin types and delivery systems have made the use of the more physiologic replacement programs more practical for an increasing number of patients. The development of smoother basal insulin analogs, the rapid-acting insulins that more precisely match the glucose pattern of incoming food, and improved insulin delivery devices such as pens, have made these physiologic insulin programs more practical for many people. Thus, the trend in recent years has been for people to move more rapidly along the spectrum to earlier usage of the more physiologic programs to achieve smoother glucose patterns and more flexibility.

Designing a Specific Insulin Program

The first step in the design of a multidose insulin program for people with either type of diabetes is to determine the structure of the program.

TABLE 10-1. Summary: Designing a Physiologic Treatment Program

1. Determine the number of daily insulin doses and timing of these doses. Decide whether or not to use have these doses adjusted each time they are given. To do so, assess the patient's:
   a. metabolic needs
   b. schedule and lifestyle
   c. willingness to self-monitor blood glucose using frequent glucose checks
   d. willingness to take injections
   e. ability to understand the complexities of an insulin treatment program
2. Initiate the program, using less than the anticipated eventual insulin quantity. This allows you to:
   a. avoid hypoglycemia and rebound
   b. clearly recognize glucose patterns
   c. adjust insulin doses to achieve smooth glucose patterns
3. Increase insulin doses to target normoglycemia

Conventional fixed dosing programs, or physiologic variable doses? How many insulin doses daily? Determining the answers to these questions requires an assessment of the patient's:

- *Metabolic needs* — is the patient newly diagnosed, implying that there is residual ß-cell function and stable patterns? Such a patient could achieve adequate control using a simpler program than one who has had diabetes for a longer period of time with less ß-cell secretory capacity.
- *Schedule and lifestyle* — does the patient live a relatively regimented life, with a daily schedule and activity level that is fairly predictable? Such a patient could achieve adequate control using a simpler program than one that has more variability and provides more flexibility.
- *Willingness to SMBG and take injections* — no matter what the result of the above assessment, ultimately the design of the program will depend on what the patient can realistically do.
- *Ability to understand the complexities of an insulin treatment program.*

Overwhelming a patient with complex instructions for adjustment may lead to dangerous mistakes.

Next, based on the above assessment, the healthcare provider should initiate the program, using a total quantity of daily insulin that one anticipates may be less than that which might eventually be needed. Keep in mind that assessing insulin quantity is often like trying to hit a moving target; it can change with time, particularly in the first months and years following the diagnosis of type 1 diabetes. Here are a couple of points to keep in mind:

- Upon initial diagnosis, hyperglycemia, and perhaps also ketonemia, increases insulin resistance. Initial insulin requirements may be higher than that which will be needed once metabolic normalcy is restored. Often, patients may eventually require 0.6 to 1.0 unit/kg body weight. Start with lower than this, perhaps 0.2 to 0.5 unit per/kg body weight, anticipating that the dose may rise higher during the next week or two of dose adjustments.
- If a honeymoon phase (described earlier in this chapter) occurs during the first few months, the insulin requirements may drop to amounts as low as 0.1 unit/kg body weight.
- After the honeymoon resolves, the insulin requirements will rise again.
- Once a patient has had type 1 diabetes long enough for the decline in pancreatic function to stabilize (on average, about 5 years, but it can vary), the typical requirement for adults is 0.5 unit/kg body weight. This quantity is higher for children and may also be greater for adolescents as they go through puberty and post-pubertal growth. These estimates are rough guides only, and many patients may have insulin requirements that differ. The quantity of insulin required may vary due to the following factors:
  - some patients may not lose all β-cell secretory capacity and thus may require less insulin
  - some patients may take longer to loose their ß-cell secretory capacity
  - some patients may have concomitant insulin resistance which would increase their insulin requirements
- The quantity of insulin that is needed may be greater when treatment programs using fewer daily injections are used. However, the

increased risk of hypoglycemia with such programs may limit how aggressively the insulin quantity can be increased. When more-physiologic insulin replacement programs are used, one can more safely increase the quantity of insulin given each day, approaching actual replacement needs, because the action pattern of the exogenous insulin matches natural requirements more precisely and imbalances of insulin quantity vs. needs are less frequent.

By starting with a dose that is below what estimated eventual needs may be, and by targeting preprandial glucose levels between about 100 to 200 mg/dl, hypoglycemia and subsequent rebound hyperglycemia are avoided. This approach allows the glucose patterns to be more easily recognized. Thus, if a glucose level at a particular time of day is consistently elevated, it *is* due to insufficient insulin — the question of whether it could be rebound is not likely to arise.

In addition, during this part of the process, the patient and his or her family are going through an intense learning process. It is helpful if they don't have to face the difficult task of treating frequent hypoglycemic reactions and determining whether hyperglycemia is due to insufficient insulin or rebound hyperglycemia following a hypoglycemic event.

Once patients are comfortable with the basic principles of diabetes self-care, they are better able to handle these more complex issues. By that time, the glucose patterns should be clear, and the balance of insulin doses among the scheduled administration times should be set. It is then time to increase the insulin doses to target desired glucose values that are as close to normal as is safely possible.

Keep in mind that the various components that entered into the decision of which initial treatment program to use can change over time:

- the diabetes will progress and β-cell secretory capacity may decline
- lifestyles and schedules will change
- patient willingness and/or ability to perform self-care functions may change

Thus, continual update and review of the treatment program is necessary to maintain the optimal level of control for that patient.

Initiation of Insulin Therapy for Type 2 Diabetes

For patients with type 2 diabetes, the particular indication for initiating insulin therapy often dictates the initial starting method and regimen. For those with residual β-cell function but who need insulin due to glucose toxicity, this need for insulin may be temporary while the cause of the hyperglycemia is resolving. However, patients with significant β-cell dysfunction will require a long-term insulin replacement program, and many of the considerations for treatment selection are similar to those for people with type 1 diabetes.

It should be noted, too, that just because a person with type 2 diabetes needs insulin, it doesn't mean that the insulin resistance disappears. Therefore, it is common to continue antidiabetes medication therapy aimed at reducing insulin resistance at the same time that exogenous insulin treatments are administered.

Recently, with the availability of new insulins and delivery systems, the question of when, in the natural progression of insulin secretory insufficiency, insulin therapy would be indicated has become quite relevant. For many years, people with type 2 diabetes were felt to need insulin once there was moderate insulin secretory deficiency, and often started with one daily injection of NPH or a basal insulin given at bedtime, or with a mixture such as 70/30 at suppertime, along with some or all of the daytime oral therapies.

However, the first defect in insulin secretion for people with type 2 diabetes is usually a loss of first phase insulin release. The defect in initial insulin secretion occurring right after ingested food reaches the blood stream often results in postprandial hyperglycemia. This glucose pattern is often the first glucose abnormality noted, and has been implicated in increased macrovascular risk. As many people with type 2 diabetes have hoped to avoid insulin injections, and many antidiabetes medications can adequately manage to return postprandial hyperglycemia close to targeted levels, the use of insulin therapy at this early stage has rarely been recommended. However, the availability of newer, more easily used and comfortable pens and other insulin delivery devices now make insulin coverage more acceptable to many who had previously been hesitant. It is therefore possible that we will see the initiation of prandial insulin coverage at these earlier stages of the progression of type 2 diabetes for people for whom this approach would be the most effective method to manage this glycemic pattern.

It is likely, however, that initiation of insulin therapy using replacement of basal insulin with a long-acting analog will remain a common starting point in the therapeutic progression when prandial coverage with insulin is not such an acute issue, particularly if an antidiabetes medication is already addressing this need. In such a circumstance, if the A1C and postprandial glycemia have been on target, the next marker of progression would be a rise in glucose levels at other times of the day. Elevations in the fasting glucose levels reflect hepatic insulin resistance in the setting of waning insulin secretory capacity leading to less effective suppression of nocturnal glucose production.

From a clinical standpoint, when the A1C levels reflect suboptimal control, and fasting glucose levels rise toward 200 mg/dl and are unresponsive to aggressive use of other therapies and appropriate lifestyle interventions, then insulin therapy must be considered.

The use of late-day insulin along with daytime antidiabetes medication therapies can be effective. Studies have suggested that at the stage of progression of type 2 diabetes where a moderate degree of insulin secretory capacity remains, although the "weak link" is the early morning, allowing antidiabetes medications to control glucose levels during the day results in control comparable to that of full multidose insulin programs without as much tendency for weight gain.

Initiation of late-day insulin may begin with a moderate estimate of total dose, say between 10–20 units depending on the size of the patient and the degree of hyperglycemia. Formulae have been suggested for calculating this dose, but ultimately the best advice is to start low but then aggressively titrate upward as needed, based on response to therapy reflected by improvements in the fasting glucose level.

A full, multidose insulin program is indicated when hyperglycemia persists throughout the day, particularly if it is accompanied by marked rises in postprandial glucose levels. Program selection and initiation are the same as for people with type 1 diabetes. People with type 2 diabetes likely have more residual β-cell function remaining than those with type 1 diabetes and may not need the complexity of a true physiologic insulin replacement program. Nevertheless, there may be some benefits to such a program, and with the availability of insulin pens, more physiologic insulin replacement programs have become more practical in this population as well. A study from Japan that was similar to the DCCT but that studied intensive insulin therapy in people with type 2 diabetes (the Kumamoto study), suggests that such treatment did reduce the incidence of complications. Therefore, it is an individual decision as to how aggressive (i.e., physiologic) a program for type 2 diabetes needs to be, considering the same factors as for type 1 diabetes:

- metabolic needs
- schedule and lifestyle
- willingness to SMBG
- willingness to take injections
- ability to understand the complexities of an insulin treatment program

The Implications of Insulin Quantity

Those unfamiliar with diabetes and its pathophysiology often mistakenly think that higher insulin doses indicate a "worse" condition. Severity of diabetes can be measured from many perspectives: the presence or absence of complications, the degree of instability of patterns and the resulting impact on lifestyle, or the A1C. In reality, the quantity of insulin needed may reflect only the presence and degree of insulin resistance, body size, or the balance of food consumption and exercise. Clinically, there are many anecdotal examples of patients for whom the clinical impact is *inversely* related to insulin dose. Therefore, the quantity of insulin required, and changes in quantity over time, may reflect the dynamics of the clinical treatment, variations in the level of diabetes control, presence of another underlying condition, or other related medical parameters. But it should not be used as a measure of "severity."

As noted previously, people with type 1 diabetes of more than about 4 to 5 years duration often need about 0.5 units of insulin per kilogram of body weight per day. This is not a precise calculation, but rather a rough estimate of insulin needs to be used when designing an insulin treatment program. This calculation is not valid for people with type 2 diabetes and insulin resistance. Nor is it valid when residual endogenous insulin secretory capacity remains as, for example, in patients with early type 1 diabetes and many with type 2 diabetes. For someone with longer-duration diabetes, for whom you are revamping an insulin program, and who is using a daily quantity of insulin that is *less* than 0.5 units/kg body weight, it is usually safer to use this lower insulin amount to calculate the new program. They may have residual β-cell function and not need as much exogenous insulin. Also, keep in mind that the quantity of insulin needed is often greater for programs using fewer daily injections, although the frequency of hypoglycemia in such programs may limit aggressive dosing.

Specific Insulin Regimens

Guidelines for some commonly-used insulin dosing patterns and their variants are described below.

I. Peakless basal insulin given once daily at bedtime (see Figure 10-1)

Example: Insulin glargine or detemir given at bedtime (Figure 10-1A)

- Nonpeaking insulin provides even coverage during most of the 24-hour day
- Lack of prandial coverage makes this program inappropriate for people with type 1 diabetes or with type 2 diabetes and significant postprandial hyperglycemia not adequately treated with other medications
- May not adequately cover variable basal insulin needs at certain times of the day:
  - Early morning due to release of counterregulatory hormones
  - Upward drift of glucose levels during the day due to insufficient meal-time insulin secretory capacity

Variations:

- *Use of basal insulin twice daily. (Some data suggests that detemir is slightly shorter acting, and may provide more complete coverage in some people if given twice daily.)* (Figure 10-1B) The basal insulin is given twice daily,

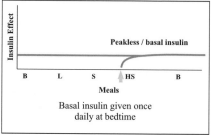

Figure 10-1A

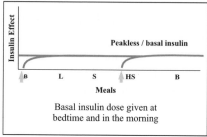

Figure 10-1B

Figure 10-1.

at bedtime and at breakfast. Doing so, with unequal doses, allows differential coverage overnight/early morning vs. later in the day

Comments:

- Appropriate initial therapy for people with type 2 diabetes if postprandial glycemia is otherwise adequately controlled
- Often used in conjunction with oral antidiabetes therapies.

II. Single, morning intermediate insulin (see Figure 10-2)

Example: NPH at breakfast

- peaks all at once in the late afternoon.
- potential for hypoglycemic reaction at peak time:
  - late afternoon "drive time"
  - if supper is delayed
  - later in the evening if insulin action is prolonged
- insufficient insulin coverage for supper and early evening.
- insufficient overnight coverage resulting in fasting hyperglycemia.
- no short- or rapid-acting insulin at breakfast to counteract carbohydrate load at breakfast and early morning release of counterregulatory hormones.

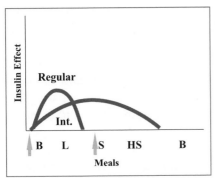

Figure 10-2A

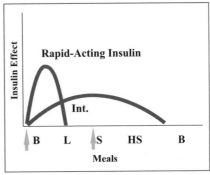

Figure 10-2B

Figure 10-2: Morning mixed insulin program of NPH and either A) regular insulin or B) rapid-acting insulin (aspart, glulisine, lispro).

Variations:

- *Adding short-acting or rapid-acting insulin with the morning NPH injection* covers the breakfast carbohydrate load. It allows somewhat less intermediate insulin to be used, reducing the risk of hypoglycemia later in the day.
- *Giving intermediate insulin before breakfast and before supper.* The second intermediate insulin dose covers overnight. It allows a reduced dose of intermediate insulin to be given in the morning, reducing the risk of hypoglycemia later in the day.

Comments:

- As has been emphasized previously, one morning injection of intermediate insulin is not ideal therapy for anyone. Thus, its use is discouraged.
- Keep in mind that intermediate insulin begins to work in about 3 hours. A person who tries a morning mixed dose of short-acting (regular) and intermediate insulin (described below) and experiences prelunch hypoglycemia may try reducing the dose of morning short-acting insulin to prevent these reactions. In reality, the hypoglycemia may not be caused primarily by the morning short-acting regular

insulin, but rather by a large dose of morning intermediate insulin that began working during the late morning. Its effect, added to that of the short-acting insulin, caused the hypoglycemia. A better dosing adjustment that would maintain smoother glucose patterns would be to reintroduce a morning mixed dose but reduce the dose of morning intermediate insulin. Also, the use of rapid-acting (aspart, glulisine, or lispro), rather than short-acting insulin may avoid as much overlap of action.

- Most patients have smoother control with more than one daily injection of insulin. Introduce or adjust insulin dose(s) later in the day if necessary to compensate for a reduction in morning intermediate insulin quantity and, conversely, when adding a second daily injection, *be sure* to reduce the morning insulin doses.

III. Mixed insulin before breakfast and before supper (see Figure 10-3)

Example: Regular or rapid-acting insulin and NPH (or premixed) at breakfast

Regular or rapid-acting insulin and NPH (or premixed) at supper

- Even distribution of insulin action throughout the day:
  - covers morning insulin needs
  - avoids excessive insulin peaks that cause hypoglycemia
  - avoids prolonged insulin action
- Suppertime short- or rapid-acting insulin covers food intake.
- Suppertime intermediate insulin provides overnight coverage
  - however, it may peak during the middle of the night (2–3 AM) resulting in hypoglycemia
  - insulin peak action does not match hyperglycemia that can occur during the waking hours (6–8 AM)

Comment:

A rough calculation of the insulin distribution for this "split/mix" program (applicable to the two injection variety or the three injection variety below) would be: Use two-thirds of the total daily insulin dose in the morning, one-third at night. Within each time (morning and evening), use one-third of the assigned quantity of insulin as short- or rapid-acting insulin, and the remainder as intermediate-acting NPH insulin. For

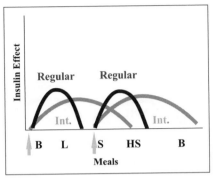

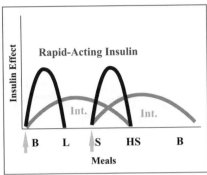

Figure 10-3A

Figure 10-3B

Figure 10-3: **Split-Mix program of 2 daily injections of NPH and either A) regular insulin or B) rapid-acting insulin (aspart, glulisine lispro or).**

example, if a total daily dose is estimated to be 36 units, give 24 as the morning dose and 12 later in the day. For the morning dose, an estimate would be 8 units of short- or rapid-acting insulin and 16 units of intermediate NPH insulin. For the remainder of the insulin, one could give 12 units of intermediate NPH insulin at bedtime, or 4 units of short- or rapid-acting insulin and 8 units of NPH at suppertime. (If the mixed dose at suppertime is split with short-acting at supper and NPH at bedtime, these ratios may need some further adjustment based on actual glucose test results.) Use of rapid-acting insulin in these programs is less likely to cause as much overlap of action with the NPH insulin at the 3-hour mark postprandially.

IV. Morning mixed insulin plus bedtime intermediate insulin (see Figure 10-4)

Example: Regular or rapid-acting insulin and intermediate NPH insulin (or pre-mixed insulin) at breakfast,
NPH at bedtime

- Even distribution of insulin action throughout the day:
  - covers morning insulin needs
  - avoids excessive insulin peaks causing hypoglycemia
  - avoids needing prolonged insulin action.

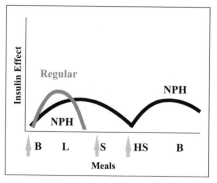
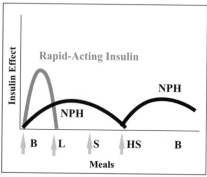

Figure 10-4A   **Figure 10-4B**

Figure 10-4: A) Prebreakfast NPH and regular insulin and bedtime NPH, B)
Prebreakfast NPH and rapid-acting insulin, and NPH at bedtime

- Lack of suppertime short- or rapid-acting insulin coverage may lead
  to bedtime hyperglycemia.
- Bedtime intermediate insulin:
  - provides sufficient overnight coverage
  - peaks when the individual is awakening which controls fasting
    blood glucose levels

V. Morning mixed insulin plus suppertime short- or rapid-acting and bedtime intermediate insulin (see Figure 10-5)

Example: Regular or rapid-acting insulin and NPH at breakfast
             Regular or rapid-acting insulin at supper
             NPH at breakfast

- Even distribution of insulin action throughout the day:
  - covers morning insulin needs
  - avoids excessive insulin peaks that cause hypoglycemia
  - avoids need for prolonged insulin action
- Suppertime short- or rapid-acting insulin covers food intake.
- Bedtime intermediate insulin:
  - provides sufficient overnight coverage
  - peaks when the individual is awakening which controls fasting
    blood glucose levels

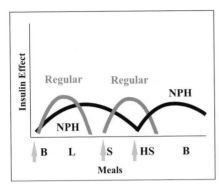

Figure 10-5A

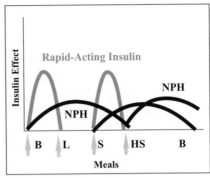

Figure 10-5B

Figure 10-5:   Multiple Injection Programs: A) Prebreakfast NPH and regular insulin, supper regular insulin, and bedtime NPH, B) Prebreakfast NPH and very-rapid-acting insulin, Presupper very-rapid-acting insulin with NPH added, and bedtime NPH

Variations:

- Small doses of intermediate NPH insulin administered along with the supper rapid-acting insulin can improve control. The rapid-acting insulin given at suppertime usually wears off before the bedtime intermediate insulin begins working. Short-acting regular may last a bit longer, but could have prolonged action into the nighttime, increasing the potential for nocturnal hypoglycemia
- Rapid-acting insulin (aspart, glulisine, or lispro) has a shorter action than regular insulin. In the morning, it will be less likely to cause overlap hypoglycemia late morning. However, at suppertime, it could run out before the bedtime NPH starts working. Mixing in a few units of intermediate NPH insulin at suppertime bridges the gap in insulin coverage between these two insulins' action times.

Intensified Conventional Therapy

A conventional insulin program can be made more responsive to daily variations in food consumption, activity, and other factors impacting the glucose levels by the use of adjustment scales known as *algorithms* or *sliding scales.* These programs provide guidelines for regular or rapid-acting insulin dose adjustments based on glucose readings, but these doses may also be adjusted based on variations in food consumption and/or activity. The terminology "intensified conventional therapy" or "physiologic conventional therapy" really just reflects another step in the spectrum of treatments starting with simple, fixed dose programs and leading to physiologic insulin replacement programs (Chapter 11).

Currently, an optimally-designed physiologic insulin replacement program would be a program that provides basal insulin coverage by use of a peakless basal insulin, a combination of intermediate-insulin doses (not used much now with the peakless basal insulins) or rapid-acting insulin infusion from an insulin pump. These programs used to be called "intensive insulin therapy." The terminology "intensified conventional therapy" isn't really a distinct category of treatment, but rather the evolutionary stage of treatment that begins to take on some of the characteristics of a physiologic insulin replacement program. In the case of intensified conventional therapy, it usually is a program that uses an adjustment scale of some sort for regular or rapid acting insulin (and sometimes for NPH) but the program does not include administration of regular/rapid insulin prior to *each* meal. Instead, it may involve a schedule of injections similar to one used for a conventional program but with the dose adjustment plan. Compared with conventional programs with *fixed doses,* these programs are more effective and flexible, but require more frequent glucose checking and attention to variations in the daily routine.

An example of the intensification of a conventional insulin program is outlined in Table 10-2. This example uses a morning mix, supper rapid-acting, and bedtime intermediate NPH insulins. Keep in mind that the numbers used in this example are hypothetical. Use the guidelines discussed above to determine actual doses. Also, making insulin dose adjustments of 1 unit for each glucose interval of 50 mg/dl is arbitrary as well. For people using smaller amounts of insulin, the incremental increase of 1 unit may occur for increases of 100 mg/dl. For people using larger amounts of insulin, the dose adjustment may be more than 1 unit of insulin for an incremental increase of 50 mg/dl of glucose.

The adjustments of regular or a rapid-acting insulin should be used to accommodate for variations in glucose values that are inconsistent from day to day. One cannot always identify, much less control, all of the fac-

TABLE 10-2. Example of Intensification of a "Conventional" (Fixed Dose) Insulin Treatment Program

61 year old male; 16 years of type 2 diabetes; insulin-treated for 5 years. BMI: 33

(Note: Based only on this information, one could conclude that this patient likely has significant insulin resistance, but with 16 years of diabetes he has significant insulin secretory deficiency as well. As this patient has insulin-treated type 2 diabetes, do not use the formula for type 1 diabetes (0.5 unit/kg actual body weight) in this case. Instead, insulin quantity estimates should be based on actual clinical response to therapy)

Current insulin dose based on fixed-quantity dosing:

Prebreakfast:	14 units of rapid-acting insulin
	36 units of NPH insulin
Presupper	8 units of rapid-acting insulin
Bedtime	12 units of NPH insulin

This patient has unstable glucose patterns, which can be caused by a number of factors. Some, such as variations of activity and food consumption, are identifiable and controllable, but many, such as variations in insulin absorption, food absorption, etc. may not be. The decision has been made to intensify the fixed-dose treatment program by providing algorithmic adjustments of the rapid-acting insulin doses. An example of an initial adjustment algorithm might be:

Intensification of a fixed insulin dose:

Regular or Rapid-acting insulin dose:

Glucose Range	Pre-breakfast	Pre-lunch	Pre-supper	Bedtime
0–50	*		*	
51–100	12		7	
101–150	14		8	
151–200	15		9	
201–250	16		10	
251–300	17		11	
301–400	18		12	
>400	20		14	
Intermediate (NPH) Insulin:	36			12

Note: Insulin amounts are hypothetical examples and should not be applied to specific patients. Determine the insulin quantity by utilizing an estimate based on methods described in the text.

*Eat and test again.

tors that can cause glucose level variations for many patients. Thus, the variable dose of insulin is used to accommodate for these factors, with some glucose values being high, and some low.

However, a sliding scale of this nature should not be used blindly to "fix" all off-target glucose values. For variations in activity or eating that can be identified and quantified before the impact on glucose levels occurs, anticipatory insulin dose adjustments are preferable. For example, if one knows that a large amount of late-day eating will occur, an increase in the morning intermediate insulin dose on that day might be preferable to letting the presupper and/or bedtime glucose level run high and then be corrected by a sliding scale insulin dose.

Similarly, if glucose values at a particular time are consistently off-target, then anticipatory adjustments factors prior to that off-target time should be examined as possible solutions to the problem. Thus, if the fasting glucose were consistently elevated, rather than letting the prebreakfast sliding scale fix the problem after the fact, an assessment of the cause leading up to the fasting reading would be more appropriate. The cause could be insufficient bedtime insulin, or conversely it could be excessive bedtime insulin and nocturnal hypoglycemia and rebound. Food consumption or exercise the day before could play a role as well. Thus, a more appropriate approach to correcting consistently elevated fasting glucose values than relying on the morning sliding scale might be an adjustment of the bedtime insulin based on an assessment of nocturnal glucose patterns, food consumption at night, and activity the day before.

Modifying the Insulin Treatment Program

Insulin treatment programs usually need modification over time. If it were the case that a program could be designed and then left to work for years without attention, diabetes treatment would certainly be a much easier! Beyond the usual day-to-day factors that impact glucose levels, there are multiple factors that can control to change over longer periods of time, necessitating adjustment in the components of a treatment program. Such factors include, but are probably not limited to:

- change from short-acting (regular) insulin to a rapid-acting (aspart, glulisine, or lispro)
- further deterioration in β-cell function

- degree of adherence to the medical nutrition and/or activity programs
- changes in the interval between injection and meals
- deterioration of injection technique or use of insulin that is outdated or has been exposed to extreme temperatures
- incorrect blood monitoring technique, monitoring equipment failure, or outdated monitoring supplies
- changes in lifestyle (timing, activity, stress, food consumption)

  - new job or change in job description/schedule
  - start of school
  - start of a new sports season with participation (ski season, summer tennis, etc.)
  - vacation
  - retirement
  - change in schedule of others in family that affects patient's schedule (e.g., child starting school, spouse starting new job)

- family or work stress (stress leads to increased epinephrine levels that can elevate glucose levels; however, more significantly, stress is a distraction from the self-care routine)
- change of season (subtle changes in activity and schedule often occur — such as going from winter evenings spent sitting, to spring evenings spent watching a child play little league baseball.)
- tasks that may be unrecognized as causing significant increases in physical exertion (ex: holidays with more exertion shopping in stores or a mall)
- birth of a child (more pronounced effect usually seen with the first child!)
- change of social habits (cessation of cigarette smoking, alcohol consumption, or drug use)
- menstrual periods
- pregnancy
- menarche/menopause
- illness or injury
- development of gastroparesis or other causes of erratic GI function

Patients should be encouraged to take an active role in the adjustment of their insulin doses. With proper education, many can provide valuable insight into the need for, and degree of, adjustment. A properly trained patient can help identify factors such as those listed above that might be affecting glucose control. Whether a patient actually adjusts his or her own doses — the preferred scenario — or just recognizes when adjustments are needed and the possible reasons for that need, he or she should be part of the process.

With proper instruction, people with diabetes can make dose adjustments themselves. Generally, they should be instructed not to adjust the insulin doses by more than 2 units at a time and not to make such changes too often without a review with the healthcare provider. The ability to self-adjust insulin doses, and the specific parameters allowed for self-adjustment before contacting the healthcare team, should be based on individual ability and interest. Some people can and will make many changes themselves, while others need the help of their physician, nurse practitioner, physician assistant, or diabetes educator.

When patients are properly taught insulin dose adjustment, many can intelligently establish their own insulin dosing program. The traditional approach to adjusting a fixed dose program has been to change the dose of insulin when abnormal blood glucose values are noted at a particular time for three days in a row. For example, if hyperglycemia occurs at suppertime for 3 days, it would be recommended to increase the morning dose of NPH insulin. However, with the increased complexity of the adjustment algorithms, patients must have a better understanding of the dynamics of insulin action, how various insulins overlap and interact, and the relationship of insulin dosing to food and activity. For people using such treatment programs, a session or two with a diabetes educator to review adjustment principles as well as work through some examples would be quite valuable. Ultimately, the solution to high or low glucose levels is often not as simple as just adjusting an insulin dose.

Special adjustment situations are "sick days." During days of sickness, extra doses of rapid-acting insulin may need to be administered in addition to the usual insulin dosing program. Guidelines for managing sick days can be found in Chapter 12.

Rebound Hyperglycemia

One of the more confusing phenomena in insulin treatment is the rebound hyperglycemia that follows a hypoglycemic event. If the glucose level drops either too low (usually under 60 mg/dl or so, but the actual level can vary) or too precipitously, it can trigger the counterregulatory mechanism. This mechanism consists of production of the counter-insulin hormones glucagon and epinephrine which mobilize release of stored glucose from muscle and liver into the bloodstream to raise the glucose level. This rise in glucose, known as the "rebound," can lead to subsequent hyperglycemia. The classic symptoms of hypoglycemia — shakiness, sweatiness, etc. — are more the result of the epinephrine effect than a direct result of the hypoglycemia. It is only if the glucose level drops extremely low — to about 20 mg/dl or below — that the direct effect of hypoglycemia will be felt — the neuroglycopenia that results in mental status changes.

If a hypoglycemic reaction is symptomatic and recognized, then the subsequent hyperglycemia can be interpreted properly by the patient. However, the symptoms of hypoglycemia may not always be recognized. People may sleep through them, may confuse them with the effects of exercise, or just may have lost the ability to develop classic hypoglycemic symptoms in the first place. The latter phenomenon, known as **"hypoglycemic unawareness,"** can be seen with long-standing diabetes and a decrease in, or loss of, the ability to actively secrete the counterregulatory hormones. Also, the smoother insulin action patterns that are obtained through the use of the newer more physiologic insulin replacement programs (not just those discussed in Chapter 11 but even conventional programs are designed to be more physiologically correct) often lead to more gentle drops in glucose levels which may not be precipitous enough to effectively stimulate counterregulatory symptoms.

Keep in mind, as well, that some of the hyperglycemia following a hypoglycemic event may result from overtreatment of the hypoglycemic reaction. Patients need to be instructed in appropriate reaction treatments so that overtreatment of hyperglycemia is minimized.

Therefore, when trying to determine the cause of hyperglycemia, one must determine whether or not it is due to insufficient insulin quantity, or excessive insulin quantity causing hypoglycemia and rebound. It is important to determine which the cause is. If there is insufficient insulin, *more* needs to be given. However, the proper adjustment for hypoglycemia and resultant rebound is a *reduction* in the insulin dose to eliminate the hypoglycemic reaction. In these circumstances, it is important to resist the temptation to increase the insulin dose in response to the hyperglycemia. Doing so would just make the situation worse.

Adjustment Guidelines

The "Guidelines for Insulin Adjustment," which can be found in Table 10-3A–F, outline insulin adjustment guidelines for commonly used insulin treatment programs described earlier in this chapter. While these tables do not outline every possible situation or adjustment consideration, they do reflect the thought process needed to determine a dose adjustment. The traditional teaching described above, which would dictate insulin adjustments should be made for a glucose test result that is off target for 3 days in a row, is not necessarily the best approach in this era of pattern recognition. It is often wise to wait longer, particularly if the aberration in glucose level is not great or dangerous and if other extenuating events could be playing a role. Also, if an algorithmic adjustment program is used, more time should be given to assess efficacy at the many dosing levels.

Also, keep in mind that these guidelines are somewhat simplistic instructions to address what is really a fairly complex dynamic interaction among insulin and the various other factors influencing glucose control. In fact, these guidelines specifically ignore the many non-insulin factors that can contribute to deterioration of an insulin treatment program. Implicitly, they suggest that if a glucose level does not come out right, it is the insulin that needs to be fixed. Of course, this is often far from the truth. DO NOT forget about the many other factors discussed earlier in the chapter that may be playing a role.

Do not let patients be caught in the trap of thinking that all problems with an off-target glucose level at a particular time relate to *one* specific insulin dose. This assumption fails to capture the complex reality of overlapping insulin action patterns. Adjustment rules such as those in this volume must address the potential role that multiple insulin doses may play in aberrant glucose levels.

This complexity stems from the fact that an insulin does not work *at its peak time*, but rather builds to its peak, and then peters out. Thus, it can have considerable hypoglycemic effect both before and after the peak. If one fails to recognize the real insulin action distribution, errors in adjustment are likely. For example, if prelunch hypoglycemia is a problem and one assumes that this is due solely to morning regular insulin, one may reduce or even eliminate this dose. Yet, the morning *intermediate* insulin may be playing a role in the hypoglycemia as well, particularly if the morning dose is given quite early in the morning. Thus, a balanced adjustment of both insulins may be more effective in solving this type of problem.

Insulin action is just not as simple as people would like to think, and if one becomes wedded only to simple adjustment guidelines, there is a tendency to follow the primrose path to poorly balanced insulin doses. Indeed, not only might they use such unbalanced doses, but they may believe that they have proven that other dosing plans or insulin ratios will not work. Properly conceptualizing insulin action and dose interactions is crucial if proper adjustment, design, and control are to be achieved. It is for these reasons that there is a sense now that the more physiologic insulin replacement programs using a basal insulin and prandial coverage are easier to use. While they involve more frequent dosing, it is often easier to sort out which insulin needs adjustment for a given problem.

The goal today is to focus on glucose patterns. To do so effectively requires conscientious self-checking of glucose levels and careful recording of the results. The computerized memories that are built into some meters often fail to provide easy input of information recording the daily life-events that must also be considered in interpreting glucose patterns. Handwritten records that include glucose levels, insulin doses, and comments on daily event variations still can provide the best visualization of the patterns for dose analysis and adjustments.

Having spent the last few paragraphs outlining the precautions to take when using the Adjustment Guidelines, it is still important to understand the basic action patterns of the various insulins. Onset and peak times are listed in Chapter 9, as are some diagrams of insulin action patterns. The overlap seen on such diagrams can be used to emphasize to patients that off-target glucose levels at times of dual or triple insulin dose effect may be influenced by any of these insulin doses. Corrective action may mean adjustments of any one of these insulins that act at that time. However, to further complicate things, each of those insulins also has effects at other times. Adjustment may fix the problem of immediate concern, but doing so could create another problem at one of those other action times, leading to the need for further dose adjustments. It is a series of overlapping action patterns, all interdependent! Sometimes it seems that the more you adjust, the more you seem to be chasing your tail!

TABLE 10-3.   Guidelines for Insulin Adjustment

Guidelines in this table apply to insulin adjustment only. Always consider non-insulin factors such as food consumption and activity as well in troubleshooting glucose levels that are not at target.

A. Present dose: INTERMEDIATE NPH insulin given before breakfast

If blood glucose results are consistently off-target at this time:	consider the following action
High or low before supper	Adjust the morning NPH insulin. If the prelunch and presupper values are high, consider adding regular or rapid-acting in the morning, and reducing the morning NPH. If the prelunch is low and presupper is high, consider hypoglycemia and rebound hyperglycemia at suppertime.
High or low before breakfast, but on target presupper	Consider using an evening insulin dose.
High prelunch, but better presupper	Consider using a morning mixed insulin dose. Morning NPH insulin may need reduction, particularly with use of regular, but also likely with use of a rapid-acting insulin.
Low prelunch	Reduce the morning NPH insulin. Once done, an evening dose, or even a morning mixed dose, may become necessary. One could also consider a midmorning snack.

B. Present dose: mixture of REGULAR OR RAPID-ACTING AND INTERMEDIATE NPH INSULINS given before breakfast

If blood glucose results are consistently off target at this time:	consider the following action
High or low before supper	Adjust the morning NPH insulin If prelunch is also high, adjust morning regular or rapid-acting insulin. If prelunch is low, consider rebound hyperglycemia at suppertime—may need reduction of either morning insulin, then possibly an evening dose when less morning insulin is being used.

High or low before breakfast, but on target presupper	Consider using an evening insulin dose of NPH.
High prelunch, but better presupper	Consider increasing the morning regular or rapid-acting insulin dose. If using rapid-acting insulin, check 1–2 hours postbreakfast and adjust accordingly. Consider increasing the morning NPH insulin if postbreakfast level is on target.
Low prelunch	Reduce the morning regular or rapid-acting insulin. If using rapid-acting insulin, check 1–2 hours postbreakfast and adjust accordingly. Consider also reducing the morning NPH insulin. If this occurs, an evening dose of NPH insulin may be necessary.

C. Present dose: INTERMEDIATE NPH INSULIN given before breakfast and again before supper

If blood glucose results are consistently off target at this time:	consider the following action
High or low before supper	Adjust the morning NPH insulin. If the prelunch and presupper values are high, consider adding regular or rapid-acting insulin in the morning, and reducing the morning NPH. If the prelunch is low and presupper is high, consider hypoglycemia and rebound.
High or low before breakfast, but on target presupper	Adjust the evening insulin dose. If supper and bedtime are high, consider using a mixed dose at suppertime.
High prelunch, but better presupper	Consider using a morning mixed insulin dose. If so, morning NPH insulin may need reduction.
Low prelunch	Reduce the morning NPH insulin. Once done, the evening dose, or even a morning and/or evening mixed dose, may become necessary.

High at bedtime, but on target fasting	If using presupper NPH insulin dose, may need presupper mixed dose. If bedtime intermediate dose, consider moving it to suppertime, or, preferentially, adding a third daily injection with regular or rapid-acting insulin at suppertime. If using regular insulin at supper with marked post-supper hyperglycemia, consider changing to rapid-acting insulin.
Low at bedtime, but on target fasting	If supper NPH insulin dose, reduce dose. This may result in elevated fasting level, in which case moving the dose to bedtime may help. This may be the best first adjustment anyway. May eventually need NPH at bedtime and then a third daily injection with regular or rapid-acting insulin at suppertime.

D. Present dose: mixture of REGULAR OR RAPID-ACTING and INTERMEDIATE NPH INSULINS given before breakfast and INTERMEDIATE NPH INSULIN given at supper or bedtime

If blood glucose results are consistently off target at this time:	consider the following action
High or low before supper	Adjust morning NPH insulin. If prelunch is also high, increase morning regular or rapid-acting insulin. If prelunch is low and presupper high, consider rebound hyperglycemia at suppertime—may need reduction of either morning insulin, then possibly increase of evening dose when less morning insulin is being used.
High prebreakfast, but evenings on target	Increase evening insulin dose. Rule out nocturnal hypoglycemia/ rebound, which would call for a reduced evening dose.

Low prebreakfast, but on target presupper	Reduce evening insulin dose
High prelunch, but better presupper	Consider increasing the morning regular or rapid-acting insulin dose. If using rapid-acting insulin, check 1–2 hours postbreakfast and adjust accordingly. Consider increasing the morning NPH insulin if postbreakfast level is on target.
Low prelunch	Reduce the morning regular insulin. If using rapid-acting insulin, consider also reducing the morning NPH insulin. If this is done, increase in evening dose of NPH insulin may be necessary.
High at bedtime, but on target fasting	If NPH insulin is presupper, change to mixed dose. If bedtime NPH dose, consider moving it to presupper or, preferentially, keep it at bedtime and add presupper regular or rapid-acting insulin. If using regular insulin at supper, consider changing to rapid-acting insulin.
Low at bedtime, but on target fasting	If supper NPH insulin dose, reduce dose. If this elevates fasting levels, move supper NPH dose to bedtime. If bedtime dose initially, reduce morning NPH insulin dose. May ultimately benefit from the more physiologic control from a more significant reduction in morning NPH, and addition of supper regular or rapid-acting insulin. Rapid-acting insulin would be less likely to extend through and cause later hypoglycemia than regular insulin, so this choice may be preferable.

E. Present dose: mixture of REGULAR OR RAPID-ACTING AND INTERMEDIATE NPH INSULINS given before breakfast and at suppertime

If blood glucose results are consistently off target at this time:	consider the following action
High or low before supper	Adjust morning intermediate NPH insulin. If prelunch is also high, increase morning regular or rapid-acting insulin. If prelunch is low, consider rebound hyperglycemia at suppertime—may need reduction of either morning insulin, then possibly increase of evening dose when less morning insulin is being used.
High prebreakfast, but evenings on target	Increase evening NPH insulin dose. If bedtime is also high, increase presupper regular or rapid-acting insulin dose. Rule out nocturnal hypoglycemia/ rebound, which would call for a reduced evening dose.
Low prebreakfast, but on target at bedtime	Reduce evening NPH insulin dose
High prelunch, but better presupper	Consider increasing the morning regular or rapid-acting insulin dose. If using rapid-acting insulin, check 1–2 hours postbreakfast and adjust accordingly. Consider increasing the morning NPH insulin if postbreakfast level is on target.
Low prelunch	Reduce the morning regular or rapid-acting insulin. If using rapid-acting insulin, consider also reducing the morning NPH insulin. If this is done, an increase in presupper dose of regular or rapid-acting insulin may be necessary.
High at bedtime, but on target fasting	Increase suppertime regular or rapid-acting insulin. If nocturnal hypoglycemia then occurs, consider moving NPH only to bedtime, keeping regular or rapid-acting

insulin presupper. If using regular insulin at supper and there is marked post-supper hyperglycemia, consider changing to rapid-acting insulin.

Low at bedtime, but on target fasting	Reduce presupper regular or rapid-acting insulin dose. If this elevates fasting levels, move supper NPH dose to bedtime.

F. Present dose: mixture of REGULAR OR RAPID-ACTING AND INTERMEDIATE NPH INSULINS given before breakfast, REGULAR OR RAPID-ACTING INSULIN presupper, and INTERMEDIATE NPH INSULIN at bedtime

If blood glucose results are consistently off target at this time:	consider the following action
High or low before supper	Adjust morning NPH insulin. If prelunch is also high, increase morning regular or rapid-acting insulin. If prelunch is low, consider rebound hyperglycemia at suppertime—may need reduction of either morning insulin, then possibly increase of evening dose when less morning insulin is being used.
High prebreakfast, but evenings on target	Increase bedtime NPH insulin dose. If bedtime is also high, increase regular or rapid-acting insulin dose at suppertime. Rule out nocturnal hypoglycemia/rebound, which would call for reduced evening doses, or use of rapid-acting insulin, if the longer tails of regular insulin are implicated in the nocturnal hypoglycemia.
Low prebreakfast, but on target at bedtime	Reduce bedtime NPH insulin dose
High prelunch, but better presupper	Consider increasing the morning regular or rapid-acting insulin dose. If using rapid-acting insulin, check 1–2 hours post-breakfast and adjust accordingly. Consider increasing the morning NPH insulin if post-breakfast level is on target.

Low prelunch	Reduce the morning regular or rapid-acting insulin. If using rapid-acting insulin, consider also reducing the morning NPH insulin. If this is done, increase in evening dose of regular or rapid-acting insulin may be necessary.
High at bedtime, but on target fasting	Increase suppertime regular or rapid-acting insulin. If nocturnal hypoglycemia then occurs reduce bedtime NPH dose. If using regular insulin presupper (with longer tail), consider changing to rapid-acting insulin.
Low at bedtime, but on target fasting	Reduce presupper regular or rapid-acting insulin dose. If this elevates fasting levels, increase bedtime NPH dose.

Redesigning an Insulin Program

For the reasons stated above, many diabetes specialists approach the frustrating situation of a patient who has poorly balanced patterns by just starting from scratch! Using tried and true dosing schedules outlined in this chapter and the next, the specialist will often redesign the program from the ground up! In redesigning a patient's program, formulas mentioned earlier that should be kept in mind for the patient with type 1 diabetes include:

- 0.5 unit per/kg body weight per day
- For split/mix type programs (2 or 3 injection varieties) use two-thirds of the daily total in the morning, one-third at night, with one-third at each time as regular or rapid-acting insulin and the remainder as intermediate acting insulin. (Other such formulas will be provided in the next chapter.)

Using such basic assumptions, you can restart the program and begin fine-tuning doses over again.

Alternatively, another approach may be tried: When a program that worked previously deteriorates for no obvious reason and numerous adjustments have been made, it is often difficult to determine what dynamic is really affecting the control pattern. Return to the *original* program that had worked initially, and start over again! (This advice is useful for both the conventional type programs discussed in this chapter and the physiologic insulin replacement programs discussed in the next chapter)

With good records that provide daily data and with the mind-set that there is a complex dynamic of insulin action that has to be balanced, appropriate insulin adjustments can be made with some success.

11

Physiologic Insulin Treatment Programs

Richard S. Beaser, MD,
Osama Hamdy, MD and
Howard Wolpert, MD

It can be argued, in this era of diabetes treatment that follows results from studies such as the DCCT, that we no longer need to separate discussions of insulin treatment into a chapter on "conventional" therapy and a chapter on physiologic "intensive" insulin therapy. The results of the DCCT and other similar studies suggest that physiologic insulin replacement therapy does reduce the risk of long-term diabetes complications. Thus, implicitly, *all* insulin therapy should be physiologic therapy.

While this theoretical argument makes sense based on results of such studies, the realities of clinical practice make it obvious that not all patients can self-manage physiologic insulin therapy, nor do all patients need it to achieve desired treatment goals. Studies such as the DCCT were "intent-to-treat" trials, and the finding of complication-risk reduction was based on treatment group analysis. However, the implicit conclusion from this study, and results of other studies, suggest that optimizing diabetes control as measured by the A1C should be the objective of therapy.

For each patient, it is important to determine how much "intensity" of physiologic replacement is needed in the program they use. Many approach this decision with this goal: Achieve the best A1C possible, using a treatment program that the patient is able to self-manage and that is safe.

What Is Physiologic Insulin Therapy?

Physiologic (in the past referred to as "intensive") insulin therapy is treatment using exogenous insulin in a manner that attempts to mimic normal endogenous insulin secretory patterns of basal and postprandial insulin secretion. The treatment program must include the following components in order to provide physiologic insulin replacement therapy:

- It must consist of multiple ($\geq$3) daily administrations of insulin doses.
- It must provide for the basal insulin effect. This is usually provided by injections of peakless basal insulin or by a constant infusion of rapid-acting insulin from an insulin pump. It could be provided by multiple injections of intermediate (NPH) insulin, but this is often less optimal.
- It must provide incremental insulin bolus doses covering food consumption by utilizing regular or rapid-acting insulin. The doses of this insulin vary, based on:
  - The results of glucose checks as part of a self-monitoring of blood glucose (SMBG) program
  - Food: type, quantity and timing
  - Physical activity: quantity, timing, frequency

It took a number of developments in diabetes treatment occurring simultaneously, beginning in the 1980s, to pave the way for the development of what we now refer to as physiologic insulin therapy. Key among these developments were:

- the glycohemoglobin (A1C) measurement
- self-monitoring of blood glucose
- human insulin and insulin analogues

A1C provides an easy measurement of the results of treatment that not only reflects glucose control, but probably also provides a gauge of the risk of complication development. Without the A1C, it would be impossible to measure the effect of intensive therapy and, frankly, it would be impossible to prove that it was worthwhile.

SMBG allows close examination of daily glucose patterns while patients live in their normal environments and with their normal lifestyle. It also provides the data needed to assess the interrelations of insulin action, food, and activity, and to determine the amount of insulin needed for variable-dose treatment programs.

The newer insulins that have been developed in the last two decades have allowed us to design insulin treatment programs that more closely mimic normal physiologic patterns of insulin action. The synthetic human insulins decrease antigenicity, which results in more precision with regard to action-times. Each insulin's action occurs more precisely during the anticipated timeframe, resulting in less dose overlap, less prolongation of action, and less confusion as to which insulin is exerting its effect at any given time.

The most recent advance is the development of insulin analogues. These altered insulins can be used to construct insulin treatment programs that even more precisely resemble natural patterns. The insulin peaks of the rapid-acting insulins (aspart, glulisine, and lispro) more closely match the times that food absorption is occurring. Long-acting peakless basal insulin effects produced by newer analogues such as glargine and detemir (which have replaced ultralente, used in the past) are smoother and more predictable. When used together, these insulins result in treatments that produce action patterns that come quite close to endogenous secretion.

Physiologic insulin therapy uses either multiple daily injections (MDI) of insulin or insulin infusion pumps, which provide a continuous subcutaneous insulin infusion (CSII). Prior to each meal, a measurement of blood glucose is performed. The glucose level obtained and the planned food to be eaten are used to determine the dose of regular or rapid-acting insulin that is administered prior to food consumption. The goal is to target normoglycemia and thus achieve an optimal glycohemoglobin level.

Conventional therapy uses a dose of insulin that is essentially unchanged from day to day. It is based on the assumption that each day is metabolically close enough to the previous days that a fixed dose of insulin is sufficient to achieve optimal control. Physiologic insulin replacement therapies, on the other hand, utilize premeal insulin doses that are adjusted based on the blood glucose level at the time of injection and on anticipated food consumption and activity. Such programs are based on the assumption that each day does not resemble the previous days and that adaptations must be made to maintain stable, targeted glucose levels.

Physiologic insulin replacement therapy is not really a different treatment of diabetes; rather, it is a different way of using the same therapies employed in conventional treatments. As a result, there are not clear dividing lines between conventional therapy, intensified conventional therapy, and physiologic insulin replacement therapies. These are merely labels for ranges on the spectrum of physiologic insulin replacement. In reality, treatments are individualized, and what may seem to be an "intense" effort to maintain normal insulin physiology in terms of effort and self-management skills for one patient may seem conventional and rudimentary for another patient. Thus, the evolution to the term "physiologic insulin replacement therapy" is considered by most to be a better description of what these programs are all about than the previous term, "intensive insulin therapy."

Why Physiologic Therapy Makes Sense

As outlined at the beginning of Chapter 9, the earliest forms of insulin were regular insulins that had a short action-time and needed to be administered several times a day. The longer-acting insulins that were developed later sought to ameliorate symptoms of hyperglycemia while providing an easier dosing program for patients. However, arguments raged as to whether symptom elimination alone was enough, or whether "tight" control should be the treatment mode to successfully avoid long-term complications. Clearly, these simplified programs using longer-acting insulins did not effectively mimic natural insulin action patterns. Physicians recommended multiple injections per day rather than just one daily injection of intermediate (NPH or lente) insulin for patients with type 1 diabetes. Many used programs with regular plus intermediate insulin ("split-mix") given in the morning and in the evening (Figure 10-3).

Although these physicians may not have fully appreciated it, these multiple injection programs were coming closer to mimicking normal pancreatic insulin "basal/bolus" secretory patterns (see Figure 11-1). One

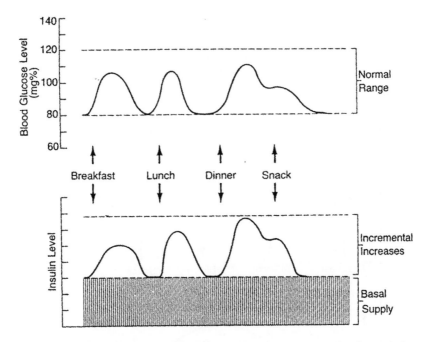

Figure 11-1. Blood glucose and insulin patterns in a person who does not have diabetes.

injection of intermediate insulin, peaking 6 to 12 hours after injection, does not produce this natural pattern (see Figure 11-2).

Some people with type 1 diabetes, and many with type 2 diabetes, still have some endogenous insulin secretory capacity remaining, so that simplified injection programs lead to targeted glucose levels. In the person with type 2 diabetes in particular, a program such as bedtime intermediate insulin and daytime coverage with antidiabetes medications can often achieve successful control. Yet, as discussed in the previous chapter, the focus on controlling postprandial hyperglycemia has lead to the consideration of initiation of prandial insulin coverage earlier in the natural history of type 2 diabetes if non-insulin therapies are ineffective in doing so.

The backbone of a conventional insulin therapy program is one of anticipation — a dose of insulin is given in anticipation of the insulin needs over the next 6 or 12 hours. For this to work, however, all of the fac-

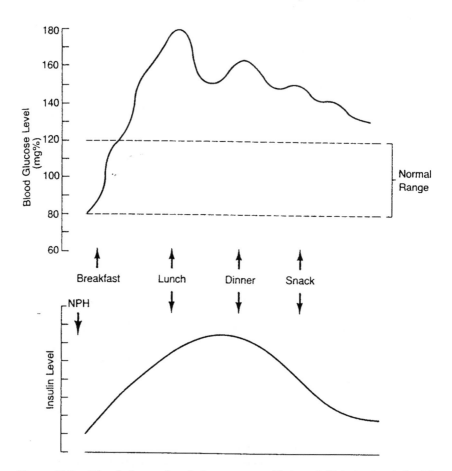

Figure 11-2. Blood glucose levels in a person with type 1 diabetes treated with one morning injection of NPH (intermediate-acting) insulin.

tors that affect blood glucose levels must be relatively predictable — consistent eating habits and predictable activity. In addition, since all factors influencing glucose levels cannot be identified, much less controlled, some endogenous secretory capability must remain if recommended glucose control is to be achieved. This is particularly true if postprandial glucose levels are to be on target.

Eventually, though, such individuals may lose much of their insulin secretory ability, and more physiologic dosing programs should then be recommended. While conventional therapy is an anticipatory program, intensified conventional and true physiologic (intensive) insulin treatment programs are responsive programs. The ability to be responsive is another characteristic of a normal pancreas. A pancreas has the ability to constantly measure glucose levels and modulate insulin production accordingly. The pancreas of someone with diabetes obviously cannot do this, and through SMBG, plus adjustment for food intake and activity, the individual with diabetes using physiologic insulin replacement therapy tries to replace this pancreatic function through his or her own efforts at self-care.

Patient Selection for Use of Physiologic Insulin Replacement Therapy

In the late 1980s, people felt that "intensive insulin therapy" was a complicated program that was not for everyone. It was typically thought that conventional therapy could adequately control the blood glucose of most patients with type 1 diabetes and all patients with type 2 diabetes. The prevailing belief was that no one who was newly diagnosed should even consider intensive therapy. Certainly most thought that for patients with frequent hypoglycemia or hypoglycemic unawareness intensive therapy was contraindicated. Intensive insulin therapy was reserved for those with long-standing diabetes or diabetes that was so unstable that no matter what was done, no matter how well patients tried to control all the variables affecting glucose levels, they could not even come close to safe or adequate control.

Many health professionals still believe that the views described above are correct. However, while they might be applicable to some patients, the thinking on intensive — physiologic — therapy has changed markedly in the last decade. Compelling reasons to undertake treatment using physiologic insulin replacement patterns, or indications for intensification of a conventional insulin therapy program to make it more responsive and physiologic, are summarized in the box below.

In light of the findings of the many studies demonstrating the benefits of achieving A1C levels at or below 7%, many people are making attempts do so. For patients with erratic patterns, either due to lifestyle issues or inherent instability, physiologic therapy is the only way to achieve such goals safely. In the 1980s healthcare professionals still were of the mind-set that to improve control, they needed to give their patients more and more insulin. Intensive therapy was merely a means to do so systematically.

However, throughout the 1990s and into the new millennium, people have come to recognize that physiologic insulin replacement therapy is really an approach to insulin treatment design that allows a more accurate reproduction of natural insulin patterns. It does not necessarily mandate more insulin, but, if more insulin is needed to lower glucose levels, it provides a means to give that insulin more safely.

In addition, the nature of the basal/bolus approach, with emphasis on shorter-acting insulins, allows more frequent adjustments of significant portions of the insulin effect. Thus, it maximizes the flexibility of lifestyle that can occur while maintaining targeted glucose levels.

Clearly, the complexity of physiologic therapy is contraindicated for those who cannot handle it, and a discussion of such issues can be found below. However, many people prefer the flexibility that such a program provides. For example, active young people who are newly diagnosed may prefer a program using four daily injections that allows the typical lifestyle of a college student to continue with minimal interference. People with type 2 diabetes requiring insulin, who work jobs with varying schedules or shifts or with unpredictable physical demands, may also choose to

---

Reasons to Utilize Physiologic Insulin Replacement Therapy

- desire to achieve standards of control (ADA, Joslin, European, other)
- desire to avoid erratic patterns
- desire for flexibility of lifestyle
- concerns regarding safety with non-physiologic treatments
- desire to optimally control postprandial hyperglycemia
- only able to achieve suboptimal control with non-physiologic treatments

adopt such a program because of the convenience and flexibility it provides.

Today, few believe that physiologic insulin replacement therapy is reserved for rocket scientists or those of that ilk, and recognize that the benefit of using physiologic insulin replacement programs can be offered to those who may not, with all due respect, quite qualify for NASA! It can be refreshingly amazing to see who takes to a physiologic insulin replacement program: some older individuals, some salt-of-the-earth types, some with minimal education, some children (with much help from their parents). Therefore, patient selection *must* be individualized, based on the criteria provided below.

Physiologic insulin replacement therapy is not contraindicated in those with hypoglycemic unawareness or for whom severe hypoglycemia might be harmful. In fact, it might be *indicated* in such people. Properly designed physiologic insulin replacement programs come closer to mimicking natural insulin secretory patterns and are therefore *less* likely to lead to hypoglycemia. Further, if they did cause hypoglycemia, since the insulin effect is spread out over more injections, the severity of the hypoglycemic reaction would be reduced.

In such cases, it is not the physiologic design of the insulin replacement program that needs to be changed, it may be just the glucose goals. If a patient wants to avoid frequent and significant hypoglycemia, he or she may adopt physiologic therapy, but set slightly higher glucose levels as targeted goals so as to maintain proper safety.

Key Considerations

There are several key considerations for selecting patients for physiologic insulin therapy. More is required of patients undertaking full physiologic insulin replacement programs than of those intensifying a conventional program by introducing an adjustment algorithm. In general, patients need:

- knowledge, judgment, skill, and willingness to self-adjust treatment parameters (insulin, food, activity)
- realistic expectations for intensification goals, including glucose and A1C levels, and lifestyle impact

- willingness and ability to:
  - frequently check glucose levels
  - maintain a diabetes monitoring program which includes detailed records of glucose levels, insulin doses, and lifestyle events that impact glucose control
  - follow medical nutrition therapy and physical activity plans
- ability to understand the dynamic interrelationships among insulin, food, and activity
- ability to utilize, and have access to, adequate medical support systems for patient care and education

Physiologic Insulin Dosing Schedules

The hallmark of physiologic insulin replacement programs is having the opportunity to adjust the prandial insulin (rapid-acting or regular) insulin doses on multiple occasions each day based on the results of frequent blood glucose checks that are part of an aggressive diabetes monitoring program, and/or in anticipation of food quantity to be consumed, targeting specific glucose levels. While most programs are similar conceptually in terms of the prandial insulin dosing, the various means of providing the basal insulin supply typically differentiates one program from another. For programs using insulin injections, basal insulin is usually provided by one of the long-acting peakless basal insulins (glargine or detemir) given according to one of the schedules that are in common usage, some of which are listed below. For insulin pump programs, which provide constant insulin infusions, the basal insulin is provided by a continuous infusion of rapid-acting insulin.

Multiple doses of intermediate insulin have also been used to provide basal insulin supplies, more so in the past before we had the peakless basal insulins available. While NPH can still work well as a basal insulin for some people, the ease of the new peakless basal insulins has lead to a predominance of usage of these insulins as injected basal insulin. Nevertheless, at times there is a need for marked variation in the basal insulin levels. Pumps are the best at accomplishing this goal. However, if the patient is not a pump candidate, multiple NPH injections could be utilized with varying doses leading to differing basal insulin levels. Alternatively,

---

Practical Means of Providing Basal Insulin in a Physiologic Insulin Replacement Program (MDI Programs)

For programs using insulin injections:
- Insulin glargine or detemir given at bedtime or before breakfast, once daily
- Insulin detemir or glargine given twice daily, before breakfast and at bedtime/or before supper
- NPH given before breakfast, before supper, and at bedtime
- NPH given in small doses before each meal, and a larger dose of NPH at bedtime

For insulin pump programs:
- A constant infusion of rapid-acting insulin

---

detemir, which has a slightly shorter duration of action in many people, if given twice daily, can provide crude variations in the basal insulin levels during parts of the day through the use of differing doses.

Each of these programs has advantages and disadvantages. One difference occurs in the control of the fasting glucose levels, particularly for those patients who experience a prominent **"dawn phenomenon."** The dawn phenomenon is a rise in glucose levels that increases insulin requirements in many people during the latter part of the nightly sleep cycle. Changes in contra-insulin hormone levels, such as growth hormone, increase insulin requirements at this time of day. People who do not have diabetes can secrete the extra insulin, but people requiring injected insulin may need to adjust the dose or timing of insulin injection to compensate for this increased insulin need.

In particular, if a person has a prominent dawn phenomenon, and using detemir with higher doses in the evening than in the morning does not work, then perhaps an NPH program might be helpful. Conversely, programs using glargine or detemir as basal insulins can be very effective at smoothing out variable glucose patterns and allow timing flexibility.

Insulin pumps utilize a continuous subcutaneous insulin infusion (CSII) that comes closest to mimicking normal insulin secretory patterns. Their capacity for the use of alternative basal doses can also be useful for patients who have difficulty controlling fasting glucose levels, particularly if these elevations are the result of a significant dawn phenomenon.

Estimating Starting Doses

When estimating starting doses for these programs, the total daily amount of insulin can be determined based on either the total amount used with the previous program or by one of the standard estimates of the daily number of units of insulin per kilogram of body weight. Use the lower amount if the amount of insulin used in the previous treatment program is lower than that which was calculated by the body weight method, unless the patient was significantly underinsulinized. If the amount calculated by the body weight method is lower than the amount used in the previous program, particularly if the patient may be overweight or have insulin resistance, then use the actual amount of the previous program or a dose in between the two. If weight loss is desired, the revision of the treatment program can be an opportunity to work on weight loss, and a revision of the nutrition plan.

It is important to note that rapid-acting or regular insulin doses, listed in the discussion of specific dosage patterns below, are for glucose levels in the targeted range, or about 100 to 150 mg/dl. Algorithmic adjustments can be stepped up or down by amounts such as 1 or more units for every 50 to100 mg/dl glucose level increment. Actual increments and adjustments are usually dependent on total daily insulin amount. Alternative methods of adjusting insulin can also be quite effective. Increasing numbers of people are now using a program referred to as "carbohydrate counting," which bases premeal insulin dose adjustments on the amount of carbohydrate consumed. Such programs usually also utilize a correction or sensitivity factor to add a further dose adjustment to compensate for a high or low blood glucose level.

Specific comments on each of these insulin patterns are provided below. Details for estimating insulin doses assume the calculations described above, unless otherwise noted. Advantages and disadvantages of each pattern are also provided. Be aware also that distribution of carbohydrates in the patient's diet may affect the standard 40%-30%-30% premeal insulin distribution noted in these examples, when carbohydrate counting is not utilized.

Descriptions of Basal Insulin Patterns

Below are descriptions of commonly-used basal insulin patterns.

1 A. Use of Peakless Basal Insulin once daily, at bedtime (Figure 11-3)

An alternative timing would be at suppertime. For once daily dosing, Insulin Glargine is theoretically preferable over insulin detemir, which has a shorter duration of action, but many report the in the clinical arena the differences in the duration are not significant, particularly at higher doses.

- ◆ **Guidelines for estimating doses:**
  - Approximately 25%–50% of daily total as insulin glargine or detemir, given at bedtime.
  - Premeal (prandial) insulin (rapid-acting or regular insulin) total is the remaining 50%–75% of the daily total, distributed as 40% before breakfast, 30% before lunch, and 30% before supper.
  - The dose of basal insulin at bedtime may need to be increased if fasting glucose levels are elevated (dawn phenomenon), or adjusted above or below the 50% ratio relative to rapid-acting or regular insulin doses based on actual glucose patterns and hypoglycemia avoidance.
  - When changing from intermediate insulin to glargine or detemir, if the previous dose of intermediate insulin was once daily, then the dose of glargine or detemir can be the same. However, if the dose of intermediate insulin was two or more daily injections, reduce the total daily total when changing to glargine or detemir by approximately 20%, then monitor and adjust as needed.

- ◆ **Advantages:**
  - The basal insulins provide a smoother basal effect than some of the intermediate insulin programs.
  - Simpler means of providing a smooth basal effect than patterns using multiple injections of intermediate insulin.
  - Programs using basal insulins provide moderate flexibility in timing of meals.
  - Very effectively mimics normal physiologic action patterns, particularly when used with one of the rapid-acting insulins.
  - Very effective in controlling the fasting glucose without increasing nocturnal hypoglycemia.

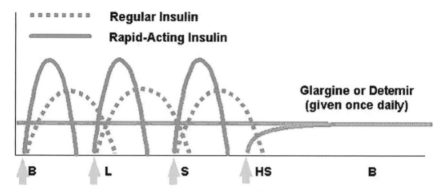

Figure 11-3:   Effect of a program using premeal rapid-acting or regular insulin at each meal, and peakless basal insulin at bedtime.

> – Basal insulins can be given via insulin pens, and also allows use of prandial insulin via insulin pen or prefilled syringe at mealtimes.
> – Less weight gain than NPH-based regimens

♦ **Disadvantages:**
> – Lack of peaking effect may be less effective against prominent dawn phenomenon than intermediate insulins given at bedtime. Detemir, with a slightly greater peak, may be used if peaking action is desired and varying basals daytime vs. nighttime are needed.
> – More difficult to make rapid changes in basal insulin supply for changes in activity, food consumption, and/or timing than a program using frequent injections of NPH or a pump.
> – As these insulins work for up to 24 hours, if dose is adjusted to target a glucose control issue at one particular time, compensatory adjustments in rapid-acting or regular insulin, or alterations in food consumption at other times may be needed to avoid hyper- or hypoglycemia.
> – Contraindicated during pregnancy and therefore cannot be used to provide physiologic insulin replacement pre-conception.

1 B. Use of Peakless Basal Insulin twice daily, given before breakfast and at bedtime/ before supper (Figure 11-4)

Insulin detemir, with the shorter duration of action and data suggesting more predictable action pattern from day to day, would theoretically be the choice with giving basal insulin twice daily. This would be particularly important if the doses were uneven, to provide differing basal rates for day vs. nighttime. In this instance, it is usually given at breakfast and at bedtime, although the second injection can be at suppertime. The goal is to have them approximately 12 hours apart. Insulin glargine has also been given twice daily, particularly if it is felt that in a given patient, it is not lasting the full 24 hours.

- ◆ **Guidelines for estimating doses:**
  - Approximately 50% of daily total as peakless basal insulin, given before breakfast and 12 hours later, either at suppertime or at bedtime.
  - Premeal (prandial) insulin (rapid-acting or regular insulin) total is the remaining 50%–75% of the daily total, distributed as 40% before breakfast, 30% before lunch, and 30% before supper.
  - The PM basal insulin dose may need to be increased if fasting glucose levels are elevated (dawn phenomenon). Either or both doses may be adjusted above or below the 50% ratio relative to rapid-acting or regular insulin doses based on actual glucose patterns and hypoglycemia avoidance.
  - When changing from intermediate insulin to detemir or glargine, if the previous dose of intermediate insulin was once daily, then the dose of detemir or glargine or detemir can be the same. However, if the dose of intermediate insulin was two or more daily injections, reduce the total daily total when changing to detemir or glargine by approximately 20%, then monitor and adjust as needed.

- ◆ **Advantages:**
  - The basal insulins usually provide a smoother basal effect than some of the intermediate insulin programs.
  - The twice-daily dosing of the basal insulin can allow differing basal insulin levels during the night vs. during the day, and with dose adjustments, raise or lower the basal over a shorter time frame than the once daily program.

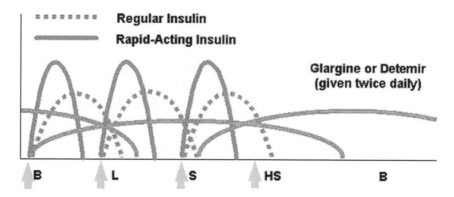

Figure 11-4. Effect of a program using twice daily injection of basal insulin in use with premeal doses of rapid-acting or regular insulin. Slightly unequal doses of the basal insulins can change the basal effect in different parts of the day.

- Simpler means of providing a smooth basal effect than patterns using multiple injections of intermediate insulin.
- Programs using basal insulins provide moderate flexibility in timing of meals.
- Very effectively mimics normal physiologic action patterns, particularly when used with one of the insulins with rapid peaks (rapid-acting insulins).
- Very effective in controlling the fasting glucose without increasing nocturnal hypoglycemia.
- Basal insulins can be given via insulin pens, and also allows use of prandial insulin via insulin pen or prefilled syringe at mealtimes.
- Less weight gain and hypoglycemia than NPH-based regimens.

♦ Disadvantages:
- Lack of peaking effect may be less effective against prominent dawn phenomenon than intermediate insulins given at bedtime. Detemir, with a slightly greater peak, may be used if peaking action is desired
- More difficult to make rapid changes in basal insulin supply for changes in activity, food consumption, and/or timing than a program using frequent injections of NPH.

- As these insulins works for 24 hours, if dose is adjusted to target a glucose control issue at one particular time, compensatory adjustments in rapid-acting or regular insulin or food at other times may be needed to avoid hyper- or hypoglycemia.
- Contraindicated during pregnancy and therefore cannot be used to intensify diabetes management pre-conception.

2. Intermediate insulin given before breakfast, a small dose of intermediate insulin given before supper, and a moderate dose of intermediate insulin given at bedtime (Figure 11-5)

Providing basal insulin using NPH was the standard for many years, but now with the availability of peakless basal insulins, NPH-basal programs are not commonly used. However, for patients who need more frequent adjustments of basal insulin effect, these still may be used. There is nothing wrong with these programs, and they may be continued for those who are still using them without difficulty, as long as the A1C is on target, postprandial glucose control is adequate, and there is no evidence of reduced safely. However, for those starting a multidose physiologic program, one of the basal programs described above is usually recommended.

◆ **Guidelines for estimating doses:**
  - Approximately 20%–25% of daily total as bedtime intermediate insulin.
  - Approximately 5%–10% of daily total as suppertime intermediate insulin.
  - Approximately 10%–30% of daily insulin total as morning intermediate insulin.
  - Remaining insulin given as premeal rapid-acting or regular insulin, with dose distributed as 40% of the **total remaining insulin** given before breakfast, 30% before lunch, and 30% before supper. Alternatively, premeal insulin doses can be calculated using carbohydrate counting and sensitivity/correction factor (see later). With a higher dose of morning intermediate insulin, a lesser percent of lunchtime premeal insulin might be used.

◆ **Advantages:**
  - Bedtime intermediate insulin effective against dawn phenomenon.
  - Insulin coverage at midnight can be improved using a small dose

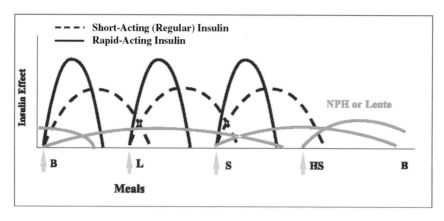

Figure 11-5. **Effect of a program using pre-meal doses of rapid-acting or regular insulin injected before meals, with three injections of NPH insulin, one at breakfast, one at suppertime, and one larger dose at bedtime providing the basal effect.**

    of intermediate insulin mixed with the rapid-acting or regular insulin at suppertime.

– Morning intermediate insulin provides basal effect during the day, which is particularly important when rapid-acting insulins are used before meals.

– Mixed insulin doses are not used at lunchtime, allowing the use of insulin pens.

– Useful for providing physiologic insulin replacement therapy during pregnancy in individuals who do not wish to use pump therapy (glargine and detemir cannot be used during pregnancy).

♦ **Disadvantages:**

– Morning intermediate insulin can peak late in the afternoon, which can have an additive effect on lunchtime premeal insulin, particularly if regular insulin is used. The risk of hypoglycemia can be increased, particularly with variable supper times. Use of lower doses of morning intermediate insulin, with a greater percentage of daily insulin as rapid-acting insulin, can reduce this risk.

- If there is a particularly long period of time between breakfast and supper (e.g., breakfast at 6:00 AM and dinner at 7:00 PM), the effect of the morning intermediate insulin may wane before supper insulin begins to work.
- The action pattern of NPH is not as predictable and consistent from day to day as the basal insulins.

3. **Intermediate insulin given in small doses before each meal, and a larger dose of intermediate insulin at bedtime (Figure 11-6)**

- **Guidelines for estimating doses:**
  - Approximately 20%–25% of daily total as bedtime intermediate insulin.
  - Approximately 25% of remaining total (15%–20% of daily total) given as premeal intermediate insulin, divided as 40% of this amount before breakfast, 30% before lunch, and 30% before supper.
  - Premeal rapid-acting or regular insulin total (daily total minus all of the intermediate doses) distributed as 40% before breakfast, 30% before lunch, and 30% before supper. Alternatively, premeal insulin doses can be calculated using carbohydrate counting and sensitivity/correction factor (see later).

- **Advantages:**
  - Frequent small doses of intermediate insulin during the day mimic basal with smooth effect that can be adjusted up or down at various times of the day by adjusting appropriate intermediate insulin dose.
  - Bedtime intermediate insulin is effective against dawn phenomenon.
  - Insulin coverage going into the nighttime is smooth when a small supper intermediate insulin dose is given to cover the time period between supper rapid-acting or short-acting insulin depletion and bedtime intermediate insulin effect onset (a key issue in particular with the use of rapid-acting insulins with the shortest duration of action).
  - Very effectively mimics normal physiologic action patterns, particularly when used with a rapid-acting insulin.

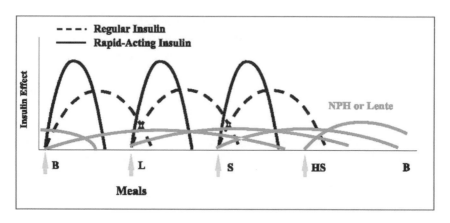

Figure 11-6.   Effect of a program using pre-meal rapid-acting or regular insulin injected before meals, and NPH also given before meals and with a fourth larger injection of NPH at bedtime.

   – Allows a moderate amount of lifestyle flexibility. Insulin doses can be adjusted to compensate for variable quantity and timing of meals and activity.

♦ Disadvantages:
   – Complexity of program makes it difficult for some patients to understand and self-manage.
   – Complexity of program can be difficult for medical professionals to understand (for example: postprandial glucose is affected by premeal prandial insulin (rapid-acting or regular), pre-next-meal affected by previous intermediate, and previous prandial insulin. Post-next meal is affected by premeal intermediate from that previous meal plus current meal prandial insulin, and possibly early onset of that meal's NPH as well).
   – Mixed doses at each meal make it difficult to use insulin pens and necessitates mixing at each dosing time. Inconvenient for those taking insulin away from home or office.
   – The action pattern of NPH is not as predictable and consistent from day to day as the basal insulins.

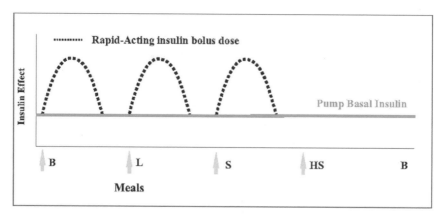

Figure 11-7.   Insulin action pattern seen with insulin pump (continuous subcutaneous insulin infusion or CSII) treatment. For clarity, the effects of basal and bolus dosing are depicted separately.

4. Insulin pump constant infusion of rapid-acting (Figure 11-7)

♦ **Guidelines for estimating doses:**
There are a number of approaches to determining pump doses. One is the traditional method using estimated doses and an adjustment algorithm. More recently, methods based on carbohydrate counting have become popular. Still others may use methods that use components of both approaches. Unlike the guidelines for multiple injection programs, determining pump doses is best not done by rote formula and better accomplished by a medical professional who is experienced with pump use and can individualize the method he or she finds most comfortable and which fits the needs of the patient. With these concerns in mind, the guidelines listed below are more of an outline of what healthcare professionals familiar with pump therapy may do, rather than providing firm recommendations for a treatment approach.

– **Total Daily Dose (TDD) [two methods of calculation]**
  ▪ *Method One:* Determination based on reducing pre-pump total daily dose by 20%–25%. If underinsulinized prior to pump start, reduce by less.
  ▪ *Method Two:* Calculate dose based on body weight, using 0.5–0.6 units/kg body weight per day.

- Typically the smaller of the above estimations is used for a new pump total daily dose.
  - **Basal Insulin:** A typical initial basal insulin uses 50% of newly determined total daily insulin quantity. Divide that number (50% of the daily total) by 24 to determine the number of units per hour.
    - Start with only one basal rate over a 24-hour time period, unless the patient has a recognized dawn phenomenon.
    - Focus first on adjusting this basal rate over time to achieve targeted fasting glucose levels.
    - Frequently, people need a lower basal during the very early morning hours, but then a higher-than-daytime basal during the latter part of the sleep cycle.
    - Next, adjust daytime basal doses and bolus doses.
  - **Bolus Insulin:**
    - *Method One:* algorithmic adjustments: initial premeal dose total is the other 50% of the daily total, distributed as 40% before breakfast, 20–30% before lunch, and 20%–30% before supper and 0–10% with snacks. This method assumes the patient typically eats meals with a consistent amount of carbohydrate and at consistent times.
    - *Method Two:* using carbohydrate counting and sensitivity factors, patients calculate premeal bolus doses based on 1) the amount of carbohydrate to be consumed, and 2) the blood glucose value at the time. This method of bolus determination is more commonly used and tends to provide better results in glucose levels since, by its nature, it incorporates a greater degree of flexibility in the plan.
  - *An insulin to carbohydrate ratio (I:Carb)* is used to determine the food bolus. It tells how many grams of carbohydrate are covered by 1 unit of rapid-acting insulin. For example, a ratio of 1:15 means that 1 unit of insulin is needed for every 15 grams of carbohydrate consumed.
  - A starting I:Carb ratio can be estimated using the "450-rule":

$$\frac{450}{Pump\ TDD}$$

  - A sensitivity factor (SF) determines the estimated blood glucose decline per 1.0 units of rapid-acting insulin. This is used to deter-

mine any necessary correction bolus to bring glucose to target range. These values are estimated at the beginning of pump therapy and adjusted once basal rates are fine-tuned.
  – A starting SF can be estimated using the "1500-rule":

$$\frac{1500}{Pump\ TDD}$$

Here is an example of how to calculate a starting carbohydrate counting program for a 60 KG person who uses an insulin pump:

- The calculation of the total daily insulin dose would be 0.5 unit per kilogram, or 30 units per day.
- The starting insulin to carbohydrate (I:Carb) ratio for this person would be: 450/30 or 1:15. The person would take one unit of insulin for every 15 grams of carbohydrate consumed.
- The sensitivity factor (SF) would be 1500/30, or 1:50. The person would take one unit of insulin for every 50 points above the target glucose level that his or her glucose was at the time of the meal.

♦ **Advantages:**
  – "Basal/bolus" provided by a pump program comes the closest of any treatment program available in clinical practice to mimicking normal physiologic insulin patterns.
  – Allows the most lifestyle flexibility.
  – Convenient to bolus insulin doses whenever food is consumed — the need to eat meals and snacks on schedule is eliminated.
  – Short-term adjustments can be made to basal rates to compensate for increased activity, illness and stress to meet unpredictable activities of life.
  – Avoids inconsistencies of peaking intermediate and long-acting insulins leading to fewer episodes of hypoglycemia.
  – Avoids large depots of long-acting insulin that can result in variable absorption — and thus unpredictable action-patterns.
  – Use of rapid insulin in pumps (all the rapid insulins have pump indication) can lead to rapid changes in insulin levels with basal adjustments and bolus doses.
  – Pregnancy and pre-conception (Glargine and detemir are contraindicated in pregnancy).

♦ **Disadvantages:**
  – If insulin delivery is interrupted, DKA can result quickly as only rapid-acting insulin is used. This problem is minimized by frequent SMBG.
  – Requires wearing an external device. A basic level of technical skill is required and technical problems are a possibility.
  – Requires use of subcutaneous infusion set, which must be maintained and changed every 2 to 3 days. Possibility of infusion set site infections or catheter kinking.
  – Requires intensive patient education, involvement and frequent SMBG (at least 4–6 times per day, and typically 8–10 times per day during initial pump start).
  – Expensive. Some insurance plans will not cover some or all of the costs, and/or make it difficult to get support for pumps and supplies.

Preparing Patients To Start Physiologic Insulin Replacement Therapy

Primary Care Provider or Specialist — or Both?

Unlike treatment with an intensified conventional insulin treatment program, successfully initiating a true physiologic insulin replacement program is often handled more effectively by enlisting the assistance of a team of medical professionals and educators experienced in managing such treatment programs. Under *no* circumstances should patients attempt to self-initiate treatment, particularly using information obtained from reading material such as this book or from friends using similar programs. Improperly designed or initiated physiologic programs — or unsupervised programs — may be more dangerous than poor conventional therapy.

Thus, it is often useful for the primary healthcare provider for whom it is impractical to have a trained diabetes educator within his or her practice setting to know what regional services are available for diabetes patients and to have a good, working relationship with a local diabetes center. It is important to develop a comfort level regarding when a diabetes patient can be successfully treated within the primary care practice and when the patient needs to be referred to a diabetes specialist and his or her team, including a diabetes educator, a registered dietitian and/or an exercise physiologist. Similar to the referral out to a cardiologist for cardiac angioplasty by a primary care provider who has diagnosed likely angina, that same clinician should understand the indications for the initiation of physiologic insulin replacement even if it takes an external consultation to make it happen.

The extent of care and education required by a patient beginning physiologic insulin therapy should not be underestimated. For example, for a successful insulin pump start, Joslin Clinic uses a program that consists of a series of patient appointments described on the following page.

A good working relationship between the diabetes specialty centers and primary care providers can result in smooth initiation and subsequent interactions through properly coordinated *collaborative care.* In such an ideal setting, primary care providers can identify patients for whom physiologic therapy would be beneficial. Such patients may be referred to the diabetes center where medical and educational support can be provided to initiate therapy. Patients then return for ongoing care from their primary care provider, with frequency of return visits to the specialty center determined by the skill and experience of the primary provider and the individual patient's care needs.

Unfortunately, such smooth interaction may be ideal, but is rarely real. Insurance regulations can present barriers to smooth collaboration and proper education. Such regulations may provide short-term economic savings, but most people in the diabetes field would argue that they probably lead to longer-term increases in healthcare expenditures.

Therefore, it often remains for the primary care provider(s) to determine when physiologic insulin therapy is indicated, and to coordinate its initiation and ongoing management. To do so effectively, it is necessary to:

- Understand what physiologic insulin replacement therapy is, and how it can benefit patients in terms of:
  - improved lifestyle flexibility and quality of life;
  - safer short-term control, including decreased risk of hypoglycemia;
  - reduced long-term complication risk through improved glucose control and, in particular, control of postprandial hyperglycemia.

Initiation of Pump Therapy at Joslin Clinic

- Information class on insulin pump therapy which discusses pros, cons and realistic expectations.
- Pre-pump assessment appointment with a pump trainer to determine the patient's appropriateness for pump therapy, and to assess education needs.
- Appointment with Registered Dietitian to learn carbohydrate counting if patient is not already effectively doing this.
- 4-hour class on pump therapy, taught by a pump trainer, prior to the pump start
- Appointment with pump trainer to begin a 'saline run' where patient will wear pump with saline for 1 week.
- Appointment with pump trainer to transition to insulin use with the pump.
- Minimum of two follow-up appointments with the pump trainer to work on troubleshooting, continued education, and basal/bolus adjustments.
- Follow-up appointment with Registered Dietitian for further nutrition education and to begin fine-tuning bolus doses.
- Appointment with exercise physiologist to begin working on basal/bolus adjustments for changes in activity.

Note: Throughout this process, the pump trainer and other members of the team, work with the physician to confer on insulin doses, goals, and adjustments. Patients typically have daily phone contact with the team during the first few days to weeks of pump therapy depending on need.

- Understand the indications for physiologic insulin replacement therapy.
- Become familiar with the parameters for proper patient selection.
- Establish a working relationship with local or regional diabetes centers for collaborative care of patients needing initiation of a more physiologic treatment program; developing routines for patient referral for initiation or maintenance.
- Develop the skills to oversee ongoing management.
- Learn to recognize signs of problems with an ongoing treatment program, and be cognizant of one's own ability to handle these issues rather than referring them back to the diabetes center.

Patients for whom physiologic insulin therapy, or in some cases even the intensification of a conventional treatment program, is being contemplated, should, ideally, start by meeting with a diabetes educator experienced in the initiation and management of such programs. Clearly, a primary care provider who is familiar with the patient can and should provide important input — the consideration of the advancement in therapy would not be occurring if that physician had not been supportive. However, proper patient assessment can be time consuming, and most physicians cannot take the time to perform this task.

The diabetes educator will be able to get a sense of how much the patient can handle, how much physiologic precision may be needed, and the lifestyle issues that might impact treatment design.

Selecting the specific treatment regimen involves an integration of the level of the patient's willingness to perform self-care tasks, his or her lifestyle and schedule, and his or her metabolic needs. With these factors in mind, a program structure can be selected from among those listed previously, or from a hybrid of them.

For whatever program is selected, initial doses of insulin are calculated based on guidelines such as those outlined earlier. Usually, the initial dose is slightly less than the amount that is ultimately expected to be needed just so as to avoid hypoglycemic reactions that can make pattern interpretation more difficult. It is important to avoid confusion as to whether high glucose levels are due to hypoglycemic reactions and rebounds, or to not enough insulin. Set the initial glucose target in a range such as 100 mg/dl to 200 mg/dl. Once the program patterns are established and the patient is comfortable with self-management, targeted glucose levels can be approached through increases in the insulin doses.

An important part of the initiation process is time. There is no need to have the glucose numbers perfect by the first week. Part of initiating physiologic insulin replacement treatment therapy is for the patient to develop the skills to self-manage his diabetes using the program design, along with an appreciation of the interrelationships of all the components affecting glucose control. Following a solid educational foundation from a skilled and experienced diabetes educator, a period of trial and error over a number of weeks is usually the best teacher.

Treatment Adjustments

As noted above, after an initial insulin dosing program is selected (see *Estimating Starting Dose* above), subsequent adjustments will undoubtedly be needed. This is certainly true for those using glucose value-based insulin dosing algorithms, but it is also true for those using carbohydrate counting and sensitivity factors to determine a dose. (See the section on pump insulin doses later in this chapter.) Insulin:carbohydrate ratios and sensitivity factors can be used with multiple-injection basal/bolus programs as well as insulin pump programs.

For those using the traditional algorithm, where doses are based on glucose test values, the doses must be designed to move a given range of blood glucose values toward the targeted blood glucose level. The use of an algorithm facilitates accommodations in insulin dose for variations in the blood glucose range at the time that the dose is to be taken. For example, using the algorithm shown in Figure 11-8, if the morning glucose level is 123 mg/dl, then 7 units of rapid-acting insulin would be taken along with the insulin glargine. However, if the fasting glucose was 223 mg/dl, the rapid-acting insulin dose would be 9 units.

In making adjustments, both early on and over time, there tends to be an undue focus on the insulin doses themselves. If the glucose levels are not at target, people often try to "fix the insulin dose!" Clearly, there can be many reasons for glucose variability, and it is important not to fall into the trap of thinking that incorrect insulin doses are the cause of all ills.

Physiologic therapy is not just "insulin," and part of the process of initiating such a treatment program is to develop an understanding of the interrelationships among all of the factors influencing diabetes control. Glucose monitoring and log-keeping is crucial if one is to successfully achieve this understanding. This discipline is an essential component of true physiologic therapy. By using a properly completed log form, other factors that influence glucose control can be detected and properly addressed.

Accepting that non-insulin factors must be addressed, it is still true that the dosing algorithm frequently needs to be adjusted. Adjusting an algorithm often requires the patient to have close contact with the healthcare team — particularly when the patient is new to this type of program. For example, using the algorithm shown in Figure 11-8, the prelunch glucose

Figure 11-8.   Physiologic Insulin Therapy Algorithm (Sliding Scale)*

Insulin Dose Schedule For: _____

Date: _____   *Patient Number:* _____

RAPID-ACTING OR REGULAR INSULIN:

Blood Glucoose	Breakfast	Lunch	Supper	Bedtime Snack
0–50	2	1	0	0
51–100	4	3	3	0
101–150	7	5	5	0
151–200	8	5	6	0
201–250	9	6	7	2
251–300	10	8	8	3
300–400	12	9	10	4
Over 400	14	10	12	5

Intermediate or peakless basal insulin (NPH/insulin glargine or detemir):

18

*The above figure represents a sample insulin adjustment algorithm, in this case illustrating an insulin glargine and rapid-acting insulin program. (Similar algorithms may be used for other physiologic insulin replacement programs.) Eighteen units of Insulin glargine are given before supper, while the blood glucose test results at the time of the injection determine the premeal rapid-acting insulin dose.

levels might *always* be above target. This pattern suggests that every prebreakfast dose — from the 2 units at a glucose level of 0 to 50 mg/dl to the 12 units for a level over 300 mg/dl — would need to be increased.

Another possibility is that only part of the scale needs to be changed. Perhaps the scale worked well if the glucose level at the time of insulin administration was under 200 mg/dl. However, if the glucose was above 200 mg/dl, the insulin dose was insufficient, and the glucose level at the next test-time was elevated. In this instance, only the insulin doses for those higher glucose levels need to be increased.

Further, keep in mind that while the pharmacokinetics of rapid-acting insulins are listed in Table 11-2, the action of rapid-acting insulin (pharmacodynamics) shows that in most people its effects begin in about $\frac{1}{2}$ hour, peak effect occurs at about 2 to 3 hours, and it is gone by about 4–6 hours. The best measure of the efficacy of the rapid-acting insulin is the postprandial glucose. The glucose value before the next meal (or bedtime) is often influenced by both the impact of the rapid-acting insulin and the basal insulin.

As one can see, in reality there are many more insulin doses to be adjusted for a physiologic insulin replacement program that uses an algorithm. For a conventional, fixed dose program, a dose of X units is given at a particular time, and if the subsequent glucose level is too high, one should increase those X units by some amount. However, with physiologic therapy, at that particular time there are multiple insulin doses, each for a specific glucose range. Similarly, food consumption and activity need to be considered. Hence, programs using adjustments based on carbohydrate counting bring this additional significant factor into the daily dose adjustment equation. Further, one should think of there being doses for each level of carbohydrate intake. Treatment adjustments require a longer period of time to gauge the efficacy of multiple doses, and then a similarly long time to assess the impact of any adjustments that were made. Keep in mind that the presence, or suspicion, of hypoglycemic reactions and resultant rebounds can increase the complexity of this process. If reactions are suspected, particularly if the evidence is circumstantial and difficult to confirm, it can often be helpful to reduce the doses so that reactions are less likely. With lower doses, most highs are presumably due to insufficient insulin action, and the patterns can be more easily interpreted.

Adjusting for Hyperglycemia

The most common cause of hyperglycemia in a person using physiologic insulin replacement therapy is insufficient insulin quantity. Having made that statement, insufficient insulin quantity is not the only cause and cannot and should not be *assumed* to be the cause. The first step in assessing causes of hyperglycemia is to consider all of the other possible non-insulin reasons that have been discussed in this chapter and throughout this book.

Particularly for people with type 1 diabetes, the glucose level at a given time of day is not usually *always* elevated. It may *often* be elevated. It may be elevated more than it is not elevated. It is rarely *always* elevated. Similarly, there is often not *a* reason for hyperglycemia. There may be multiple reasons for a given elevated glucose. Or there may be essentially one reason on a given day, but multiple reasons causing the variability over a period of time. The point is, one should always look for a reason. You may find a possibility. You may find a likely probability. You may even find a confirmed reason on occasion. But rarely will there be a simple explanation. The importance of this concept is that rather than *changing* insulin dose, patients are often encouraged to *adjust* a dose on a given day when there is a circumstance known to affect glucose control in a known manner. This recommendation carries with it an implicit suggestion that they must *pay attention* to all of those factors that *could* impact glucose control. (All too often, particularly when people use algorithms or carbohydrate counting, there is a tendency to think that the adjustment scale or the Insulin:Carbohydrate ratio will put the diabetes on "autopilot," eliminating the need to pay attention to other factors.) People should adjust their dose for that Thanksgiving meal or on the day that they are working hard to clean out the cellar. The basic dose does not change, but the amount of insulin administered on a given day is adjusted because of variations in the usual routine. Thus, many of the multiple reasons for off-target glucose control can be addressed without "changing" *the* basic insulin dose.

There *are* times when there is consistent hyperglycemia, not caused by rebound or other factors that clearly cause glucose elevations, and such times indicate the need for an upward adjustment of the insulin dose. Of course, the basic rule to correct blood glucose levels that are too high is to increase the insulin dose that affects that particular time period in the day. That used to be simple! With some of the complex programs using overlapping or superimposed insulin action patterns, however, it can be much more challenging.

With traditional intensive programs that use premeal regular insulin, the relatively long duration of action for regular insulin makes assessment simpler, even though the control is less precise. The broad "brush stroke" of regular insulin action usually extends out to 6 hours or beyond. As a result, measuring the glucose level before subsequent meals or at bedtime reflects the adequacy of the previous premeal dose. Basal doses can be adjusted based on fasting glucose levels and also if the glucose levels are generally high throughout the day.

With the advent of the rapid-acting insulin analogs with faster time to peak action and shorter duration of action that are used in today's physiologic insulin treatment programs, the prandial coverage is more precise. However, as noted above, these newer insulins have also brought with them an increased dependence on a basal insulin effect to extend coverage until the next dosing and mealtime. Therefore, one cannot gauge insulin efficacy by looking at premeal glucose levels alone.

To exemplify how to approach this problem, let's think of a patient using premeal mixtures of rapid-acting insulin and NPH outlined in example No. 3 from the section earlier in this chapter titled *Descriptions of Basal Insulin Patterns*. If a prelunch glucose level is on target, but the presupper value is too high, and both rapid-acting insulin and NPH are given at lunchtime, which needs to be increased? The following information will be helpful in assessing this problem:

- How many hours is it from lunch to supper?
- How much of a glucose rise was seen between the prelunch value and value obtained 1 to 2 hours after lunch?
- What was the glucose value mid to late afternoon?

The shorter the interval between lunch and supper, the more likely it is that the rapid-acting insulin plays a significant role in determining the presupper value. Conversely, if there is a long duration, such as well over 6 hours, then the intermediate insulin probably is more influential in determining the presupper glucose level.

With a prelunch value on target and the presupper value too high, the postlunch value can be useful. A post-lunch value that is too high suggests that an increase in the prelunch rapid-acting or regular insulin might be the best first step. However, a postlunch value that is on target would suggest that increasing the longer-acting NPH insulin might be best.

Finally, the glucose level mid to late afternoon should be examined. A very low value suggests that there might be true hypoglycemic reactions and rebounds. However, lower values in the absence of true hypoglycemia could become much lower and evolve into true hypoglycemia if either of the prelunch insulin doses are increased. Snacking may prevent such a problem, although it would promote weight gain. Alternatively, you could reduce a prebreakfast dose of NPH, which extends its effect into the midafternoon time period.

More people are now using the basal insulins glargine or detemir (see example 1A & 1B in the earlier section of this chapter titled *Descriptions of Basal Insulin Patterns*). The regimen may be simpler with the bedtime glargine or detemir, and premeal rapid-acting insulin, but the solutions to problems outlined above may be less easily accomplished, as this insulin is given but once or twice daily. Reliance on compensation adjustments of the rapid-acting insulin and/or snacking may be the rule if the glargine or detemir dose needs to be adjusted. Keep in mind that the premeal dose of rapid-acting insulin starts things off at a given level, high if insufficient, on target if proper, and heading downward too rapidly if excessive. This trajectory of glucose movement is then acted upon by the basal later on after the meal. Thus, both come into play in determining the glucose level before the next meal.

These examples utilize some of the more complex treatment designs intentionally to demonstrate how to sort out the interacting and overlapping insulin action patterns. Nevertheless, one cannot always be certain which insulin is having the predominant effect at a given time, and trial and error often is needed to find the best balance of doses.

Fasting Hyperglycemia

Elevations of fasting blood glucose levels are handled differently. It is usually the "basal" insulin — glargine, detemir, overnight NPH, or pump basal infusion — that controls the fasting glucose level. Food consumption, unless markedly greater than usual or of significantly higher fat content, has less influence over the fasting glucose level than many people would imagine. Elevated fasting glucose levels are more likely to result from one of the following:

- insufficient quantity of overnight insulin (either injected insulin or from the nocturnal basal insulin dose quantity in an insulin pump program)
- the dawn phenomenon — an increase in the amount of insulin required during the latter part of the sleep cycle due to circadian

changes in anti-insulin hormone levels — probably predominantly growth hormone

- insufficient duration of action of the overnight insulin (injected insulin)
- incorrect timing of basal dose increases to accommodate for increases in insulin requirements due to the dawn phenomenon (pumps)
- nocturnal hypoglycemia (the so-called "Somogyi" phenomenon) and subsequent hyperglycemic rebound hyperglycemia
- insulin resistance due to dietary fat in the supper meal
- late supper with glucose absorption after bedtime

The actual adjustments for fasting hyperglycemia depend on which of the common causes above is the most likely explanation. Deciding which of these possibilities is the actual cause can be difficult. Common teaching suggests that patients monitor their blood during the night so that patterns obtained can tell which explanation is most likely. However, patients are not always lucky enough to set their alarm clock for the precise time that the glucose level is just right to give them clear evidence of one explanation or another. Usually, the results are equivocal, are not reproducible, or the patient gets fed up and turns off the alarm clock. Often, the cause is the result of multiple factors and may differ from night to night. Nevertheless, some nocturnal monitoring can provide suggestive evidence, and once there is enough proof to warrant a dose change, do so. Ultimately, whether or not this is the correct change will become evident once enough time has passed to tell whether the change corrected the problem or not.

For the possible explanations for fasting hyperglycemia listed above, there are patterns that might classically indicate a specific etiology. *Insufficient quantity of overnight insulin* is suggested by glucose levels that are on-target around the bedtime hour but rise steadily starting in the early part of the night after the patient has gone to sleep. If this elevation in glucose extends during the night, up to and including the end of the sleep period, then increasing the dose of nocturnal insulin coverage would be the desired maneuver.

Insufficient overnight insulin quantity, however, may be impossible to differentiate from the dawn phenomenon, which, many might argue, is the other side of the same coin. One has insufficient quantities of overnight insulin action *because* of the effects of the dawn phenomenon.

Merely increasing bedtime insulin doses may help, but it also may increase the likelihood of reactions occurring either during earlier parts of the night when less insulin is needed, or during the next morning, overlapping the effect of prebreakfast insulin.

Of course, duration of action may also be playing a role, and it might be considered seriously if a program is being used in which the late-day NPH is given at suppertime and thus is peaking early during nighttime, and with a duration that might not extend through into morning. Patterns can again be confusing. Here, the nocturnal glucose might drift upward. Theoretically this pattern, caused by insufficient nocturnal insulin duration, might result in a gentler glucose upswing than would be seen if caused by the dawn phenomenon. It would begin earlier during the sleep hours than would be seen with insulin insufficiency. Unfortunately, clear patterns are rarely evident and intuitive interpretations are often needed to determine the problem.

Insulin adjustments for fasting hyperglycemia due to insufficient insulin quantity or duration overnight would focus on the proper amount of insulin action at the time of need — the end of the sleep cycle. This must be done without having too much insulin action during the earlier part of the night as this could cause hypoglycemia. Possible maneuvers would include:

- **For programs using multiple doses of intermediate NPH insulin as basal:** shift some of the suppertime NPH insulin to the bedtime dose.
- **For programs using a peakless basal insulin (glargine or detemir) at bedtime:** increase the bedtime basal insulin dose. This may necessitate a reduction in premeal rapid-acting insulin doses.
- **For programs using twice daily peakless basal insulin (detemir or glargine):** increase the quantity of basal insulin given late in the day (bedtime or suppertime) relative to the morning dose.
- **For pump programs:** adjust the basal doses overnight, increasing the quantity of insulin infused toward the end of the sleep cycle.

The problem of nocturnal coverage is one of the more significant reasons people may choose to use an insulin pump. The ability to program alternative basal rates during the night allows for proper insulin quantities early, and then safely initiates a dose step-up precisely when needed.

Another pattern to watch for that is suggestive of nocturnal hypoglycemia is the "high-low" pattern. Some days, the glucose value drops low enough to trigger a rebound. In this case, the fasting glucose is high. Other days, the glucose level is not low enough to trigger rebound and remains low into the morning hours. Values falling into the middle ground are much less common.

Insulin adjustments for fasting hyperglycemia due to nocturnal hypoglycemia would most likely be a reduction of the insulin dose having predominant effect overnight. However, as noted above, *shifting* units of insulin from an earlier dose of intermediate insulin to a later dose would push some of that insulin action to later in the sleep cycle, and could also ameliorate the problem.

Regardless of the pattern seen, or whether any is seen at all, the best advice is to make the best guess as to the explanation and make an adjustment accordingly. Then see if the problem is fixed.

Keep in mind that you might be fooled by patterns also. For example, for hypoglycemia caused by an insulin dose in considerable excess, reducing the dose might not eliminate the hypoglycemic reaction but instead remove some of the insulin effect that extends into the next morning. If a hypoglycemic reaction still occurs, but there is less insulin during the latter part of the sleep cycle, the rebound may appear to be higher. One might mistakenly interpret this response to the dose adjustment to suggest that the patient needed *more* insulin, rather than the correct answer which is that he or she needed an even *greater* reduction in the evening dose. It is in this circumstance that a nocturnal test suggesting a dip in the glucose pattern — even if true hypoglycemia was not demonstrated — could be enough evidence to continue reducing the dose rather than increasing it.

Adjusting for Hypoglycemia

Hypoglycemia can be a common problem for people using an intensive treatment program. However, it is a common misconception that intensive therapy *automatically* means more hypoglycemic reactions. Clearly, if someone has an A1C of 11% and initiates physiologic therapy, achieving an A1C of 7%, they are more likely to experience more hypoglycemia merely on the basis of the improved control. A properly constructed program, designed to mimic normal insulin action that is monitored properly by the patient should actually produce less hypoglycemia than a program achieving the same A1C level that is not constructed in a physiologic manner.

Many people will point to the DCCT results, which demonstrated more frequent hypoglycemia in the "experimental" (intensive) group than in the "control" (conventional) group. The DCCT was similar to the above scenario — suboptimal control improving to very aggressive control. In fact, for the DCCT patients, the goal was extremely aggressive treatment, whereas in usual clinical practice now, the level of "aggressiveness" is more commonly tempered by safety. In addition, it was the sense of many investigators, this author included, that much of the hypoglycemia occurred early in the study. Intensive therapy was a new concept for the DCCT, and patients *and* the healthcare team were learning how to use it. With practice came more skill in treatment design and avoidance of hypoglycemia.

The early symptoms of hypoglycemia are primarily the indirect effect of the adrenergic response to hypoglycemia, and not the direct effect of the hypoglycemia itself. One of the factors that leads to adrenergic stimulation is a rapid drop in the glucose level. Therefore, in less physiologic programs designed with less frequent, but larger, individual doses of intermediate insulin, the more rapid glucose drops can stimulate more noticeable symptoms. The gentler undulations of glucose levels seen with a physiologic replacement program can lead to more gradual drops in the glucose level, and, thus, fewer symptoms. Patients need to be cognizant of this difference. Some may even benefit from specific training to recognize hypoglycemia, such as a "Blood Glucose Awareness Training" course (BGAT) that trains patients who can no longer feel adrenergic responses to recognize cognitive changes in behavior.

The approach to hypoglycemia for patients using physiologic insulin replacement therapy should not differ greatly from the approach used by *any* patient using insulin therapy. Every attempt should be made to document hypoglycemic glucose levels to be sure that the suggestive symptoms were not caused by something else. Rapidly dropping — but not truly low — blood glucose levels, while less likely with a properly constructed program, are still possible if there is a particularly significant imbalance of activity, food, or insulin. Certainly, anxiety, a significant stimulator of adrenergic discharge, may also be playing a role.

Clearly, if there is true hypoglycemia, immediate treatment should be sought. However, making a subsequent attempt at determining the cause is the essential next step. All too often, the approach of medical care personnel unfamiliar with the patient, unable to get a proper history, or unskilled in diabetes management is to drastically reduce an insulin dose that they think is the culprit. Worse, they might tell the patient to stop taking one of his or her injections. Further discussions of the approach to hypoglycemia can be reviewed in the chapter on acute complications (see Chapter 13). Suffice it to say, such recommendations drastically upset the delicate balance of an insulin program. They can lead to compensatory increases in other doses, which further unbalance the program and can lead to even more difficulty with reactions.

Use a Systematic Approach to Determine Cause

As with conventional programs, a systematic approach to determine the cause of the reaction is usually the best approach. As you — and the patient — go through the mental exercise of trying to determine the cause of the reaction, think of reactions being categorized into two groups:

- explained reactions — the cause of the reaction can be identified with reasonable certainty
- unexplained reactions — where the cause cannot be determined

Keeping meticulous records of blood glucose monitoring, insulin doses, and activities can make this task much easier.

When hypoglycemic reactions occur and present no obvious explanation, it is possible that an insulin dose is too high. However, unexplained reactions may also be due to a confluence of factors, which, on that particular day, happened to all converge and result in a low blood glucose level.

When the hypoglycemic reaction is severe, with mental status changes, or with real or potential injury or harm, the insulin that has the most predominant action at the time of the reaction should be reduced the next day. In reality, it might not be this insulin dose that is primarily the cause, but safety must come first.

If the reaction is mild, however, and there have been no problems in the past using the same dose, then the dose should not necessarily be changed. Careful monitoring should be performed over the next few days to ensure that the hypoglycemic reaction was, indeed, just a one-time occurrence. The patient should keep track of food consumption, activity, timing, and any other factor suspected to have played a role. If repeated hypoglycemic reactions occur, or there is a clear dip in the glucose level at that particular time, then the dose should be reduced.

Keep in mind that occasional, mild hypoglycemic reactions or dips in the glucose levels are to be expected with intensive therapies, but the risks of these mild reactions should be outweighed by the benefits of this type of program.

Determining Which Insulin to Reduce

If the patient is using one of the more complex treatment designs, it may not always be obvious which insulin is best to reduce. As should be obvious from the earlier discussion, it may not be the insulin that peaked closest to the time of the hypoglycemia but, perhaps, one that worked during a previous time period and started a downward trend that may have been too steep. It could just be too much downward trajectory from an earlier dose of rapid-acting insulin, carried forward by the ongoing effect of the basal insulin.

This phenomenon, often referred to as a "crisscross" or "piggyback" effect, and more commonly seen with programs using NPH than a basal insulin, is another possibility. This phenomenon occurs when the apparent effect of one insulin dose is increased because there is additional insulin left over from the tail-end of a previous insulin dose or coming on at the beginning of the next. For a physiologic insulin program, it might be that the insulin providing the basal level could be in excess. For example, when adjustment of the morning rapid-acting or regular insulin dose does not stop frequent late-morning hypoglycemic reactions from occurring, another insulin may be the cause. This may be particularly true for programs using rapid-insulins, as the action is mostly dissipated by late morning. It could be the basal insulin (NPH, glargine or detemir) that is responsible for the hypoglycemia.

Frequently, when trying to be a hypoglycemia detective, one finds that the patient's SMBG record is full of scattered low glucose levels, often with subsequent highs. These low glucose test results are common at various times of the day or night, not just at the time of the reaction in question. The tendency for overinsulinization can occur with intensive programs, as patients and healthcare professionals alike may be more likely to chase high glucose levels than to recognize subtle hypoglycemic reactions.

In such an instance, it is usually wise to reduce the insulin doses throughout the day — not necessarily all of them, but many of them — in order to eliminate the hypoglycemia. This is much like the approach to the newly initiated program. Let the glucose levels run a little high, eliminate hypoglycemia, and then re-adjust the insulin doses in the proper, balanced patterns.

Weight Gain/Loss on Physiologic Insulin Replacement Therapies

Physiologic therapy, it is hoped, will result in an improvement in diabetes control. When diabetes control is improved by any means, fewer calories are lost through glycosuria. Thus, more calories are available for use as energy or to be stored as fat.

Weight gain is frequently noted after initiation of physiologic therapy as a result of the fluid retention seen with sudden control improvements and as a result of the retention of additional calories. It is important to be sure that the program is properly balanced without excess insulin, avoiding the hypoglycemia that necessitates consumption of additional calories and stimulates the appetite. It may be helpful for the patient to review his or her nutrition program with a registered dietitian. In addition to weight gain from fluid retention, people on insulin pumps may gain weight simply because it is so easy to take additional insulin to compensate for larger meals and snacks.

On the other hand, many patients who employ physiologic insulin therapy may find that they are able to meet their weight loss goals. When glucose levels are stabilized on pump therapy, for example, patients may be able to forgo snacks that they used to need to consume to prevent hypoglycemia when intermediate insulin was peaking. Similarly, they may find that they consume fewer calories since they don't need to treat hypoglycemia as often. The use of the basal insulins with rapid insulin, combined with carbohydrate counting, has proven to be improvements over intermediate insulin programs with respect to weight loss. Studies with detemir have shown it to be particularly good in this regard.

Insulin Pump Therapy

Treatment using continuous subcutaneous insulin infusion (CSII) therapy, commonly referred to as an insulin pump, comes closest to mimicking normal endogenous insulin patterns. Insulin pumps use only one type of insulin, usually a rapid-acting insulin (aspart, glulisine and lispro have an FDA indication). Due to the unique mode of insulin delivery afforded by insulin pumps, people who use them can have the ability to live a more flexible lifestyle than those using injections. CSII is an alternative treatment to MDI for people who desire excellent glucose control but are either unable to obtain this with injections or for those who simply want to achieve maximum flexibility with regard to meals, exercise, and daily schedules. Since it is the most physiologic of commonly used insulin programs, it also requires the greatest self-care effort from the patient and requires mastery of the most self-care principles. Pumps need to be worn at all times; interruption of insulin delivery for more than 1 to 2 hours without substitute injections will put the patient at risk for hyperglycemia and ketoacidosis.

Insulin pumps are small mechanical devices, typically the size of a beeper. Insulin is contained in a reservoir inside the pump. These disposable insulin reservoirs are regularly filled by patients and can hold up to 300 units of insulin. The insulin reservoir is connected to plastic tubing called an infusion set. Infusion sets, another disposable insulin pump supply, are changed every 2 to 3 days. Today's most common infusion sets use a guide needle for subcutaneous insertion, but only a soft, flexible cannula actually remains under the skin. Most infusion sets today also have a "quick-release" feature that allows a patient to easily disconnect from the pump for showering, exercise, or intimate moments. The most common site for insertion of the infusion set is the abdomen, though the hip and thigh areas may also be used.

Pumps deliver insulin in two different modes: basal and bolus. *Basal insulin,* or the insulin delivered in a slow continuous rate, is designed to mimic the basal insulin released by a nondiabetic pancreas. Basal insulin controls blood glucose in the fasting state. Basal rates are measured in terms of "units per hour" reflecting the number of units of insulin infused over a 1-hour period. Basal rates can typically vary from less than 0.4 units/hour to as much as 2 units/hour or more. Basal rates are programmed typically in 0.10 unit increments/hour. Some newer pumps on the market can deliver basal rates to the level of 0.05 unit increments. Pumps can be programmed to vary the basal insulin infusion rates for various intervals over 24 hours. While today's pumps can accommodate up to 48 separate basal rates in a 24-hour period, typically patients will only require 2 to 4 rates a day and certainly not more than 6 or 8. The most common use of the alternative basal rates is to accommodate for the differing basal insulin needs seen at the end of the sleep cycle, the so-called dawn phenomenon.

Bolus insulin doses are larger "bursts" of insulin used to cover food and to correct high blood glucose. Bolus doses can be determined using algorithmic adjustments or by using insulin:carbohydrate ratios and sensitivity factors. This second method is the most common and typically leads to better glucose control and enables lifestyle flexibility to be maximized. Bolus doses can be fine-tuned to levels of 0.1 of a unit, and some of today's pumps have features that can alter the way a bolus is delivered. For example, an "extended" or "square wave" bolus may be used to cover higher-fat foods/meals. Since a high-fat meal will delay the glucose response, an extended bolus can be programmed to deliver the insulin over a designated period of time instead of all at once.

The Decision to Use a Pump

Newer model insulin pumps are easier to use than ever before, opening up this form of treatment to more individuals. However, the decision to embark on pump therapy should still not be taken lightly, and such a decision must be made with specific goals and objectives in mind. It must be evident to both the patient and the healthcare provider or team that pump therapy will provide some improvement in therapy as compared with previous therapies. Improvement may not necessarily be measured in terms of A1C, as other parameters for improvement may be sought. Patient selection criteria for pump use are the same as for selection of patients to undertake any physiologic insulin replacement therapy — and then some. Compared to multiple injection physiologic therapy, pump use requires even more motivation, dexterity, judgment, insight, psychological stability, and self-management skills. Unfortunately, finances maybe a consideration as well, as some insurance plans will not cover some or all of the costs of pump therapy. Support from family and/or friends is also important. Pump therapy can be challenging, and having someone close to the pump user who can help and provide emotional support is often a great benefit.

Patients, and those close to them, should have clear and realistic expectations about what pump therapy can and cannot do. Many people have the misconception that a pump will measure glucose levels and normalize them around-the-clock and allow patients to return to a lifestyle that resembles that of a person who does not have diabetes. Closed-loop implantable pumps that can accomplish this feat may someday be widely available. However, at the writing of this book, such devices are still under development. Many people falsely believe that pump therapy will eliminate out-of-range blood glucose values. It should be emphasized that though most likely they will experience *fewer* glucose excursions than before pump therapy, they should still expect some highs and lows. This often needs to be reinforced during the first few weeks of pump therapy when patients are typically monitoring glucose levels more than ever before. For example, they may never have measured glucose values at certain time intervals, such as 2 hours after meals. These numbers, which may be higher than those they are used to seeing, need to be put into perspective. People considering pump therapy should also understand that the pump education required to successfully get them started is extensive. They may need to put some thought into the best time, in terms of other events in their personal lives, to begin the training for pump therapy. They need to be committed to the time investment required to safely and successfully begin this new therapy.

Assessment of Potential Candidates for Pump Therapy

Diabetes centers providing support for insulin pump therapy usually require that potential candidates for treatment undergo a preliminary assessment before the decision to initiate pump therapy is finalized. A certified diabetes educator usually performs this assessment. Nevertheless, it is often useful for the referring primary care provider to perform a similar preliminary assessment which can both prevent referrals of patients who are, in fact, inappropriate pump candidates as well as target educational deficiencies that must be addressed.

What follows is a general list of indications for CSII and specific characteristics of optimal pump candidates:

Indications:

  ♦ Medical need
    – Suboptimal glycemic control: A1C >7–8% on a multiple daily injection program, A1C in target range but experiences marked glucose fluctuations, significant dawn phenomenon, extreme insulin sensitivity
    – Recurrent episodes of severe hypoglycemia and/or has hypoglycemia unawareness
    – Recurrent DKA
    – Planning conception and has suboptimal glycemic control

  ♦ Need for lifestyle
    – Unpredictable schedules, shift-work, frequent travel

Patient Characteristics:
  ♦ Regular SMBG: minimum of 4 times per day and willing to monitor more frequently (up to 8–10 times/day) during pump start and periodically.
  ♦ Motivated and responsible; keeps regular medical appointments.
  ♦ Knows, or is willing to learn, carbohydrate counting.
  ♦ Has proper understanding and acceptance of appropriate goals of pump therapy.
  ♦ Has the intellect and physical capability to learn pump treatment regimens:
    – the technical components of using an insulin pump, including physical acuity and manual dexterity
    – appreciation of the interrelationships among insulin action, activity, food consumption, and any other daily factors impacting glucose control.
    – ability to problem solve in a logical manner

Oftentimes patients may *seem* to be appropriate candidates, yet they do not meet all of the above patient characteristics. It is common for patients who have not met with a diabetes educator and/or a physician in some time to fall into a bit of a rut with their diabetes self-care habits. These patients may in fact *become* good pump candidates after working with a diabetes educator and/or dietitian to upgrade their self-care routine. Only once the patient has proven to the healthcare team, and perhaps, to himself as well, that such behaviors are feasible as components of the long-term treatment routine will pump therapy be considered.

In addition to the criteria above, part of a pre-pump assessment should include an evaluation of the patient's ophthalmologic status and clearance by an ophthalmologist for potential short-term retinopathic progression due to intensification of therapy.

Initiation of Pump Treatment

Most pump treatment programs can be initiated on an outpatient basis. Education and medical support provided by a diabetes treatment program are usually sufficient to provide adequate support. However, participation in an intensive outpatient education or treatment program or hospitalization (though rarely) are not unreasonable venues to begin pump therapy. A patient beginning pump therapy will require a substantial amount of support from the healthcare team initiating the therapy. They should have phone contact the first few days to review blood glucose values and to begin initial insulin pump dose adjustments. The patient should also have 24-hour access to the healthcare team for any emergencies. Typically, pump manufactures have 24-hour customer-support numbers for technical pump questions.

Initiation of pump therapy needs to begin with patient education. Ideally, this education will occur just prior to and at the time of the pump start. Components of this education program involve instruction on how to use the pump itself and how to effectively and safely manage diabetes using insulin pump therapy. The recommended components of the education plan are listed in the box on the following page.

Obviously the list of topics to be covered is extensive and therefore several visits with a diabetes educator who specializes in pump therapy should be expected in order for pump therapy to be successful. Some pump trainers may be found at larger diabetes referral centers. In addition, some pump manufacturers make pump trainers available in certain areas. Having the patient wear the pump with saline for a few days to a week prior to starting insulin in the pump can be an extremely effective way to begin to teach pump therapy. The patient will gain confidence in his ability to operate of the pump so that when he begins insulin in the pump, he can turn his attention to the diabetes management issues involved. After the pump start, several follow-up visits with the pump

---

Education for Insulin Pump Therapy

- Pump mechanics
  - pump programming
  - catheter insertion, site selection, rotation, management/maintenance
  - troubleshooting pump problems
- Diabetes management using a pump
  - carbohydrate counting and using insulin:carbohydrate ratios
  - insulin sensitivity factors and how to use them to correct out-of-range blood glucose
  - use of SMBG and proper record-keeping to track pump treatment
  - adjustment for lifestyle variations like exercise
  - management of hypo- and hyperglycemia
  - sick-day management
  - day-to-day living with an insulin pump; practical issues
  - guidelines for basal rate and bolus adjustments

---

trainer will be needed to continue education and to begin to fine-tune pump doses.

Pump Insulin Doses

Guidelines for determining the initial pump basal and bolus doses are outlined earlier in this chapter (see the section *Physiologic Insulin Dosing Schedules*). Many patients will start pump therapy based on such a dose-estimate formula, and adjustments upward or downward are made subsequently as the program is used.

While extreme glucose excursions may prioritize the order of insulin dose adjustments, the usual approach is to first adjust the basal rates and then to adjust the bolus doses. Basal rates are more important for initial control since they are responsible for overnight and fasting glucose levels.

Patient involvement in this process is crucial. He or she must take frequent SMBG readings and chart them along with insulin doses and keep records of any other lifestyle variations that might have had a significant impact on glucose levels.

Basal Rates

General guidelines for evaluating and adjusting basal rates include:

- Divide the day into four segments (overnight, breakfast time, lunch time, dinner time) and evaluate one segment at a time.
- Begin with the overnight basal evaluation. Evaluations of the other time frames require skipping meals/snacks in order to isolate the effects of the basal insulin.
- Basal rate evaluations can begin 4 to 5 hours after the last bolus dose was taken.
- Blood glucose should be between ~100 to 150 mg/dl at the beginning of the evaluation in order to proceed.
- Basal rate evaluations should end in the event of a low blood glucose or high blood glucose that requires treatment.
- During a basal rate evaluation: no food, alcohol, or exercise.
- During a basal rate evaluation, generally blood glucose should be checked every 1 to 2 hours. For the overnight timeframe, blood glucose should be checked before bedtime, at midnight, at 2 to 3 AM and upon waking.
- Basal rates adjustments should be made when the blood glucose trends up or down more than 30 mg/dl during the timeframe being evaluated.
- Remember to look for repeated patterns before making adjustments in basal rates.
- Basal rate adjustments should be made in small increments (0.05 or 0.10 units depending on the pump) and then reevaluated.
- Change the basal rate 1 to 2 hours before the time that the blood glucose begins its upward or downward trend.

Bolus Doses

Evaluate bolus doses (insulin:carb ratios [I:Carb] and sensitivity factors) once basal rates are evaluated and adjusted. To test I:Carb ratios patients should check their blood glucose before a meal. If blood glucose is within their target range, they can proceed with the test. They would add up the grams of carbohydrate they plan to eat and divide it by the number of grams of carbohydrate they expect a 1-unit bolus to cover. They should then bolus that amount. For example, if they are planning to eat 60 grams of carbohydrate and their I:Carb ratio is 1:15, they would bolus 4 units. To evaluate the effectiveness of the bolus, they would check their glucose 2 to 3 hours after the meal. An appropriate blood glucose at that point would be 40 to 80 mg/dl above the glucose before the meal (the bolus is still working at this point). If their blood glucose did not rise by this amount, their ratio should be adjusted upward (meaning the bolus would be less for the same amount of carbohydrate). If their blood glucose rose by too much, adjust the ratio down.

To evaluate the sensitivity factor or correction doses, the patient should take a correction bolus at a time when their glucose is elevated and they are not planning to eat for awhile. They should check their glucose following the correction bolus to see if they come close to their glucose target by 3 to 4 hours after the bolus was taken. Assume the sensitivity factor is correct if blood glucose is within 30 mg/dl from target at this point.

Potential Problems with Pump Therapy

There are two main problems associated with pump therapy: infusion-site infections and unexplained hyperglycemia leading to DKA. With proper attention, and appropriate self-care habits and routines, these risks can be virtually eliminated. Once again, proper education is key to a safe insulin pump initiation.

To prevent skin infections at the infusion site, patients need to learn proper skin care and sterile techniques for filling their insulin cartridge and inserting their infusion sets. The following guidelines should be followed to prevent problems:

- Infusion sets should be changed every 2 to 3 days. The new set should be placed at least 1-inch from the previous site.
- Hands should be washed and a clean area used to work with the pump supplies when changing a cartridge and/or infusion set. An ideal time to change an infusion set is after bathing.
- Soap and water cleansing is usually adequate to prep the skin prior to inserting an infusion set. Skin should be cleansed with an antiseptic cleanser in those patients who are prone to skin infections.
- Wipe the skin with an adhering agent with antibiotic properties such as IV Prep™ prior to inserting an infusion set.
- Infusion sets should feel comfortable at all times. If pain, discomfort, redness, warmth, or swelling occur, the infusion set should be

removed immediately. If the area appears to be infected, a topical antibiotic should be applied. The patient should be instructed to call their healthcare team if there is no improvement in 24 hours.

The second risk, or complication, of pump therapy is ketoacidosis. Since pumps use primarily rapid-acting insulin alone, even a short interruption in insulin delivery may lead to elevated blood glucose and ketoacidosis in a matter of hours. For this reason, hyperglycemia should be treated seriously by pump users. Unexplained hyperglycemia, or a glucose reading of >250 mg/dl without any known association to food, stress, illness, or insulin omission, should especially be treated seriously and promptly. Urine ketone levels should be checked in the case of unexplained hyperglycemia. If moderate to large ketones are present, it should be assumed that there was an interruption in insulin delivery and supplemental insulin should be taken via injection (not a pump bolus). The dose of insulin should be 20% of the average total daily dose of insulin. The infusion set and site should subsequently be changed. Blood glucose and urine ketones should be rechecked every 2 to 3 hours and supplemental insulin should be taken until levels are acceptable. If no ketones are present, a pump bolus can be used for the correction dose, but blood glucose should be checked in 1 to 2 hours to assure that the glucose is decreasing and the problem is being resolved. If blood glucose is not decreasing, supplemental insulin should be taken via injection and the infusion set and site should be changed.

Insulin pump users should be well versed in procedures to troubleshoot their pump to assess any problems. The following list should be considered when unexplained hyperglycemia occurs:

- Bolus memory — was the last bolus inadvertently missed
- Basal rates — are they programmed correctly?
- Batteries — pumps typically alarm when they are low and/or expired.
- Insulin — was an old vial used or was the insulin pump exposed to extremes in temperature?
- Infusion set tubing — are there air bubbles or air spaces, blood, or "clumps"; was the tubing primed (filled with insulin)?
- Insulin cartridge — is it empty? Pumps typically alarm when they get low.
- Connections — is there any leaking?

- Infusion site — is there redness, pain, or discomfort. Is the catheter dislodged or kinked?

Problems related to interrupted or partial insulin delivery are more commonly related to the infusion set or site as opposed to a true pump malfunction. If a pump malfunction is suspected, the primary care provider or healthcare team should be contacted for alternative insulin injection plans (see below) until the problem is resolved or the pump replaced. The pump manufacturer's technical support department should also be contacted.

Sick-Day Pump Adjustments

The principles used to determine sick-day insulin coverage rules for people treated with insulin infusion pumps are, with some exceptions, similar to those treated with any other physiologic insulin replacement program. The key point is that people often need more insulin during times of illness. Many times, they need quite a bit more insulin. Patients should be instructed to monitor their blood glucose during illness every 2 hours and to check for ketones if blood glucose exceeds 250 mg/dl. The amount of supplemental insulin, and the mode of delivery (pump bolus versus injection), will depend on the presence of ketones. If moderate to large ketones are present, a correction dose of approximately 20% of their average total daily dose should be taken by injection.

On clearly defined sick days, when blood glucose is consistently running high, the following parameters should be followed:

- Increase the basal infusion rate by 20%–50%. It is not uncommon for the higher percent increase to be needed. Temporary basal rate features of pumps can be used to easily accomplish this.
- The bolus doses may need to be increased as well. Changing the Insulin:Carb ratio and sensitivity factor for the duration of the illness is an easy way to do this. For example, if a patient normally uses an Insulin:Carb ratio of 1:15, he or she might try 1:10 during illness to allow more insulin to cover the same amount of carbohydrate.
- The blood glucose level should be checked regularly and extra bolus insulin doses should be given:
  - If the glucose reading is over 250 mg/dl without urine ketones, the patient's sensitivity factor can be used to determine a correction

bolus or it can be determined to be equal to approximately 10% of his or her average total daily dose.

- If the glucose reading is over 250 mg/dl with urine ketones, or over 400 mg/dl regardless of ketone status, a correction dose of approximately 20% of the average total daily dose should be used at the time of the glucose check. This dose should be taken as an injection rather than a pump bolus.

• The pump insulin supply should be checked more frequently during sick-day management as increased quantities of insulin are being used.

When patients are using an adjustment algorithm, the hyperglycemia accompanying an illness will lead to the use of a supplemental insulin bolus dose that is determined based on glucose levels and the presence or absence of ketonuria, according to standard sick-day rules. However, with illness-induced hyperglycemia, the insulin requirements are increased, and thus when the sick-day monitoring coincides with a usual premeal bolus time, incremental insulin should be added to the algorithm-designated bolus dose.

Patients should know their sick-day rules well before they get sick. If, after increasing both the basal and the boluses, the blood glucose level does not come into an acceptable range in a period of 2 to 3 hours, the pump should be removed and injected insulin should be used, with the alternative off-pump dose being used along with sick-day rules. Sick days are not times to troubleshoot, and if there is any question whether the pump is functioning properly, injected insulin should be used.

If these sick-day rules do not maintain reasonable glucose control or suppress ketones or if the patient becomes very symptomatic, particularly if unable to hold down nutrients, hospitalization will be necessary. Ketoacidosis can develop quite rapidly, and any suggestive symptoms should prompt the immediate switch to injected insulin plus a trip to the physician or emergency room.

Also, insulin therapy — with pumps in particular — is best individualized. This is never so true as for sick days on pumps. The above guidelines are for general information. However, all people using pump therapy should receive specific sick-day instructions designed for them from their own doctor or pump management team.

Exercise Adjustments with Pumps

With individual variations in exercise quantity and response, trial and error is often the best way to determine how best to make changes. A number of possible adjustments can be made for exercise. The overriding guiding principal should be to decrease insulin levels during exercise using the higher percent decrease so as to prevent hypoglycemia and subsequently decrease the amount of the reduction in future exercise sessions if the glucose levels ran high the first time. Basal rate adjustments and/or bolus adjustments can be used depending on the timing of the exercise. Below are some options for handling exercise for patients treated with an insulin pump:

- For short duration activities (1/2 hour or less), often no change in the insulin dose is needed.
- For intermediate duration exercise (30 to 60 minutes) occurring within 2 hours after a meal, the meal bolus can be reduced by 5% to 20%. If the exercise occurs more than 2 hours after a meal, a temporary basal rate reduction of 5% to 20% should be used.
- For longer duration and high intensity exercise, decrease the basal rate by 30% to 50%. Again, consider bolus adjustments when the activity is close to a mealtime.
- Basal rate reductions should begin 30 to 60 minutes prior to the activity so that insulin levels are decreased by the time the activity starts.
- Keep in mind that the lag effect — hypoglycemia for a prolonged period following an exercise period — may necessitate extended periods of time during which the reduced basal is utilized.
- The pump can be disconnected for a short time. This is particularly useful for periods of strenuous exercise, contact sports, or water sports.
- Additional food may also be consumed in addition to, or in lieu of basal/bolus adjustments. Combining extra food with a reduction or temporary suspension of basal infusion may be used for extremely strenuous exercise, for day-long events, or for exercise that has not been planned or compensated for in advance.

Each situation needs to be individualized. If exercise is performed within 3 hours of an insulin bolus, hypoglycemia is more likely. Additional food is more likely to be needed. Alternatively, if the activity is anticipated, a reduction to about 50% of the usual premeal bolus is another means of compensation. This would be preferable if weight loss is a goal. For prolonged, less strenuous exercise, such as 2 to 3 hours of bicycling or walking, reducing the basal rate by 30% to 50% may be preferable.

Generally, it is recommended that pump management teams be consulted for advanced training and guidance in determining dose adjustments for exercise. If the primary care provider or diabetes center works with an exercise physiologist, consultative assistance can also be quite valuable. Careful record keeping is key, allowing later review of the efficacy of adjustments. Records should be kept on the dose adjustments that are made, how long and how strenuous the activity is, adjustments of food, and the ultimate effect on the blood glucose levels. Monitoring blood glucose level before, during, and after exercise is recommended to get a more complete picture of the effect on glucose levels.

Going Off the Pump

There are times when a patient may want to go off the pump for a short time or need to because of pump malfunction. If a patient needs an off-pump program and does not have one, calculation of a program using any of the guidelines outlined for intensive programs earlier in this chapter may be adapted. If all else is impractical, below are guidelines for an off-pump treatment programs:

- The quantity of insulin given as the pump basal over a 24-hour period should be determined and given as multiple injections of NPH insulin, or 1–2 injections of peakless basal insulin (detemir or glargine).
- If NPH insulin is used, doses should be divided so that the amount of NPH given at breakfast is equal to basal insulin delivered by the pump from breakfast till lunch, the amount of NPH given at lunch is equal to basal insulin delivered by the pump from lunch till supper, the amount of NPH given at supper is equal to basal insulin delivered by the pump from supper till bedtime, and the amount of NPH given at bedtime si eaul to 1.2–1.5 times the amount of basal insulin delivered by the pump from bedtime till breakfast.
- If detemir is used, start initially with half in the morning and the other half in the evening. However, if the basal doses were markedly

    unbalanced favoring either night or daytime, similar adjustments of
the detemir dose can be made.

- If glargine is used, the 24-hour total basal insulin quantity is given as
  bedtime glargine.
- Occasionally a 10–20% reduction is made, particularly if the patient
  had difficulty with frequent hypoglycemia while using the pump, or
  if there is reason to think that hypoglycemia might be a concern.
- The same plan used for pump bolus doses is used for doses of rapid-
  acting insulin doses, given before meals, with adjustments as needed
  based on actual usage.

Further dose adjustments beyond those outlined above may be necessary if the pump vacation is to be prolonged, if activity differs from normal, or if the vacation is due to a prolonged illness or severe injury. Keep
in mind that when returning to pump use, the prolonged effect of previous intermediate insulin doses, or, in particular, glargine may overlap
the initial pump doses. Therefore, start pump doses gradually and with
caution.

Pramlintide

There is another new injectable hormone, pramlintide, which can be used
in conjunction with insulin therapy. It is a synthetic analogue of a natural
occurring substance, amylin. Amylin was first discovered in 1987 from
pancreatic amyloid deposits. It is a 37 amino acid polypeptide related
structurally to calcitonin and adrenomedullin. It is found in the pancreatic
β-cell secretory granules that also contain insulin and seems to be co-se-
creted with insulin in response to rising glucose levels in the same pattern
of insulin secretion. Like insulin, it seems to be absent in people with type
1 diabetes. Although it does not appear to be deficient in people with type
2 diabetes, its serum level does not increase in response to meals.

    Amylin receptors have been identified in a number of tissues, and this
hormone appears to have multiple physiologic effects. It predominantly
functions as a neuroendocrine peptide, binding to receptors in the brain,
promoting feelings of satiety and slowing of gastric emptying. It also appears to have an inhibitory effect on glucagon secretion. The serum

glucagon level is always high in the postprandial period in people with untreated type 1 or type 2 diabetes. Amylin, together with insulin, suppresses the postprandial glucagon secretion in healthy people, a process that is deficient in diabetes patients leading to high glucagon in the post meal period. One impact of this effect is to suppress the tendency of unopposed glucagon to deplete glycogen stores in the liver. Amylin, therefore, would help promote hepatic glycogen storage and reduce hepatic glucose production. It should be emphasized that the delicate balance between glucagon on the one hand, and both insulin and amylin from the other, maintain the normal response of the liver in providing glucose supply to protect against low glucose levels during the fasting state.

In addition, amylin has an affect on gastric emptying through its neuroendocine effect. People with diabetes *who do not have gastroparesis* (a neuropathy affecting neural function of the stomach, leading to slowed stomach emptying) have a tendency to have more rapid gastric emptying. Amylin slows gastric emptying and, in theory, better coordinates it with the action of the secreted insulin. This mechanism has a significant impact on the postprandial blood glucose level.

Curiously and fortunately, many of these affects are overridden when other abnormalities are superimposed. For example, amylin's effect on the gut requires intact neural control. People with diabetes who develop gastroparesis have derangements of the neural control of the gut, and thus amylin does not seem to further slow gastric emptying in these individuals. Similarly, when a patient has a hypoglycemic event, the response of more rapid gastrointestinal glucose absorption, needed to counter that hypoglycemic reaction, seem to occur, overriding any amylin affects.

It has been postulated that the absolute or relative deficiency of amylin in type 1 and 2 diabetes respectively contribute to the characteristic postprandial glucose abnormalities. This is the rationale behind the development of the synthetic form, pramlintide, which is structurally slightly different from the natural molecule: its absence contributes to the abnormalities, and its replacement should help ameliorate them.

Amylin in its natural form is quite "sticky" and could not be produced and used as a pharmaceutical agent. (In fact, one theory is that the hypersecretion of insulin in early type 2 diabetes is accompanied by hypersecretion of amylin. This sticky amylin builds up in the pancreas, leading to the amyloid deposits seen in later type 2 diabetes that accompany β-cell

TABLE 11-1 Dosing of Pramlintide using U-100 insulin syringes

Dosage Prescribed (µg)	Increment using a U-100 Syringe (Units)	Volume (mL)
15	2.5	0.025
20	5.0	0.050
45	7.5	0.075
60	10.0	0.100
120	20.0	0.200

dysfunction.) A slight alteration in few amino acids of the amylin polypeptide chain lead to the production of more soluble and thus usable form, pramlintide.

Pramlintide is administered by subcutaneous injection, similar to insulin, into the abdomen or thigh immediately prior to a major meal ($\geq$ 250 Kcal or $\geq$ 30 g of carbohydrate). Sites should be rotated regularly. It is indicated for people with either type 1 or type 2 diabetes who use mealtime insulin therapy but have not yet achieved optimal diabetes control. For those with type 2 diabetes treated with insulin in this manner, they may also be using concurrent sulfonylurea and/or metformin therapy. Pramlintide is a clear solution supplied in 5 mL vials containing 0.6 mg/mL Pramlintide and is usually injected using a U-100 insulin syringe, preferably with a total capacity of 0.3 mL to make dosing more accurate. The conversions for dosing using a U-100 syringe are listed in Table 11-1. Unopened vials should be stored in a refrigerator, but not frozen. Vials exposed to freezing or persistent temperatures over 77° F (25° C) should be discarded. Opened in-use vials can be kept for up to 28 days in a refrigerator or at room temperature (<77° F (25° C)).

The use of pramlintide can lead to reductions in insulin requirements, so it is recommended that the preprandial rapid-acting or regular insulin (or premixed insulin) be reduced by 50% initially to avoid postprandial hypoglycemia. The duration of action of pramlintide is similar to rapid acting insulin.

For people with type 1 diabetes, pramlintide dose should be titrated gradually to reduce the incidence of nausea, which is the commonest side event. The initial dose of pramlintide should be 15 µg (2.5 units) before each meal. Once there has been no clinically significant nausea at this starting dose for 3 days, the dose should be titrated upward in 15 µg (2.5 units) increments to a maintenance dose of 30 µg (5 units), 45 µg (7.5 units), or 60 µg (10 units) as tolerated. If nausea persists at a given dose, it should be reduced and maintained at the previous dose for a longer period before attempting to increase the dose again. The ultimate goal is to reach the 60 µg (10 units) dose before each meal. Most type 1 patients tolerate the 15 and 30 µg dose very well with minimal or no nausea, but nausea becomes obvious at 45 µg and 60 µg dose. If 30 µg cannot be tolerated because of severe nausea or vomiting, it should be discontinued. Once the maximal dose of pramlintide is achieved, the premeal insulin may be adjusted back to maintain a reasonable postprandial blood glucose level.

For people with type 2 diabetes, the usual starting dose is 60 µg (10 units) before each meal. Preprandial insulin doses should similarly be reduced by 50% to avoid hypoglycemia. When there has been no nausea for 3–7 days, the dose should be increased to 120 µg (20 units) before each meal. If there is significant nausea at this higher dose, reduce to 60 µg. Again, once the dose of pramlintide is set, the insulin doses should be adjusted to optimize glucose control.

The possible postprandial hypoglycemia is likely to be insulin-induced. The risk of hypoglycemia is minimized by the recommendation of a reduction in the premeal insulin doses by 50% at initiation of pramlintide therapy. However, the eventual premeal insulin dose may end up being titrated upward above that after pramlintide is titrated.

If pramlintide is discontinued for any reason such as illness or surgery, it should be reinitiated using the same method described above for initiation. Pramlintide cannot be mixed with insulin, as the pH of the two makes them incompatible. Therefore, they should be given in separate injections using different syringes. The sites of injections should be at least 2 inches apart. Missed doses should not be made up. If premeal blood glucose is too low, or the patient has an acute illness that affects appetite, pramlintide dose may be omitted.

Pramlintide can produce a modest lowering of A1C (0.4–0.6%). However, equally as important, it may blunt some of the high and low glucose excursions seen in insulin-treated patients, having particularly significant glucose stabilizing effects in the postprandial period. It also has modest effect on body weight due to suppression of appetite and increased sensation of fullness after meals due to slowed gastric emptying. This effect is particularly important in overweight and obese type 2 diabetic patients on insulin therapy. It may also reduce the tendency for weight gain in intensively treated type 1 diabetic patients.

Pramlintide use needs a higher degree of compliance and frequent blood glucose monitoring, especially after meals. For this reason, it may not be suitable for patients who are poorly compliant to their insulin, blood glucose monitoring or regular follow up. Patients with gastrointestinal problems or on medications that may slow gastric emptying (e.g. metoclopramide or erythromycin) are not suitable for pramlintide use. Pramlintide is particularly unsuitable for patients with hypoglycemic unawareness or patients with recent history of frequent severe hypoglycemic episodes that required assistance.

So far it is not recommended for pediatric use or for use in gestational diabetes. Patients with liver impairment do not need to alter the pramlintide dose as pramlintide is mainly metabolized by the kidneys. No change in dose is even required in patients with moderate to severe renal impairment (creatinine clearance between 20–50 mL/min), but the drug has not been tried in patients on dialysis.

No drug interaction was seen with either metformin or sulfonylureas, but patients on medications that require timely absorption (e.g. antibiotics, analgesics), should be cautious as absorption of these medications may be delayed. It is advisable that these medications should be taken one hour before pramlintide or 2 hours after its injection. If such medications are required to be given with meals, a small snack may be sufficient.

The major side events of pramlintide are nausea and postprandial hypoglycemia. Nausea is usually mild to moderate. It occurs mainly in type 1 diabetic patients during the titration period and usually decreases with time. It is less frequent in type 2 diabetes patients.

Conclusion

The popularity of physiologic, and intensified conventional insulin replacement therapies is increasing. Numerous recent studies have demonstrated that physiologic therapy does reduce the risk of the chronic complications of diabetes. Therefore, for people with type 1 diabetes, as well as many with type 2 diabetes requiring insulin, designing physiologic insulin replacement programs is becoming increasingly popular. Yet, physiologic insulin replacement therapy is not appropriate for everyone. And not everyone choosing physiologic therapy needs to use a pump. Developing a proper routine for, and method of, physiologic insulin replacement therapy takes time and effort. It also requires a major, long-term commitment on the part of the patient and medical and educational support from a skilled healthcare team.

So how should the primary care provider approach physiologic insulin replacement therapy?

1. First, it is important that each primary care provider understand why physiologic therapy is important, what it is, and for whom it should be recommended.
2. Next, the practitioner must decide to what degree his or her practice can initiate and manage physiologic insulin replacement programs itself versus how much should be referred out.
3. A local or regional diabetes center should be identified that can provide consultative services for the primary care provider, assessing patient need for physiologic insulin replacement, and providing services to help initiate such programs.
4. A decision should be made as to whether, or to what degree, ongoing monitoring of therapy will be provided by the primary care provider versus the consultative specialty center.
5. The primary care provider must be comfortable, at minimum, recognizing when problems arise with the treatment program. This does not just refer to the obvious problems of ketoacidosis. It also includes suboptimal control as reflected by above-targeted A1C levels or variable or dangerous glucose level fluctuations. In such instances, a determination must be made as to whether the patient should see the primary provider or the diabetes center.

It may be that a consultative relationship between the primary care provider and a specialty center may be the best approach for the patient. However, this construct occurs less often than one may imagine, as it is stifled by economic restraints, managed-care restrictions, lack of awareness of the need and benefit of intensive therapy, or plain old inertia.

Yet, with growing evidence that physiologic therapy does impact long-term complications — and by implication, probably long term costs — the effort must be made to work past the obstacles and allow any patient who would benefit from physiologic insulin replacement therapy to have the support and care needed to utilize this treatment approach.

12

Patient Education

Elizabeth Blair, MSN, APRN, BC, CDE*

Introduction

Optimizing diabetes management requires that people with diabetes have the basic skills and knowledge to monitor glucose levels and to adjust medications, dietary intake and activity. Because diabetes is a multi-system disease and not just an abnormality of blood glucose levels, people with diabetes must also be knowledgeable about, as well as actively involved in, risk factor reduction. The process of learning about glucose control and risk factor reduction must be a joint effort between the person with diabetes and the healthcare team. Ultimately, the role of the healthcare team is to help the patient develop self-care and problem-solving skills so that he or she can be as independent as possible and achieve positive health outcomes.

The Emotional Component

Before an education plan can be completely implemented, feelings about the diagnosis of diabetes as well as the burden of its everyday diabetes

* This chapter was adapted from The Joslin Way, A Health Care Professional's Guide to Diabetes Patient Care. *Adaptation and revision by Elizabeth Blair.*

management, need to be acknowledged. For a patient to hear that he or she, a significant other, or a child, has diabetes is a significant life event. The patient's knowledge about, and experience with, diabetes must be assessed. Incorrect information — or no information — is often scarier than the facts. It can be overwhelming to add the time and the emotional burden of caring for diabetes to the day-to-day stress of contemporary life. Before teaching patients and others about the pathophysiology of diabetes, answer the patient's questions, then add to the person's knowledge and skill base.

Some of the initial questions you may hear patient ask include: Will I lose my vision? Will I lose my legs or feet? Will I be able to continue to work? A young woman may wonder about childbearing potential and have concerns of "passing" diabetes on to the next generation. Patients may have questions about nontraditional treatments and purported cures based on information obtained on the internet or from other sources. Some questions may not be directly asked, but may be alluded to instead. Careful listening can help elicit these concerns, giving the healthcare team an opportunity to clarify and educate.

Take time to ask the patient what came to mind when they were told they had diabetes. Discuss their experiences with friends or relatives who have diabetes. To help explore and resolve issues related to having a chronic illness, many people with diabetes benefit from group education and from support groups. Groups allow interaction with other people with diabetes who have experienced similar issues and, in many instances, have overcome obstacles. Some people will also benefit from a referral to a mental health professional for individual counseling. (See Chapter 23 for more information about the psychological issues surrounding diabetes.)

Evaluation, Negotiation and Goal-Setting

Because so many issues face the patient and the healthcare team, priorities for interaction and education need to be negotiated. Ideally, all patients should have a thorough assessment of their past and present diabetes treatment and education programs. Sort out what worked, what didn't work, and why. Barriers to medical care and to education need to be identified and evaluated. Familiarity with the patient's cultural and religious beliefs will also help the healthcare team tailor education strategies. When developing educational and treatment priorities, goals need to be agreed upon and established for *and with* the patient. Together, the team and the patient should develop a plan for action if goals are not met.

Examples of goal-setting for glucose control include establishing:

- Frequency and timing of glucose monitoring
- Fasting and post-prandial glucose targets
- A1C goals
- Weight targets, both the amount of weight change and the time frame for the change
- Activity goals, including frequency, duration and intensity

Self-Management Education

Successful management of diabetes is primarily dependent upon the patient's understanding of diabetes principles and the ability to make informed decisions on a daily basis. Learning occurs over time. It is unrealistic and unfair to expect a patient to learn everything about diabetes self-care in one or two sessions. Prioritizing education is determined by what the patient *needs* to learn to be safe and by what the patient *wants* to learn.

Survival Skills

"Survival skills" are the minimal skills required to maintain safe, but not necessarily optimal, glucose control for the short term. In general, when faced with limited time, ensure that the patient knows the following:

- When and what to eat
- When and how to take diabetes medication
- The major side effects of their diabetes medication
- How and when to check blood glucose levels
- How to detect and treat hypoglycemia
- When to call the healthcare team to report high glucose levels
- When to call the healthcare team with questions or concerns

The Complete Program

The National Standards for Diabetes Self-Management recommend that self-management classes for people with diabetes include the following content areas:

1. A description of the diabetes disease process and treatment options
2. Appropriate nutritional management
3. How to incorporate physical activity into lifestyle
4. Utilization of medications
5. Glucose and ketone monitoring and use of the results
6. Prevention, detection, and treatment of acute complications (hypoglycemia, hyperglycemia, sick days)
7. Prevention, detection, and treatment of chronic complications
8. Goal-setting to promote health and problem-solving for daily living
9. Integrating psychosocial adjustment into daily life
10. Promotion of preconception care, gestational diabetes information and diabetes management during pregnancy.

Effective Diabetes Education

Effective diabetes education requires an ongoing relationship between the patient and the healthcare team. The effectiveness of education is maximized when the healthcare provider:

- understands the characteristics of the learner
- incorporates the special needs of each individual
- develops specific, realistic goals with each patient
- delivers the message in a creative, interactive and memorable way
- anticipates patient challenges and obstacles that may impede behavior change
- prepares the patient for situations that may cause a lapse into old behaviors

The education process begins with an assessment, and is followed by establishing priorities, setting goals, and then evaluating outcomes and process.

Assessment

Assessment is a crucial first step to any successful intervention. It provides an opportunity to explore the patient's expectations and past experiences, to determine the feasibility of treatment plans, and to anticipate potential barriers to successful change.

When conducting an assessment, help the patient feel comfortable. Establish privacy and physical comfort. Let the patient know that you want to learn something about him or her, the nature of his or her diabetes and the particular challenges that it presents. Listed below are seven areas to explore when assessing a patient's readiness to learn:

1. *Ask about the patient's experience with diabetes and about personal goals.*
   Use past experiences as "data" to learn how the patient views diabetes as well as what behaviors have been easiest and most difficult to change or maintain over time.
2. *Ask about current habits.*
   Build on current accomplishments by setting realistic short and long-term goals for behavioral change.
   Example: In the past week, what has been your routine for checking your blood glucose, taking medication(s) and getting physical activity?
3. *Find the preferred style of learning.*
   While active learning is the most effective learning style, individuals differ in their comfort level with various modes of teaching. Ask the patient how he or she best learns material (e.g., books, discussion, videos, etc.).
4. *Inquire about psychological status.*
   Moods and feelings can have a powerful impact on a patient's readiness and ability to change. Life events can interfere with the patient's ability to focus on the education session. Patients who experience "burn-out" with their diabetes or who are feeling depressed may not be ready to make major changes.
   Sample question: What's going on in your life? How does diabetes change the way you live? What are your thoughts about that?
5. *Assess cultural and economic background.*
   Culture and economics influence daily interactions, thoughts and feelings. Areas to evaluate include: cultural expectations patients may have about visiting their healthcare provider; role expectations or

function of the patient within the family and how diabetes impacts the roles; financial resources available to the patient — does the patient have access to health insurance, money for diabetes supplies or for transportation?

    Sample questions: How do you support yourself? How does diabetes impact this?

6. *Assess literacy.*

   Printed educational materials are often at an 8th grade reading level. If you are unsure of the patient's reading ability, ask them if they understand the information or have them read instructions back to you. If needed adjust teaching techniques/materials.

7. *Assess physical health and impairments.*

   Fundamental to learning is feeling well enough to absorb new information. For some patients, physical illness may require limiting educational interventions until they feel better. For other patients, a recent acute illness (e.g., a cardiac event or foot infection) may provide high motivation to learn lifestyle changes. Assess the impact of the patient's illness on readiness to learn, and adjust teaching techniques to accommodate physical challenges. Explore the patient's prior and current coping strategies and ways to incorporate diabetes self-care using these strategies.

Goal-Setting

Once the assessment phase has been completed, it is important to set goals. Goals provide the patient and healthcare team with concrete behavioral objectives and a way to evaluate change. Behavioral goals or objectives are simple statements that define what the patient will do. Goals must be concrete, realistic, and measurable at a later date. After discussing their goals, most patients will benefit by having the goals written down so that they can be taken home. Asking a few key questions will help determine the patient's understanding, willingness and interest in making the necessary behavior changes. Here are some questions you might ask:

- What is the most important goal for you in managing your diabetes?
- What are some changes you could make to your present meal plan to more closely follow the diabetes nutrition goals we discussed?

- You said you wanted to begin walking. What time of the day would you do that?

Goals or objectives should be *measurable* and *realistic*. The goal should include an action verb such as "demonstrate," "identify," "choose," or "state," as opposed to verbs like "know" or "understand." An example: "I agree to check my blood glucose before breakfast, lunch and supper on Monday, Thursday and Sunday."

Evaluation

Follow-up appointments should include an evaluation of the patient's behavior changes. This enables both the patient and the team to track the progress towards each behavioral goal. The evaluation helps determine if the goal is feasible for *this* patient at *this* particular time in his or her life, as well as to reinforce progress being made. Evaluation can take a variety of formats:

- Patients may self-report information about what actions they have and have not been able to initiate, as well the barriers and successes they encountered.
- The provider may examine logs such as meal planning records or blood glucose monitoring diaries.
- The provider may measure related clinical outcomes such as weight, blood pressure, lipids, or glycohemoglobin.

Encouraging patients' feedback enhances the patient-provider relationship by providing interactive support, motivation, and strategies to enhance current progress. In addition, old goals may be modified and new goals established.

What about the patient who does "nothing" between your encounters?

You may discover at a follow up visit that none of the behavior changes have been implemented, even though they were concrete and were agreed to by the patient and team. It's not uncommon for patients to ask for advice and not use it, or agree to recommendations but then not implement them. These behaviors are not a cause for a "scolding" from the provider, but an indication of the need for reassessment. Consider finding the answers to the following questions.

- Did both the patient and provider share these goals?
- Did the patient understand them? Was there miscommunication between patient and provider?
- Were the goals realistic and feasible?
- Did the patient feel the need to please the provider during the last visit?
- What about the plan was difficult for the patient to implement?

Understanding Behaviors

It is important to remember that patients' behaviors are *in part* the result of their attitudes about diabetes, beliefs about treatment, degrees of success with blood glucose management, and their experiences with medical care. Intervening variables such as major life events, other competing priorities (such as tension between work demands and self-care), or conflicting messages from the healthcare team or from home (e.g., lack of support from family members for nutritional recommendations) can also affect the patient's ability to follow through on goal setting. The patient may not be ready to make changes because of denial or other psychological factors or obstacles. These variables require the provider to renegotiate goals, pay attention to negative feelings about diabetes, assist in conflict resolution and actively engage the patient in problem solving. To help more fully understand behaviors, consider the following:

Motivation
The reasons underlying most human behaviors are complex and not readily recognized by outside observers. For example, insulin omission may at first appear foolhardy to the provider but, to the young woman who is distressed about gaining weight, it makes sense because omitting insulin results in weight loss. It is important to realize that behavior is not random but is the result of a series of active choices. *The healthcare provider needs to put aside judgment, inquire about what lies behind a patient's choice or behavior, and modify the treatment program and/or goals to address the patient's primary motivations.*

Ambivalence

It is important for the provider to realize that indecision, reluctance, or resistance to clinical recommendations is not uncommon. Patients have mixed feelings about being in control of their self-care and about needing help. Patients also fear the potential of unknown side effects from medications and are not willing to completely trust current research recommendations. These issues and feelings need to be openly discussed.

Provider behavior

Communication, trust, respect, acceptance and support are elements that help create a positive climate for patients to learn and to ultimately change behaviors. It is important to respect the patient's choices even when such decisions conflict with recommendations made by the health team member.

Expectations

The patient brings expectations to the patient/provider relationship based on need, knowledge level, attitudes, preconceptions and past history. In some cases there may be unrealistic expectations of the health-care team. This can lead to conflict and/or disappointment. For example, the patient may expect that after one visit with the diabetes educator glucose levels will be perfectly controlled. The healthcare provider needs to ask the patient about expectations of the visit and treatment program and if necessary clarify and negotiate realistic goals and expectations. *All patients are looking for a cure for their diabetes, or at least perfect treatment leading to perfect diabetes management. It is important to acknowledge the imperfection of available treatment modalities.*

Enhancing the Learning Process

The ability of the provider and patient to relate to one another facilitates successful learning. Without warm human interest and responsive rapport, teaching can be done *to* patients, but not *with* them. The following concepts help facilitate learning:

The need to know — When patients want to learn, particularly when they come to a healthcare provider on their own initiative, the success of learning is enhanced. Individuals who initiate contact for education are more likely to participate in their education. Patients who receive education as part of their hospital care may not have a specific agenda for learning about their diabetes. Asking a patient, "What would you like to learn?" can help you to better identify how engaged this person is in the education process. The provider must balance what patients say they *want* to know with what they *need* to know.

Personal relevance — Learning is a process of assimilating or taking in new information and linking that information with existing knowledge. It is important to assess what the patient knows and has experienced in the past in order to determine a starting point. Using past experience as a platform of learning provides continuity for patients and allows the healthcare team to better understand potential barriers to learning and doing. Minimize teaching of abstract and theoretical information and emphasize knowledge and skills that are tangible and that will be personally useful to the patient. A good way to begin a session is to simply ask, "What are you most concerned about?"

Self-confidence and a desire to learn — Continually reinforce the idea that the patient can master the skills and knowledge needed to control diabetes. Simple statements like, "I know you can do it!" can help reinforce self-confidence. A patient's confidence in making and maintaining changes is predictive of success in making the change. This process is enhanced when the education program builds on a series of carefully planned successful experiences that lead to achieving short-term goals. Guide the patient with poor confidence in making positive self-talk statements such as "I can do it." Anticipate and acknowledge problems that the patient might encounter as he or she begins to change behaviors.

Active learning — Patients will acquire and retain knowledge and skills better if they are given opportunities to be active participants in the learning process rather than passive recipients of information (such as reading or lecture). Engaging the patient in a conversation about the topic area, having the patient take notes about key concepts, or encouraging interaction with others in a group setting help promote active learning.

Apply learning immediately — Patients will retain knowledge and skills longer if they have opportunities for frequent application and repetition. Offer "homework" assignments, such as looking for a particular food label, so the patient can apply new knowledge. Having opportunities to practice what one has learned not only reinforces the concepts, but also promotes mastery of the material.

Keep it simple and short — Deliver only one or two main messages at a time. Staging the learning and setting priorities will enhance the learning. Remember the K.I.S.S. principle of education, "Keep It Short and Simple." When a patient accomplishes a measurable, small goal (and that goal is acknowledged), self-confidence will increase, increasing the likelihood that other goals will be successfully met.

Example:
Weight control is a good example for goal setting. The initial goal should not be pounds lost, but perhaps keeping a food diary for 3 days or controlling portions during the after-dinner hours.

Adjust the pace — Patients usually do not learn at a constant rate. The pace of education and goal setting may need to be adjusted to accommodate variations in the patient's ability to absorb and retain information. Be prepared to adjust your goals for the patient to match his or her readiness to learn. When people are ill, it makes learning and retention of material much more difficult. Be sensitive to the physical as well as psychological effects of illness on motivation and learning.

Make it an enjoyable experience — A warm smile and a good sense of humor on the part of the provider can go a long way in enhancing learning. Think about your patients as "customers." If they don't find the education session enjoyable, they will not want to hear more or come back.

Review, reinforce and repeat — Learning is enhanced when it is practiced and reviewed. Not only do repetition and review help to solidify understanding, they provide opportunities for success and building confidence. Having the patient practice and review information provides valuable information about the areas that may be problematic for the patient.

People forget what they have learned as time passes. Level of education, profession, or the length of time living with diabetes does not necessarily correlate with *knowledge* of diabetes. Core diabetes knowledge and skills should be reviewed and updated on an annual basis.

The following management areas should be reviewed annually:

- Blood glucose monitoring technique and schedule
- The use of and interpretation of monitoring results
- Medication dosing and schedule

- Meal planning
- Hypoglycemia plan and practices
- Sick-day plan
- Foot care

Educational materials — Use of written materials, handouts, discussion or other educational interactions can be used to refresh diabetes self-care knowledge. Learning is enhanced when it is fun, personlly relevant, necessary, interactive, goal-oriented, short and repetitive.

Written patient education materials or audiovisual aids such as videotapes, should enhance but not replace individualized attention from a healthcare provider. Patient education videos can be a helpful way to "teach" basic diabetes information. Here are a few tips for enhancing the use of patient education materials:

- Make sure the print size and reading level is appropriate for your patient. Ask the patient: "Do you need glasses to see this better?" Use a non-threatening approach to identify a reading or vision problem.
- Personalize the written piece by writing the following on it: your name, phone number, patient's name and date.
- Use a colored pen or highlighted marker when reviewing a tool with the patient. Have the patient use the marker to circle or underline key information.
- Encourage the patient to write down his or her own behavioral goals as well as follow-up plan.

Group vs. individual teaching sessions — Traditionally, education has been conducted in individual sessions. Studies, however, have shown that group sessions are at least as effective as individual educational sessions. In the current healthcare climate of cost-containment, group sessions can provide effective education in a cost-effective format.

Lifelong Learning

As a life-long chronic condition, diabetes requires ongoing care for patients as they progress from childhood, to adolescence, to adulthood and to the older adult. The needs and life demands of each of these populations are rich and varied. Each population has different learning styles.

Children and adolescents can benefit from visits with a pediatric diabetes educator.

Children

Teaching children about their diabetes involves not only teaching the child, but teaching family members as well. Early in the course of care, it is important to identify which adult is primarily responsible for the care of the child. The primary care giver may be the mother, father, grandparents or other.

The most important concept in childhood diabetes education is understanding the developmental level of the patient. Childhood is a time rich in cognitive, emotional, and physical growth and changes. It is important to be attuned to the developmental level of the child so that the healthcare team can connect in meaningful ways. Moreover, the way children learn about their diabetes and the ways to assist in their self-care can have important positive effects on their self-care as adults. Diabetes education in childhood plays an important role in both the short and long-term care of the person with diabetes. Following, are four concepts for teaching children:

1. **Make it developmentally relevant.** Based on the age and demonstrated competencies of each child, adjust teaching strategies to the strengths and capabilities of that child. For example, when teaching blood glucose monitoring to a 5 year old, you can engage the child by letting her choose which finger will be used for the test, but you should actually instruct the parents. For a 13 year old, the parents would observe while the teenager receives the instructions and demonstrates skills. Teaching tools you can include dolls, plastic foods, puzzles, and, for older children, games.
2. **Make it enjoyable.** Children, like adults, learn best when they are engaged in what they are doing and when it is fun. Open communication about the experience of diabetes coupled with smiles can turn a potentially frightening visit with healthcare team into a great learning opportunity. Additionally, using multiple teaching aides such as games, examples and rewards will increase the "fun" factor.
3. **Make it concrete.** Abstract thinking normally develops during late childhood and early adolescence. As with adults, making examples

and teaching aids as concrete as possible will ensure that a complex idea is understood.

4. **Provide positive reinforcement.** Children are best motivated when they are told they are doing well. Using simple behavioral aids such as stickers for a job well done gives children the emotional boost they need to continue to accomplish simple as well as complex self-care tasks.

Adolescents

Adolescents, almost by definition, are undergoing a time of physical, emotional and social transition as they mature beyond childhood into young adulthood. This period poses special physical challenges for blood glucose control and heightened social and emotional pressures as adolescents move away from their families and toward peer relationships. Several concepts are important when working with adolescent patients/ learners:

- **Developmental relevance** — There is considerable variability in the emotional and cognitive maturity of adolescents. Negotiating roles for self-care behaviors between family members and adolescents based on the cognitive and emotional maturity of the adolescent creates a more successful diabetes management plan.

  Teens also need an opportunity for frank discussions about some of the most pressing topics of this developmental period: drugs, alcohol, dating and sex. None of these topics can be raised without a trusting, supportive relationship. Exploring how teens manage diabetes around these issues will be more meaningful to them and increase their willingness to listen and learn if the discussion is presented in an honest, open, nonjudgmental forum.

- **Engage in conversation** — Adolescence can be a time of shyness or awkwardness, especially when it comes to visits with a doctor or other healthcare provider. Engage the adolescent in a dialogue about what diabetes means to him or her, difficulties in balancing diabetes self-care with peer relationships, or the impact of physical changes on insulin administration, self-monitoring, or meal planning. Ask questions! Listen not only to the words the teen uses, but also pay attention to his or her body language and emotional responses. The more actively the adolescent is involved, the greater the chances are of using the information you impart. Confidentiality between teen and provider must be emphasized. Spend part of a visit alone with the teen. Having a parent in the room will alter the educational process. If a parent is part of an education intervention, a teen may feel less committed to listening. End a visit by including parents in the wrap-up so that they are informed.

- **Make the learning experience enjoyable.** Vary the way the information is conveyed as well as the context. Diabetes camps, science clubs, and teen support groups can provide important access to learning self-care skills in a fun and engaging way. Be sensitive to modes of education that may feel too "condescending" to the maturity level of your adolescent patient.

Adult Learners

With the benefit of maturity, most adult learners are capable of advanced skills in reading, listening, focusing attention on relevant tasks, problem solving and assimilating information. Tap into these traits by noting these four characteristics of adult learners:

- **Self-direction** — Adult learners can be self-directed in teaching themselves beyond the patient education session. Provide adult patients with the resources and tools they will need to continue their own efforts at education. Resources such as support groups, reading lists, and relevant organizations (e.g., American Diabetes Association) can be valuable tools to the adult learner.
- **Problem orientation** — Discussing concrete, realistic problems that are easily applicable to the individual patient are excellent teaching strategies for all ages. Adults in particular are well acquainted with problem solving. Giving homework such as case histories or situations for patients to solve, promotes greater assimilation of material and useful problem solving techniques that can be applied quickly.
- **Using experience** — Adults learn better when their own experiences are incorporated into education. Using the patient's frame of reference increases understanding of concepts and the relevance of new information. Use analogies from work or hobbies to help incorporate information.

- **Participation in the learning process** — Active participation in the learning process not only enhances understanding of the material, but also engages the patient to use the information right away.

The Older Adult

Older adults present a diverse and unique set of developmental and social needs. Older adults face greater challenges due to an increased number and frequency of illnesses, the increased demands of self-care, the need for multiple medications, changes in social interactions (or isolation), and differing expectations about the utility of self-care efforts. While some older adults have multiple medical issues and cognitive impairment, others are very capable of incorporating complex and necessary self-care tasks into their daily regimen. An individualized teaching plan drawing on the strength of the older adult will help meet the needs of such diversity. Consider the following when working with the elderly:

- **Co-morbid health issues** — Older adults frequently present with additional medical conditions that require on-going professional care and self-care. Such co-morbid healthcare issues may make it even more burdensome to learn about or follow diabetes management principles. Be aware of how diabetes education can overlap or contradict self-care recommendations for other conditions. Integrate and prioritize teaching objectives to cover the diabetes and other medical information most essential to the patient. Be mindful of the use of other medications so that interactions can be avoided.
- **Sensory changes** — Identify and clearly communicate physical challenges to other team members. For patients with low vision, use larger print and black ink on white paper to make written materials easier to see. For patients with impaired hearing, an individual appointment in a quiet location rather than a group session may enhance understanding.
- **Need for the opportunity to practice self-care behaviors** — Research has found that many older adults are highly motivated to learn about their diabetes. Taking advantage of such motivation allows patients to practice what they have learned during educational sessions. Observing skills gives the healthcare team an opportunity

to assess cognitive ability and pace, literacy, and perceived ability to perform tasks appropriately.

- **The power of self-confidence** — A common misperception of older adults is that "you can't teach an old dog new tricks." It is important to dispel such myths among healthcare professionals and patients alike by presenting material in a relevant and confidence-building way. Older patients bring a lifetime of experiences with them. Draw on their ability to adapt and meet challenges.

- **Need for sensitivity to social and financial issues** — Limited social support and financial resources play an important role in the continued success of self-care behaviors. Access to family members, food preparation, financial resources, and medications may pose important daily challenges for an older person. Discuss financial constraints that may impact self-care. Referral to a social worker may be appropriate so that older adults get connected to relevant agencies and programs.

See Chapter 22 for additional discussion about diabetes and the older adult.

Strategies for Relapse

Even with all these tools and strategies, behavior change and lifestyle maintenance are fundamentally difficult. Feeling discouraged, "burned out" or hassled by diabetes is common among newly diagnosed and long-duration patients alike. Reversing course and reverting to old patterns of behavior or old habits of self-care is a common phenomenon.

Relapse is usually defined as a period of time when an individual stops behavior change and returns to familiar habits of the past. While feelings of failure are common for both providers and patients, relapse is not a return to a previous state. Whenever an individual has worked to make any kind of change, he or she will retain the knowledge and experience from that attempt, regardless of the ultimate outcome. For example, an individual who returns to smoking after quitting for 6 months has learned more about the strategies that work and don't work. Whether the individual continues to smoke or tries to quit smoking again, she will be able to use her experience as a tool the next time she wants to make a change.

Relapse is a natural part of change. It is estimated that most patients will relapse at least three times while attempting to make a behavioral change. Relapse is most common during high-risk or high-stress situations such as:

- physical illness
- emotional stress
- changes in routine (e.g., eating out)
- social situations (e.g., hanging out with friends)
- special occasions (e.g., holidays)
- boredom or burn-out
- negative feedback or lack of positive reinforcement.

The healthcare provider should discuss the potential for relapse with the patient. Discussing the potential for relapse can help the patient anticipate challenges as well as have consider possible solutions ahead of time.

Conclusion

Diabetes education is not a one-time experience where everything can be learned at once. Diabetes is a chronic illness, and because patients change physically and emotionally over time, the skills and knowledge that patients need to provide the best self-care will also change. To be most effective, education needs to be tailored to the patient.

Diabetes self-management education begins as a relationship between the healthcare team and the person with diabetes. While providing this care the diabetes team weaves sensitivity, curiosity, and compassion into the interaction as behavioral goals are jointly decided and barriers to change are anticipated. Both the healthcare provider and the patient are part of an ongoing learning process that may span several developmental periods of life and require a continuous flow of new information. Thus, providers and patients have an opportunity to be dynamic and thoughtful in their teaching. Ultimately, the role of the healthcare team is to help the patient develop self-care and problem-solving skills so that he or she can be as independent as possible and achieve positive health outcomes.

13

Acute Complications

Ramachandiran Cooppan, MD,
Richard Beaser, MD, and
Greeshma K. Shetty, MD

Introduction

It is quite reasonable to expect that a person who develops a chronic disease like diabetes mellitus will experience an acute complication during his or her lifetime. Most often, and especially for an insulin-treated patient, this will be an acute hypoglycemic event. For others, it may be a presenting symptom of the disease such as diabetic ketoacidosis. These acute complications can be life-threatening, and it is extremely important to make the patient aware of them while at the same time putting them in their correct perspective. Too often, either the patient or a member of the patient's family has knowledge of someone else who may have experienced one of these events and had a poor outcome. Fear of hypoglycemia, for example, can become a major reason that a patient would resist using insulin when it is necessary even though by doing so he or she compromises control of the diabetes and risks long-term complications. By addressing these problems with care and understanding, and by teaching patients the skills needed to take care of them when they do occur, much of the morbidity, and even the mortality, associated with complications can be reduced.

The acute complications of diabetes can be categorized as relating to either very high glucose levels (hyperglycemia) and their consequences, or very low glucose levels (hypoglycemia):

- diabetic ketoacidosis (DKA)
- hyperosmolar hyperglycemic state (HHS)
- lactic acidosis (LA)
- hypoglycemia

Very high glucose levels usually result from a reduction in the effect of circulating insulin plus an elevation of counterregulatory hormones, including glucagon, catecholamine, cortisol, and growth hormone. Reduced effective circulating insulin can result from either a deficiency of endogenous insulin secretion or a lack of exogenous insulin, particularly in a situation where insulin needs may be increased (e.g., during the stress of another acute medical condition, such as an infection). Low blood glucose — hypoglycemia — usually results from excess insulin, either due to insulin administration/calculation errors or an improper balance among the various components impacting glucose levels. In addition, lactic acidosis must be included in this list of potentially life-threatening conditions, particularly if a patient with ketoacidosis does not respond to therapy or a sudden deterioration occurs during therapy.

Diabetic Ketoacidosis (DKA)

Diabetic ketoacidosis is an acute event that is a result of acute insulin deficiency. It is often associated with type 1 diabetes and, may, in fact, be the presenting event for this condition. Fortunately, however, this dangerous metabolic condition is usually preventable, even in someone not yet known to have diabetes. While it is increasingly rare that DKA is the first sign of diabetes, it still can result if the classic signs are not recognized, and even today, people still die due to misdiagnosis. In the United States, it is estimated that up to 100,000 patients a year are seen in emergency rooms for it. Accurate estimates of the problem are hard to come by, but one review from the Regional Medical Center of Memphis estimated that DKA was the diagnosis in 34.9% of all primary diabetes admissions. The prevention of DKA on presentation of diabetes is dependent upon the greater awareness in the population about diabetes and the tendency of people to seek medical attention sooner. While the overall mortality of this condition is < 5%, it still has the real potential to result in mortality. Risk for mortality is higher for older patients and those presenting with coma, hypotension, or other co-morbid conditions. Thus, it must be thought of in the differential diagnosis in acutely presenting patients with suggestive signs and symptoms.

The syndrome itself consists of hyperglycemia, ketosis and acidemia. Often, the blood glucose is quite elevated — greater than 400 — but it can be between 250 and 300 mg/dl, especially in patients who may have taken some insulin. This is an important point to remember because the tendency is to think that glucose values have to be much higher for DKA to occur. Valuable time can be lost and delays in treatment can have very serious consequences. The arterial pH is usually less than 7.3 and the bicarbonate value less than 15 mEq/l.

Setting for DKA

The precipitating factors for DKA are mainly infection, concurrent illness, and omission of insulin or inadequate coverage for sick days. Many patients are seen because they have not been taught how to take care of their diabetes during a concurrent illness, and DKA often precipitates rapidly, so hesitation in self-treatment can be problematic. Even patients who have received education and have had diabetes for many years can make errors in handling sick days. It is not uncommon for patients to state that because of anorexia or poor appetite, they felt it was not necessary to take insulin. This is a major error, especially for a patient with type 1 diabetes who relies completely on exogenous insulin. In fact, during this time of increased stress, patients will often need more insulin due to elevations of counterregulatory hormones, such as adrenalin, which cause glucose elevations and the catabolic effect of the illness and infection. Factors associated with DKA are most commonly infection (40%), especially of the urinary tract, and omission of insulin (25%).

It is important to note that even after many years of diabetes and previous episodes of poorly treated sick days, adult patients can still continue to make mistakes. Myocardial infarction, cerebrovascular accident, trauma, stress, surgery or undiagnosed hyperthyroidism can all also precipitate the problem. Similarly, use of medications which can impact carbohydrate metabolism such as corticosteroids, thiazides, or sympathomimetic agents can contribute. Nonetheless, in about 20% to 30% of cases, there is no obvious cause, though it is likely due to an increased insulin requirement for some unidentifiable reason.

It is worthwhile to mention one setting in which iatrogenic DKA can occur in patients with type 1 diabetes who may be hospitalized for some other cause. It is tempting for such patients to be managed by a "sliding scale" of insulin coverage — an approach that has some convenience but a great deal of risk as well. A common scenario is that of a patient who is not eating — either at all or very much. As this patient has diabetes, there is a fear of giving him or her dextrose in the intravenous solution. To compound the error, the sliding-scale insulin coverage is written so that no longer-acting insulin is given (fearing that, without eating, hypoglycemia could occur) and the rapid-acting insulin coverage isn't invoked until the glucose level is relatively high, perhaps about 200 or 250 mg/dl. Thus, with no food or intravenous glucose and depleted glycogen stores, the glucose level rarely rises high enough to trigger insulin administration. Yet, there is nevertheless an insulin deficiency, made worse if there is an elevation of the contra-insulin hormones. With surprising rapidity and reliability, such patients can slip into DKA under the eyes of the hospital staff.

The simple solution to a scenario like the one described above is to use dextrose in intravenous solutions when patients with type 1 diabetes have insufficient oral intake. Doing so allows the use of a modest dose of long-acting insulin (NPH, glargine or detemir), which shuts off ketogenesis. Adjustable doses of regular or rapid-acting insulin may then be used to correct glucose elevations. If there is still fear of hypoglycemia with long-acting insulin, and rapid-acting or regular insulin is felt to be preferable, then the use of intravenous dextrose will still allow insulin coverage to be given safely at much lower glucose levels.

Keep in mind that the newer rapid-acting insulin analogs have a shorter duration of action than regular insulin. Thus, their effect runs out sooner than regular insulin. Therefore, in the care of an ill patient, the effect of insulin to suppress counterregulatory hormones due to the stress of the illness will run out sooner with rapid-acting insulin analogs than with regular insulin. Thus, glucose checks and insulin coverage should be more frequent (every 3 hours may be needed) when these analog insulins are used. However, the advantage of these insulins is the ability to change course in the coverage more rapidly if the patient's condition changes.

Repeated episodes of acidosis in adolescent patients may be a clue to underlying psychological issues and noncompliance. Here again, the pattern of the events, such as repeated DKA, or DKA when family, school or social stress is greatest, should alert the provider that something is amiss.

In the last few years, the use of subcutaneous insulin infusion pumps (CSII) has emerged as another important factor affecting the incidence of ketoacidosis. Since these devices infuse small amounts of rapid-acting insulin, any interruption of the insulin delivery can result in acute insulin deficiency and ketoacidosis. This may be particularly true with pumps because no longer-acting insulin is used, and once the rapid-acting insulin is gone, there is no "safety-net" provided by residual NPH or glargine or detemir. Pump patients should be taught vigilance for situations in which insulin delivery can be interrupted, such as tubing kinks and insertion-site inflammation or infection.

While DKA is most often associated with type 1 diabetes, some type 2 patients can present with it also. Many of these patients can have a slowly evolving form of type 1 diabetes. When studied, it can be seen that some may have markers of autoimmune β-cell destruction. These patients actually have reduced insulin secretory reserve, and under stress can develop an acute deficiency.

Pathogenesis

Patients develop DKA because of three factors:

1. insulin deficiency
2. increased counterregulatory hormones
3. dehydration.

Appropriate insulin secretion is necessary for the body to utilize glucose and maintain normal glucose homeostasis. It also plays a major role in fat and protein metabolism. Insulin deficiency is associated with hyperglycemia and an increase in counterregulatory hormone secretion, as noted above. This increase in glucagon, catecholamines, cortisol and growth hormone also contributes to a further elevation in glucose levels from increased glycogenolysis and gluconeogenesis. In addition, there is increased lipolysis with an increased concentration of free fatty acids, which undergo beta oxidation by the liver and increase ketogenesis. Consequently, ketone bodies, acetoacetate (AcAc) and β-hydroxybutric acid are increased in the blood, causing the acidosis. The ratio of these two is normally 1:1, but in ketoacidosis the levels of β-hydroxybutyric acid increase to a greater extent than acetoacetate so that the ratio can reach as much as a 10:1 β-hydroxybutric acid predominance, decreasing the bicarbonate level.

Acetoacetic acid and acetone react very vividly with nitroprusside on urine "acetone" test strips, while the β-hydroxybutyric acid does not. During treatment of DKA, the conversion of β-hydroxybutyric acid to acetoacetic acid increases as a result of insulin and fluid replacement. Therefore, the nitroprusside reaction in the blood and urine remain at a plateau, suggesting a lack of reduction in acetone levels despite improvements in other measures of the patient's metabolic state.

Dehydration occurs in these patients because of the marked hyperglycemia with concomitant polyuria, as well as from nausea and vomiting. In severe DKA, the fluid deficit can be as much as seven liters. Hydration is therefore critical, especially early on in the treatment.

Clinical Presentation

Patients with DKA can present with the classical symptoms of diabetes, including polyuria, polydipsia and weight loss. Vomiting may also be part of the picture about 25% of the time and may show evidence of blood. They can also complain of generalized weakness, lethargy and malaise, nausea with the accompanying vomiting, and abdominal pain. The abdominal pain could be a result of the DKA or an underlying condition which is causing it. In severe cases there are mental status changes such as confusion. Acidosis can result in a compensatory rapid and shallow respiration. On physical examination, patients may exhibit poor skin turgor, orthostasis or frank hypotension from the dehydration, tachycardia, and rapid "Kussmaul" respirations. Sometimes the patient's breath has a fruity smell that is associated with ketones. Body temperature may be misleadingly low, even in the setting of an infection, due to peripheral vasodilation. Patients may drift slowly into DKA over hours and days if the cause is a relatively mild insulin deficiency, but DKA can develop very rapidly in the setting of a more significant insulin deficit and/or an acute illness.

Patients may delay going to the hospital or may know that repeated vomiting and diarrhea are signs that immediate medical attention is needed. There is even greater urgency if ketones are present in the urine. If patients call in with some of these symptoms late at night, a trip to the emergency room for intravenous fluids and further treatment should be recommended.

When faced with a patient with severe acidosis, the differential diagnosis has to include a number of other conditions that may either be a *precipitating cause* of DKA or may be *mistaken for* ketoacidosis but are really another metabolic abnormality.

Other metabolic conditions that may be mistaken for DKA might include:

- alcoholic ketoacidosis
- hyperosmolar hyperglycemic state (HHS)
- high-anion gap acidoses such as lactic acidosis, ingestions

If the patient is known to have type 1 diabetes and is young, DKA should easily and rapidly be confirmed as the etiology. Then, the primary focus other than correcting the metabolic abnormality is to seek the precipitating cause. In this setting, infection or insulin omission are the usual culprits.

In an older person with confirmed DKA, however, the list of potential causes may be longer. Depending on the clinical situation, the following might be considered as possible precipitating causes of DKA:

- acute appendicitis
- myocardial infarction
- shock, sepsis or other systemic events
- urinary tract infection
- pneumonia
- oral or dental infections
- in an immunocompromised individual, any other occult infection must be considered gastrointestinal infection (often confusing — DKA can cause GI symptoms or be caused by a GI infection.)

This list includes common precipitating factors but is not meant to be a complete listing of all possible causes. Careful clinical examination, appropriate laboratory testing, and good clinical judgment are important tools when trying to determine the cause of DKA.

Alcoholic Patients

Alcoholic patients presenting with ketoacidosis often do not have the smell of alcohol on their breath. They present with abdominal pain, nausea and vomiting. Poor general nutrition and signs of liver disease may be present. Presenting symptoms are often attributed to gastritis, pancreatitis or hepatitis. These patients are prone to aspiration pneumonia, bacterial infections, subdural hemorrhages and rhabdomyolysis. In general, the blood glucose is not increased (usually < 250 mg/dL) and may even be low. While the patient is acidotic, the bicarbonate tends not to be under 18 mEq/l. Lactic acid levels are elevated and the serum potassium, magnesium and phosphate are low. Serum alcohol levels may be low or absent if the patient has been anorexic. Dehydration is present and must be treated, and glucose is often needed to stimulate endogenous insulin secretion and inhibit the ketogenesis that is occurring.

Diagnosis of DKA

While it is important to obtain a good history, it is likely that more than 50% of patients will not be able to provide one because of their illness. If the patient cannot communicate, then relatives or friends can be very important in providing some details of the events leading to the problem. If the patient is comatose, the situation is much more serious and attention must be paid to keeping an open airway and a nasogastric tube should be placed to avoid the dangers of aspiration from gastric dilatation that may be present.

Laboratory Tests

After the physical examination, the following testing should be performed:

- *Glucose.* A fingerstick can be done while awaiting the chemistry profile. Do not be surprised if the glucose seems low, perhaps as low as 250 mg/dl.
- *Electrolytes.* In DKA, fluid and electrolyte losses per kilogram body weight are, in general, 100 ml water, 7 to 10 meq of sodium, 3 to 5 meq of potassium, 5 to 7 meq of chloride, 1 mmol of phosphorous and 0.5 to 0.8 meq of magnesium. Note that the serum sodium values can be factitiously low because of the hyperglycemia and

TABLE 13-1. Diagnosis of Diabetic Ketoacidosis and Hyperosmolar Hyperglycemic states

	DKA			
	Mild	**Moderate**	**Severe**	**HHS**
Plasma glucose (mg/dl)	>250	>250	>250	>600
Arterial pH	7.25–7.30	7.00–7.24	<7.00	>7.30
Serum bicarbonate (mEq/l)	15–18	10 to <15	<10	>15
Urine ketones*	Positive	Positive	Positive	Small
Serum ketones*	Positive	Positive	Positive	Small
Effective serum osmolality (mOsm/kg)†	Variable	Variable	Variable	>320
Anion gap‡	>10	>12	>12	Variable
Alteration in sensoria or mental obtundation	Alert	Alert/ drowsy	Stupor/ coma	Stupor/ coma

* Nitroprusside reaction method;
† calculation: 2[measured Na (mEq/l)] + glucose (mg/dl)/18;
‡ calculation: $(Na^+) - (Cl^- + HCO_3^-)$ (mEq/l). See text for details.
Copyright © 2007 American Diabetes Association, from Diabetes Care®, Volume 27, Suppl.1, 2004; S94–S102. Reprinted with permission.

hyperlipidemia. The correct sodium level can be estimated by adding 1.6 meq to the reported sodium value for every 100 mg of glucose over 100 mg/dl. The bicarbonate is used to calculate the anion gap. AG = Na-(Cl+HCO3) and is normally 8 to 16 mM.

- *Complete Blood Count.* High white counts of over 15,000 with a left shift may suggest an underlying bacterial infection, but can be seen with DKA without infection.
- *Arterial Blood Gas (ABG).* The pH is usually less than 7.3.
- *Ketones.* Acetest and Ketostix measure blood and urine acetoacetic acid. They do not measure the beta-hydroxybutyrate. During treatment, the latter is converted to the former, so the ketone measurements may paradoxically worsen.
- *Electrocardiogram.* There is a high risk for cardiac events, especially in older patients.

- **Urine Analysis and Culture.** Evaluate for possible urinary tract infection.
- **Osmolality.** Measured by formula. DKA patients in coma usually have osmolality of 330 mOsm/kg water. If it is less than this and patient is obtunded, search for other causes for obtundation.
- **Phosphorous.** Levels may be low. Be particularly cautious if the patient is at risk for hypophosphatemia due to chronic alcoholism or poor nutrition. Levels should be checked.
- **Hyperamylasemia.** Levels are rarely in range of acute pancreatitis.

It is important to check the lab values repeatedly. The potassium must be checked every 1 to 2 hours during the initial stages, as rapid drops can occur with treatment. Glucose and other electrolytes can be checked every 2 hours or so in the initial stage when aggressive volume, glucose and electrolyte management takes place.

Imaging Studies

The following imaging studies should be performed:

- *Chest X-ray.* Pneumonia may not be clinically evident with dehydration.
- *CT scan.* May be needed to assess altered mental status and to check for cerebral edema.
- *Telemetry.* Needed to monitor for ischemia and hypokalemia.

Procedures

Adequate IV access is essential. A #18 catheter or larger is recommended. An adequate airway must be maintained and intubation undertaken when indicated. A nasogastric tube should be placed in comatose patients to prevent aspiration. Consider treatment with anti-emetics. A urinary catheter may also be needed.

Management

In the emergency room, intensive fluid resuscitation is critical. General guidelines are provided in Table 13-2. Fluid is generally given in the first hour at the rate of at least 15–20 ml per kg body wt per hour, targeting at least 1 litre in that time period. The IV solutions replace fluid loss and electrolytes, lower the glucose and dilute the counterregulatory

TABLE 13-2. Suggested Fluid Amounts

May need to adjust the type and rate of fluid administration in the elderly and in patients with CHF or renal failure. KCL should be added to the IV fluids once urination is established. If patient is severely hypovolemic or in shock, initiate fluid resuscitation before commencing insulin.

Administer NS as indicated to maintain hemodynamic status, then follow general guidelines:

- Administer normal saline (NS) for the first 4 hours
- Then consider ½ NS X 4 hours
- Then D5/½ NS when plasma glucose is < 250 mg/dL.

Hour	Volume
1st ½–1	1 Liter
2nd hour	1 Liter
3rd hour	500 ml–1 Liter
4th hour	500 ml–1 Liter
5th hour	500 ml–1 Liter
Total 1st 5 hours	3.5–5 Liters
6–12th hours	250–500 ml/hr

Joslin Diabetes Center. *Guideline for Management of Uncontrolled Glucose in the Hospitalized Adult.* 2007.

hormones. The amount of fluid needed depends on the severity of the dehydration and is based on the blood pressure, pulse, urine output and mental status. After initial stabilization with normal saline (up to about 4 hours), a switch to 0.5 normal saline at 200 to 1000 cc/hr can be continued.

The other additional, immediate need is insulin to stop the catabolic process, inhibit lipolysis, and thus lower free fatty acids and promote glucose disposal into tissues. Guidelines for insulin therapy are provided in Table 13-3. The standard practice now is to use an insulin infusion. Studies have shown that an intravenous loading dose followed by continuous infusion is the best overall. A loading dose of 0.1 units/kg of body weight is reasonable, followed by 5 to 7 units/hour. The hourly dose is adjusted based on the glucose levels. The insulin loading dose and insulin infusion with aggressive fluid replacement may result in a 10% drop in

TABLE 13-3. Insulin Management

- Aim for target plasma glucose between 100–200 mg/dl
- Administer regular insulin 10 units IV STAT
- Start Regular insulin infusion at 5 units/hour or 0.1 units/kg/hour
- Assess possible causes for lack of adequate decrease in plasma glucose
- Increase Regular insulin by 1 unit/hr q 1–2 hours if <10% drop in glucose or no improvement in acid-base status
- Decrease insulin by 1–2 units/hr when glucose ≤250mg/dl and/or progressive improvement and anion gap closing
- DO NOT decrease insulin infusion to <1 unit/hour
- If plasma glucose initially drops to <100 mg/dl on insulin infusion, add glucose to IV as D5 or D10 at sufficient rate
- Check plasma glucose every 30 minutes if plasma glucose drops to <100 mg/dl
- If plasma glucose continues to drop consistently on IV D5 consider change to IV D10 to maintain glucose at 100–200 mg/dl while on insulin infusion
- Once patient can eat and anion gap is resolving, consider change to subcut insulin (continue IV insulin infusion for 1 hour **after** starting subcut insulin)
- For patients previously managed on insulin: re-evaluate insulin regimen before returning to prior dose
- For patients new to insulin, consider a regimen including a mixture of rapid- and long-acting insulin.

Joslin Diabetes Center. *Guideline for Management of Uncontrolled Glucose in the Hospitalized Adult.* 2007.

the glucose level. Once the blood glucose drops to 200 to 250 mg/ dl, the fluid can be changed to 0.5 normal saline with 5% dextrose.

Potassium replacement is critical in managing these patients. Guidelines are outlined in Table 13-4. If the initial K^+ is less than 3.5 mEq/l, indicating severe potassium deficiency, add 40 mEq KCl to the hydrating fluid as soon as the result is known. Otherwise, add 10–20 mEq/l of KCl to each liter of fluid once the K^+ is under 5.5 mEq/l. The potassium can be given two-thirds as KCl and one-third as KPO_4, particularly if the patient is comatose.

TABLE 13-4. Potassium Replacement

Do not administer K⁺ if K⁺ > 5.5 or if patient is anuric	
Serum K⁺ *(mEq/l)*	**Additional K⁺ *required***
<3.5	40 mEq/L
3.5–4.4	20 mEq/L
4.5–5.5	10 mEq/L
>5.5	Stop infusion

If there is persistent acidosis due to hyperchloremia, consider using K⁺ phosphate or K⁺ acetate instead of KCL as replacement. Can consider oral K⁺ replacement, as needed.

Joslin Diabetes Center. *Guideline for Management of Uncontrolled Glucose in the Hospitalized Adult.* 2007.

Bicarbonate therapy has been controversial. It is generally agreed that it is not usually needed unless the pH is less than 7.0. In this case, consider giving 100 ml $NaHCO_3$ over 45 minutes. Check the acid-base status 30 minutes later, and repeat this dose if the pH < 7.0. Bicarbonate should not be given if the potassium level is< 3.5 mEq/L.

Phosphate and magnesium are also not routinely needed and losses are replaced once the patient starts eating. However, careful phosphate replacement may occasionally be indicated in the setting of cardiac dysfunction, respiratory depression, anemia, or with serum phosphate concentration <1.0 mg/dl. In such instances, 20–30 mEq/l potassium phosphate is added to the IV fluids.

It is important to treat any infection present and to maintain adequate oxygenation. Constant monitoring is the key, and all severely ill patients must be admitted to the intensive care unit. The use of data flow sheets to monitor the timing of labs and the therapy is essential.

Complications of Therapy

Cerebral Edema. This is a rare event, but it can be fatal or result in serious neurologic damage. It is most often seen in children and adolescents, and in many patients who have undiagnosed diabetes. The etiology of the condition is still speculative. Brain edema without overt clinical signs during treatment of DKA appears to be a fairly common finding. The use of CT scans facilitates this finding. If there are sudden changes in the mental and neurologic status of the patient during the treatment of DKA, it is best to assume this possibility and immediately start mannitol therapy. A dose of 1 to 2 g/kg body weight is recommended. If the patient is comatose, intubation with hyperventilation should be instituted.

Hyperchloremic Acidosis. Patients recovering from DKA may commonly develop a non-anion gap hyperchloremic metabolic acidosis. This phenomenon may have a number of causes. Loss of ketones via ketonuria that results from fluid therapy can be a cause, as ketones would otherwise be used as a substrate for bicarbonate regeneration. The amount of bicarbonate in the proximal tubule may also be reduced, resulting in increased chloride reabsorption. Finally, both plasma bicarbonate and total buffering capacity are reduced, leading to hyperchloremic acidosis.

It is important clinically to distinguish these potential causes of hyperchloremic acidosis, which are routinely seen as part of the overall clinical picture, from a persistent low serum bicarbonate level due to an inadequacy of insulin treatment for the DKA itself. Clearly, this latter cause would warrant more aggressive insulin administration. When the pH rises to 7.30 or above, the glucose is controlled, and the patient is clinically recovered, oral intake is usually resumed and one can be reasonably comfortable that the insulin treatment has been sufficient. Nevertheless, the patient usually takes several days to recover from the hyperchloremic metabolic acidosis that results from these other causes, as the kidneys must readjust bicarbonate production and acid secretion.

Pulmonary Edema. If fluid replacement is vigorous, pulmonary edema may occur, particularly if the patient has underlying cardiac disease. However, with more tempered fluid replacement and/or adequate cardiac function, pulmonary edema is rare. Similarly, *aspiration of gastric contents* is another potential problem. While also rare, it can be prevented by the placement of a nasogastric tube with suction in all obtunded patients. The hypokalemia seen with DKA can worsen gastric atony and dilatation, further increasing the possibility of an adverse gastrointestinal event.

Education

Early and appropriate therapy can reduce the morbidity and mortality from DKA. Most patients with known diabetes will recover from the metabolic derangements without permanent sequellae and resume their normal insulin programs.

However, when patients present with DKA as the first indication of diabetes, they will need the same educational interventions offered to people who are diagnosed as having type 1 diabetes in another, non-DKA setting. While the team approach to diabetes management and education is the ideal, rapid initiation of an educational intervention by whatever means are available is important. These patients have not just had the diagnosis of type 1 diabetes, but have just recovered from a potentially fatal metabolic condition that must be prevented from recurring. Thus, initial teaching for new patients should address basic survival skills as plans are made to implement a more comprehensive and integrated treatment and education program.

Another sign that intervention may be needed is repeated episodes of DKA in adolescents. These young patients will need careful assessment for psychosocial problems that often are in the background.

One important way to reduce the burden of this complication is to educate patients with type 1 diabetes about managing sick days appropriately. Make sure that patients understand that acute complications can always occur but that with proper attention to the basics of good diabetes self-management, they will be able to recover from them without additional or secondary complications.

Hyperosmolar Hyperglycemic State (HHS)

The key etiologic difference between DKA and the hyperosmolar hyperglycemic state (HHS) is that with HHS, insulin is present. This acute hyperglycemic state occurs in people with type 2 diabetes who still have insulin secretion. The presence of insulin prevents the production of ketones, and thus the development of ketoacidosis. As with DKA, a physiologic stress leads to worsening hyperglycemia. However, unlike DKA, the mere omission of insulin does not usually lead to HHS; it takes the superimposition of a significant physiologic stress to cause this condition to occur.

When HHS is present, one has extreme hyperglycemia, profound dehydration (up to 10 liters deficit) and increased serum osmolarity. Osmolarity is calculated as follows: $2(Na)(mEq/l) + glucose (mg/dl)/ 18 +$

BUN (mg/dl)/2.8, with normal values being 290 ± 5 mOsm/kg water. In general, with HHS, the glucose is over 600 mg/dl and the bicarbonate concentration is over 20 mEq/l. Anion gap is usually normal. The sensorium is depressed more and coma is present in 10% of patients. HHS is seen more frequently in elderly patients and those with newly diagnosed type 2 diabetes. Many patients have a preceding illness and other chronic co-morbid conditions that contribute to the illness, e.g., mild renal insufficiency, dementia, immobility or vomiting. In many cases infections, such as pneumonia, uremia or viral syndrome result in the acute event, which develops gradually. The mortality is high — estimated anywhere between 10–50% — on the higher end of this scale for older patients. Many of these patients are from nursing homes.

It is important to note that certain drugs that inhibit insulin secretion can contribute to this state. Examples are diuretics, β-blockers, as well as dialysis and total parenteral nutrition with glucose-and dextrose-containing fluids. The major finding is severe dehydration with changes in mental status from confusion to deep coma, and various neurologic findings mimicking a cerebrovascular accident. The neurologic signs tend to improve with therapy. The profound dehydration predispose these patients to thrombosis. Diagnosis is made by the high glucose level, with increased serum osmolarity, absence of ketonemia, bicarbonate >20 mEq/l and minimal or negative urine ketones. Treatment is mainly aggressive volume replacement similar to that for DKA (normal saline and later 0.5 normal saline) with careful monitoring of the cardiovascular status of the patient. Note that these people are usually more dehydrated than those with DKA. If the patient survives the acute state, then the diabetes can usually be managed with either oral medication or small doses of insulin.

Lactic Acidosis

Lactic acidosis has number of different causes and is often an indicator of a very serious problem in a critically ill patient. A working criteria for this diagnosis is a blood lactate level of 7 mM or greater with arterial pH lower than 7.35. Lactate is normally cleared by the liver, kidney and skeletal muscles; hyperlactemia exists if the level is 2.5 mm/l or higher (normal <2 mm/l). Lactic acidosis is classified into two categories: type A and type B. Type A is associated with hypoxia or hypoperfusion and is more common. It can occur with hemorrhage, myocardial infarction, congestive heart failure, cardiogenic shock, anemia, carbon monoxide poisoning, profound sepsis, and *grand mal* seizures. Type B is associated with many diseases (diabetes mellitus, liver disease, renal failure, malignancy, sepsis, thiamine deficiency, severe hypoglycemia, and pheochromocytoma), drugs (alcohols, biguanides, cyanide, isoniazid, salicylates and aceto-aminophen) and toxins.

The occurrence of type B lactic acidosis is low with biguanide therapy (10X lower with metformin than phenformin). It usually is not due to the drug, but to predisposing conditions such as hepatic, renal or cardiac disease. The incidence of *any* type of lactic acidosis in patients with DKA is quite low. Once the diagnosis is made, the focus has typically been on the correction of the arterial pH, as the increase in lactic acid level can account for the reduced cardiac output, reduced response to catecholamines, abnormal hepatic metabolism, and arrhythmias. However, the underlying disease, often multiple organ failure, is frequently playing a significant role in the vascular collapse, and the presence of increased levels of lactic acid can actually increase cardiac output and decrease systemic vascular resistance. In fact, there is an argument against using bicarbonate infusion because of the potential for worsening pulmonary edema, hypertonicity, hypokalemia, hypocalcemia and rebound alkalosis. In general, as these patients have all the hallmarks of severe vascular collapse, primary attention should be paid to maintaining cardiac output, blood pressure, oxygenation, renal perfusion, and treating any infection or other underlying factors precipitating the metabolic derangement.

Hypoglycemia

Hypoglycemia is the most common acute complication in type 1 diabetic patients. It can, however, also be seen in type 2 patients being treated with insulin and, less commonly, in patients being treated with antidiabetes medications for hyperglycemia. The symptoms can range from minor (tremor, palpitations and hunger) to severe (mental changes, convulsions and coma). It can even result in death, especially if it occurs while driving, or during deep sleep, and especially in a patient with hypoglycemic unawareness. It is estimated that 4% of deaths of patients with type 1 diabetes can be attributed to hypoglycemia. In general, the milder episodes are associated with glucose in the 50 to 60 mg range and the more severe episodes with glucose levels of less than 40 mg. The milder cases can be managed with oral carbohydrate treatment, but severe cases will need either glucagon injection or intravenous glucose. Recurrent hypoglycemia can be associated with major morbidity and even psychological morbidity that can be persistent.

The symptoms of hypoglycemia are categorized as either neurogenic or neuroglycopenic.

Neurogenic:

- diaphoresis
- tremor
- palpitations
- pallor
- arousal/anxiety
- hypertension

Neuroglycopenic:

- cognitive impairment
- fatigue
- visual changes
- hunger
- paresthesias
- inappropriate behavior
- focal neurologic deficits
- seizures
- loss of consciousness
- death

Incidence and Precipitating Factors

As noted above, it is almost impossible to avoid hypoglycemia when using our current methods of insulin replacement, because insulin therapy is affected by many factors that influence the response to daily doses. These are discussed in greater detail in the chapters on insulin therapy; however, they include variations of absorption, particularly with rotation of injection sites, combinations of insulins, variations in food consumption and activity that was not properly anticipated, and errors made by the patient, especially when mixing insulins.

Glucagon and epinephrine are counterregulatory hormones and normally serve as the major defenses against hypoglycemia. Patients who have had type 1 for a long time develop progressive loss of counterregulatory hormone response, and as a result may become unaware of early sympathetic symptoms that serve as an early warning of impending hypoglycemia. Lack of glucagon and reduced epinephrine responses can result in a marked increase in the frequency of severe hypoglycemia.

It has traditionally been said that the more aggressive the insulin therapy, the more risk there is of hypoglycemia. In the DCCT, the incidence of severe hypoglycemia in the intensive treatment group was 6%, which was greater than that in the conventionally treated group. This finding seemed to confirm what people had believed for years — that intensive therapy caused more hypoglycemia.

However, as the impact of time and experience has allowed us to contemplate these DCCT findings, another conclusion seems to be evident: attempting to be aggressive with control by increasing insulin quantity in a *nonphysiologic* insulin treatment program is *more* likely to cause hypoglycemia than similar attempts at aggressive therapy using a physiologic program, where insulin quantities more accurately match actual needs. Much of the hypoglycemia in the DCCT may have been due to the inexperience of both the healthcare professionals (intensive insulin therapy was a new concept at the time of the study) and the patients, combined with the mandate of the study to target normoglycemia.

Now, with more experience using physiologic insulin replacement therapies of multiple injections and pumps, their physiologic design may actually allow more aggressive therapy while actually *reducing* the risk of hypoglycemia. Also, when hypoglycemia occurs, it may be milder because a lesser quantity of insulin is peaking than might occur with a conventionally designed program. In particular with pump therapy, the use of a single type of rapid-acting insulin actually reduces the hypoglycemic risk. The basal infusion rate allows constant insulin availability without the irregularities associated with intermediate-acting preparations given subcutaneously. In addition, the growing popularity of using rapid premeal insulin in physiologic insulin replacement programs has been shown to reduce the number of hypoglycemic reactions, particularly at night.

Clinically significant hypoglycemia appears most often in people using insulin to treat their diabetes. However, it can occasionally be seen in those using oral therapy, particularly among those using some of the longer-acting oral sulfonylureas. A typical candidate for clinically significant hypoglycemia is in an elderly patient who may not eat on time or who has a problem with access to food. Similarly, hypoglycemia can occur in patients using antidiabetes medications to treat their diabetes who have other co-morbid illnesses requiring multiple therapies leading to polypharmacy. Certain drug interactions can potentiate the hypoglycemic effects or impair symptoms, such as is seen with the use of β-blockers. (More detail about such interactions can be found in the chapter on oral treatment of diabetes.) Specific medications or the use of multiple medications can also affect appetite and further potentiate hypoglycemia.

When hypoglycemia occurs due to the use of sulfonylureas, it can potentially be prolonged and lead to the need for hospitalization and treatment with intravenous glucose. Mild hypoglycemic episodes may be treatable with simple carbohydrates and a meal if it is close to that time, but beware of repeated hypoglycemia over the next few hours. Once again, monitoring blood glucose is the key to treatment.

Keep in mind, as well, that some patients taking sulfonylureas who experience hypoglycemia may not present with the classic symptoms. In particular, an elderly patient's hypoglycemia may present as unexplained mental or behavior changes. In severe cases in this older group, there may be hypothermia.

Understanding the pharmacology and clinical effects of the various antidiabetes medications is extremely important today because of the increasing number of classes of drugs available for use. Delayed-release sulfonylureas or the shorter-acting non-sulfonylurea insulin secretagogues such as repaglinide and nateglinide can reduce the risk. Similarly, the glucose-dependent mechanism of action of the GLP-1 agonist and DPP-IV antagonists also have reduced hypoglycemia risks. Drugs which trigger the more rapid glucose-dependent postprandial insulin release targeting postmeal glucose elevations have an effect which dissipates once the postprandial glucose rise resolves, and they are thus less likely to cause late hypoglycemia.

In general, it is a good rule to regard all insulin secretagogues as having the potential for hypoglycemia and to inform patients accordingly. Because there is a trend now to use combination oral therapies in patients with type 2 diabetes, it must be noted that any combination of medications in the right setting, such as that of decreased food intake, has the potential for causing hypoglycemia, although rare. The best way to avoid the problem is to educate patients about their therapies and the risks of hypoglycemia occurring, and to emphasize the importance of self-monitoring of blood glucose. If in doubt, it is always better to treat for a low glucose than to ignore the possibility. Sometimes circumstances will not be ideal for checking or the equipment to do so may not be available. These are appropriate times for empirical treatment and to check on the real situation with a blood test as soon as is feasible.

Hypoglycemia can be a special problem in children with diabetes who are using insulin. The young child may not be able to understand or describe what is going on, but may behave differently. Parents must test the child's blood glucose if they are not sure. In the event that it is not possible to check the blood glucose, they should treat the child for a low glucose.

Women with diabetes using insulin can also experience more low glucose during their menstrual cycle. The rapid drop in levels of progesterone and estrogen may be involved in this process.

Hypoglycemic Unawareness

One of the major problems in diabetes treatment today is the issue of *hypoglycemic unawareness*. As noted above, with increasing duration of diabetes there is a loss of normal counterregulatory response. With a drop in blood glucose there is a release of glucagon and epinephrine, which are the acute response hormones. They increase the rate of glycogenolysis and gluconeogenesis by the liver and this reverses the hypoglycemia. In patients with hypoglycemic unawareness, the secretion of these hormones are blunted and, as a consequence, symptoms are reduced and the resulting increase in glucose is also limited. Patients may still have some symptoms but they occur at much lower glucose levels, so the window of warning is compromised. This results in a lack of timely corrective action and thus more severe reactions.

In the past, it was believed that the problem of hypoglycemic unawareness was due to an autonomic neuropathy, but now research has shown that it is in large part due to a lack of adaptation by the body to previous hypoglycemia. It is not unusual for one low glucose to be followed by another because of the further blunting of the already impaired counterregulatory response. With the development of the unawareness, the neurogenic symptoms are generally lost and more of the neuroglycopenic ones dominate the event. Studies have also shown that careful treatment programs designed to avoid hypoglycemia can restore the counter-regulatory response, especially in patients without any autonomic neuropathy.

Treatment

Treatment principles are summarized in Table 13.5. Once detected, hypoglycemia can be easily be treated by the patient or parent of a child with diabetes. The main determinant of how aggressive treatment should be is how low the glucose level has dropped. Mild hypoglycemia (50–60 mg/dl) can usually be adequately treated by the patient using 15 grams of simple carbohydrate. This can be 4 oz. of unsweetened fruit juice or a nondietetic soft drink. Another option is the use of three glucose tablets (5 gm of glucose per tablet) by mouth.

It is important not to overreact and over-treat hypoglycemia, which is a common error many patients make. It can result in subsequent hyperglycemia, which can be difficult to differentiate from the rebound hyperglycemia caused by a counterregulatory response.

However, more severe hypoglycemic symptoms are associated with lower glucose levels and should be treated with 25–30 grams of simple carbohydrate followed by 15–30 grams of more complex carbohydrate like crackers or bread in order to sustain the hyperglycemic effect.

Patients who are unconscious should never be given any liquid orally because of the danger of aspiration. Viscous sources of sugar such as honey, sugar gels or icing sugar from cakes can be carefully placed inside of the cheek or side of the tongue. However, when a patient's mental status and ability to swallow are impaired, the best option, if available, is to use a glucagon injection — 1 mg should be given intramuscularly and will raise the blood glucose through its direct effect on the liver. Glucagon kits are available by prescription, and patients who are even remotely at risk for hypoglycemia should always have a fresh one handy. Relatives and/or friends should be instructed on their use, as clearly patients themselves will not be self-administering this drug, and must therefore rely on others.

For severe hypoglycemia, calling for transport to a hospital is usually not a bad option prior to attempting other maneuvers. It is obviously not wise to have a well-intentioned relative administering multiple injections

Table 13-5. Treatment of Hypoglycemia in People with Diabetes

- If patient is symptomatic or unable to confirm hypoglycemia with SMBG, or if blood glucose levels are <70 mg/dl (<90 mg/dl at bedtime or overnight), treat it as mild-moderate hypoglycemia.
- Caution patient to avoid alternate site testing with blood glucose meter.
- For mild to moderate hypoglycemia (plasma glucose 51–70 mg/dl), begin with 15–20 gm carbohydrate (See Table 13-4). If glucose level is ≤50 mg/dl, consume 20–30 grams carbohydrate.
- Recheck blood glucose after 15 minutes.
- Repeat hypoglycemia treatment if blood glucose does not return to normal range after 15 minutes.
- Follow with additional carbohydrate or snack if next meal is more than one hour away.
- If hypoglycemia persists after second treatment, patient or companion should be instructed to contact healthcare provider.
- In event of severe hypoglycemia (altered consciousness, unable to take carbohydrate orally, or requiring the assistance of another person) treat with glucagon and/or intravenous glucose.
- For patients with hypoglycemia unawareness, the threshold for treatment of hypoglycemia needs to be individualized.

of glucagon to no avail and thus delay hospital treatment if a stroke had really been the cause of the coma. In the hospital setting or with the emergency medical response team, hypoglycemia can be confirmed. Intravenous dextrose (D50) can be given if appropriate, and other conditions can be addressed if present.

Education

In order to avoid serious problems with hypoglycemia, patients must be educated about the issue, taught how to prevent it, and how to treat an event if it does occur. As noted above, every patient on insulin should have an emergency kit of glucagon at home, and someone must know where it is kept and when to use it. An identity bracelet indicating that the patient is on insulin can be critical if the patient is in an automobile

Table 13-6.   Foods Equal to 15 Grams of Carbohydrate that Can Be Used to Treat Hypoglycemia

3 Glucose tablets or 4 dextrose tablets
4 ounces of fruit juice
5–6 ounces (about ½ can) of regular soda such as Coke or Pepsi
7–8 Gummy or regular Life Savers
2 Tbs. raisins
1 Tbs. sugar or jelly

accident. Prompt recognition of the possibility of hypoglycemia can avert delay in treatment and avoid serious neurologic damage.

The need to avoid overtreatment must be stressed and the importance of regular blood testing repeatedly emphasized. A blood test should be done if symptoms are occurring or before driving. In the latter situation if the sugar is less than 125 mg/dl a small amount of carbohydrate should be ingested before the drive starts. This is especially important for patients using an aggressive treatment program such as an intensive treatment program with multiple injections or insulin pumps. In general, if the patient is well-educated about avoidance of and treatment of hypoglycemia, the risk is reduced. Nevertheless, repeated hypoglycemia must be assessed carefully. The insulin program and the overall treatment plan have to be evaluated. Psychological issues also need to be ruled out. Patients with type 1 diabetes can develop an autoimmune polyglandular syndrome with hypothyroidism and/or adrenal insufficiency that can result in increased insulin sensitivity and more hypoglycemia. Advancing renal disease can also do this. In the postpartum state repeated severe hypoglycemia can be a sign of pituitary damage from postpartum bleeding.

Conclusion

Today the patient who has to live with a chronic disease like diabetes has a very good chance of living a long life, especially if he or she has good glycemic control. However, it must be stressed that acute complications can occur with very little warning and the best approach is for the patient to be aware of these. With good education and follow-up most of our patients will survive these problems, especially hypoglycemia and diabetic ketoacidosis. As new therapies are developed and with better self-glucose-monitoring methods, we can look forward to a time when we can recommend intensive therapy to most of our patients. At the same time, we will be able to reduce their risks for long-term microvascular complications and acute problems.

Suggested Reading:

American Diabetes Association. Position Statement on Hyperglycemic Crises in Diabetes. Diabetes Care 27:S94-S102, 2004

Joslin Diabetes Center. Guideline for Management of Uncontrolled Glucose in the Hospitalized Adult. Accessible on line at from Joslin's website: www.joslin.org

Joslin Diabetes Center. Clinical Guideline for Adults with Diabetes. Accessible on-line at www.joslin.org

14

Microvascular Complications

*Jerry D. Cavallerano, OD,
PhD and
Robert M. Stanton, MD*

Introduction

Once glucose is controlled to a sufficient degree to avoid the acute effects of hyper-or hypoglycemia, the ultimate goal of diabetes treatment is to prevent the chronic complications of this condition. The efforts made to safely achieve the best possible A1C level stem from the growing evidence that better control improves the odds of avoiding these complications for people with either type of diabetes. Landmark studies in recent years demonstrating this point include the Diabetes Control and Complications Trial (DCCT), the United Kingdom Prospective Diabetes Study (UKPDS), the Kumamoto Study from Japan, and numerous epidemiologic studies such as the Wisconsin Epidemiologic Study of Diabetic Retinopathy (WESDR).

While it is likely that the etiology of the diabetic macrovascular complications are multifactoral (see Chapter 15), the risk of developing diabetic neuropathies (see Chapter 16) and the microvascular complications of diabetes seem to be directly related to the degree of glucose control. In addition to glucose control, aggressive efforts to reduce the impact of other risk factors, as well as careful screening for early signs of complications, round out the challenge to the primary care provider in maintaining good health for his or her patients with diabetes.

For years many healthcare providers felt that bad things would inevitably befall those with diabetes no matter how well glucose levels were controlled. Therefore, many felt that they shouldn't burden people's good years of life with the rigors of aggressive glucose control, as it didn't matter anyway. Many patients who then developed early signs of diabetic complications turned to the specialists to whom they were referred to stop the disease progression before it impacted their quality of life. Now we know that aggressive efforts, starting with the primary care providers, can often have a tremendous impact on the long-term health of their patients with diabetes and prevent the need for specialty care of complications.

The role of the primary care provider literally begins at the beginning. As has been noted, many people with type 2 diabetes go undiagnosed for long periods of time. While much attention has been paid to the impact of the accompanying macrovascular risks of hypertension, dyslipidemia, abdominal adiposity, and hypercoagulability that often accompany type 2 diabetes, the untreated hyperglycemia can also give a head start to the development of other complications such as retinopathy, nephropathy, and neuropathy. Thus, the first job in ameliorating the risk factors for microvascular — and all other chronic complications — is to diagnose diabetes early.

Diabetic Eye Disease

Diabetic Retinopathy

While diabetes can have a number of effects on the eye, the one that most people think of is retinopathy because it is the complication that causes vision loss and blindness. It is the leading cause of new blindness among adults aged 20 to 65 years and results in about 24,000 new cases of blindness per year. For this reason, when the diagnosis of diabetes is made, many patients become quite concerned that they will lose their vision. This concern is heightened by the possible development of blurred vision shortly after initiation of treatment. This initial blurriness is common; it

TABLE 14-1. Characteristics of Stages of Diabetic Retinopathy (DR)

Levels of DR	Symptoms	Characteristics
Nonproliferative (NPDR) Mild to very severe	Generally none	- dot and/or blot hemorrhages - microaneurysms - cotton wool spots (soft exudates) - intraretinal microvascular abnormalities - hard exudates - venous caliber abnormalities
Proliferative (PDR)	frequently none, floater, **reduced vision**	- vascular proliferation - fibrous tissue proliferation - preretinal hemorrhage - vitreous hemorrhage
Diabetic macular edema (DME)	frequently none, blurred vision, distortion of straight lines	- macular hard exudates - retinal thickening in the macula

results from fluid changes in the lens within the eye that accompany improving glucose control, and usually clears up within a matter of days or weeks.

Diabetic retinopathy is a specific vascular complication seen with both types of diabetes, typically progressing through a number of stages (see Table 14-1) each with characteristic findings on examination. In type 1 diabetes, observable retinopathy usually does not occur until after the patient has had diabetes for about 5 years, and is present to some degree in 50% of patients with diabetes at 10 years. At 20 years diabetes duration, over 90% of patients with type 1 diabetes, and more than 60% of patients with type 2 diabetes have some findings of diabetic retinopathy. Retinopathy is usually not seen in patients with type 1 diabetes before puberty.

Classification of Diabetic Retinopathy

Diabetic retinopathy is broadly classified as nonproliferative diabetic retinopathy (NPDR) and proliferative diabetic retinopathy (PDR). Generally, diabetic retinopathy progresses from mild nonproliferative disease, through moderate and severe nonproliferative disease, to proliferative diabetic retinopathy. The level of NPDR establishes the risk of progression to sight-threatening retinopathy and appropriate clinical management. The ETDRS clinical levels of DR (Table 14-2) is useful in monitoring progression of DR and the need for follow-up and treatment. Recently, a simplified DR scale was proposed (Table 14-3) that simplifies the description of the levels of DR and provides a convenient classification for correspondence between eye specialists and other care providers.

In its earliest stages, *nonproliferative diabetic retinopathy* usually causes no symptoms, but there are signs of retinopathy noted on examination. These signs or lesions of NPDR include dot and blot hemorrhages and/or microaneurysms, cotton wool spots, hard exudates, venous caliber abnormalities, and intraretinal microvascular abnormalities (IRMA). Based on the presence and extent of these retinal lesions, NPDR is further classified as mild, moderate, severe, or very severe. *Proliferative diabetic retinopathy* is characterized by new vessels growing on the optic disc (NVD) or new vessels growing elsewhere on the retina (NVE) away from the optic disc. The new vessels are fragile and may rupture, causing preretinal hemorrhage (PRH) or vitreous hemorrhage (VH) within the eye, resulting in significant loss of vision. Furthermore, the new vessels may be accompanied by growth of fibrous tissue. The fibrous tissue may cause traction or pulling on the retina, resulting in traction retinal detachment. New vessels on or within one disc diameter of the optic disc that are 25 to 30% of the disc area in size, or new vessels on or within one disc diameter of the optic disc that are less than 25 to 30% of the disc area in size when there is vitreous or preretinal hemorrhage, or new vessels elsewhere when there is vitreous or preretinal hemorrhage heighten the concern and are characterized as high-risk proliferative diabetic retinopathy. Eyes that are approaching or at the high-risk stage generally should be treated with scatter (panretinal) laser photocoagulation.

Diabetic macular edema (DME) results from leakage of fluid from retinal vessels that accumulates in the macula of the eye. The macula is responsible for our sharp, discriminating vision, color vision, reading vision, etc. Diabetic macular edema can be present with any level of nonproliferative or proliferative diabetic retinopathy. This condition usually requires stereoscopic examination for diagnosis. Macular edema that involves or threatens the center of the macula is termed clinically significant macular edema (CSME). When CSME is present, focal laser photocoagulation is usually indicated.

TABLE 14-2:   Levels of Diabetic Retinopathy

Nonproliferative Diabetic Retinopathy (NPDR)	Characteristics
Mild NPD	• At least one microaneurysm • Characteristics not met for more severe DR
Moderate NPDR	• Hemorrhages and/or microaneurysms (H/Ma) of a moderate degree (i.e., ≥ standard photo 2A*) and/or • Soft exudates (cotton wool spots), venous beading (VB), or intraretinal micro-vascular abnormalities (IRMA) definitely present • Characteristics not met for more severe DR
Severe NPDR	• One of the following: – H/Ma ≥ standard photo 2A in 4 retinal quadrants – Venous beading in 2 retinal quadrants (e.g., standard photo 6B) – IRMA in 1 retinal quadrant ≥ standard photo 8A – Characteristics not met for more severe DR
Very severe NPDR	• Two or more lesions of Severe NPDR • No frank neovascularizations

Proliferative Diabetic Retinopathy (PDR)	Characteristics
Early PDR	• New vessels definitely present • Characteristics not met for more severe DR
High-risk PDR	• One or more of the following: – Neovascularization on the optic disc (NVD) ≥ ¼ to ⅓ disc area; i.e., NVD ≥ standard photo 10A – Any NVD plus vitreous or preretinal hemorrhage – Neovascularization elsewhere on the retina (NVE) ≥ ½ disc area + vitreous or preretinal hemorrhage

Clinically Significant Macular Edema (CSME)
(May be present with any level of DR)

Any one of the following lesions:

* Retinal thickening at or within 500 microns (1/3 disc diameter) from the center of the macula
* Hard exudates at or within 500 microns from the center of the macula with thickening of the adjacent retina
* A zone or zones of retinal thickening ≥ 1 disc area in size, any portion of which is ≤ 1 disc diameter from the center of the macula

Standard photographs refer to the Modified Airlee House Classification of Diabetic Retinopathy.

TABLE 14-3.   International Clinical DR and DME Scale (1;2)

Level of DR	Findings
No apparent retinopathy	No abnormalities
Mild NPDR	Microaneurysms only
Moderate NPDR	More than microaneurysms but less than severe NPDR
Severe NPDR	Any of the following: • >20 intraretinal hemorrhages in each 4 retinal quadrants • definite VB in 2+ retinal quadrants • prominent IRMA in 1+ retinal quadrant and no PDR

PDR	One or more of the following:
	  • neovascularization
	  • vitreous/preretinal hemorrhage

Level of DME	**Findings**
DME apparently absent	No apparent retinal thickening or hard exudates (HE) in posterior pole
DME apparently present	• **Mild DME:** some retinal thickening or HE in posterior pole but distant from center of the macula • **Moderate DME:** retinal thickening or HE approaching the center but not involving the center • **Severe DME:** retinal thickening or HE involving the center of the macula

DR = diabetic retinopathy; NPDR = Nonproliferative diabetic retinopathy; PDR = Proliferative diabetic retinopathy; DME = diabetic macular edema; HE = hard exudates; CSME = clinically significant macular edema

Table 14-3 Legend

The International Classification of Diabetic Retinopathy and Diabetic Macular Edema simplifies descriptions of the categories of DR and communications among care providers, but is not a replacement for ETDRS levels of DR in large-scale clinical trials or studies where precise retinopathy classification is required.

Risk Factors for Developing Diabetic Retinopathy

There are a number of factors that increase the risk that a person with diabetes will develop diabetic retinopathy:

1. *Duration of diabetes* — The longer a person has diabetes, the more likely he or she will develop some type of retinopathy.
2. *Degree of diabetes control* — Poor diabetes control increases the risk of development and progression of diabetic retinopathy. The glycohemoglobin (A1C) levels are often used as a measure of chronic hyperglycemia, reflecting this risk. This correlation has been demonstrated in a number of studies including the DCCT for type 1 diabetes, and the Kumamoto, WESDR, and UKPDS for type 2 diabetes.
3. *Hypertension* — elevated systolic and diastolic pressures increase the risk of development and progression of diabetic retinopathy. Hypertension itself, even in the absence of diabetes, can lead to hypertensive retinopathy.
4. *Proteinuria and renal disease* — Proteinuria and elevated serum creatinine levels are often associated with retinopathy. Retinopathy in diabetic patients experiencing renal failure can result in significant retinal changes and edema that becomes difficult to manage.
5. *Hypercholesterolemia* — There is an association between hyperlipidemias and the development of hard exudates (lipid deposits) and macular edema.
6. *Anemia* — There is an association between anemia and the progression of diabetic retinopathy.
7. *Abdominal obesity* — There is an association between abdominal obesity and presence of diabetic retinopathy in type 2 diabetes.
8. *Puberty* — Diabetic retinopathy is rarely seen in prepubertal patients with type 1 diabetes. Patients with diabetes should have a complete dilated retinal examination at the onset of puberty.
9. *Pregnancy* — Diabetic retinopathy can progress during pregnancy, particularly in the first trimester. Women contemplating pregnancy should have a dilated eye examination prior to conception, and women who are pregnant should have a dilated eye examination early in the first trimester. Simultaneous control of diabetes and blood pressure are important. Pre-pregnancy counseling should include a discussion of the risk of the progression of retinopathy.

10. *Cataract surgery* — Patients undergoing cataract surgery may experience a worsening of diabetic retinopathy or diabetic macular edema.
11. *Sudden improvement in diabetes control* — Sudden improvement of control, often seen with the initiation of intensive insulin programs such as the use of insulin pumps, can sometimes lead to a transient worsening of retinopathy. While these therapies are usually beneficial in the long run, this period of transient worsening may precede evidence of the beneficial effects of improved control. Therefore, patients initiating intensive diabetes therapies or even just significant changes in therapy leading to marked improvement in control should have a dilated retinal examination prior to these changes, and again after they are in place, to monitor the level and change of retinopathy.

Preventive Strategies

Primary care providers can play an important role in the prevention of diabetic retinopathy through their efforts to encourage and achieve optimization of glucose control. Recognizing that the hand-held funduscopic examination is often suboptimal, the practitioner needs to encourage regular comprehensive examinations by an eye care professional skilled in caring for people with diabetes.

Much can be done early-on in the progression of diabetic ophthalmologic disease, prior to the development of significant symptoms. It is only through regular ophthalmologic examinations that the need for intervention can be determined. For example, scatter (panretinal) laser photocoagulation has been demonstrated to reduce the risk of severe vision loss in high-risk patients to less than 2% over a 5-year period; and for those with diabetic maculopathy, focal laser photocoagulation reduces the risk of vision loss from over 30% to less than 15%. With vitreous hemorrhage or retinal detachment, vitrectomy may restore useful vision or prevent catastrophic loss of vision.

A general strategy for ophthalmologic care recommendations by the primary care provider is outlined below:

- Insist that patients have regular eye examinations, based on recommendations below, that include a dilated exam.
  - People with type 1 diabetes should start having annual examinations within 3 to 5 years of the diagnosis of diabetes and at puberty.

- People with type 2 diabetes should have annual examinations starting at the time of diagnosis.
- Women who have diabetes before pregnancy should have an examination prior to conception; during the first, second and third trimesters; and 6–8 weeks postpartum.
- Patients desiring pump therapy (as well as any significant intensification of therapy using multiple insulin injections) should consult with their eye doctor prior to and after initiating such therapy.
- Patients with diabetes should have their eyes examined more often if they experience visual changes.
- Patients with diabetes who have any other medical conditions that might affect vision may need more frequent examinations.
- Make sure that aggressive medical care has been initiated for the following conditions:
  - hyperglycemia
  - hypertension
  - dyslipidemia
  - proteinuria (microalbuminuria and gross proteinuria)
  - anemia
- If active proliferative diabetic retinopathy is present, suggest activities not involving the Valsalva response. Encouraged activities might include stationary cycling, low-intensity rowing, swimming, and walking.
- Encourage patients with any significant ophthalmologic condition to undergo treatments aimed at prevention or containment of the process:
  - Laser surgery would be indicated for prevention of severe visual loss from PDR and moderate vision loss from macular edema.
  - Vitrectomy surgery would be indicated to restore useful vision for some patients who have lost vision from PDR or have the threat of traction retinal detachment.
- Patients with significant vision loss should be referred to vision rehabilitation services that enhance independent life skills.

Treatment of Diabetic Retinopathy

It has been demonstrated that scatter (panretinal) photocoagulation (laser) therapy significantly reduces the risk of severe visual loss from proliferative diabetic retinopathy (see Table 14-4). Furthermore, studies such as the Early Treatment Diabetic Retinopathy Study (ETDRS) and the

Diabetic Retinopathy Vitrectomy Study (DRVS) have helped determine the proper time in the natural history of this condition to begin such treatments. Therefore, any patient with diabetic retinopathy should be under the management of an eye care professional experienced with diabetic eye diseases.

Other Eye Diseases

People with diabetes can develop conditions other than retinopathy. Two key conditions are *glaucoma* and *cataracts*.

Glaucoma

Many people over age 40 can develop open-angle glaucoma. Some studies suggest higher prevalence of glaucoma in persons with diabetes. Therefore, screening for this condition should occur every year. Glaucoma is initially asymptomatic, so that is another good reason for regular eye examinations. With more advanced and untreated glaucoma, symptoms may develop, including visual field loss.

Treatments for open-angle glaucoma can be quite effective, but must be chosen with care. Beta-blockers, oral and topical carbonic anhydrase inhibitors and other typical medications are available. Argon laser trabeculoplasty can be used if medical therapies are ineffective.

Narrow-angle glaucoma and acute angle-closure glaucoma, medical emergencies, are not usually more common in people with diabetes. Glaucoma resulting from hemorrhage in the eyeball is, fortunately, unusual.

Cataracts

Cataracts, the clouding of the lens that is one of the most common eye problems in older people, can occur earlier in life and progress more rapidly in people with diabetes. Cataracts are 1.6 times more common in the diabetic population, including those with both type 1 and type 2 diabetes. Factors contributing to cataract formation include duration of diabetes and degree of diabetes control. Cataract extraction with intraocular lens implant is usually highly successful in the restoration of vision.

Other Lenticular Changes

Other lenticular changes can occur as well, and usually are refractive changes related to blood glucose changes. As patients are often keenly aware that diabetes can cause visual problems, the changes in refraction seen soon after diabetes diagnosis, during a period of acute glucose control improvements, can cause high levels of concern. Acute hyperglycemia, improvements of control, and variable glucose patterns can all lead to variations in visual acuity. The cause of these changes is probably due to fluid absorption by the crystalline lens.

The major treatment of such refractive changes is primarily glucose control and reassurance. It is usually recommended that patients do not purchase new eyeglasses until glucose control stabilizes. However, if visual problems have enough of an impact on a patient's day-to-day function, interval refractions and eyeglass prescriptions, in spite of the cost, might be needed. Stabilization of vision typically takes 1 to 2 months after diagnosis of diabetes and initiation of treatment, but this timeframe may vary depending on the severity of the glucose abnormalities upon diagnosis and the ease with which glucose control can be achieved.

Effect on the Iris

The major effect of diabetes on the *iris* is rubeosis iridis, or neovascularization of the iris (NVI) — the growth of new blood vessels on the iris. Retinal venous obstructive disease is another major cause of this problem. In this condition, a fine network of vessels can grow over the iris tissue and into the filtration angle of the eye. Neovascular glaucoma may result. Treatment includes laser surgery to the retina and other glaucoma medications. NVI is usually first seen in the area of the pupillary margin and must be detected through the use of a slit-lamp microscope. Thus, screening for this condition is part of a thorough eye evaluation.

Ophthalmoplegia Mononeuropathy

Ophthalmoplegia mononeuropathy, or ophthalmic mononeuropathies of the third, fourth, or sixth cranial nerves, can occur in patients with diabetes. These mononeuropathies are often of great concern to patients and a diagnostic challenge to clinicians, as strokes are often initially thought to be the cause in many such cases. Ruling out such other neurologic events or other causes of mononeuropathies is quite important before assigning such abnormalities to this category of classic diabetic complications. Conversely, mononeuropathies can be the initial presenting sign of diabetes.

- Third-nerve palsies are the most common, with presence of characteristic physical changes such as ptosis of the affected eye often

TABLE 14-4. Recommended General Management of Diabetic Retinopathy

Level of DR	Natural Course — Risk of Progression to PDR 1 yr	PDR 5 yr	Evaluation Color photo	FA	Laser Treatment Scatter lsr (PRP)	Focal lsr	Follow-up (months)
Mild NPDR	5%	15%					
-No ME			No	No	No	No	12
-ME			Yes	Occ	No	No	4–6
-CSME			Yes	Yes	No	Yes	2–4
Moderate NPDR	12–27%	33%					
-No ME			Yes	No	No	No	6–8
-ME			Yes	Occ	No	Occ	4–6
-CSME			Yes	Yes	No	Yes	2–4
Severe NPDR	52%	60%					
-No ME			Yes	No	Rarely	No	3–4
-ME			Yes	Sometime	OccAF	OCC	2–3
-CSME			Yes	Yes	OccAF	Yes	2–3
Very Severe NPDR	75%	75%					
-No ME			Yes	No	Occ	No	2–3
-ME			Yes	Sometime	OccAF	Occ	2–3
-CSME			Yes	Yes	OccAF	Yes	2–3
PDR < high-Risk		75%					
-No ME			Yes	No	Occ	No	2–3
-ME			Yes	Sometime	OccAF	Occ	2–3
-CSME			Yes	Yes	OccAF	Yes	2–3
High-Risk PDR							
-No ME			Yes	No	Yes	No	2–3
-ME			Yes	Yes	Yes	Usually	1–2
-CSME			Yes	Yes	Yes	Yes	1–2

NPDR = nonproliferative diabetic retinopathy; PDR = proliferative diabetic retinopathy; ME = macular edema; CSME = clinically significant macular edema; FA = fluorescein angiography; Occ = occasionally; OccAF = Occasionally after focal.

The first two columns describe the risk of PDR and high-risk PDR based on a baseline level of diabetic retinopathy. Early detection and treatment can reduce the number of patients who progress to this level.

- In patients with mild NPDR, 5% of patients will naturally progress to PDR in 1 year and 15% to high risk PDR within 5 years.
- Fifty-two percent of patients with severe NPDR will develop PDR within 1 year and 60% develop high risk PDR within 5 years.

The third and fourth columns list the types of evaluations needed. Most patients require color photo evaluations while others with more advanced macular edema require fluorescein angiography. Newer technologies, such as optical coherence tomography (OCT) are valuable in assessing diabetic macular edema and vitreo-retinal traction.

The last three columns outline when laser therapy is needed. Laser treatment can consist of focal laser or scatter laser. Treatments such as intravitreal injection are now used clinically, but their safety and efficacy are undergoing clinical trial. Recommendations for follow-up are outlined in the very last column.

leading to patient presentation. The eye is typically in an exotropic and hypotropic (down and out) posture, and pain may also be present. In third nerve palsies, pupillary function is usually not affected; presence of pupillary involvements suggests a nondiabetic etiology.

- Sixth-nerve palsies usually are brought to the care provider's attention by patient complaints of horizontal diplopia, some times only on extreme lateral gaze to the side of the affected eye. Again, nondiabetic etiologies of this abnormality may be the cause — some life-threatening, such as space-occupying lesions — so diabetes should not be assumed to be the cause unless these other conditions are ruled out.
- Fourth-cranial-nerve (trochlear) palsies can occur but are less likely to be of diabetic origin.

Mononeuropathic palsies are usually self-limited and usually clear spontaneously in a period of from 2 to 6 months. Treatments include eye patching to ameliorate diplopic symptoms and analgesia as needed.

Renal Complications of Diabetes

The Scope of Diabetic Nephropathy

Traditionally, the focus of diabetic renal disease has been on the classic microvascular complication, nephropathy. In 1936, Kimmelstiel and Wilson first described the classic pathologic lesion of diabetic kidney disease, the nodular intercapillary lesion, that now bears their names. By the 1950s, as the longevity of people with diabetes was improving, numbers of patients with diabetic renal disease due to this Kimmelstiel-Wilson lesion were increasing. The classic Kimmstiel-Wilson lesion currently comprises only a small percentage of all cases of diabetic nephropathy, as diabetic nephropathy is most commonly characterized by mesangial expansion and sclerosis with no antibody staining. At that time, clinicians could only address the challenge of diabetic nephropathy by treating hypertension in an effort to slow the destructive process and by measuring proteinuria to gauge it. Time would pass, and in some patients the excretion of protein would begin and inevitably increase. Physicians would try to predict the timing of renal failure and the need for dialysis and/or transplantation.

While end-stage renal failure has by no means been eliminated, the focus for the clinician has broadened in some significant ways. The ability to measure micro-amounts of protein excreted, the microalbumin measurement, and the growing understanding of the significance of its presence, have provided a preventive tool that was not previously available. Similarly, the implications of the presence of hypertension have moved beyond its directly damaging renal effects and into consideration as a component of the insulin resistance syndrome that ties together type 2 diabetes and various other clinical abnormalities. Thus, it appears that treatment of hypertension has an increasing impact on long-term health.

Clinically, the arena for caring for these newly recognized issues is often that of the primary care provider. Therefore, rather than assuming the development of renal disease and subsequent progression to end stage disease is unavoidable endpoint for many unfortunate patients, primary care providers can significantly impact outcome by early attention to conditions that are quite amenable to treatment.

Diabetic nephropathy is first manifest as microalbuminuria. In patients with type 1 diabetes, the development of nephropathy usually begins after 5 years of diabetes duration, with an increasing incidence of nephropathy over the next decade of duration to a peak at about 15 to 17 years of having had diabetes. It then begins to decline in annual incidence thereafter.

Risks for developing nephropathy are increased by:

- increasing duration of diabetes
- poor control of diabetes (elevated A1C)
- family history of nephropathy (particularly in a sibling)
- hypertension
  - poorly controlled hypertension
  - a genetic predisposition for hypertension, as signified by a family history of hypertension
  - smoking

However, it has been evident for years that there are many people whose risk profile does not reflect actual disease development, and there are clearly other less easily identifiable or well understood factors that may also play a role in determining nephropathy risk. Other factors increasing risk have been suggested, such as male gender or development of diabetes after puberty. Similarly, while many clinicians assume the close relationship between insulin resistance and hypertension, this really applies most strongly to Caucasians; it is less so for African Americans and Pima Indians.

For patients with type 2 diabetes, studies have suggested that the prevalence of proteinuria ranges from about 12 to 16%. Men seem to have a greater prevalence than women, and prevalence increases with duration of diabetes. Similar risk factors and considerations as for type 1 diabetes seem to hold for type 2 diabetes. While the prevalence of renal disease in type 2 diabetes is less than for type 1 diabetes, as there are many more people with type 2 diabetes, the actual numbers of people with type 2 diabetes-induced nephropathy are considerable.

The Natural Progression of Diabetic Nephropathy

The classic view of the natural history of diabetic kidney disease is as follows. The *early phase* of diabetic nephropathy is clinically silent. During this phase, the glomerular filtration rate (GFR) can be elevated by about 20 to 40% reflecting a state of hyperfiltration.

During this early "silent" phase, there is no overt proteinuria (>300 mg/24 hours). However, there may be a significant increase in albumin excretion rate (AER), and now, with the ability to measure micro-albumin levels, this increase of AER can be clinically apparent. The presence of microalbuminuria is often referred to as a state of *early nephropathy*. The presence of microalbuminuria may also signal an increased risk of coronary artery disease. The level of microalbuminuria reflecting significant microalbuminuria would be >30 mg/day, 20 μg/min, or in terms of the albumin/creatinine ratio, 30–300 mcg albumin/mg creatinine.

Microalbuminuria is also a very important risk factor for coronary artery disease. Patients with microalbuminuria should also have an assessment of macrovascular risk factors, including lipid status, presence of hypertension, smoking status, and weight and exercise levels.

In recent years, it has become clear that kidney function can deteriorate even if there are normal urine albumin levels. Thus it is very important to follow kidney function. It is best followed by measuring serum creatinine and using a formula to estimate glomerular filtration rate (GFR). Because of the many variables associated with serum creatinine, assessing renal function on serum creatinine alone can be very misleading. Currently, the most accurate formula is the MDRD formula. *(Formula available at www.kidney.org — the National Kidney Foundation website).* The National

Kidney Foundation (NKF) strongly recommends that all physicians use the MDRD formula to estimate GFR and to treat and refer accordingly. Use of the MDRD allows the primary care physician to both recognize disease progression and to be aware of when to look for complications of kidney disease such as anemia and hyperparathyroidism, which can be seen at GFR of <60 ml/min (Stage 3 kidney disease — as per NKF guidelines). Of note the MDRD is less accurate if GFR is >60 ml/min but quite accurate below 60 ml/min.

The **late phase** of nephropathy is heralded by the appearance of persistent proteinuria and is often referred to as *overt nephropathy*. Clinically, this is represented by a total protein excretion of ≥0.3 g/day, corresponding to an AER of ~200 μg/min or ≥300 mg/day. In terms of an albumin/creatinine ratio, this would be at a level of about 300 mcg albumin/mg creatinine. As patients progress to this phase, there is a progressive, linear decline in the GFR toward end-stage renal failure. At this stage, the degree of hypertension control seems to slow the progression of nephropathic development, but the degree of glucose control probably has a lesser impact on progression. In the past, the development of persistent proteinuria indicated a 7-year interval to end-stage renal failure, however, with clinical strategies to prevent and slow the progression of renal failure, this estimated interval is probably more than doubled.

End-stage renal disease (ESRD) represents the development of uremia as the GFR has declined to critically low levels. Fluid retention and edema are seen. Other coexisting medical conditions such as cardiac insufficiency can be impacted. Decreased water and solute disposal occurs, and pulmonary edema can develop. Hyporeninemic hypoaldosteronism can lead to hyperkalemia, further worsening the metabolic acidosis. With development of all of these conditions, the prognosis becomes quite poor.

For patients with type 1 diabetes who have overt nephropathy, 50% will develop end-stage renal failure within 10 years, and more than 75% by 20 years. However, for patients with type 2 diabetes, only about 20% will have developed ESRD after 20 years of overt nephropathy.

Summarizing the **clinically important points along the progression of diabetic renal disease,** the following should be kept in mind:

- The earliest sign of diabetic nephropathy is usually the detection of microalbuminuria.
- Estimated GFR using MDRD formula should be done routinely.

- Microalbuminuria indicates the presence of microvascular involvement of the kidney. The presence of microvascular involvement of the retina, retinopathy, should also be suspected and a retinal examination should occur.
- 80% of people with type 1 diabetes who develop microalbuminuria will develop diabetic nephropathy in the next 10 to 15 years unless specific interventions are undertaken.
- For patients with type 2 diabetes, the presence of microalbuminuria may be less specific a predictor for subsequent renal disease; approximately 10 to 25% of patients with type 2 develops overt nephropathy.
- Hypertension in patients with microalbuminuria contributes to the progression to overt nephropathy.
- Microalbuminuria is a marker for cardiovascular morbidity and mortality in patients with type 1 and type 2 diabetes; aggressive screening and management of coexisting vascular risk factors is important.
- It has been suggested that treating hyperlipidemia slows the progression of renal disease.
- The presence of micro-or macroproteinuria indicates the need for aggressive treatment and control of blood glucose and blood pressure.
- Intermittent to sustained hypertension in the late phase of renal failure indicates increased risk for further deterioration of renal function.
- Reduced creatinine clearance is a manifestation of late diabetic nephropathy.

The Diagnosis of Diabetic Renal Disease

The diagnosis of diabetic renal disease is made by the documentation of increasing urinary microalbumin or albumin (protein) excretion and increasing serum creatinine levels. As the development of nephropathy is asymptomatic, detection requires lab screening (see Table 14-5). The first sign of diabetic nephropathy is seen with the detection of micro-albuminuria (see Table 14-6). The diagnosis is confirmed when two out of three tests within 3 months are positive. Once microalbuminuria is found to be present, it is also important to document levels of serum creatinine and creatinine clearance.

Microalbuminuria is rarely present until diabetes has been present for

TABLE 14-5. Tests Used to Assess Renal Function

Test	Values and Implications
Albumin excretion rate (AER)*	Normal <30 mg/24 hr of protein in urine Microalbuminuria = 30–300 mg/24 hr Proteinuria >300 mg/24 hr (24-hr collection, which allows for simultaneous measurement of creatinine clearance) OR Normal < 20 mcg/min. Microalbuminuria = 20–199 mcg/min. Proteinuria = ≥ 200 mcg/min. (Timed collection - i.e., 4 hr or overnight) OR Normal < 20 mcg/mg creatinine Microalbuminuria = 30–300 mcg/mg creatinine Proteinuria = > 300 mcg/mg creatinine (spot collection)
Serum Creatinine	A marker of renal function: every doubling of the serum creatinine indicates a loss of 50% of renal function. For example, a rise in creatinine from 0.8 to 1.6 represents a loss of 50% of renal function.
Estimated GFR	Use MDRD formula to measure GFR. (Formula available at *www.kidney.org* — the National Kidney Foundation website).
Creatinine Clearance	24-hr urine collection measuring urinary volume and creatinine excretion. As renal function deteriorates, the creatinine clearance will as well.

* Factors that cause transient elevations in microalbumin and albumin levels:
- urinary traction infection
- short-term hyperglycemia
- illness (acute, febrile)
- heart failure
- marked hypertension
- strenuous exercise
- pregnancy

TABLE 14-6.   Comparison of Measurements of Albumin Excretion

Category	24-hr collection (mg/24 hr)	Timed collection (μg/min)	Spot collection (μg/mg creatinine)
Normal	<30	<20	<30
Microalbuminuria	30–299	20–199	30–299
Clinical albuminuria	≥300	≥200	≥300

Adapted with permission from Diabetic Nephropathy, Table 1 — Definition of abnormalities in albumin excretion; *Diabetes Care* 24: (Suppl 1), S70, 2001.

some time, or before puberty. Therefore, postpubertal individuals should be screened for microalbuminuria after they have had diabetes for 5 years. For patients with type 2 diabetes, who often have an uncertain date of onset of diabetes, screening should begin at the time of diagnosis. The following is a summary of the methods of measurement, with comparative interpretations found in Table 14-6:

- **Albumin-to-creatinine ratio:** This can be measured on a random spot urine. This is the easiest measurement in the office setting. First void or morning collections are preferred, as there are diurnal variations in albumin excretion. However, if this is impractical, comparing comparably timed samples would maximize accuracy.
- **24-hour urine collection:** This is for the measurement of microalbumin excretion. If taken along with a serum creatinine level, a creatinine clearance measurement can also be determined. The disadvantage of this is the cumbersome nature of urine collection.
- **Timed urine collection:** This collection is usually made either overnight or over a 4-hour period.

The albumin/creatinine ratio is the preferred measurement as it is accurate and convenient. Nephrologists routinely use the a/c ratio and rarely order 24 hour urines or timed collections.

Transient elevations in albumin levels, and thus inaccuracies in interpretations of the microalbumin measurement, can occur in the following situations:

- urinary tract infections
- acute febrile illness
- exercise
- short-term hyperglycemia
- marked hypertension
- heart failure

Prevention of Diabetic Renal Disease

In recent years, studies have demonstrated that improved glucose control will slow down the progression of renal damage. The DCCT, the UKPDS, the Kumamoto Study, and the Stockholm Intervention study, among others, have highlighted this clinical recommendation. The first, best way to prevent or at least slow down the progression of diabetic renal disease is to control the diabetes.

Control of hypertension has also been a traditional method of reducing the risk of the progression of renal disease. However, in recent years, evidence that use of certain antihypertensive agents in normotensive patients to treat microalbuminuria has refocused attention on this treatment option. Restriction of dietary protein may also reduce hyperfiltration and intraglomerular pressure, slowing renal disease, although the benefits of this approach have been inconsistent. Currently, the recommendation is to prescribe restrictions in protein intake for patients with overt nephropathy only when the GFR begins to fall. At this point, the ADA recommends a restriction of protein intake to 0.6 to 0.8 g/kg per day. The benefits of this approach should be weighed against the nutritional deficits that might result. Consultation with a registered dietitian for initiation of such a diet is thus strongly recommended.

The current approach to preventing renal disease includes:

- tight glucose control
- hypertension control
- use of ACE inhibitors and angiotensin receptor blockers and/or low protein diet

The first item is discussed extensively in other sections of this book. Protein restrictions are reviewed above and in Chapter 5. Detailed below is a recommended approach to the treatment of hypertension and the use of pharmacologic agents to prevent renal disease.

Treatment of Hypertension and Pharmacologic Interventions

In recent years, two findings have revolutionized the preventive strategies for diabetic renal disease: 1) reduction of microalbuminuria does retard the progression of diabetic renal disease, and 2) specific hypertensive medications, in particular the angiotensin-converting enzyme (ACE) inhibitors, will effectively reduce the progression of microalbuminuria.

The etiology of hypertension in people with diabetes is multifactoral. Certainly, atherosclerosis plays a role in many patients, particularly those with preexisting risk factors. However, in the non-atherosclerotic patient, hypertension seems to result from factors including expanded plasma volume, increased peripheral vascular resistance. Certainly, superimposed renal insufficiency reduces the water excretion, leading to increased vascular volume, further aided by the osmotic effects of hyperglycemia or sodium excess.

Within the kidney, it has been postulated that the damage to some of the glomeruli results in changes in the microcirculation to cause hyperfiltration in the remaining glomeruli and resultant increases in the intraglomerular pressure. This intraglomerular hypertension can be damaging to those remaining glomeruli. Much of this effect reflects sensitivity to angiotensin II.

ACE inhibitors exert their action on this mechanism. They probably act by reducing this effect of angiotensin II and reducing interglomerular pressure. The result is a reduction in hypertension and microalbuminuria. While these effects are clearly beneficial to patients with diabetes who have coexisting microalbuminuria and hypertension, benefit has also been demonstrated for patients with diabetes who have only microalbuminuria and who are normotensive.

Treatment with ACE inhibitors can have the significant clinical impact of slowing the progression of renal disease. Once lifestyle modifications are deemed inadequate, these agents are recommended as first-line pharmacotherapy for people with diabetes who have hypertension and/or microalbuminuria. Their use has proved to be extremely effective in many patients with these conditions. Use of angiotensin receptor blockers (ARBs) in the setting of proteinuria has also been shown to reduce progression of renal disease. The current ADA position statement on diabetic nephropathy treatment with ACE-I and ARBs states: "In hypertensive and nonhypertensive type 1 diabetic patients with any degree of albuminuria, ACE inhibitors have been shown to delay the progression of nephropathy. In hypertensive type 2 diabetic patients with microalbuminuria, ACE inhibitors and ARBs have been shown to delay the progression to macroalbuminuria. In patients with type 2 diabetes, hypertension, macroalbuminuria and renal insufficiency (serum creatinine >1.5mg/dl), ARBs have been shown to delay the progression of nephropathy."

The most common side-effect of ACE inhibitor therapy is a dry cough. ARBs, less likely to cause the cough, constitute an alternative therapy. There is some evidence that combined use of ACE inhibitors plus ARBs, each having separate mechanisms, *do provide added benefit.*

ACE inhibitors should be used with caution in patients with advanced renal disease. In such patients, and in those with significant hyporeninemic hypoaldosteronism, hyperkalemia may result. Also, in patients with advanced renal disease or bilateral renal artery stenosis, use of ACE inhibitors may result in rapid deterioration of renal function. For these reasons, it is important to monitor renal function and electrolytes after initiating ACE inhibitor therapy. It is usually recommended that these parameters be measured within 4 to 7 days after initiation of such therapy, particularly when at high risk.

Currently, the use of ACE inhibitor therapy is recommended for any patient with type 1 diabetes who has confirmed microalbuminuria. ACE inhibitor therapy is less clearly advantageous for patients with type 2 diabetes and confirmed microalbuminuria, as the risk of progression to ESRD is less clear. In this setting, ARBs have been used as well. However, with growing evidence of benefit, and clearly if hypertension is present, treatment would be recommended.

The newest class of antihypertensive agents is renin blockers. The first drug to be marketed is aliskiren. Renin is released by the juxtaglomerular apparatus (JGA) of the nephron, which are special cells located in the afferent arteriole that is the conduit for blood flow to the glomerulus. When the JGA senses low blood pressure, renin is released which catalyzes the conversion of angiotensinogen to angiotensin I (AI). AI is converted to AII by the enzyme angiotensin converting enzyme (ACE). AII is a vasoconstrictor (as noted above) that acts both in the kidney (on the efferent arteriole to raise intraglomerular pressure) and systemically to raise systemic blood pressure. Among other actions, AII stimulates aldosterone. The so-called RAA (renin-angiotensin II-aldosterone) axis is a very important regulator of blood pressure and other actions. The success of ACE-inhibitors, angiotensin receptor blockers (ARB), and aldosterone inhibitors in treating blood pressure as well as helping to prevent progression of kidney and cardiovascular disease is well-documented as noted above.

The addition of a renin inhibitor to the treatment armamentarium occurred just as the writing of this book was being completed, and time will tell how this new class of medications fits into the antihypertensive treatment paradigm. This class is certainly an intriguing addition. Studies on aliskiren have shown it to be an effective once a day antihypertensive with few side effects. Yet, some unanswered questions remain. Will additional blockade of the RAA axis offer even more protection than what is provided by ACE inhibitors and ARBs? Renin inhibitors are unique in that renin levels are lower whereas ACE inhibitors and ARBs raise renin levels. So does lowering renin offer a unique protection to kidney or cardiovascular disease? Studies are yet to be done on these issues. Nevertheless, another antihypertensive is always appreciated as the achievement of the blood pressure goal (usually <130/80) offers proven health benefits. In that many patients need multiple medications to achieve the blood pressure goal and that patients often cannot tolerate certain medications, another option is very welcome.

People with diabetes of either type may develop hypertension. Hypertension in people with either type of diabetes needs aggressive treatment, underscored for patients with type 2 diabetes by the recent UKPDS results. Much of the hypertension in these people may be part of the insulin resistance syndrome of macrovascular disease-promoting conditions and is present at the time of diabetes diagnosis in about one-third of patients. Other causes must also be considered, including renovascular disease, essential hypertension, or any other cause. Mechanisms that may be responsible for the hypertension include increased peripheral vascular resistance and expanded plasma volume.

Aggressive treatment of hypertension is therefore recommended for all people with diabetes. Often, multidrug therapy is needed, and timely advancement to this level of therapy is recommended if needed. Recommended goals of treatment are listed below:

GOALS OF TREATMENT FOR HYPERTENSION

- Goal for adults: decrease blood pressure to at least $<130/80$ mmHg. Goal is $\leq 125/75$ if proteinuria is present.
- For isolated systolic hypertension of ≥ 180 mmHg, the goal is a blood pressure <140 mmHg.

Hypertension treatment should consist of the following components:

- Lifestyle changes, including:
  - low-fat, high-carbohydrate (or lower carbohydrate with monoun-saturated fat) diet
  - sodium intake ≤ 2400 mg/day
  - limited alcohol use, <1 oz ethanol (8 oz wine, 24 oz beer, 2 oz 100-proof spirits)
  - regular physical exercise
  - smoking cessation
- If lifestyle changes do not achieve desired goals, pharmacotherapy is indicated.
  - **Medications with specific advantages for people with diabetes:**

    ACE inhibitors have become the most widely used class due to their clearly demonstrated benefits in reducing microalbuminuria and slowing the progression of renal disease. They also have no detrimental effects on lipids or glucose control. Serum creatinine and potassium levels should be monitored shortly after initiating therapy, as hyperkalemia accompanied by renal failure can occasionally occur. The cough, previously discussed, is an occasional side effect.

    ARBs are also useful in the treatment of hypertension, particularly if the patient has a cough with ACE inhibitors. Also for unclear reasons, ARBs tend to cause less hyperkalemia than ACE inhibitors.

    Thiazide diuretics had fallen into disfavor due to a tendency to promote dyslipidemia and worsened glycemia, hyperinsulinemia, hypokalemia, hypomagnesemia, and hyperuricemia. They may promote impotence. However, as people with diabetes have high-volume hypertension, these agents, in small doses (e.g., 12.5–25 mg hydrochlorothiazide or chlorthalidone 12.5–25 mg daily) have recently been recognized to be effective therapy and an important component of a multidrug treatment program. Do not use if creatinine is .2.0 mg/dl.

α-Blockers can be effective in patients with diabetes, and may help lower lipids and increase insulin sensitivity. A side effect can be orthostatic hypotension.

Nondihydropyridine calcium antagonists (verapamil and diltiazem) have been shown to have some beneficial effect on micro-albuminuria as well as being an effective treatment of hypertension. The extent of long-term renal protection is unclear. They do not adversely affect lipids or glucose control. They can cause peripheral edema.

- **Medications to be used with caution (But all can be used to lower blood pressure if blood pressure goals have not been achieved):**

  α-and β-Blockers can have cardioprotective properties. However, they can worsen glycemia and dyslipidemia. β-Blockers can impair awareness of impending hypoglycemia, impair insulin release in response to hyperglycemia (type 2 patients), and can reduce peripheral blood flow. They may cause impotence. Cardioselective β-blockers are preferable.

  Other classes of medications to be used with caution include: centrally acting a_2-agonists, sympathol\ytic agents (less effective, poorly tolerated due to orthostasis), and potassium-sparing agents (greater risk of hyperkalemia in diabetic patients, also impotence and gynecomastia).

- **Agents whose use is minimally affected by the presence of diabetes include:** direct vasodilators (can cause fluid retention) and loop diuretics (useful in patients with reduced renal function suggested by creatinine >2.0 mg/dl.)

Multiple drug therapy is quite effective for patients whose diabetes cannot be adequately controlled with one of the above agents alone, and is often needed for people with diabetes. Drug class selection should be individualized based on patient needs, other medication conditions, and demonstrated drug-class efficacy for that patient. Refractory hypertension certainly warrants evaluation for other etiologies. Significant hypertension may have adverse effects on other conditions such as advanced retinopathy or cerebrovascular disease, and when present concurrently with these conditions should be treated as aggressively as possible.

Once hypertension control has been established for a period of at least 6 months, reduction of the number of drugs (if multiple) or drug dosage can be attempted.

Orthostatic Hypotension

This condition may occur in patients who have autonomic dysfunction. Antihypertensive therapy may exacerbate this problem. Support hose and increased sodium intake can help reduce some symptomatology. However, some patients may need pharmacologic intervention to reduce the orthostasis, particularly if the need for multiple antihypertensive medications is present; 9 beta-fludrohydrocortisone and midodrine are commonly used agents for use in this setting.

Other Urinary Tract Conditions

Other conditions that affect the urinary tract can occur in people with diabetes, and some can impact renal function.

Urinary tract infections (UTIs), particularly if repeated, or severe, can damage the kidneys. UTIs are said to be more common in people with diabetes, although in the modern era of better glucose control, this may not really be true. Certainly, bacteriuria is a frequent incidental finding with urine screening during routine office visits. However, they can be asymptomatic in many people, particularly women. UTIs are associated with deterioration of diabetes control as well as worsening of renal function. Aggressive screening for UTIs is often the only way to detect them and initiate timely therapy.

Neurogenic bladder resulting from neuropathic involvement can also occur. It is often insidious at onset, with the first detectable symptom being a subtle decrease in awareness of bladder distention. Therefore, as this condition progresses, the patient feels the need to urinate with progressively greater bladder volumes, and a resulting weaker bladder contraction. In these early stages, the only clue of the developing neuropathic condition might be an amelioration of nocturia or decreased voiding frequency, information that needs to be carefully elicited during a systems review interview.

Difficulties that can occur as a result of a neurogenic bladder include increased likelihood of urinary tract infections due to reflux or retained urine post-voiding. Other symptoms of voiding dysfunction might also be seen. Early in the course of neurogenic bladder dysfunction, scheduled voidings, perhaps with external manual pressure, can be helpful in preventing excessive expansion of the bladder. Further intervention with parasympathomimetic drugs and/or self-catheterization may become necessary. At these stages, consultation with a urologist is strongly recommended.

Radiocontrast-Induced Acute Nephropathy

Radiocontrast-induced acute nephropathy is a concern for many patients with underlying diabetic renal dysfunction. By definition, acute nephropathy is defined as a post-exposure rise in the serum creatinine by beta 1.0 mg/dl. The risk does not seem to be dose dependent. This complication can be quite common after intravenous pyelography and is seen as well after angiography. Avoidance of such nephrotoxic dyes in diabetic patients is recommended whenever possible. If the study is needed, adequate hydration before and after such procedures is strongly recommended as a prophylactic maneuver. When such patients are using medications that are excreted by the kidney, increased caution should be exercised, monitoring renal status carefully for signs of acute renal failure. Many of these medications are stopped during and right after such procedures. Of particular concern in this group is metformin, with increased risk of lactic acidosis in patients with renal dysfunction. This medication should be stopped at the time of the procedure, and then restarted 48 hours later once stability of renal function is ascertained.

References:

For Table 14-2. Levels of Diabetic Retinopathy:

Early Treatment Diabetic Retinopathy Study Research Group. Fundus photographic risk factors for progression of diabetic retinopathy: ETDRS rport number 12. Ophthalmology 1991;98 (5)(Suppl):823–33.

For Table 14-3. International Clinical DR and DME Scale (1:2):

Wilkinson, C. P., Ferris, F. L., III, Klein, R. E., Lee, P. P., Agardh, C. D., Davis, M., Dills, D., Kampik, A., Pararajasegaram, R., and Verdaguer, J. T. Proposed International Clinical Diabetic Retinopathy and Diabetic Macular Edema Disease Severity Scales. Ophthalmology 2003;110(9):1677–82.

Chew, E. Y. A Simplified Diabetic Retinopathy Scale. Ophthalmology 2003;110(9):1675–6.

Suggested Reading

The Diabetes Control and Complications Trial Research Group. The effect of intensive treatment of diabetes on the development and progression of long-term complication sin insulin-dependent diabetes mellitus. N Engl J Med. 1993; 329:977–986.

Ohkubo Y, Kishikawa H, Araki E, et al. Intensive insulin therapy prevents the progression of diabetic microvascular complications in Japanese patients with non-insulin[dependent diabetes mellitus: a randomized prospective 6-year study. Diabetes Res Clin Pract. 1995; 28:103–117

UKPDS Group. Effect of intensive blood-glucose control with metformin on complications in overweight patients with type 2 diabetes (UKPDS 34). UK Prospective Diabetes Study (UKPDS) Group. *Lancet.* 1998; 352:854–865.

American Diabetes Association:Diabetic Nephropathy (Position Statement). *Diabetes Care* 26 (Suppl 1): S94–S98, 2003. American Diabetes Association: Diabetic Retinopathy (Position Statement). *Diabetes Care* 26 (Suppl 1): S94–S98, 2003.

ALLHAT Collaborative Research Group. Major Outcomes in High-Risk Hypertensive Patients Randomized to Angiotensin-Converting Enzyme Inhibitor or Calcium Channel Blocker vs Diuretic. *JAMA*. 2002; 288:2981–2997

Brenner BM et al. Effects of Losartan on Renal and Cardiovascular Outcomes in Patients with Type 2 Diabetes and Nephropathy. N Engl J Med 2001; 345:861–869.

Poggio E, Wang X, Greene T, et al. Performance of the modification of diet in renal disease and Cockcroft-Gault equations in the estimation of GFR in health and in chronic kidney disease. J Am Soc Nephrol 16: 459–466, 2005.

15

Macrovascular Complications

Richard S. Beaser, MD and
Michael Johnstone, MD

Introduction

While diabetes is a result of a metabolic dysfunction resulting in hyperglycemia, complications make diabetes mellitus a vascular disease. Diabetes is implicated in both microvascular and macrovascular diseases. Diabetic microvascular diseases are covered in Chapter 14. Macrovascular disease, which includes coronary artery disease, peripheral vascular disease and stroke, is more prevalent in people with diabetes than in the general population. However, only in recent years have we begun to understand the magnitude and implications of the association between macrovascular disease and diabetes. Both type 1 and type 2 diabetes increase macrovascular risk, and, after glucose control itself, reducing the risk of macrovascular disease is probably the greatest challenge facing the clinician caring for people with diabetes.

Compared to the general population, macrovascular disease tends to occur at a younger age. In addition, the protection imparted by female gender (particularly being a premenopausal female) in the general population disappears when diabetes is present.

The likelihood of macrovascular disease among those with diabetes is two to three times that of the nondiabetic population. This risk of developing atherosclerosis only increases with the presence of frequently con-current risk factors including hypertension, smoking, sedentary lifestyle, family history, or dyslipidemia. Macrovascular disease accounts for 65% of the deaths in patients with diabetes. The risk of death from cardio-vascular disease is twice as high for males with diabetes than the non-diabetic male and up to four times higher among females with diabetes than the non-diabetic female. Cerebrovascular accidents are also more fre-quent in the diabetic patient than the non-diabetic.

Most of the macrovascular complications occur in patients with type 2 diabetes. The underlying cause of type 2 diabetes is insulin resistance and has been referred to as the *insulin resistance syndrome (IRS)*.

Clinical Manifestations:
- central obesity
- glucose intolerance/type 2 diabetes
- atherosclerosis
- hypertension
- first degree relatives with type 2 diabetes
- history of gestational diabetes
- polycystic ovary syndrome
- acanthosis nigricans

Biochemical Abnormalities:
- carbohydrate: glucose intolerance, hyperinsulinemia, insulin resis-tance
- lipid: high triglycerides, low HDL-cholesterol, small, dense LDL par-ticles
- fibrinolysis: increased PAI-1 level

The *metabolic syndrome,* a subset of measurable components in the insulin resistance syndrome, includes:
- abdominal obesity (men >40 in, women >35 in)
- elevated triglycerides (≥150 mg/dL)
- low HDL-cholesterol (men <40 mg/dL, women <50 mg/dL)
- elevated Blood pressure (≥130/≥85 mm Hg)
- *fasting glucose* ≥ 100 mg/dL*

---

* ATP III definition is ≥110 mg/dL, but revised definition of diabetes uses the 100 mg/dL value which we have listed here.

People with 3 or more of these have metabolic syndrome.

People with insulin resistance often have hyperinsulinemia, an attempted compensatory response to the insulin resistance. After some debate as to whether insulin plays a direct role in the etiology of atherogenesis, it is now believed that the hyperinsulinemia should be viewed primarily as a metabolic marker of this syndrome and the process leading to atherogenesis, rather than as playing a direct causal role in the pathogenic process. It is the many related conditions such as glucose intolerance and the others listed above that are manifestations of metabolic syndrome and the constellation of findings often related to insulin resistance that are probably more directly linked to the atherogenic process. Therefore, **from a clinical standpoint, it is imperative that these macrovascular risk factors be identified and treated as aggressively as possible.** Many treatments directly targeting various of these abnormalities have been shown to reduce some atherosclerotic endpoints. However, taking it one step further, it has been speculated that treatments reducing the insulin resistance itself may have similar beneficial effects, although less evidence for this theory has been accumulated as yet.

RISK FACTORS FOR DIABETIC CARDIOVASCULAR DISEASE

Hypertension

Hypertension is discussed in detail in Chapter 14. It often occurs as a result of renal disease in people with type 1 diabetes. Among those with type 2 diabetes, hypertension is very prevalent whether renal disease is present or not. Macrovascular disease can cause, and in turn can be caused by, hypertension. The development of type 2 diabetes was found to be almost two and a half times higher in patients with hypertension than their normotensive counterparts after adjustment for age, sex, race, adiposity and physical activity level. Hypertension in the patient with diabetes has several unique features. Supine hypertension with orthostatic hypertension is not uncommon as a result of autonomic neuropathy. Furthermore many diabetes patients do not have the usual nocturnal drop in blood pressure. Aggressive treatment of hypertension must be part of an overall strategy for diabetes management, both to protect renal function and to preserve vascular patency.

Dyslipidemia

It has become increasingly apparent that the dyslipidemia that is often seen in people with diabetes significantly increases the risk of athero-sclerotic cardiovascular disease. The pattern of lipoprotein abnormalities most commonly seen in people with diabetes includes:

- elevated total cholesterol
- decreased high-density lipoprotein (HDL) cholesterol levels
- increased small, dense low-density lipoprotein (LDL)
- elevated triglyceride levels

There seems to be a direct correlation between the triglyceride level and the degree of insulin resistance. In addition, this classic pattern of abnor-malities described above may be altered by other factors, such as the de-gree of glucose control, obesity, physical inactivity, use of alcohol, use of medications that might affect lipid patterns, and genetic lipid abnormali-ties.

The presence of these lipid abnormalities (increased triglycerides and decreased HDL) is thought to be a marker for increased risk of coronary artery disease (CAD). It is not uncommon to find this pattern of lipid ab-normalities present in people at the time they are diagnosed with type 2 diabetes, or even in those who do not currently have type 2 diabetes but who later develop it. However, whether or not these lipid alterations di-rectly impact CAD risk has been the subject of debate. This pattern of ab-normalities, it has been suggested, may really represent a measure of the severity of insulin resistance or perhaps a marker for the insulin resistance syndrome rather than a direct causal factor for macrovascular disease.

In fact, much of the focus of therapy has been on lowering the choles-terol levels of those with diabetes. While cholesterol and LDL cholesterol levels in people with diabetes are similar to those seen in the nondiabetic population, the Multiple Risk Factor Trial (MRFIT), a study examining the impact of macrovascular risk factors on the development of atherosclero-sis, has clearly demonstrated the relationship between elevations of these levels and CAD risk in both populations. However, the baseline risk for the diabetic subgroup was two to four times greater, suggesting that there must be other factors in the diabetes population that further raise the frequency of this complication. These might include renal disease, hypertension, glucose control, and the presence of advanced glycation end products (AGEs), hypercoaguability, and obesity. In addition, people with diabetes, particularly type 2 diabetes, tend to have increases in the small, dense LDL particles which are thought to be more atherogenic.

In addition, clinical intervention to lower LDL cholesterol levels has been demonstrated to reduce CAD endpoints in a number of clinical trials that looked at treatment in a general population but also showed benefits in the diabetic subgroups. The Scandinavian Simvastatin Survival Study (4S), a secondary prevention trial, demonstrated that treatment to reduce elevated LDL cholesterol levels with an HMG CoA reductase inhibitor resulted in a decrease in incidence of, and mortality from, CAD. These benefits were also seen in the diabetic subgroup in this study. The Cholesterol and Recurrent Events (CARE) study showed similar results in patients with lower LDL levels, with a study population having more patients with diabetes. The Heart Protection Study (HPS), the largest study to date, confirmed these results in the subgroup analyses of 6000 patients with diabetes, > 90% of whom had type 2 diabetes. More recently, the PROVE-IT and TNT trials suggest that a lower LDL level, that is, less than 70 mg/dl, for all patients with coronary artery disease is preferred. Since diabetes is considered to be a risk equivalent for coronary artery disease, lower LDL goals are likely to be indicated, particularly if accompanied by multiple other risk factors

Goals of Treatment

The CAD risk with elevated cholesterol levels has undergone numerous revisions in the last few years. As recently as the late 1970s, medical schools were still teaching the "normal" cholesterol levels based on the standard bell-shaped curve of the general population. However, during the ensuing decades, we learned that these so-called normal levels were not necessarily healthy, and thus desirable targets for lipid levels have decreased. In addition, the therapeutic focus has shifted to LDL cholesterol.

The LDL cholesterol levels at which therapeutic intervention is recommended have undergone downward revisions. The current recommendations of the ADA, based on the presence or absence of existing macro-

TABLE 15-1.   ADA Lipid Treatment Recommendations

- **Individuals without overt CVD**
  - Primary goal : LDL-C <100 mg/dl
  - If age >40 yr, statin therapy to reduce LDL by 30–40% regardless of baseline LDL-C
  - If age <40 yr but other CVD risk factors, consider drug therapy to achieve goals
- **Individuals with overt CVD**
  - Statin to achieve LDL-C reduction of 30–40%
  - LDL-C goal of < 70 mg/dl with high dose statin
- **Additional goals and recommendations**
  - Triglycerides goal <150 mg/dl; HDL-C >40 mg/dl (men), > 50 mg/dl (women)

Combination therapy to achieve lipid goals may be needed but outcome studies pending

Adapted from American Diabetes Association: Prevention and management of diabetes complications; Diabetes Care 30 (Suppl 1): S17, 2007.

vascular disease, are listed in Table 15-1. In May, 2001, the National Cholesterol Education Program (NCEP) published the "Third Report of the NCEP Expert Panel on Detection, Evaluation, and Treatment of High Blood Cholesterol in Adults" (Available on line at www.nhlbi.nih.gov or as NIH publication No. 01–3670, May 2001), which included an update in the approach to treatment of dyslipidemia in people with diabetes. This report makes the following points:

- People with diabetes who do not have coronary heart disease (CHD), many of whom display multiple risk factors, are equivalent in risk of CHD to those without diabetes who have CHD.
- Persons with multiple metabolic risk factors (metabolic syndrome) are candidates for intensified therapeutic lifestyle changes.
- An LDL cholesterol remains the primary goal of therapy, with optimal target for people with diabetes <100 mg/dl.
- The category of low HDL has been raised from <35 mg/dl to <40 mg/dl.
- Treatment beyond LDL-lowering for persons with triglycerides ≥ 150 mg/dl is recommended.

- The complete lipoprotein profile (total cholesterol, LDL cholesterol, HDL cholesterol, and triglycerides) is the preferred initial screening test, rather than just screening with total cholesterol and HDL alone.

Clearly, the downward trend of LDL goals continues. As suggested above, PROVE-IT and TNT suggest that the goal for LDL should be 70 mg/dl in patients with coronary artery disease.

A second therapeutic goal should be raising the HDL level, although available tools — primarily lifestyle changes, glucose control, and nicotinic acid, are often either less effective than those for lowering LDL cholesterol or relatively contraindicated (nicotinic acid at high dose) in people with type 2 diabetes. Triglyceride lowering is also recommended by the ADA, although direct impact of this intervention on clinical outcomes is less well demonstrated.

Nonpharmacologic Treatment

As with treatments to control glucose levels, the first-line therapy for dyslipidemias is medical nutrition therapy (MNT) and physical activity, with a focus on weight loss. These interventions can effectively impact the typical dyslipidemic pattern seen in diabetes by lowering triglyceride levels and raising levels of HDL cholesterol, as well as by lowering LDL cholesterol.

The recommended nutritional adjustments for people with dyslipidemia include reductions in the proportions of saturated fat and a compensatory increase in the carbohydrate and/or monounsaturated fat levels. Keep in mind, however, the difficulty and limitations of this approach. The challenges of maximizing and sustaining patient compliance aside, the American Heart Association suggests that such interventions may reduce LDL cholesterol by up to 15–25 mg/dl. Therefore, if the LDL is greater than this interval above target, the likelihood of achieving desired improvements with lifestyle changes alone is small.

However, the impact of nonpharmacologic interventions on triglyceride levels may be more significant. A reduction in total calorie intake and initiation of an exercise program in an overweight person that leads to a reduction of even 5 to 10 pounds can substantially reduce triglyceride levels.

TABLE 15-2. Treatment Summary for Dyslipidemia in Adult Patients With Diabetes

---

First Priority Treatment: Lowering LDL Cholesterol

1. First-line therapy:

HMG CoA Reductase Inhibitors ("Statins")

• Primary effect	Very effectively lowers LDL
• Secondary effects	May raise HDL
	May lower triglycerides

2. Second line therapies:

Bile acid binding resin ("resin")

• Primary effect	Lowers LDL
• Secondary effects	May raise triglycerides
	May raise HDL
	Some (Cholesevelam) can improve glycemic control

Impacting GI absorption of Cholesterol: Ezetimibe

• Primary effect	Lowers LDL by blocking cholesterol absorption

Fibric Acid Derivatives
- Effects: see below

Second Priority Treatment: Raising HDL Cholesterol

1. First-line therapy

Lifestyle changes (medical nutrition therapy, exercise, weight loss, smoking cessation)

• Efficacy	Variable

Glucose Control

•Efficacy	Variable

2. Second line therapy

Nicotinic Acid (relatively contraindicated for people with diabetes)

• Primary effect	Lowers LDL
• Secondary effects	Effective at raising HDL
	Effective at lowering triglycerides

3. Third-line therapy

Fibric acid derivatives
- Effects: see below

Third Priority Treatment: Lowering Triglyceride:

1. First-line therapy

Glucose control

• Efficacy	Variable

2. Second-line therapy

Fibric acid dervatives (gemfibrozil, fenofibrate)

• Primary effect	Very effectively lowers triglycerides
• Secondary effects	Can raise HDL
	Variable effect on LDL cholesterol

3. Third-line therapy

HMG CoA reductase inhibitors ("statins" — use at moderate to high dose when elevated LDL is also present)

• Efficacy	See above

Pharmacologic Treatment

The pharmacologic treatment approach to dyslipidemias in patients with diabetes is summarized in Table 15-2. There are a number of choices within each group, particularly the HMG CoA reductase inhibitors ("statins"). While the similarities within these groups outweigh the differences from a clinical standpoint, individualized choices are often made on the basis of slight differences in effect, dosing, or cost. For the statins in particular, higher doses may also have a significant effect in lowering triglycerides.

While the majority of the patients with diabetes and dyslipidemia have type 2 diabetes, much of the advice given also applies to those with type 1 diabetes. In particular, patients with type 1 diabetes may also benefit from the effects of improved glucose control.

Monitoring Lipids

For people with diabetes and no history of dyslipidemia, monitoring their lipid levels yearly should suffice. If values are at desirable levels, then this frequency should be sufficient to pick up changes soon enough to initiate appropriate treatment. However, there are a number of considerations that might suggest the need to monitor more often. Certainly, values suggestive of the development of the early stages of the diabetic dyslipidemic pattern might warrant increased frequency. Evidence of end-organ effects in this setting would lend further weight to this approach. Changing glucose control would also warrant more frequent testing. In particular, a patient with suboptimal glucose control and elevated lipids might achieve some lipid improvement just from the establishment of a proper diabetes management program. Thus, the initial therapeutic focus for patients with poorly controlled diabetes accompanied by dyslipidemia is often improvement of glucose control. Concurrent monitoring of lipid levels will determine whether or not the lipid-lowering response to improved glucose control is sufficient to avoid the need for additional pharmacologic intervention.

Monitoring should be done by way of a fasting test for serum total cholesterol, triglycerides, and HDL cholesterol. Newer methodology for a direct LDL cholesterol measurement has increased the accuracy of this determination. However, if this measurement is not available or convenient, the LDL cholesterol can be calculated indirectly via the following Friedwald formula:

$$\text{Total cholesterol} - [(\text{triglycerides}/5) + \text{HDL cholesterol}] = \text{LDL cholesterol estimate}$$

Note: This formula is not valid if the triglyceride level is >400 mg/dl.

Hypercoagulability

There are three disorders of coagulation and fibrinolysis that have been associated with the resistance syndrome and which further increase the risk of developing macrovascular disease:

- increased levels of plasminogen activator inhibitor (PAI-1)
- increased levels of von Willebrand factor and factor VII
- increased levels of fibrinogen and C-reactive protein (CRP)

How these coagulation findings relate to, and are perhaps caused by, insulin resistance and/or endothelial damage is the subject of much academic discussion. They clearly have an impact on coagulability. There is also an increased platelet aggregability in people with diabetes. The increase on PAI-1 probably has the direct effect of decreasing fibrinolysis. Increased Von Willebrand factor implies endothelial damage. Elevated fibrinogen and CRP levels may result from endothelial damage or proinflammatory cytokines. Nevertheless, regardless of the mechanism, the resulting increase in coagulability seen in people with type 2 diabetes clearly increases their risk for macrovascular disease.

Preventive Strategies

The cornerstone of therapy aimed at reducing hypercoagulability is aspirin therapy. Aspirin has been used in both primary and secondary prevention for people with and without diabetes. The current recommendation by the ADA for people with diabetes is to use aspirin therapy as a secondary therapy for people who already have evidence of macrovascular disease. In addition, it is recommended that aspirin be considered for use as primary preventive therapy in those people with diabetes who are at high risk for macrovascular disease. This category includes people with:

- a family history of CAD
- hypertension
- obesity (>120% ideal body weight (IBW) or body mass index (BMI) >28 in women, >27.3 in men)
- cigarette smoking
- microalbuminuria or macroalbuminuria
- dyslipidemia
- age >30 years

Traditionally, the recommended aspirin dose has been 81 mg (a "low dose") of enteric-coated aspirin. However, more effective risk reduction has been seen with increased doses, up to a full enteric-coated aspirin tablet (325 mg) daily. Some experts suggest that the higher the risk factor profile, the higher the aspirin dosage. An alternative to aspirin therapy is clopidogrel (75 mg daily).

The major risk of aspirin therapy is bleeding, particularly from the upper gastrointestinal tract. Enteric-coated aspirin preparations may reduce this risk. Contraindications to aspirin therapy largely relate to this bleeding risk and include other bleeding disorders, anticoagulant therapy, history of recent gastrointestinal bleed, clinically active hepatic disease, or aspirin allergy. Aspirin therapy does not seem to increase the risk of retinal bleeding.

Obesity

Obesity is also a macrovascular risk factor. Obesity is defined as being >20% over IBW. It has been estimated that about 80% of all people with type 2 diabetes are obese at the time of diagnosis or have a history of obesity. There are two classic patterns of obesity. One is the android, "apple" shape, or central obesity, which represents increased intra-abdominal fat and is associated with type 2 diabetes and insulin resistance. Alternatively, the gynoid or "pear" shape represents increased fat in the hips and thighs, classically seen in women. The treatment of obesity using medical nutrition therapy is discussed in detail in Chapter 5.

Diabetes as a Macrovascular Risk Factor

Having diabetes does seem to increase the chances of developing macro-vascular disease. However, the exact relationship has not been clearly demonstrated. Although the insulin resistance syndrome itself, with the associated conditions such as dyslipidemia and hypercoagulability, does seem to be a macrovascular risk factor, is the hyperglycemia of type 2 dia-betes itself a direct risk factor as well? Many would argue that it is, but this association remains controversial until more direct data has been ac-cumulated.

Clearly, hyperglycemia is a microvascular risk factor, so aggressive glu-cose control is still appropriate for all people with diabetes. While proof that hyperglycemia, per se, is a macrovascular risk remains elusive, it has been demonstrated or suggested that hyperglycemia is associated with multiple abnormalities that lead to an increased incidence of macro-vascular disease. In the UKPDS study, the relationship between glucose control and macrovascular endpoints just missed statistical significance. Two other studies from Finland do suggest a weak but significant rela-tionship for people with type 2 diabetes. A stronger relationship between glucose control and macrovascular disease has been noted for patients with type 1 diabetes in a number of observational studies. More recently, the DCCT/EDCIC study did show that glucose control does reduce the likelihood of clinical macrovascular events in patients with type 1 diabe-tes. To date, there are no studies that demonstrate that tight glucose con-trol in patients with type 2 diabetes reduces cardiovascular events.

Nevertheless, having diabetes clearly correlates with a worse overall risk of problems associated with coronary disease. In fact, a study by Haffner *et al* demonstrated that having diabetes is equal in conferring sub-sequent risk for an MI to having already had an MI but not having diabe-tes. Further, individuals with diabetes who have heart disease are at much greater risk for:

- congestive heart failure
- a second heart attack
- involvement of multiple coronary arteries

Therefore, it seems reasonable to state that the benefits of aggressive glucose control have been demonstrated for all patients, but whether these benefits include a clear reduction of macrovascular risk, independ-ent of other risk factors, are not yet clearly proven.

The reduction of macrovascular risk is clearly an important imperative in the approach to treatment of people with diabetes. With the trends seen in recommendations such as the new NCEP guidelines, it is clear that diabetes itself, independent of the specific risk factors that accompany it, is being thought of as a risk factor for macrovascular disease. Indeed, many consider diabetes itself a disease entity that is a precursor to macrovascular disease, and thus approach people with diabetes as if they already have commenced the pathophysiologic process that results in atherosclerosis.

Classic evidence supporting this approach was demonstrated in the HOPE (Heart Outcomes Prevention Evaluation) study and the substudy, MICRO-HOPE, that looked at a diabetic subpopulation. The MICRO-HOPE trial showed that patients with diabetes who were treated with an ACE inhibitor, ramipril, 10 mg daily, showed an overall reduction in the risk of MI of 22%, reduction of cardiovascular death of 37%, and stroke of 33%. Treatment with ramipril was independent of the traditional indications, hypertension or microalbuminuria. This study suggests that pharmacologic intervention in people over 55 with diabetes and one other cardiac risk factor (criteria for the Micro-Hope population) may have a significant impact in reducing macrovascular risk. In the HOPE trial itself, people 55 years or older who had a history of CAD, Stroke, or PVD and were thus at high risk of having a major cardiovascular event showed similar reductions in events, plus had a 34% lower risk of developing diabetes. Ramipril is now indicated for use as part of preventive strategies in patients with these risk profiles. Whether or not these benefits are shared by other ACE inhibitors will have to await confirmatory data.

Gender Issues in Assessing Macrovascular Risk Factors

Premenopausal women with diabetes lose the natural protection from the development of macrovascular disease that their female gender would otherwise have conferred. The Framingham Heart Study data suggest that, correcting for all other risk factors, diabetes doubles a woman's risk of developing coronary heart disease. In addition, women with diabetes are more likely to die after a myocardial infarction, with a marked increased incidence of congestive heart failure, than either diabetic men or nondiabetic women. As a result, the focus on macrovascular risk reduction for women with diabetes should be as aggressive as for men, and symptoms suggestive of macrovascular end-organ damage should be taken very seriously.

Cigarette Smoking

The fact that cigarette smoking can be hazardous to one's health is a fact that should be known to everyone by now. Nevertheless, many people still smoke and others are affected by second-hand smoke. Smoking can increase macrovascular risk as well as increase the risk of diabetic retinopathy.

The focus on diabetes healthcare interventions is most often on glucose control, lipid management, treatment of hypertension, and dyslipidemic therapy, with time remaining dealing with foot care, insuring ophthalmologic exams have occurred, and the like. The chance to address cigarette smoking cessation is often squeezed into the ever-shortening time allotted for primary care visits. Yet, if successful, this change in personal habits can often impact health and longevity as much, if not more, than interventions aimed at some of the other risk factors.

Specific actions focusing on smoking cessation that a healthcare professional can take include:

- Taking a detailed smoking history at each visit, including the amount smoked and ongoing efforts to stop. This attention reinforces the importance of smoking as a health risk.
- Counseling people about the negative impacts of smoking on overall health and, in particular, on diabetes and its complications.
- Recommending smoking cessation medications or patches, or referring people to formal cessation programs, if other efforts have been unsuccessful.

Macrovascular End-Organ Damage

The end-organ damage resulting from macrovascular disease is the leading cause of death for people with diabetes. While preventive strategies aimed at risk factor reduction are theoretically the best approach, many people still present with the results of atherosclerosis. After prevention, early detection of end-organ damage is the next best thing.

Coronary Artery Disease

Coronary artery disease (CAD) is common in people with both type 1 and type 2 diabetes. Underlying abnormalities at presentation can include angina, congestive heart failure (CHF), myocardial infarction, or sudden cardiac death. On the other hand, the presenting symptoms may by atypical, or absent altogether. The underlying pathology in a person with diabetes is similar to that in a person without diabetes, although in the diabetic person the distribution of disease is often more diffuse and involves more of the smaller coronary vessels. This diffuse distribution of coronary involvement has been implicated as a cause of the increased incidence of CHF seen in this population. Impaired ventricular function in the absence of significant atherosclerotic disease has suggested however that a cardiomyopathic process specific to diabetes may also be present.

The onset of CAD in people with diabetes occurs at a much younger age than in those people who do not have diabetes. Trends toward earlier intervention in the diabetic population as suggested by the HOPE and MICRO-HOPE trials will undoubtedly continue.

Autonomic Neuropathy

Autonomic neuropathy can also affect the heart. Initial manifestations may include increased resting heart rate and a decrease in the beat-to-beat interval variation with inspiration and expiration, progressing to loss of variation with Valsalva or postural change. Autonomic cardiac neuropathies increase the risk for sudden cardiac death. Diabetic cardiac neuropathies have also been implicated as the cause for the loss of classic anginal pain. Thus, clinicians must approach these patients with heightened scrutiny. He or she should carefully seek hints of "anginal equivalents," which might include jaw or tooth pain, indigestion, arm or shoulder pain, increased fatigue, or decreased exercise tolerance.

Early Diagnosis Essential

The benefits of making an early diagnosis of coronary artery disease are multiple, and thus early recognition of signs and symptoms of CAD is important. Symptoms of CAD in people with diabetes may be subtle. The presence of microalbuminuria should be a marker for the increased likelihood of coronary artery disease. Initiation of earlier, more aggressive risk factor reduction programs may significantly slow the progression of the atherosclerotic process. In particular, lipid-lowering has been demonstrated to have significant impact on disease progression and mortality in a number of trials as reflected in the guidelines. Hypertension treatment, demonstrated to be beneficial in the UKPDS, can also be approached more aggressively. Early intervention using an ACE inhibitor (ramipril) to reduce progression to macrovascular disease seems to be gaining acceptance. Aspirin therapy should also be initiated.

Treatment aimed at the coronary ischemia can also be initiated once the diagnosis is established. Initiation of therapies with medications such as ß-blockers might be indicated and can be quite beneficial in reducing the impact of ischemia.

Further cardiac testing may be indicated in patients with diabetes who have underlying CAD. As classic coronary symptoms may be absent in people with diabetes, the ADA has recommended that testing be initiated in patients with specific indications that would indicate an increased cardiac risk (see Table 15-3).

Selection of the modality for further cardiac testing must be individualized based on specific patient considerations. When cardiac disease is suspected, but the patient's electrocardiogram (EKG) is normal, an exercise tolerance test may be an appropriate first step. If this patient had multiple risk factors, an abnormal ECG, or had more typical anginal symptoms with a normal EKG, then stress perfusion imaging or a stress echo might be an appropriate initial choice. Evidence of more significant cardiac disease such as clear ischemia or a myocardial infarction (MI) on EKG, unstable angina, or congestive heart failure (CHF) would warrant referral to a cardiologist for evaluation and possible angiography. Follow-up evaluation of exercise tolerance testing based on findings and risks should follow the recommendations of the ADA (Table 15-4). When making such decisions, the patient's overall condition, including the presence of other complications, must be considered as well.

TABLE 15-3. Indications for Cardiac Testing in Patients with Diabetes

Testing for coronary artery disease (CAD) is warranted in patients with the following:

1. **Typical or atypical cardiac symptoms**
   NOTE: May include: "anginal equivalents," such as jaw or tooth pain, indigestion, arm or shoulder pain, increased fatigue, or decreased exercise tolerance.

2. **Resting electrocardiograph suggestive of ischemia or infarction**
   NOTE: Look carefully for evidence of silent, past myocardial infarctions

3. **Peripheral or carotid occlusive arterial disease**
   NOTE: Look for history of transient ischemic attacks (TIA's) or claudication. Palpate peripheral pulses. Check for carotid bruits.

4. **Sedentary lifestyle, age ≥35 years, and plans to begin a vigorous exercise program**

5. **Two or more of the risk factors listed below in addition to diabetes:**

   a. **Total cholesterol ≥240 mg/dl, LDL cholesterol ≥160 mg/dl, or HDL cholesterol <35 mg/dl**

   b. **Blood pressure >140/90 mmHg**

   c. **Smoking**

   d. **Family history of premature CAD**

   e. **Positive micro/macroalbuminuria test**

Adapted with permission from American Diabetes Association: Consensus Development Conference on the Diagnosis of Coronary Heart Disease in People with Diabetes, Table 1—Indications for cardiac testing in patients with diabetes; *Diabetes Care* 21: 1551–1559, 1998.

Peripheral Vascular Disease

Like CAD, the symptoms of peripheral vascular disease may be variable. Activity-induced pain in thighs, buttocks, or calf that is relieved by rest may represent peripheral vascular disease. However, unlike CAD, a physical examination is often much more revealing. Decreased pedal pulses, a dusky blue color or dependent rubor of the feet, or decreased hair growth on the feet are suggestive findings. A full review of the prevention, diagnosis, and treatment of peripheral vascular disease in people with diabetes can be found in Chapter 17

TABLE 15-4. Follow-Up After Screening Exercise Treadmill Test in Asymptomatic Diabetes Patients Based on Pre-Test Risk and Exercise Tolerance Test (ETT) Results

Pretest Risk		ETT Results		
	Normal	Mildly Positive	Moderately Positive	Markedly Positive
HIGH 4–5 risk factors	XX	XXX	XXXX	XXXX
MODERATE 2–3 risk factors	X	XXX	XXX	XXXX
LOW 0–1 risk factors	X	XXX	XXX	XXXX
X	Routine Follow-up (Ann. Symptom review, CXR, ECG; ETT in 3–5 yrs.)			
XX	Close Follow-up (More frequent evaluations & ETT in 1–2 yrs.)			
XXX	Imaging			
XXXX	Cardiology referral / Possible Catheterization			

Adapted with permission from American Diabetes Association: Consensus Development Conference on the Diagnosis of Coronary Heart Disease in People with Diabetes; Figure 3; *Diabetes Care* 21: 1551–1559, 1998.

Cerebrovascular Disease

Cerebrovascular disease may be more common in people with diabetes than may be evident from easily recognizable symptoms. Clearly, once a stroke or transient ischemic attack (TIA) occurs, the diagnosis is strongly suggested. However, the clinical challenge is to determine the presence of cerebrovascular disease prior to these events. The presence of carotid bruits, while not always reliable indications of vascular occlusions, certainly provide enough suggestive evidence to justify non-invasive Doppler testing of carotid circulation. Carotid endarterectomy may be indicated if this test shows a significant stenosis, even if the patient is asymptomatic. Prophylactic aspirin may be effective as a preventive strategy, while coumadin anticoagulation is often prescribed once a neurologic event has occurred. Some of the newer studies have shown a reduction in the risk of stroke or TIAs by LDL cho-lesterol-lowering drugs, particularly statins, in patients with pre-existing macrovascular disease. Clopidogrel may also reduce the risk of stroke. The HOPE and MICROHOPE trials also suggested the benefits of ACE inhibitor (ramipril) treatment.

Major Psychoses and Increased Risk of Diabetes and the Metabolic Syndrome

It has been recognized that people with major psychoses such as schizophrenia have an increased risk of developing diabetes and the metabolic syndrome. It seems that the increased risk is related to schizophrenia itself, and it has been suggested that it could be due to either a genetic relationship and/or a reflection of the typical lifestyle (sedentary, poor nutritional habits, smoking) of these individuals. Obesity, which certainly contributes, is increased in this population.

There is also an apparent increase in the risk of developing these metabolic abnormalities with use of some of the antipsychotic medications. Case reports and minimal comparative studies suggest clozapine and olanzapine may more significantly increase the metabolic risk, although counterarguments look to the increased risk in the population as still being the key factor. However, growing evidence does point to some drug involvement, particularly with an increased risk for diabetic ketoacidosis, suggesting a possible drug effect on ß-cell function as well. Lesser risk is seen with newer agents ziprasidone and aripiprazole.

The evidence is still being collected to understand more fully the relationship between psychoses and their treatments with diabetes and the metabolic syndrome. Until the full story is understood, increased vigilance in this population is recommended, particularly if patients are using one of the medications implicated as a possible contributor to the problem. Antipsychotic medication selection based on metabolic risk profile should be considered. Interventions to reduce or treat macrovascular risks would be the same as for the non-psychotic population, but recognizing that most lifestyle and many pharmacologic interventions are more difficult to initiate and manage in this group.

Dental Disease — Its Role in Diabetes and Implications for Macrovascular Disease

Dental and periodontal diseases have long been recognized as being more common in people with diabetes. In addition, the prevalence of diabetes is higher in people who have periodontal diseases than in those who don't. Conditions include dental abscess, gingivitis, and severe periodontitis with tooth loss. Oral conditions such as candidiasis, lichen planus, xerostomia, burning mouth syndrome, angular cheilitis and taste dysfunction are more commonly seen with poorly controlled diabetes. Oral conditions, particularly abscesses, can also lead to higher glucose levels, which may be the first or only manifestation of the oral condition. Oral candidiasis is associated with hyperglycemia, and can result from xerostomia, salivary hyperglycemia, and impaired immune function. More recently, there has been a suggestion that the inflammatory process seen in the mouth, particularly the gums, may relate in some way to the inflammatory process that is seen as a contributing factor in endothelial dysfunction. Some studies show that dental caries is more prevalent in people with diabetes, as well.

Routine dental examinations are therefore recommended for all people with diabetes. At an initial visit, the presence of diabetes should be discussed with the dentist, with consideration of visits every 6 months. People with a history of poorly controlled diabetes and periodontal diseases may need dental visits even more frequently. The exam should include specifically screening for the common dental and oral complications seen in people with diabetes as noted above. Non dental clinicians caring for people with diabetes should encourage dental consultations, particularly if symptoms of the above conditions are noted, such as sore, swollen, or bleeding gums, loose teeth, or persistent mouth ulcers. The healthcare team should reinforce the importance of proper oral health care, which includes tooth and gum cleaning and visits to the dentist at least twice a year, brushing at least twice a day, flossing at least once a day, use of fluoride-containing toothpaste, and smoking cessation. With sudden deterioration of glycemic control without any other obvious explanation, dental conditions should be considered.

Suggested Reading

American Diabetes Association. Standards of medical care in diabetes — 2007. Diabetes Care. 2007 Jan;30 Suppl 1:S4–S41.

Stern M.Natural history of macrovascular disease in type 2 diabetes: role of insulin resistance. *Diabetes Care* 22 (Suppl. 3):C2–C5, 1999.

Steiner G. Risk factors for microvascular disease in type 2 diabetes. *Diabetes Care* 22 (Suppl. 3): C6–C9, 1999.

Beaser R, Levy P: The Metabolic Syndrome: A Work In Progress, But A Useful Construct . *Circulation*. 115: 1812–1818, 2007

Kahn R: Metabolic Syndrome: Is It a Syndrome? Does It Matter? Kahn *Circulation*. 115: 1806–1811, 2007

Yusuf S et al. Effect of potentially modifiable risk factors associated with myocardial infarction in 52 countries (the INTERHEART study): case-control study. Lancet.364:937–952, 2004.

American Diabetes Association position statement: Dyslipidemia Management in Adults With Diabetes *Diabetes Care* 27 (Suppl. 1):S68–S71, 2004.

Haffner SM.Management of dyslipidemia in adults with diabetes (Technical Review). *Diabetes Care* 21:160–178, 1998.

Stamler J, Vaccaro O, Neaton JD. Diabetes, other risk factors, and 12-year cardiovascular mortality for men screened in the Multiple Risk Factor Intervention Trial. *Diabetes Care* 16:434–444, 1993.

Sacks FM, Pfeffer MA, Moye LA, Roleau JL, Rutherford JD, Cole TG, Brown L, Warnica JW, Arnold JM, Wun CC, Davis BR, Braunwald E: The effect of pravastatin on coronary events after myocardial infarction in patients with average cholesterol levels. *N Engl J Med* 335:1001–1009, 1996.

4S Study Group: Randomized trial of cholesterol lower in 4444 patients with coronary heart disease: the Scandinavian Simvastatin Survival Study (4S). *Lancet* 344:1383–1389, 1994.

Grundy SM, Balady GJ, Criqui MH, Fletcher G, Greenland P, Hiratzka LF, Houston-miller N, Kris-Etherton P, Krumholz HM, LaRosa J, Ockene IS, Pearson TA, Reed J, Smith SC,

Grundy S. et al. for the Coordinating Committee of the National Cholesterol Education Program Endorsed by the National Heart, Lung, and Blood Institute, American College of Cardiology Foundation, and American Heart Association. Implications of Recent Clinical Trials for the National Cholesterol Education Program Adult Treatment Panel III Guidelines. Circulation. 110:227–239, 2004.

Yudkin JS: Abnormalities of coagulation and fibrinolysis in insulin resistance. *Diabetes Care* 22 (Suppl. 3): C25–C30, 1999.

American Diabetes Association position statement: Aspirin Therapy in Diabetes

Diabetes Care 27 (Suppl. 1):S72–S73, 2004.

Colwell JA: Aspirin therapy in diabetes (Technical Review). *Diabetes Care* 20:1767–1771, 1997.

American Diabetes Association Consensus Development Conference Report: Consensus Development Conference on the Diagnosis of Coronary Heart Disease in People with Diabetes. *Diabetes Care* 21: 1551–1559, 1998.

Pyörälä K, Pedersen TR, Kjeksus J, Faergeman O, Olsson AG, Thorgeirsson G: Cholesterol lowering with simvastatin improves prognosis of diabetic patients with coronary heart disease: a subgroup analysis of the Scandinavian Simvastatin Survival Study (4S). *Diabetes Care* 20:614–620, 1997.

Sacks FM, Pfeffer MA, Moye LA, Fouleau JL, Rutherford JD, Cole TG, Brown L, Warnica JW, Arnold JMO, Wun C-C, Davis DR, Brunwald E: The effect of pravastatin on coronary events after myocardial infarction in patients with average cholesterol levels. *N Engl J Med* 335:1001–1009, 1996.

Haffner SM et al. Mortality from coronary heart disease in subjects with type 2 diabetes and in nondiabetic subjects with and without prior myocardial infarction. N Engl J Med 339: 229–234, 1998.

American Diabetes Association Consensus Development Conference Report: Consensus Development Conference on the Treatment of Hypertension in Diabetes. *Diabetes Care* 16:1394–1401, 1993

HOPE Study Investigators. Effects of ramipril on cardiovascular and microvascular outcomes in people with diabetes mellitus: results of the HOPE and MICRO-HOPE substudy. *Lancet* 355:253–259; 2000.

HOPE Study Investigators. Effects of an angiotensin-converting-enzyme inhibitor, ramipril, on cardiovascular events in high-risk patients. *N Engl J Med* 342–145–153; 2000.

16

Diabetic Neuropathy

Roy Freeman, MD

Diabetic neuropathy impacts the health, longevity, and quality of life for many people with diabetes. The diabetic neuropathies include several distinctive syndromes with differing clinical manifestations, anatomic distributions, clinical course, and pathophysiology. While the pathogenic mechanisms that underlie diabetic peripheral neuropathy remain incompletely understood, the challenge to the clinician is to ameliorate the often debilitating symptoms.

Classification

Since our understanding of the etiology and pathophysiology of the diabetic peripheral neuropathies is incomplete, current classifications of the many manifestations of diabetic neuropathies are based on clinical presentation. Making this challenge even more difficult is the fact that many patients do not manifest a single type of diabetic neuropathy but rather a mixture of neuropathic features often dominated by one subtype.

Perhaps the simplest and most useful classification divides the diabetic neuropathies into symmetrical polyneuropathies and asymmetric or focal neuropathies. A modification of this classification is shown in Table 16-1.

Symmetrical Neuropathies

Generalized Polyneuropathy

Epidemiology

Predominately sensory or sensorimotor distal polyneuropathy is the most common of the diabetic neuropathies. Epidemiologic studies indicate that the prevalence of diabetic peripheral neuropathy ranges from 5% to100%. This range is in large part a consequence of variations in the study population, the diagnostic criteria for diabetes and peripheral neuropathy and the duration of diabetes. Diabetic peripheral neuropathy is more prevalent in tertiary care centers and diabetes clinic populations than in the community. The prevalence of neuropathy also increases with increasing duration of diabetes.

Other factors that are associated with the presence of diabetic peripheral neuropathy include age, hypertension, quality of metabolic control, height, the presence of background or proliferative diabetic retinopathy, cigarette smoking, high-density lipoprotein cholesterol, and the presence of cardiovascular disease and microalbuminuria.

Clinical Features

Numbness and paresthesias begin in the toes and gradually and insidiously ascend to involve the feet and lower legs. The sensory deficit usually occurs symmetrically in the distal territory of overlapping nerves, but not infrequently asymmetric patterns of sensory loss in root or nerve distribution may be superimposed on this distal symmetrical pattern of sensory loss. As the distal portion of longer nerves are affected first, the feet and lower legs are involved before the hands, producing the typical "glove and stocking" pattern of sensory deficit. Sensory symptoms and signs are commonly accompanied by mild distal weakness and features of autonomic neuropathy. In more severe cases, distal portions of thoracic intercostal nerves are affected, producing an asymptomatic midline sensory loss in a teardrop distribution over the anterior thorax and abdomen. A similar pattern of deficits may occur on the vertex of the scalp and the central aspect of the face.

In most patients the symptoms of polyneuropathy are mild and consist of numbness or paresthesia of the toes and sensory perception disturbances. In more severe cases, "positive" symptoms develop. These include superficial burning, paresthesiae, deep, aching pains, dysesthesia,

TABLE 16-1. Classification of Diabetic Neuropathy

Symmetrical Neuropathies
Distal symmetrical sensorimotor polyneuropathy
Autonomic neuropathy
Acute painful neuropathy
Hyperglycemic neuropathy
Treatment-induced neuropathy
Chronic inflammatory demyelinating polyneuropathy
Symmetrical proximal lower extremity neuropathy
Focal and Multifocal Neuropathy
Cranial neuropathy
Diabetic amyotrophy
Thoraco-abdominal neuropathy
Focal limb neuropathy

contact-induced discomfort, and paroxysmal jabbing pains. These symptoms are typically more severe at night.

Both lightly myelinated and unmyelinated small nerve fibers and the myelinated large nerve fibers are affected. Small and large fiber dysfunction occurs in varying combinations, however, in most cases the earliest deficits involve the small nerve fibers. Features characteristic of a small fiber peripheral neuropathy include deficits in pain and temperature perception, paresthesias and dysesthesias, pain, deficits in the perception of visceral pain, dysautonomia and predisposition to foot ulceration. Sensory and motor nerve conduction velocities are only mildly slow, since they are dependent on conduction in the surviving large myelinated nerve fibers. This presentation, which resembles the deficits that accompany a syrinx, has been described as pseudosyringomyelic.

In contrast, features that are characteristic of large fiber peripheral neuropathy include loss of position and vibration perception sense and loss of deep tendon reflexes. Nerve conduction studies are usually abnormal. This presentation, which resembles the pattern of deficits that are associated with *tabes doralis*, has been termed pseudotabetic. Marked distal muscle weakness may occur occasionally, although usually this is due to mononeuropathy multiplex involving the peroneal, tibial, median or ulnar nerves. A pure or predominantly motor polyneuropathy with few or no sensory symptoms or signs is rarely due to diabetes and should trigger a search for alternative causes of weakness.

Pathogenesis

The etiology of diabetic neuropathy is incompletely understood. Several different mechanisms, most likely acting in combination, play a role in the pathogenesis of diabetic peripheral neuropathy.

It is likely that metabolic factors play a central role in the pathogenesis of neuropathy. Hyperglycemia produces several metabolic changes, including increased tissue levels of sorbitol and fructose, decreased concentrations of intraneuronal myoinositol and taurine, decreased Na^+/K^+ adenosine triphosphatase (ATPase) activity, impaired protein kinase C activity, and nonenzymatic glycosylation of proteins. Some or all of these metabolic abnormalities may be responsible for pathologic changes in nerve fibers.

Oxidative stress is also implicated in the etiology of diabetic neuropathy. There is evidence that oxygen-free radical activity is enhanced and antioxidant defense mechanisms are compromised in diabetes. The mechanism whereby oxidative stress gives rise to nerve damage is unknown. Oxygen-free radicals may give rise to nerve damage directly or indirectly, operating via a vascular mechanism.

There is also evidence that neurotrophic support failure is implicated in the pathogenesis of diabetic polyneuropathy. In experimental diabetic neuropathy, there is evidence of decreased growth factor expression in skin, sympathetic ganglia, and submandibular glands and impaired retrograde axonal transport from the target tissues to the neuronal cell body. In addition, it is likely that vascular factors play an important contributory role. Animal models of diabetic neuropathy have demonstrated that the neuropathy is accompanied by reduced endoneurial blood flow, increased endoneurial vascular resistance and reduced endoneurial oxygen tension. In human sural nerve biopsy specimens the pathologic changes that are consistent with this hypothesis include basement membrane thickening and duplication, endothelial cell swelling and proliferation, intimal and smooth muscle cell proliferation and vascular occlusion.

Autonomic Neuropathy

The autonomic manifestations of diabetes are responsible for the most troublesome and disabling features of diabetic peripheral neuropathy and result in a significant proportion of the mortality and morbidity associated with the disease. A broad constellation of symptoms occur, affecting cardiovascular, urogenital, gastrointestinal, pupillomotor, thermoregulatory and sudomotor function. The impairment is usually gradual and progressive, although rarely severe autonomic dysfunction may occur shortly after the diagnosis of type 1 and type 2 diabetes.

Cardiovascular System

The cardiovascular autonomic neuropathy has diverse manifestations. An increased resting heart rate is observed frequently in diabetic patients most likely due to the vagal cardiac neuropathy that results in unopposed cardiac sympathetic nerve activity. The tachycardia may be followed by a decrease in heart rate and, ultimately, a fixed heart rate due to progressing cardiac sympathetic nervous system dysfunction.

Orthostatic hypotension, the most incapacitating manifestation of autonomic failure, is a common feature of diabetic cardiovascular autonomic neuropathy. This is a consequence of efferent sympathetic vasomotor denervation that causes reduced vasoconstriction of the splanchnic and other peripheral vascular beds. Diminished cardiac acceleration and cardiac output, particularly in association with exercise, also may play a role in the presentation of this disorder

Several authors have drawn attention to the association between increased mortality and cardiovascular autonomic dysfunction in diabetics. Estimates for the mortality associated with cardiovascular autonomic neuropathy range form 27 to 56% over 5 to 10 years. There is also an increased frequency of sudden death in patients with autonomic neuropathy. Proposed mechanisms whereby the autonomic nervous system may result in sudden death or influence the outcome of diabetic patients with cardiovascular disease include the absent or altered perception of myocardial ischemia and infarction; deficient hemodynamic response to cardiovascular stresses such as surgery, infection and anesthesia; increased predisposition to cardiac arrhythmias due to QT interval dispersion and alterations in sympathetic-parasympathetic cardiac innervation balance.

Urogenital System

Symptoms of bladder dysfunction are reported in 37% to 50% of diabetic patients and there is physiologic evidence of bladder dysfunction in 43% to 87% of patients. Bladder symptoms associated with autonomic neuropathy include hesitancy, poor stream and a sense of inadequate bladder emptying. These symptoms may be followed by urinary retention and overflow incontinence.

Erectile dysfunction is a frequent and disturbing symptom in male diabetes patients. Reported incidence has ranged from 30–75%. Impotence may be the earliest symptom of diabetic autonomic neuropathy, although vascular, hormonal, and psychogenic etiologies, alone or in combination, may also be implicated. Impotence due to autonomic neuropathy progresses gradually but is usually permanent two years after onset. Sympathetically mediated ejaculatory failure may precede the appearance of impotence, although impotence can occur with retained ability to ejaculate and experience orgasm. Retrograde ejaculation will occur if the bladder neck fails to close. There are few studies of genital autonomic neuropathy in female diabetic patients.

Gastrointestinal System

Autonomic dysfunction occurs throughout the gastrointestinal tract, producing several specific clinical syndromes. Gastrointestinal autonomic neuropathy results in disordered gastrointestinal motility, secretion, and absorption. The term *gastroparesis diabeticorum* is used to describe the altered gastrointestinal motility in diabetics. Food residue is retained in the stomach due to absent or decreased gastric peristalsis compounded by lower intestinal dysmotility. Diabetic gastroparesis may manifest as nausea, postprandial vomiting, bloating, abdominal distension and pain, belching, loss of appetite and early satiety. Many patients, however, are asymptomatic despite impaired gastric motility. Gastroparesis may impair the establishment of adequate glycemic control by mismatching plasma glucose and insulin levels. The absorption of orally administered drugs may also be affected. Recent studies have implicated hyperglycemia as a cause of impaired gastric and small intestinal motility during fasting and after food intake.

Diarrhea and other lower gastrointestinal tract symptoms may also occur. Diabetic diarrhea manifests as a profuse, watery, typically nocturnal diarrhea, which can last for hours or days and frequently alternates with constipation. Abdominal discomfort is commonly associated. The pathogenesis of diabetic diarrhea includes reduced gastrointestinal motility, reduced receptor-mediated fluid absorption, bacterial overgrowth, pancreatic insufficiency, co-existent celiac disease and abnormalities in bile salt metabolism. Fecal incontinence, due to anal sphincter incompetence or reduced rectal sensation, is another manifestation of diabetic intestinal neuropathy. Incontinence is often exacerbated by diarrhea.

Sudomotor System

Sudomotor dysfunction is a common feature of diabetic autonomic neuropathy. This generally manifests as anhidrosis of the extremities, which may be accompanied by hyperhidrosis in the trunk. Initially, patients display a loss of thermoregulatory sweating in a glove and stocking distribution, which, with progression of autonomic neuropathy, extends from the lower to the upper extremities and to the anterior abdomen, conforming to the length dependency of diabetic neuropathy (distal portions affected first). This process ultimately may result in global anhidrosis.

Hyperhidrosis may also accompany diabetic autonomic neuropathy. Excessive sweating may occur as a compensatory phenomenon involving proximal regions such as the head and trunk that are spared in a dying-back neuropathy (also a neuropathy that affects distal portions first). Gustatory sweating, the abnormal production of sweat that appears over the face, head, neck, shoulders and chest after eating even non-spicy foods, is occasionally observed.

Acute Painful Neuropathy

Acute painful neuropathy is a is a variant of sensory polyneuropathy in which severe, burning pain of the extremities is combined with deep aching pain in proximal muscles, jabs of pain radiating from the feet to the legs, and striking hypersensitivity or allodynia of the extremities and trunk to touch, clothing, or bed sheets that is often likened to sunburn. Objective sensory deficit is surprisingly mild in comparison with the painful paresthesia and dysesthesia. Depression, anorexia, and weight loss are often so prominent that the term "diabetic neuropathic cachexia" has been used to describe this syndrome. Prognosis may be good in some patients with gradual recovery over a period of months, particularly if the onset of symptoms follows a metabolic disturbance.

Hyperglycemic Neuropathy

"Hyperglycemic" neuropathy refers to widespread paresthesias of the extremities and trunk that occasionally occur in patients with newly diagnosed or poorly controlled diabetes and that rapidly improve with control of hyperglycemia. Similar symptoms sometimes appear following recovery from ketoacidosis. The unique reversibility of this form of neuropathy and the diffuse rather than distal distribution of paresthesias suggest a pathophysiologic basis that differs from that for later-appearing diabetic sensory neuropathy.

Chronic Inflammatory Demyelinating Polyneuropathy

Chronic inflammatory demyelinating polyneuropathy (CIDP) may be more prevalent in diabetic patients. These patients present clinically with a subacute progression of symmetrical motor weakness with loss of reflexes. A study suggested that the odds of CIDP occurring was 11 times greater among patients with diabetes mellitus than among those without. Treatment of 26 such patients with 5 days of intravenous immune globulin (IVIG) produced significant improvement at 4 weeks. Eighty percent of the patients responded to IVIG and the mean neuropathy impairment score (NIS) decreased significantly from baseline. Electromyographic studies are necessary to identify these patients. Characteristic features of CIDP seen on electromyographic studies include nerve conduction velocity slowing, temporal dispersion and conduction block.

Treatment-Induced Neuropathy

Sensory neuropathy sometimes appears for the first time coincident with treatment with insulin or antidiabetes medications and has been referred to a treatment-induced neuropathy. Although the cause is unknown, it has been suggested that improved glycemic control may initiate regenerating axonal sprouts, which generate ectopic nerve impulses. There is usually gradual improvement as treatment continues and glycemic control is maintained.

Clinicians are often confronted with patients complaining of this type of neuropathy, further frustrated because they have recently increased their efforts to control glucose levels. Often, the patient's complaints are as much a reflection of frustration as a reaction to pain. Reassurance that, with continued optimization of glucose control, the discomfort will subside is often sufficient medicine. Just knowing what is going on often can make the patient more accepting of the situation and able to tolerate the often relatively mild discomfort until enough time has passed.

Focal and Multifocal Neuropathy

Cranial Neuropathy

The majority of diabetic cranial neuropathies affect the third and sixth cranial nerves. Onset of diplopia is followed by complete opthalmoplegia within several days. In cases of third-nerve involvement, there may be complete ptosis, but the pupil is typically spared. Weakness involves all extraocular muscles except the lateral rectus and superior oblique muscles. Pain, which is characteristically in the frontal and periorbital region, accompanies opthalmoplegia in about 50% of cases. Differentiation from a neoplastic or vascular lesion should be made with brain-imaging studies such as magnetic resonance imaging (MRI). A vascular cause of diabetic opthalmoplegia is strongly supported by postmortem studies.

Proximal Motor Neuropathy

An array of terms have been used for this syndrome, including diabetic amyotrophy, asymmetric motor neuropathy, subacute proximal diabetic neuropathy, proximal mononeuropathy multiplex, and diabetic polyradiculopathy.

This neuropathy typically occurs with a peak incidence in the fifth or sixth decade in patients with type 2 diabetes. Many patients have mild or unrecognized diabetes at the time of diagnosis. The clinical picture is one of acute or subacute pain, weakness and atrophy of the pelvic girdle and thigh musculature. The iliopsoas and quadriceps are usually involved, producing weakness of hip flexion and knee stabilization within several weeks of onset of pain. As a result, buckling of the knee and difficulty climbing stairs are typical symptoms. In some cases, coexistent weakness of the glutei, hamstrings, thigh adductors, and, less commonly, the peroneal and tibial muscles is present, which indicates a more widespread distribution of the disorder. Symptoms may have a monophasic or stepwise progression. While the initial presentation is usually unilateral, symptoms usually involve the contralateral leg within 3 months. Substantial weight loss may be present and patients may appear cachectic. The extent of the weight loss highlights the systemic nature of the disorder. The weight loss may be compounded by anorexia caused by reactive depression or the use of narcotic analgesics.

Subtle sensory symptoms and signs may be present in the form of paresthesias and sensory disturbance in the anterior thigh and anteromedial aspects of the lower leg, typically in the anterior femoral cutaneous and saphenous nerve distribution. The knee jerk is nearly always reduced or absent on the affected side, whereas ankle jerks may be preserved unless compromised by a coexistent distal polyneuropathy.

Deep, aching pain that is unrelieved by rest is localized to the hip, buttock, and anterior thigh. Pain is typically worse at night than during the day, and is not increased with straight leg raising or other mechanical maneuvers. The process is typically unilateral in onset, but subsequent involvement of the opposite leg occasionally occurs within 3 to 4 months.

Prognosis is usually good, with most patients showing resolution of pain, followed later by gradual return of strength over a period of 6 to 18 months.

Recent studies have emphasized the likelihood that this disorder has a vascular basis. Biopsy of the intermediate cutaneous nerve of thigh and sural nerve has revealed the presence of an inflammatory infiltrate in the epineurium, perineurium and endoneurium. In select cases, vasculitis of the epineurial and perineurial blood vessels has been observed.

The possibility that this disorder has an inflammatory etiology has lead to the use of immune modulating therapies. Intravenous immunoglobulins, plasmapheresis and cortiocosteroids have all been used in open-label uncontrolled studies. A controlled study using intra-venous cortico-steroids confirmed the observed improvement in pain but did not show a greater improvement in motor strength on active drug compared to placebo.

Thoracic Radiculopathy

This entity, also known as thoraco-abdominal neuropathy, also occurs in middle-aged patients and often in those who have relatively mild diabetes. Some patients with this syndrome have had previous or concomitant painful lumbar root syndromes in the lower extremities.

Onset of pain is usually acute, and the pain may be located in the back, chest or abdomen. The character of the pain resembles that of herpes zoster and is usually deep and aching with some elements of superficial sharp or burning pain. Changes in pain with alterations of position or physical activity are variable. Paresthesia and cutaneous hypersensitivity are usually present but may be mild or absent, sometimes causing failure to recognize the neuropathic basis for the pain. The pain is usually unilateral but may occasionally be bilateral. It may also be distributed over more than one dermatomal segment, and often does not have a classic girdling radicular distribution. There may be an accompanying area of sensory loss or dysesthesia in the distribution of one or more adjacent intercostal nerves, the dorsal or ventral rami, or their branches. There is often no impairment of light touch or hypersensitivity to pin stimulation. In severe cases, weakness and laxity of segmental paraspinal and abdominal muscles are present and abdominal hernia may even occur.

Electromyography of paraspinal, intercostal, and abdominal muscles is diagnostically helpful and usually shows changes of acute denervation. As with proximal lower extremity motor neuropathy, weight loss may be prominent, and, because of the frequent absence of definite neuropathic symptoms and signs, exhaustive, unfruitful searches for an intrathoracic or intraabdominal neoplasm often are undertaken. The finding of electromyographic abnormalities usually leads to the correct diagnosis. Cases in which the distribution of symptoms and signs conforms to a single thoracic root should be evaluated with x-ray and MRI studies of the thoracic spine to exclude a compressive radiculopathy. The prognosis is usually better for the lower extremity radiculopathies, with a gradual recovery within a matter of months to a year.

Limb Mononeuropathy

Mononeuropathy is particularly common in persons with diabetes and may occur on the basis of focal ischemia, entrapment, compression or trauma to superficially placed nerves. Any of the major peripheral nerves may be affected. Symptoms may present suddenly or gradually. When several nerves are involved simultaneously, the disorder is referred to as mononeuropathy multiplex. Many patients with diabetic polyneuropathy have electrophysiologic or clinical evidence of superimposed focal mononeuropathy at various common sites of entrapment or nerve injury, such as the median nerve at the wrist, ulnar nerve at the elbow, peroneal nerve at the fibular head, radial nerve above the elbow, and lateral cutaneous nerve of the thigh. This may be because nerves affected by segmental demyelination are known to be particularly sensitive to the effects of compression and anoxia.

Carpal tunnel syndrome caused by median-nerve entrapment in the wrist beneath the transverse carpal ligament is particularly common among persons with diabetes. The symptoms and signs are similar to those in persons without diabetes. Occasionally, however, distal median-nerve mononeuropathy may occur in the absence of the usual pain and sensory symptoms of carpal tunnel syndrome. Although entrapment is still possible in such cases, coexistent distal ulnar neuropathy and bilateral involvement may suggest distal polyneuropathy rather than nerve entrapment. Nerve-conduction studies showing prolonged distal latencies in multiple nerves rather than limited to the median nerve will serve to distinguish distal polyneuropathy from entrapment.

Peroneal mononeuropathy is the most common lower extremity focal neuropathy. This disorder typically presents with sudden painless foot drop without sensory features. Vascular factors and trauma, because of the superficial location of the nerve at the fibular head, are most likely responsible for this neuropathy.

Ulnar mononeuropathy is probably also related to the vulnerable position of the nerve at the elbow. This disorder characteristically presents with pain, paresthesias and dysesthesias in the distribution of the fourth and fifth fingers. Local discomfort in the region of the medial epicondyle may also be present. The symptoms usually appear insidiously and may be due to chronic compression or trauma rather than to acute injury or entrapment. Progressive wasting and weakness of ulnar nerve innervated intrinsic hand muscles occurs.

Evaluation of Diabetic Peripheral Neuropathy

Clinical Examination

The standard clinical evaluation of a patient with diabetes includes the medical and neurologic history and physical examination. The scope and aim of the evaluation from the perspective of neuropathic assessment is outlined in Table 16-1. Table 16-2 provides a checklist for the evaluation of a diabetes patient with neuropathy.

The physical examination can be particularly useful in the characterization of and explanation for patient complaints or abnormalities of function. For example, the motor examination focusing on weakness, wasting or fasciculations may reveal that these findings are present in the distribution of one or more nerves, nerve roots, plexuses or in a distal to proximal distribution. Atrophy of foot intrinsic muscles may lead to foot deformity and predispose diabetic individuals to foot ulceration. The deep tendon reflexes should be measured in both the upper and lower extremities. The knee deep tendon reflex is frequently absent or decreased in patients with diabetic amyotrophy or femoral neuropathy. The reflexes are reduced symmetrically with a distal to proximal gradient in a generalized polyneuropathy. The ankle reflexes are affected first.

The sensory examination should encompass an assessment of both large and small fiber modalities. The small fiber modalities include pin sensation (assessed with a disposable pin) and temperature sensation (assessed with a cold tuning fork). The large fiber modalities include vibration sense (measured with a 128 Hz tuning fork) and position sense (determined by quantifying the patient's response to minute excursions of the distal phalanx of the great toe and first digit).

The autonomic assessment of supine and standing blood pressure and heart rate should be measured one and three minutes after standing. Pupillary evaluation should include assessment of the size, shape, symmetry and response to light of the pupil. The presence or absence of a Horner's syndrome should be documented. Abnormal patterns of sweating should be determined, which is especially important on the feet where the absence of sweating is a predisposing factor to the development of foot ulceration.

A careful foot examination is an important component of a complete neurological evaluation. Particular attention should be paid to the presence of findings listed in Table 16-2. The much-dreaded foot complications of diabetes often result from multiple abnormalities, and an examination for the presence of any or all of these can help gauge the etiology of the patient's current difficulties, and/or the risk for future problems.

Electromyogram and Nerve Conduction Studies

The electrodiagnostic examination is also used to confirm a clinical diagnosis, quantify the pathophysiologic process, and provide a measure of disease progression or response to therapeutic intervention. In addition, patients who present with atypical features such as prominent motor abnormalities, upper extremity greater than lower extremity involvement, predominantly large fiber sensory findings, or asymmetry on examination should also have an electrodiagnostic examination performed.

The amplitude of the evoked sensory and motor action potential of the standard nerve-conduction studies provides an index of the number of

**TABLE 16-2. Focused Evaluation of the Patient With Diabetic
            Neuropathy**

- **Characterize and quantify the neuropathy,** providing baseline measurements against which progression or improvement can be compared
- **Exclude other potential causes** of the neuropathy
- **Assess the relevant components** of diabetes control as they relate to the neuropathy, including:
  - duration of diabetes
  - quality of diabetes control
  - presence of other microvascular or macrovascular complications
- **Focused physical examination**
  - *Motor examination*
    - weakness
    - wasting
    - fasciculations
    - atrophy of foot intrinsic muscles
    - deep tendon reflexes
  - *Sensory examination*
    - small fiber
      - pin sensation
      - temperature sensation
    - Large fiber
      - vibration sensation
      - position sense
  - *Autonomic evaluation*
    - supine and standing blood pressure and heart rate
    - pupillary response to ling
    - sweating patterns
  - *Foot examination*
    - presence of calluses or blisters
    - skin color
    - presence of infection
    - status of intrinsic musculature, noting presence of any atrophy
    - deformities
    - loss of sweating
    - temperature
    - pedal pulses and overall vascular status
    - loss of joint mobility

functioning axons in the large myelinated nerves and the number of muscle fibers innervated. These parameters correlate well with clinical deficits. The distal latency and conduction velocity depend on fiber size, myelination, and internodal length. They do not correlate as well with symptoms or neurologic deficits.

Needle electromyography (EMG) assesses electrical activity generated by muscle fibers at rest and with activity. Early EMG abnormalities seen with axonal neuropathic processes include the appearance of fibrillations and positive sharp-waves, followed by abnormalities of the motor unit potential such as prolonged duration, polyphasia, and increased amplitude.

The nerve conduction velocity may be decreased slightly at the time that the diabetes is diagnosed and usually declines progressively with increased disease duration. Nerve conduction velocity may show a slight improvement with the institution of therapy to control glucose and declines with the withdrawal of such therapy, suggesting a reversible metabolic component.

The electrodiagnosis of diabetic proximal motor neuropathy rests on needle EMG more than on nerve conduction studies. The EMG usually reveals fibrillation potentials in proximal lower extremity muscles, particularly the quadriceps, iliopsoas, adductor, and gracilis muscles. There are usually fibrillation potentials in paraspinal muscles extending through multiple spinal levels. Abnormalities of motor unit potentials are typically mild.

Electrodiagnostic examination is of particular help in separating pain caused by thoracic, abdominal, or pelvic disease from pain caused by diabetic truncal neuropathies or radiculopathies, in which sensory findings on the trunk may be subtle or absent. Patients with diabetic thoracoabdominal neuropathies of radiculopathies will demonstrate fibrillations at multiple segmental levels in paraspinal muscles, rectus abdominus, and the external oblique muscles.

Quantitative Sensory Testing

Information derived from the sensory examination is inherently subjective. In order to provide a more precise and reproducible examination, quantitative sensory testing has attained widespread use in both the clinical evaluation of patients with neuropathy and also to measure the response to therapy in pharmacologic trials. A standardized, quantifiable sensory stimulus is delivered to the patient so that precise thresholds for sensory perception can be established in order to accurately determine the presence and extent of a sensory deficit. Standardized algorithms are used for both the stimulus delivery and the expected response. The sensory perception threshold is compared to an age-based database of normative values. Nevertheless, the measurements remain subjective and are dependent on the attention and motivation of the patient. The instruments available for quantitative sensory testing provide warm, cold and vibratory stimuli.

Autonomic Function Testing

The laboratory evaluation of autonomic function in patients with diabetes involves the assessment of both sympathetic and parasympathetic nervous system function. The complete assessment includes the evaluation of cardiac vagal function, sympathetic adrenergic function and sympathetic cholinergic function.

Cardiac Vagal Function

The laboratory evaluation of the cardiac vagal function includes the assessment of measures of heart rate variation in response to deep respiration, following a Valsalva maneuver and in response to postural change. Heart rate variability with deep respiration, the respiratory sinus arrhythmia, is regarded as the most sensitive and specific of the measures of autonomic function. Measures of respiratory sinus arrhythmia include the peak to trough amplitude, the standard deviation, the mean square successive difference, the expiratory-inspiratory ratio (E:I ratio), and the mean circular resultant.

The autonomic response to a Valsalva maneuver is complex and provides a measure of sympathetic, vagal and baroreceptor function. The maneuver is typically performed by blowing for 15 or 20 seconds through a mouthpiece that is connected to a mercury manometer. The mercury column of the manometer is maintained at 40 mmHg. The Valsalva ratio, derived from the ratio between the tachycardia during the maneuver and the post-maneuver bradycardia, provides an index of cardiac vagal function.

Analysis of the heart rate response to postural change also provides a measure of sympathetic nervous system, parasympathetic nervous system and baroreceptor function. Active standing results in an increase in heart rate that peaks at approximately 12 to 15 seconds after standing. The heart rate and blood pressure return to a new baseline after approximately 30 seconds. The "30:15 ratio" assesses this physiologic response by measuring the ratio of the heart rate increase that occurs at approximately 15 seconds after standing to the relative bradycardia that occurs at approximately the 30 seconds after standing. This ratio provides a measure of cardiac vagal function.

Evaluation of Sympathetic Adrenergic Function

The most frequently performed test of sympathetic nervous system function is the blood pressure response to postural change (active standing or passive tilting). When severe autonomic dysfunction is present, blood pressure abnormalities are apparent after 5 to 10 minutes of head up-tilt or active standing. Early or mild adrenergic failure may require a longer period of standing or duration of tilt.

The blood pressure and heart rate changes induced by a sustained handgrip have been used as a clinical test of sympathetic adrenergic function. The response to this test is subject to marked variability due in part to difficulty standardizing muscular effort. The test has limited sensitivity and specificity.

A direct measure of the hemodynamic response to the Valsalva maneuver can be made with a noninvasive beat-to-beat blood pressure monitor. There is a fall in blood pressure during phase II and an increase in blood pressure during phase IV of the Valsalva maneuver. The measurement of these blood pressure changes during phase II and phase IV of the Valsalva maneuver provide a measure of vasomotor adrenergic function.

Tests of Sympathetic Cholinergic Function

The cholinergic sympathetic system is assessed by measuring eccrine sweat glands function. Several methods may be used to test sudomotor function. Thermoregulatory sweating can be tested by raising the body temperature with an external heating source. This test evaluates the distribution of sweating by measuring the change in color of an indicator powder such as iodine with starch, quinizarin or alizarin-red in response to a rise in core body temperature. The quantitative sudomotor axon reflex test (QSART) provides a quantitative measure of post-ganglionic sudomotor function. The sudomotor response measured by the QSART is mediated by an axon reflex that is elicited by iontophoresis of a cholinergic agonist. A similar method involves the formation of a sweat imprint, formed by the secretion of active sweat glands into a plastic or silicone mold, in response to iontophoresis of a cholinergic agonist. A further method involves the assessment of electrodermal activity that is generated by the sweat glands and overlying epidermis. This response, which occurs spontaneously and can be evoked by stimuli such as respiration, cough, loud sounds, startle, mental stress and electrical stimuli, is referred to as the sympathetic skin response or the peripheral autonomic surface potential. The sympathetic skin response can be measured with surface electrodes connected to a standard EMG instrument.

Treatment of Peripheral Neuropathy

Hyperglycemia

Management of diabetic neuropathy, whether painful or painless, begins with treatment of hyperglycemia. The Diabetes Control and Complications Trial (DCCT) conclusively demonstrated the important benefits of intensive control of hyperglycemia in people with type 1 diabetes. Intensive, physiologically-based therapy administered either with an external insulin pump or by three or more daily insulin injections delayed or prevented the appearance of clinically evident diabetic polyneuropathy in patients with type 1. Intensive therapy reduced the development of clinical neuropathy conformed with neurophysiologic investigations by 64% after 5 years of follow-up. Nerve conduction velocities generally remained stable with intensive therapy but decreased significantly with conventional therapy. Smaller trials of a similar nature have confirmed these findings in those with type 2 diabetes.

Autonomic Dysfunction

Orthostatic Hypotension

The removal of potential reversible causes of orthostatic hypotension is the first and most important management step. Medications such as diuretics, antihypertensive agents, anti-anginal agents, and antidepressants are the most common offending agents. Numerous agents from diverse pharmacological groups have been implemented in the treatment of orthostatic hypotension. 9-a-fluorohydrocortisone (fludrocortisone acetate), a synthetic mineralocorticoid, is the medication of first choice for most patients with orthostatic hypotension. Treatment is initiated with a 0.1-mg tablet and can be increased to 0.2–0.5 mg daily. Treatment may unfortunately be limited by supine hypertension so lower doses of this medication are preferable. Other side effects include ankle edema, hypokalemia and, rarely, congestive heart failure. Potassium supplementation is usually required, particularly when higher doses are used.

A sympathomimetic agent can be added to fludrocortisone acetate should the patient remain symptomatic. The peripherally-acting selective a-agonist midodrine, which recently is approved by the FDA to treat orthostatic hypotension, is the most widely used of these pressors. Patient sensitivity to this agent varies and the dose should be titrated from 2.5 mg to 10 mg three times a day. Potential side effects of this agent include pilomotor reactions, pruritus, supine hypertension, gastrointestinal complaints, and urinary retention. Other sympathomimetic agents used include, ephedrine and pseudoephedrine

Gastroparesis Diabeticorum

Frequent small meals and pharmacotherapy are standard treatments for gastroparesis diabeticorum. The dopamine agonist, metoclopramide, continues to be the first line of therapy for this gastroparesis. Given in doses ranging from 5 to 20 mg orally, 30 minutes before meals and at bedtime, metoclopramide accelerates gastric emptying and has a central antiemetic action. It also may release acetylcholine from intramural cholinergic neurons or directly stimulate antral muscle. Erythromycin and related macrolide compounds may have motilin agonist properties. Intravenous and oral erythromycin (250 mg three times a day) improve gastric-emptying time in diabetes patients with gastroparesis and are frequently used to treat this disorder. Gastric antisecretory agents such as the H2 antagonists and proton-pump inhibitors may be used as supplementary agents to treat the symptoms of gastroesophogeal reflux. The majority of patients can be treated with these medical interventions and jejunostomy tube placement is rarely necessary. Severe cases with intractable vomiting may benefit from nasogastric suctioning.

Erectile Dysfunction

Medications influencing autonomic function such as psychotropic and antihypertensive agents should be discontinued. Oral therapy with the selective phospodiesterase 5 inhibitors, is now the first-line therapy for male erectile dysfunction. Unfortunately, some men with diabetes do not respond satisfactorily to this intervention. Furthermore, the medication is contraindicated in patients treated with nitrates and agents that compete with or inhibit the cytochrome P-450 system. Angina, hypertension requiring treatment with multiple medications and congestive heart failure are also contraindications. Other therapies include the injection of vasoactive substances such as papaverine, phentolamine, and prostaglandin E1 into the corpus cavernosum, transurethral delivery of vasoactive agents, and the use of mechanical devices such as the vacuum erection device or constricting rings. Penile prosthetic implants may be used if these therapies fail or are not tolerated by the patient. A more detailed discussion of erectile dysfunction and gender-related issues can be found in Chapter 19.

Painful Neuropathy

Pain is one of the more distressing and difficult to manage symptoms of diabetic neuropathy and occurs in both focal neuropathy and symmetric polyneuropathy. In polyneuropathy, the incidence, severity, and duration of pain are quite variable, whereas in focal mononeuropathy and radiculopathy, pain is usually more severe but temporary. The pathophysiologic basis for the pain of diabetic neuropathy has not been established. Several investigators have attempted to define the structural basis of painful diabetic polyneuropathy. Morphologic abnormalities that have been associated with neuropathic pain include axonal sprouting, acute axonal degeneration, active degeneration of myelinated fibers, and disproportionate loss of large caliber nerve fibers. Recent controlled studies, however, have failed to support these associations.

Treatment of pain requires attempts at strict control of blood glucose levels, as there is evidence that hyperglycemia may reduce the pain threshold. Should this intervention fail, a variety of agents from diverse pharmacologic classes, the so-called adjuvant analgesics, have been used to treat neuropathic pain. The antidepressants and anticonvulsants are the agents used as first-line therapy for the treatment of neuropathic pain.

TABLE 16-3. Medications for Use in Pharmacotherapy of Neuropathic Pain

Agent	Initial dose	Dose increment	Effective dose
Duloxetine	20–60 mg qd	20–30 mg q 1–3 d	120 mg qd (or 60 mg bd)
Pregabalin	50–150 mg qd	25–50 mg q 3 d	50–200 mg tid or 75–300 mg bid
Gabapentin	100–300 mg qd	100–300 q 3–5 d	300–1800 mg tid
Tricyclic antidepressants	10–25 mg qd	10–25 mg/week	25–150 mg
Tramadol	50 mg qd	50 mg qd	50–100 mg qid
Venlafaxine	37.5 mg qd	37.5 q 3–5 d	75–150 mg bid
Carbamazepine	100–200 mg bid	100–200 mg q 2d	200–400 mg tid
Lamotrigine	25 mg qd	25–50 mg q week	200–400 mg bid
Topiramate	50 mg qd	50 mg qd	200 mg bid
Topical lidocaine	Up to 3 patches for 12 of 24 hours		Up to 3 patches for 12 of 24 hours
Capsaicin	0.075% qid		0.075% qid
Mexilitine	150 mg	150 mg qd	150–300 mg tid

Tricyclic and Other Antidepressants

The tertiary amine, amytriptyline, is the best studied of these agents and has been shown in several randomized, blinded clinical trials to significantly improve neuropathic pain.

The side-effect profile that includes include drowsiness, confusion, constipation, dry mouth, weight gain, orthostatic hypotension and cardiovascular morbidity and mortality limits the use of this agent, particularly in the elderly. The secondary amines, nortriptyline and desipramine, have a less troublesome side-effect profile. A meta-analysis of antidepressant use in randomized placebo-controlled trials revealed that tricyclic agents provided at least a 50% reduction in pain intensity in 30% of individuals with neuropathic pain. Because of possible cardiotoxicity, tricyclic antidepressants should be used with caution in patients with known or suspected cardiac disease. The selective norepinephrine and serotonin reuptake inhibitors duloxetine and venlafaxine have proven efficacy in of neuropathic pain. These agents inhibit reuptake of serotonin and norepinephrine without the muscarinic, histaminic and adrenergic side-effects that accompany the use of the tricyclic agents. Duloxetine, a secondary amine, is a balanced norepinephrine and serotonin reuptake inhibitor. This agent is FDA approved for the treatment of neuropathic pain in diabetes. In doses of 60 and 120 mg/day duloxetine showed efficacy in the treatment of neuropathic pain due to diabetic peripheral neuropathy.

Anticonvulsants

Anticonvulsants from several classes have been used to treat painful diabetic neuropathy. The α_2-δ ligands, gabapentin and pregabalin, have shown efficacy in a number of clinical trials of the treatment of neuropathic pain associated with diabetic peripheral neuropathy. Both agents do not bind to plasma proteins. There is no hepatic metabolism and these agents do not compete for or inhibit the cytochrome P-450 system. There are few clinically important drug-drug interactions. Both agents are excreted unchanged by kidneys. The clearance of pregabalin and gabapentin is reduced in patients with impaired creatinine clearance and dose adjustment is required.

There are potential clinically important differences between these agents. Pregabalin, in contrast to gabapentin, has linear and dose proportional absorption in the therapeutic dose range (150–600 mg/day) due to a non-saturable transport mechanism. In addition, there is an effective starting dose, a more rapid onset of action and well defined dosage range that requires minimal titration (gabapentin requires gradual titration to the clinically effective dose of 1800–3600 mg). Pregabalin may also be effective in a twice daily dose. Side effects of these agents includes dizziness, somnolence, peripheral edema, headache and dry mouth.

The mechanism of the analgesic action of these agents is not fully elucidated. A proposed mechanism of action, based on the observation that these agents bind to the α_2-δ subunit of the voltage-dependent calcium channel, is that they modulates neurotransmission in the central nervous system.

Anti-Arrhythmics

The class 1b antiarrhythmic agent, mexiletine, a sodium channel blocker, has been studied in the treatment of DPN. The rational for sodium channel blockers in the treatment of DPN is that they inhibit neuron depolarization and thereby impair spontaneous firing of regenerating fibers that have a low threshold for depolarization. The results with this anesthetic anti-arrhythmic that is structurally similar to lidocaine have been inconsistent and this agent is rarely used to treat neuropathic pain. Side effects of this agent were frequent and include gastrointestinal disturbance, headache, dizziness, and tremor. Use of this agent is contraindicated in patients with second-and third-degree heart block. It may worsen cardiac arrhythmias.

Topical Agents

The use of topical agents to treat DPN offers several theoretical advantages. There are minimal systemic side effects, no drug interactions, and usually no need for drug titration. Also, the pharmacotherapeutic effect is applied directly to site of pain generation, although chronic neuropathic pain usually results in changes at more proximal sites in the peripheral and central nervous system. Capsaicin, an extract of chili peppers, is the most widely used of these agents and is available in cream form. This TRPV1 receptor agonist initially activates and then depletes substance P from the terminals of unmyelinated C fibers. The results of treatment trials using this agent have been inconsistent. Side effects include cutaneous burning, erythema, and sneezing. Topical lidocaine may be effective in the treatment of diabetic neuropathic pain. In post-herpetic neuralgia, this agent is most effective in patients with allodynia. Adverse effects include mild skin reactions such as erythema and edema. Systemic absorption is minimal provided the patches are not placed over broken or inflamed skin.

Typical and Atypical Opioids

There is evidence that the "atypical -opioid" analgesic tramadol may be effective in the treatment of painful diabetic peripheral neuropathy. This agent which is a mixed opioid agonist, exhibits low-affinity binding to the μ opiate receptor. It is biochemically distinct from other opioids in that analgesia is only partially antagonized by naloxone. Tramadol inhibits reuptake of norepinephrine and serotonin. Side effects of this medication include dizziness, nausea, constipation, and drowsiness. This agent has a low potential for abuse but should be avoided in opiate-dependent patients and patients with a tendency to abuse drugs. Several randomized controlled trials have shown opioids such as CR-oxycodone, controlled release morphine, and levorphanol can effectively treat neuropathic pain due to diabetic peripheral neuropathy. Opioids may also have a dose sparing effect; gabapentin and SR morphine combined achieved better analgesia at lower doses of each drug than either as a single agent, with constipation, sedation, and dry mouth as the most frequent adverse effects. Adverse effects of opioids include constipation, nausea, dizziness, drowsiness, cognitive difficulties and dry mouth. The long-term use of opioids in the treatment of neuropathic pain remains controversial. These agents should be used cautiously and monitored closely, particularly in patients with a history of substance abuse.

Conclusion

Neuropathies can be significant contributors to the morbidity and mortality associated with diabetes, as well as severely impact quality of life for diabetes patients. To further the challenge for the practitioner, the clinical presentations of neuropathies can be widely variable, often mimicking other conditions. Similarly, and because of the diagnostic confusion that often occurs, many frustrated clinicians, when confronted with a person with diabetes who has confusing symptoms or signs, are often tempted to ascribe the finding to the diabetes without adequate evaluation. The risk, and the clinical challenge, is that people with diabetes *can* develop other conditions, many totally unrelated to diabetes. To ascribe confusing or atypical clinical findings to diabetes can be a disservice to the patient, or even a serious medical mistake.

Therefore, it is important that each symptom be carefully evaluated to the extent warranted by the clinical circumstance. Often, when life-threatening conditions are ruled out, but no diagnostic conclusion is reached, symptomatic treatments and optimizing glucose control is all that can be offered initially. However, with time, the condition may either resolve or manifest its true nature. Clearly, as much as with any aspect of the care of people with diabetes, the clinical approach to neuropathies — or symptoms and signs suggestive of neuropathies — requires skills of the art, as much as the science, of medical practice.

17

The Foot: Clinical Care and Problem Prevention

*Richard S. Beaser, MD and
John M. Giurini, DPM*

The stereotypic image of a person with diabetes who suffers from its complications usually includes amputation of a lower extremity. In fact, more than half of the nontraumatic amputations performed in the United States are performed on people with diabetes. Here are some additional statistics:

- 15% of persons with diabetes will develop foot ulcers
- 50% of the patients with foot ulcers will have recurrence within 2 years
- 20% of patients with foot ulcers will undergo amputation
- 50% of amputations are preventable
- About 8% of diabetes admissions are for foot problems, which contribute to $1.8 billion dollars in direct medical care costs.

Risk Factors for Foot Wounds

It has been said that the foot is often the "Achilles' heel" for those with diabetes. Factors that contribute to the vulnerability of the foot of someone with diabetes include:

505

- peripheral neuropathy due to excessive hyperglycemia
- peripheral vascular disease, a result of both the aging process and the impact of diabetes (both its duration and the degree of metabolic abnormalities such as hyperglycemia and dyslipidemia)
- decreased ability to fight infection due to the hyperglycemic effect on leukocyte function
- altered biomechanics or foot integrity due to previous injury or infection which has altered foot shape, health of foot skin, or walking dynamics

The *peripheral neuropathy* affecting the foot, described in more detail in Chapter 16, is characterized by a number of features:

- Patients experience destruction of motor, autonomic, and sensory nerve fibers.
- Destruction is slowly progressive, promoted by sustained hyperglycemia.
- Patients may report symptoms of paresthesia (often described as "shooting pains" or "pins and needles sensation"), dysesthesia (often described as pain resulting from contact of the foot by items such as bed linen or hose) or a decreased temperature sensation.
- Symptoms can vary from mild to severe.
- In those patients with poorly controlled diabetes with predominant hyperglycemia, improvement of control may lead to a period of worsened symptoms. However, eventually, improved control should lead to diminution of the discomfort.
- Peripheral neuropathy can lead to anesthesia (loss of sensation all together) resulting from nerve destruction. Loss of sensation prevents the brain from directing the body to avoid continued pressure on inflamed areas, resulting in tissue breakdown, ulcer formation ("neuropathic" ulcers) and, if untreated, limb-threatening infections or development of Charqot foot deformities.
- The patient with peripheral neuropathy is at increased risk for injury, falls and further debilitation.

The *peripheral vascular disease* that affects the foot is characterized by a number of features:

- Diabetes increases the risk for developing peripheral vascular disease.

- Compromised circulation and oxygenation to the lower extremities, as well as decreased ability of white cells to get to the site of infection, increases the risk of lower extremity infections and poor wound healing.
- Smoking is a factor that contributes to peripheral vascular disease.
- It is peripheral vascular disease rather than just microangiopathy that is felt to be needed to result in significant increase in risk for infection.
- Early symptoms of peripheral vascular disease include feet that are cold to the touch, dependent rubor, and intermittent claudication. In many instances the pedal pulse will be faint or absent on palpation.
- Untreated cuts or abrasions can lead to limb threatening infections.

The degree and mechanism of the decrease in the ability to fight infection in people with diabetes is poorly defined and controversial. For years, it has been said that people with diabetes cannot fight off infection as well as those who do not have diabetes. However, studies looking at specific cellular action and function have found little specific evidence pointing to a mechanism. There is some evidence that people with diabetes in extremely poor control have decreased polymorphonuclear leukocyte (PMN) chemotaxis, decreased PMN adherence, decreased PMN bactericidal activity, and, for patients in ketoacidosis, decreased phagocytotic ability. Monocytes in people with diabetes have also demonstrated reduced phagocytosis. However, most of these studies were conducted in the setting of very poor glucose control. Although no one would argue that such deterioration of diabetes control should be avoided, mild hyperglycemia, in typical clinical settings, rarely seems to produce discernable deterioration in immune response. Probably a more significant factor is vascular disease which prevents adequate blood flow from reaching the affected area.

The *altered biomechanics or foot integrity* affecting the foot can be caused by:

- corns
- calluses
- bone deformities, fractures
- altered joint mobility
- nail pathology (thickening, loss)

- breaks in the skin (e.g., wounds or athlete's foot)
- poorly fitting shoes

In this setting, any precipitating infection or mechanical impediment may create a portal of entry for infection. Infection precipitates inflammation and edema, leading to increased demands for blood flow, which may not be available. Thus, the infection is allowed to increase. This vicious cycle allows the infection to spread, aided by inadequate circulation. Add to this scenario diminished pain sensation due to neuropathy; since the patient cannot rely on painful sensation as a warning of danger, he or she continues to walk on the injured foot. Further compounding the problem is difficulty seeing the foot due to decreased vision or a rotund abdomen, preventing proper inspection of the lower extremity.

The Foot Examination

The primary care provider is in a position to identify early signs of foot problems. Therefore, the foot examination must be a regular part of the care of people with diabetes.

A thorough foot examination should occur no less frequently than once a year. However, more frequent opportunities to look at the feet not only will identify problems at an earlier stage, but will emphasize to the patient the importance of regular foot inspection. In particular, people with high risk characteristics such as those identified above should have their feet examined more frequently, usually with every visit to the healthcare professional.

The ADA recommends that a foot examination of the low-risk foot of a person with diabetes should include the following:

- Neuropathy screening using a quantitative somatosensory threshold test: the Semmes-Weinstein monofilament and vibratory testing using a tuning fork.
- Peripheral vascular screening:
  - history, seeking symptoms of claudication
  - examination of pulses
  - examination of the skin integrity (between toes and under metatarsal heads) looking for erythema, warmth, or callus formation.

- Examination for structural abnormalities, including:
  - bony deformities
  - limited joint mobility
  - problems with gait or balance
  - interruption in skin integrity
  - significant foot deformity suggestive of Charcot joint disease

Charcot Joint Disease

Charcot joint disease was described in 1868 by the French neurologist J. M. Charcot. It occurs in anyone who has a condition affecting the posterior column of the spinal cord, including diabetes, but also seen with conditions such as alcoholism, spina bifida, cerebral palsy, myelodysplasia, poliomyelitis, and syphilis. The actual pathophysiology is probably multifactoral. Theories suggest that these factors include the spinal cord lesion noted above, as well as repeated trauma to neuropathic, and thus insensitive, joints. A vascular component has also been suggested.

Charcot disease is most often seen in one of three locations:

- the forefoot, phalanges, and metatarsalphalangeal joints
- the midfoot or arch
- the rear foot, ankle, and heel

Patients usually present with a unilateral swelling of the foot, without necessarily having an ulcer or obvious deformity. The foot is often warm to the touch. Manipulation of the foot may elicit crepitus. Classic deformities may be seen, such as the "rocker-bottom" foot, a foot that has lost its arch, and instead is convex and resembles a rocker. This and other deformities will show up as characteristic bony destruction and fractures on x-ray. When ulceration is also present, there may be some concern due to resemblance between these Charcot changes and osteomyelitis. Bone biopsy should be avoided so as to prevent introduction of infection into the area — an MRI may be preferable.

The focus of treatment is to keep the patient off the foot. Non-weight bearing allows fractures to heal. This usually takes 8 to 12 weeks, and progress is followed radiographically. Non-weight-bearing casts may be used to stabilize the foot. Surgical intervention to alleviate bony pressure points may be needed. Amputations may occur if the foot becomes infected or if the ankle becomes so destroyed that it is frail and cannot be reconstructed. Once healed, these feet still must be cared for meticulously, avoiding excessive trauma. The healing process usually involves joint fusion, limiting foot function. Special shoes are often required. Exercise involving the feet should be avoided. In addition, the other foot should be watched and protected; there is a 30% to 40% chance that Charcot changes will develop on that other foot as well.

Preventive Strategies for the High-Risk Patient

Patients with high-risk characteristics need preventive care specific to the abnormalities noted. Often, many of these are best initiated by podiatric physicians, particularly those experienced in working with people who have diabetes. Such condition-specific preventive strategies might include:

- For *neuropathy* — Well-cushioned shoes or athletic shoes to reduce plantar pressure. Footware such as this will cushion and redistribute impact so as to avoid development of neuropathic ulceration at points of excessive, repeated pressure. Soft orthotic devices may be helpful in adding to cushioning, providing proper support, and properly distributing pressure more evenly throughout the foot. Rigid orthotic devices should be avoided.
- For *sensory neuropathies* — Socks should be worn that serve to absorb moisture and keep it away from the skin. The use of cotton and wool socks has been a traditional recommendation; however, socks made from some of the newer synthetic materials may serve as well or better. Socks with added padding can be helpful in distribution and softening of pressures. Changing socks frequently is also recommended to avoid dampness. Patients with a Charcot deformity are often told to wear a thin sock under a thicker sock to provide an interface for friction between the two socks, reducing the chances of blistering. (In the past, it was recommended to wear white socks only so that cleanliness can be more easily determined and foot drainage can be more easily detected. However, today's colored socks are

usually acceptable if they meet the criteria outlined above. White socks are still preferable if there is any defect in skin integrity.)

- For *calluses* — Careful debridement only by professionals skilled in such treatments.
- For *bony deformities (e.g., bunions, hammertoes)* — Special, extra-wide, or extra-depth shoes. These often must be custom made. Occasionally custom-molded shoes are needed.
- For *peripheral vascular disease* — Evaluation by a vascular specialist.
- For *foot ulcers, history of or present manifestation* — Evaluation of causes, including bony abnormalities, neuropathies, interruption of skin integrity, infections. Often, podiatric evaluation for special shoeing or use of a shoe-insert device may be warranted. More extensive or chronic ulcers may warrant more extensive treatment such as off-loading dressings or even surgical intervention, and surgical professionals skilled in this type of treatment should be consulted.

Patient Education and Self-Care

The person with diabetes really represents the first line of defense against foot problems. When properly educated and using proper self-care techniques, many foot problems can be avoided. Of course, achieving the best possible metabolic control should be paramount for all patients!

Primary care providers should assess the patient's current level of knowledge and self-care. Many people erroneously assume that if they have good circulation and no neuropathic defects, they do not have to worry about foot care. While it might be true that a patient with intact sensation and good circulation, need not be quite as fastidious about checking his or her feet daily as those with neuropathy or vascular insufficiency must be, still, vascular and neuropathic changes are insidious, so patients may be lulled into a false sense of security and only realize their folly after they have developed problems. Therefore, while a patient might be pleased to learn that his or her feet seem normal at present, all patients should develop the mindset that they are not, and adopt levels of vigilance accordingly. *All* patients should know the guidelines to follow so they are prepared in the event they do develop problems.

The ***educational goals*** for people with diabetes to prevent problems and/or detect them early include:

- demonstration of foot care inspection
- understanding of basic hygiene guidelines
- identification and treatment of minor problems
- awareness for when to contact the doctor or other healthcare provider for treatment

This last item is crucial. It is unfortunately an all-to-common scenario that a patient will develop a small ulcer and not realize the seriousness of the injury or try to self-treat for too long. The presence of any ulcer is serious, particularly in the setting of a neuropathic foot, and self-treatment can worsen the condition and delay necessary intervention.

Foot Inspection

The importance of daily foot inspection cannot be overemphasized; foot problems can literally develop overnight. Discuss the importance of daily foot inspection with the patient and/or family member. Demonstrate how to check the feet. Have the patient remove his socks and shoes and, using his own foot show the patient where and how to look at his foot. Guide him in getting to know what his feet and toenails usually look like so that he can figure out when something is wrong.

A mirror is a useful foot inspection tool, particularly for patients with limited mobility. Some patients may need assistance with this daily inspection from a family member or friend.

Patients should be instructed to check their feet daily for the following:

- cuts, blisters or sores
- change in temperature (hot or cold)
- change in color (pale, red, blue)
- swelling
- pain
- dry cracking skin
- sweaty skin
- athletes foot or other rashes

- signs and symptoms of infection
- corns and calluses

Patients should be instructed to **check their toe nails daily** for:

- ingrown toe nails
- chipping, splitting
- loss of feeling of adjacent skin

Guidelines for Washing Feet

Washing the feet is important but must be done properly. A few simple precautions can prevent serious injuries. Therefore, careful instruction in bathing techniques should be part of the foot education program. Actual demonstration of these principles during the instruction will further enhance the learning process. Proper attention to protecting the integrity of the skin will help reduce the risk of infection.

Listed below are recommended patient guidelines for washing the feet:

- Wash feet gently every day with soap and warm water. Always check the temperature of the water with the elbow before putting the feet in the water. *Decreased sensation in the feet can make it difficult to estimate the water temperature and may result in serious burns.*
- Do not soak feet. Soaking only promotes softening of the tissue and makes it more susceptible to breaks and tears.
- Do not scrub or use abrasive cloths or loofas.
- Use a soft towel to gently dry feet. Take time to carefully dry between toes. *Moisture between the toes can provide a friendly environment for bacteria and fungus to grow.*
- Use lotion daily if feet and legs are dry. Avoid applying lotion between toes as this adds to excess and unwanted moisture and may promote skin breakdown.
- For optimal results, apply small amounts of lotion after bathing while the skin is still moist. Lotion may also be applied at bedtime followed by the patient putting on clean, dry socks to promote absorption of the lotion.
- Lotions that do not contain alcohol or perfume are preferred. Examples of some preferred lotions include: Eucerin, Lubriderm, or

Vaseline Intensive Care. For specific skin problems, patients should ask their physician or podiatrist or other healthcare provider about recommended lotions.

- If feet tend to sweat, apply small amounts of talcum powder to hands and pat on feet. Avoid putting powder in shoes or between your toes as they may cake and cause friction.

Nail Care

It is also important that patients take proper care of their nails. This includes the proper way to trim toenails and care for minor problems. Generally, it is safe for patients to file their nails, especially after they have bathed. The nail is softer and easier to file.

Patients should be assessed for their ability to treat minor problems and trim toenails. In some cases a physician, podiatric physician or other member of the healthcare team should provide treatment. For persons with poor vision, circulation, or neuropathy, a podiatric physician may be needed to perform routine nail care and to treat minor problems such as corns and calluses. In addition, those patients with thick, difficult-to-cut nails or nails with fungus need the expertise of a podiatric physician.

Listed below are recommended patient guidelines for nail care:

- File toenails after a bath or shower. The nail will be softer and easier to work with.
- File toenails straight across taking care not to file shorter than the ends of the toes.
- Shape the toenails according to the contour of the toes and the toes next to them.
- Do not use a razor blade or knife to trim nails.
- Do not use "over-the-counter" treatments for tough toe nails
- A podiatric physician or trained physician should trim nails on a regular basis:
  - when the nails are extremely thick and difficult to cut
  - if the person has vascular insufficiency or neuropathy
  - if the person has retinopathy or other conditions causing decreased visual acuity

  - if the person has a history of ulcers or infections, structural deformities or nail abnormalities
  - if the person has difficulty reaching her feet

Callus, Corn and Wart Care

Untreated or mistreated corns, calluses, or warts can lead to possible infection. These conditions can act like foreign bodies, stuck to the foot. Their pressure can cause bleeding in the tissue beneath them, providing a nidus for infection. Too often patients will perform "bathroom surgery" using razor blades, sharp objects, and harsh over-the-counter medications to treat corns and calluses. These methods can exacerbate existing problems and create new, often more serious, conditions.

Listed below are recommended patient guidelines for treating calluses, corns, and warts:

- Do not use "over-the-counter" medications to care for calluses, corns, or warts. These medications may contain acids that can damage the skin. When such products are used improperly or on persons with decreased feeling in the feet, they can cause serious injury and/or burns.
- Never attempt to trim calluses, corns, or warts. Use a fine emery board or pumice stone to gently rub down calluses after bathing.
- Consult with a podiatric physician to receive individualized recommendations and treatment for calluses, corns and/or warts.

Treatment of Minor Foot Infections and Abrasions

Prompt treatment and monitoring of skin and foot problems can prevent severe infection and loss of limb. While patients must know what they can treat, and when they should seek professional help, certain guidelines are useful for patients in their approach to caring for any foot wound:

- Stay off feet as much as possible.
- Clean wound with soap and warm water or normal saline twice a day or as otherwise directed.

- Keep feet dry and apply a wet to moist dressing with antibiotic ointments such as Bacitracin, Polysporin, and Neosporin.
- Apply normal saline or a hydragell dressing directly on the wound and cover with sterile gauze. Do not use a plastic bandage as this does not allow enough air exchange.
- Change the dressing at least twice a day or as otherwise directed. Check the wound for healing, drainage or other signs and symptoms of infection.
- Use paper tape. Avoid adhesive tape, as this can tear surrounding skin when tape is removed.
- Monitor blood glucose levels and report elevations to the healthcare team.

Patients should be advised to call their physician, podiatric physician or other healthcare provider if:

1. a wound has not improved in a designated period of time. Call if there is no improvement in two days if no specific time interval is indicated
2. drainage is noted
3. the area around the injury becomes red or very warm or if there are any questions

Other, general indications for patients to contact the physician, podiatric physician or other member of the healthcare team:

- Routine foot care such as toenail trimming
- Treatment for warts, corns, or calluses
- For any of the following conditions:
  - cuts (break in skin) that has not healed in 2 days
  - blisters or sores
  - infection
  - change in temperature of the skin or tissue
  - swelling
  - pain
  - changes in skin color

Athlete's Foot

Athlete's foot (dermatophytosis) is a common fungus infection of the feet and is not limited to athletes. It may remain scaly, dry, and unnoticed or can break out as an inflamed area with broken skin, often between the toes. Feet that perspire heavily are more susceptible. The fungus can be acquired in locker rooms or from bathroom floors.

For people with diabetes, athlete's foot represents a potentially serious condition, as it can create a portal of entry for further infection. The treatment of athlete's foot includes the following measures:

- Treat both the skin area involved and the insides of shoes. Wet footwear can be a source of reinfection.
- Use antifungal ointment (e.g., Lotrimin and Tinactin) on the affected skin for an extended period of time. Antifungal powder can be used in shoes as a general preventative at least twice a week after the acute infection has ended.
- Wear clogs or thongs in the bathroom or shower rather than walking barefoot, especially in gyms and health clubs.
- Keep feet dry with regular powder, especially when feet are likely to perspire profusely.

Instructions for Selecting Footwear

Improper fitting shoes and hosiery can contribute to foot problems. Shoes that are too tight may cause corns and calluses, while tight fitting hose can restrict blood flow and circulation to the feet. The following guidelines should be given to patients regarding shoeing and shoe selection:

- Patients should be instructed NOT TO GO BAREFOOT and to:
  - wear closed toe footwear at all times to prevent injury;
  - keep slippers at the bedside to wear when getting up at night;
  - wear protective shoes when at the beach and swimming. Sand can burn and shells and other beach debris can cut the feet.
- Purchase new shoes toward the end of the day. The foot size tends to be larger later in the day due to swelling. Try on shoes with socks of

similar thickness to those which will be routinely worn with the shoes. Tie shoes are preferable to loafers. Crepe or vibram are preferred over leather.

- Break new shoes in gradually. Start by wearing them one hour at a time each day until the shoes are broken in.
- Purchase leather or breathable material shoes. These materials allow moisture to evaporate and absorb perspiration. Avoid shoes constructed of "man-made" materials or "imitation leather."
- Change shoes twice a day to minimize pressure points on the feet.
- Check the inside of your shoes for sharp seams, small stones and other objects before putting on.
- Do not use shoe inserts or pads without seeking medical advice.
- Avoid wearing socks and knee high hose that are too tight.
- Do not wear shoes without socks.
- Wear socks made of materials that wick moisture away from the skin. Today's fibers, i.e. codmax and polypro blends, do a better job of wicking moisture away from skin. The new generation fibers are far superior to cotton socks.

NOTE: If patient has impaired sensation of the foot, shoes should be fitted by a professional to assure proper fit. Patients often buy shoes that are too tight, and this is particularly dangerous for people with neuropathy and/ or vascular insufficiency.

Conclusion

We have made great strides in the foot care for people with diabetes! Damaged feet that once were lost are now being saved through better care of diabetes, more aggressive patient self-care and preventive strategies, the aggressive use of antibiotics, and improved podiatric and surgical techniques. Yet, still, *the best treatment is prevention!*

Suggested Reading

American Diabetes Association Position Statement: Preventive Foot Care in Diabetes. *Diabetes Care* 27 (Suppl. 1): S63–S64, 2004.

Giurini JM: The Diabetic foot: Strategies for treatment and Prevention of ulcerations, in Kahn CR, Weir GC, King GL et al., *Joslin's Diabetes Mellitus*, 14th ed. Philadelphia, Lippincott Williams & Wilkins 2005.

Akbari CM, LoGerfo FW. Vascular Disease of the lower extremities in Diabetes Mellitus: Etiology and Management. in Kahn CR, Weir GC, King GL et al., *Joslin's Diabetes Mellitus*, 14th ed. Philadelphia, Lippincott Williams & Wilkins 2005.

American Diabetes Association, Standards of Medical Care in Diabetes — 2007. Diabetes Care 30 (Suppl. 1):S4–S41, 2007.

18

Surgical Management of the Patient with Diabetes

Richard S. Beaser, MD and
Elizabeth S. Halprin, MD

When one looks back to the early and mid years of the 20th century, it becomes apparent that the outlook for people with diabetes who face surgery has dramatically improved. Advances in anesthesia, antibiotics, intravenous fluid treatment, blood transfusions, and surgical technique clearly have played a role. Improvements in our understanding of diabetes as well as our treatment tools have also played a significant role. The concern of earlier times that people with diabetes were at a much greater risk of adverse perioperative events reflects the level of care in those times. Today, with proper care and precautions, the surgical risk for the person who has diabetes is often comparable to the risk for the person who does not.

General Approach to Surgical Management

In order to accommodate changes in medical care brought about by economic forces and the focus on cost-effectiveness that we are seeing in this era of managed care, much of what used to be done in an inpatient setting must now take place either on an outpatient basis or in an abbreviated form. The expansion of "outpatient surgery" has so distanced us from the luxury of prolonged inpatient preoperative evaluations that they seem like relics of a past era, tantamount to the "rest cure" hospitalizations of the 1920s and 1930s. Today, efforts to perform much of the management of surgical patients in the outpatient setting has forced more careful planning and coordination of strategies.

Therefore, in approaching the development of cost-efficient yet medically sound management strategies for surgical patients with diabetes, it is useful to set some clear goals and objectives for the process. The focus for the primary care consultant's management can usually be categorized into three areas:

- glucose control
- cardiac risk
- renal function/blood pressure control

Preoperative Evaluation

Glucose Control

How tightly should diabetes be controlled in the perioperative period? Evidence clearly exists that long-term diabetes management should aim for near-normoglycemia; there is now mounting evidence in support of near-normoglycemia in the *perioperative,* and immediate postoperative period as well. This is particularly true for cardiac surgery. We know that we need to avoid marked hyperglycemia in order to promote:

- proper wound healing
- improved ability to fight infection
  - decreased risk of thrombosis
  - central nervous system injury
- proper nitrogen balance
- patient comfort

Traditional teachings that "diabetics don't heal well" and "diabetics are more prone to infections" certainly have a real basis. However, such fears of the effects of hyperglycemia reflect an era before the newer insulins and insulin regimens, oral medications, and glucose control measurements. In the past, the average control of people with diabetes was much poorer than it is today. Nonetheless, the question is often asked: How aggressive at maintaining tight blood glucose control do we need to be immediately before, during, and after surgery when targeting normoglycemia can be more difficult — and more dangerous — than usual?

In the past most studies have been uncontrolled and observational; more recently there have been interventional studies that have shown an improvement in clinical outcomes when hyperglycemia is treated aggressively, particularly in acute myocardial infarction, cardiac surgery, infection and critically ill patients. With particular attention to cardiac surgery, hyperglycemia is an independent predictor of infection in patients with diabetes. Additionally, if hyperglycemia persists in the first 48 hours of the postoperative period these studies show a twofold increased rate of surgical site infection compared with the subjects' counterparts who were maintained closer to normoglycemic. Further studies using the continuous insulin infusions compared to subcutaneous injection showed a 57% reduction in deep sternal wound infection, and a 66% reduction in mortality, the lowest mortality being in those patients with a postoperative average blood glucose of <150 mg/dl.

In studies of mixed medical and surgical ICU patients, the use of physiologic insulin replacement therapy to achieve arterial whole blood glucose levels between 80–110 mg/dl reduced mortality by 34%, sepsis by 46%, renal failure requiring dialysis by 41%, blood transfusion by 50%, and critical illness polyneuropathy by 44%.

In vitro evidence suggests that insufficient response to infection due to white blood cell dysfunction occurs when average glucose levels are above 200 mg/dl. However, many feel that the glucose level should be the targeted at less than 150 mg/dl for perioperative and immediate postoperative control given the more recent studies. This approach is particularly important for patients who present with marked levels of hyperglycemia due to an active infectious process.

Glucose control goals would thus be summarized as follows:

- average glucose levels should be below 150 mg/dl
- recurrent hypoglycemic reactions should be avoided, or at least minimized
- stability of glucose levels should be sought, with most values falling between 100 to 150 mg/dl.

- adequate insulin supply (endogenous or exogenous) should be insured
- proper fluid and electrolyte balance should be established

It is important to also consider the safety of the patient with regard to both over- and under-treatment of hyperglycemia. Institution-wide systems must be in place to avoid errors. Common errors are:

- discordance between feeding and insulin administration
- infrequent blood glucose monitoring
- unclear insulin orders
- homogeneous insulin orders without regard to patient's characteristics or possible change in status (i.e., age, renal failure, liver failure, steroid, NPO, etc)

Keep in mind that if the reason for the surgical intervention is debridement or amputation of an infected foot, the treatment of the hyperglycemia may be surgical rather than medical. Once the infected tissue is removed, glucose levels may become much more manageable. In such situations, the decision needs to be made to move forward with surgery in spite of the significant hyperglycemia.

Nutritional status and hydration should also be reviewed. Malnourished patients have reduced ability to fight infections and heal wounds. Therefore, they are at greater risk for any surgical procedure. If possible, a nutritional assessment should be performed prior to a surgical procedure. Certainly, for elective procedures, this should be possible. Even for semi-urgent procedures, some nutritional supplementation may be necessary.

Proper hydration is also important. While much attention is paid to patients who are fluid overloaded, particularly if they are at risk for congestive heart failure, the dehydrated patients can also be a significant risk for perioperative difficulties such as hypotension. Patients may be at increased risk for hypovolemia if they have an infection with an accompanying fever.

Cardiac Risk Assessment

As cardiac disease is the leading cause of mortality in people with diabetes, it is particularly important to carefully assess cardiac risk when surgery is anticipated. Risk of death from cardiovascular complications, particularly those stemming from ischemia, increases with age, may be more likely if peripheral vascular or cerebrovascular disease is present, and is considerable whether the patient has type 1 or type 2 diabetes.

For patients with diabetes, symptomatology may not be an accurate gauge of the presence or severity of coronary artery disease. Patients with diabetes often have blunted symptoms — so-called silent ischemia. In addition, the concomitant presence of peripheral vascular disease, neuropathy, and/or other podiatric abnormalities may limit the physical exertion to levels less likely to elicit anginal pain.

Therefore, the cardiac risk evaluation for patients with diabetes must be a careful process, influenced by a high index of suspicion. A detailed history should include particular attention to:

- symptoms that suggest the presence of vascular disease (cardiac, but also peripheral or cerebral)
- specific cardiac history, including past episodes of ischemia, infarction, failure, or procedures
- cardiac risk profile, including dyslipidemias, hypertension, family history

Recent cardiac events significantly increase the risk of postoperative cardiac death, and the more recent the event, the more risk:

Cardiac history	Risk of postoperative cardiac death
None	0.13%
> 6 months previous	4–6%
3–6 months previous	up to 38%

Only emergency surgery should be performed on patients with a cardiac event in the past 3 months.

The physical examination should seek to elicit signs of cardiac disease such as valvular disease or congestive heart failure. However, it should also look for evidence of vascular impairment in other areas, particularly the lower extremities. An electrocardiogram should also be performed to look for typical abnormalities.

Suggestive evidence, even the most minimal, should trigger a more extensive cardiac evaluation. Methods for further testing, as suggested by evidence elicited on the initial screening, might include:

- echocardiography, looking at valvular function and wall motion.
- exercise testing to detect ischemia, often done with thallium imaging to increase accuracy. Concurrent administration of dipyridamole may also increase the sensitivity.
- multiple gated acquisition (MUGA) can assess myocardial wall kinetics and ventricular ejection fraction.
- stress echocardiography can help detect motion abnormalities indicative of ischemia.

Positive findings in tests such as those listed above may justify a preoperative cardiac catheterization to further assess problems. For ischemic disease, angioplasty or even cardiac surgery may be indicated prior to other less urgent surgery. In such circumstances, the risk of cardiac events can be significantly reduced.

Assessment of Renal Function

As renal impairment is a recognized complication among people with diabetes, careful preoperative assessment of renal function should also occur. With use of medications such as metformin requiring renal monitoring, and the advent of microalbumin screening and possible renoprotective therapy, the awareness among clinicians of renal status in diabetic patients has increased in recent years. Nevertheless, in patients with diabetes and normal renal function in the recent past, the potential for sudden deterioration is significant enough that a fresh assessment in the preoperative period is often indicated.

Preoperative screening for renal impairment significant enough to affect planned surgery should include the following:

- serum creatinine level
- blood urea nitrogen (BUN) level
- urinalysis.

If renal impairment is suggested, a 24-hour urine collection should occur to measure creatinine clearance and protein excretion. The perioperative period, with acute illness, is not the ideal setting for a measurement of routine microalbumin levels.

The presence of impaired renal function has several implications for the patient with impending surgery. Angiographic fluids, which can be nephrotoxic, should be used with caution or avoided altogether. Fortunately, diabetes patients with normal renal function should not be at increased risk for acute renal decompensation when such substances are used. However, even in these patients, and particularly in patients with some renal impairment, proper hydration should be maintained, as well as furosemide and mannitol used as necessary, to avoid damage. Treatment of hypertension is also important, maintaining existing therapy as close to schedule as possible.

Perioperative Management

The debate on how tightly to control preoperative glucose levels has extended into the perioperative period as well. It is likely that the findings in the more critically ill patient will soon apply to those undergoing elective surgeries. Generally we aim for blood glucose levels of 180 mg/dl with a target of 110 mg/dl in the critically ill and in noncritical care patient we aim for 90–130 mg/dl preprandially and <180 post prandially. Aiming for lower values is reasonable as long as they can be achieved safely.

Capillary glucose testing can be used in the perioperative period to monitor control. Patients with a history of glucose instability — such as those with type 1 diabetes — may need more frequent monitoring than those with more stable patterns such as patients with type 2 diabetes.

Intravenous Glucose

Intravenous glucose is recommended in the perioperative and postoperative period, as it helps maintain glycogen stores and avoids hypoglycemia. This approach is particularly important for patients with type 1 diabetes. The temptation is to think that a person with diabetes should not get glucose. However, under the stress of surgery, contra-insulin responses make insulin administration all the more important if ketogenesis and potential ketoacidosis is to be avoided. For the person with type 1 diabetes who is not eating, the intravenous glucose is all the more important as a substrate for the insulin that is given. Thus, the approach is:

- give intravenous glucose — minimum 100 to 150 grams glucose per 24 hours at a rate of about 100 ml/hour
- begin the intravenous glucose prior to surgery and maintain until the patient is again able to eat
- for patients requiring insulin, intravenous glucose should be administered in the perioperative and post operative period

Glucose Management for the Non-Insulin-Treated Patient

Glucose management for the non-insulin-treated patient is often determined by the treatment that he or she was on prior to surgery. This treatment may, in reality, however, not always be an adequate guideline. Patients' preoperative therapy may have been insufficient — perhaps contributing to the events leading to the surgery itself. Also, if infection is involved in the illness, more aggressive glucose control may be needed as well. Therefore, close monitoring and ongoing reassessment of treatments may be needed. While the approach to each patient must be individualized, general guidelines are listed below for non-insulin-treated patients with type 2 diabetes:

- *Previously using nonpharmacologic (medical nutrition therapy and exercise) treatment only:*
    - monitor glucose values closely
    - maintain nutritional status with gentle glucose infusion
    - if glucose levels remain in acceptable range, continue to monitor
    - if glucose levels rise above 180 mg/dl, insulin coverage should be initiated
- *Previously using oral therapies:*
    - monitor glucose values closely
    - maintain nutritional status with gentle glucose infusion
    - for short procedures, hold oral medication
    - if glucose control remains within acceptable range, resume oral therapy once patient resumes eating (for metformin, hold for 48 hours, monitoring renal status to ensure continued proper function.)
    - if perioperative glucose levels rise above 180 mg/dl, initiate insulin therapy

Invariably, the patient with type 2 diabetes who is not being treated with insulin in the immediate preoperative period will fall into one of three categories:

- *Good control preoperatively.* Glucose control is maintained throughout the operative and perioperative period with continued oral therapy, perhaps only needing an occasional injection of insulin to cover a lone high glucose value.
- *Fair control preoperatively.* Mediocrity may be due entirely or in part to common factors such as stress of illness, inactivity, effects of other medications, disturbances in eating patterns, less than optimal advancement of oral medication dose, and/or glucose toxicity due to hyperglycemia from other causes. It is important to determine wither one of these explanations is the cause, or if they are truly insulinopenic. If the former is determined to be the explanation, then these patients may require insulin perioperatively, but upon recovery often return to oral treatments.
- *Poor control preoperatively.* Will need insulin therapy perioperatively, and likely permanently. Most patients in this category probably should have been on insulin therapy preoperatively anyway.

Glucose Management for Patients Requiring Insulin Therapy Preoperatively

Glucose management for patients requiring insulin therapy preoperatively includes those people with type 1 diabetes, and the many with type 2 diabetes who use insulin to control glucose levels. For patients requiring insulin therapy during surgery, there are more similarities in the approach to patients with type 1 and type 2 diabetes than there are differences.

Type 1 diabetes used to be called "insulin-dependent diabetes" for a reason! These people *require* insulin. In particular, during the stress of surgery, insulin is definitely required. However, insulin administration can be tricky in a situation where a patient is NPO (not permitted to eat) for a period of time. To compound the challenge, significant hypoglycemia can create significant difficulty during surgery. Anesthesiologists, in particular, often go to great lengths to avoid hypoglycemia during surgical procedures.

Yet it would not be appropriate to omit the insulin. Without insulin, patients with type 1 diabetes become ketogenic, producing ketones as fat is metabolized, and ketoacidosis often results. In fact, the stress of surgery may create a need for increased insulin at a time when no nutrition is being consumed orally.

Therefore, the answer is to give intravenous glucose and cover with appropriate amounts of insulin. The presence of glucose allows sufficient insulin to be given to suppress ketone production without causing hypoglycemia. Many people automatically think to avoid glucose in the intravenous fluid when they see diabetes on the diagnosis list. In this instance, they could not be more wrong!

Type 2 diabetes that is insulin-treated needs similar vigilance. Keep in mind that while these individuals are not thought of as being as significantly insulinopenic as people with type 1 diabetes, the stress of surgery may make manifest an absolute insulin insufficiency leading to ketogenesis. Therefore, as a general rule, these individuals should be covered with intravenous glucose in the same way as is recommended for people with type 1 diabetes. Remember that a patient previously under adequate control using oral medications may be just at the cusp of insulin deficiency, and the stress of surgery may push him or her over the edge. Always be watchful for the signs of insulin deficiency:

- consistently elevated glucose levels
- ketone production

While these two signs usually go hand in hand, they may not always do so. Either one alone should still prompt increased attention to insulin treatment.

Methods of Insulin Treatment during Surgery

Methods of insulin treatment during surgery usually fall into two categories:

- subcutaneous insulin
- intravenous insulin

Subcutaneous Insulin

Subcutaneous insulin therapy is usually regarded as the easiest and most preferred therapy for shorter procedures when the patient is likely to be able to eat shortly after the surgery is completed. This approach also works the best if the surgery is performed early in the day and is therefore convenient for outpatient surgery.

The insulin dose is usually determined by using one of a number of formulas to split the usual insulin dose into a portion given before surgery, and a portion given after, just before the patient is to eat. The advantages and disadvantages of this approach can be summarized as:

Advantages:

- the patient is certain to get the full administered dose of insulin
- the insulin dose can be based on an established and proven dosing program
- it is perceived by many as being simpler to manage

Disadvantages:

- the insulin is given irrevocably all at once and cannot be removed or reduced if hypoglycemia ensues
- difficult to manage for longer surgeries or patients who may be NPO for extended periods

Many formulas for splitting insulin doses have been published over the years, and none are particularly right or wrong. In general, you should use an approach that you, and your surgical team, feel comfortable with. Most formulas assume morning surgery and are based on traditional insulin treatment programs that utilize a prebreakfast mixture of rapid acting plus intermediate insulin. Commonly used approaches include:

(R = prebreakfast dose of regular or rapid-acting insulin;
N = NPH (intermediate) insulin)

Option 1:   (R + N)/2 given as N or N/2

- *To use:* Calculate the dose using the formula, give as NPH insulin only in the morning when the intravenous glucose infusion is initiated.
- *Advantages:* No regular or rapid-acting insulin is used, reducing risk of morning hypoglycemic reactions. Emphasis on NPH insulin,

along with a steady infusion of glucose, works more smoothly over the day.

- *Disadvantages:* More than half of the usual NPH insulin dose is given, increasing the risk of hypoglycemia later in the day. Lack of morning regular or rapid-acting insulin could result in hyperglycemia at the start of morning surgery.
- *Note:* if basal insulin (glargine or detemir) is used, give ⅔ of the usual dose the night before surgery instead of the morning NPH dose.

Option 2:   ½ R + ½ N

- *To use:* Calculate the dose using the formula, give as regular or rapid-acting plus NPH insulins in the morning when intravenous glucose infusion is initiated.
- *Advantages:* Regular or rapid-acting insulin reduces the morning glucose levels more effectively. Less emphasis on NPH insulin reduces the risk of hypoglycemia later in the day.
- *Disadvantages:* Regular, and particularly rapid-acting insulin used in the morning can cause hypoglycemia if adequate intravenous glucose is not given.
- *Note:* if basal insulin (glargine or detemir) is used, give ½ of the usual basal insulin dose plus the regular or rapid-acting insulin dose as calculated above.
- People not using fixed doses of insulin, but rather using rapid-acting insulin with correction doses and carbohydrate counting would not require any insulin for food coverage. These people would use a correction dose if the blood glucose is >180 mg/dl, with a goal of 150 mg/dl.

Variation: ¼ R + ½ N: Ameliorates some of the fears of initial
                hypoglycemia

In practice, practical considerations often dictate how these formulas are used. People usually using Option 1, but faced with preoperative hyperglycemia, may add in some regular or rapid-acting insulin as in Option 2. Similarly, people preferring a version of Option 2, but concerned about the possibility of dropping glucose levels, may reduce or eliminate the regular or rapid-acting component as in Option 1. Note also that people with type 2 diabetes who are treated with insulin may have been overeating preoperatively. In the hospital setting, particularly when NPO, their insulin doses may need significant reductions.

For surgery later in the day, adjustments in the above recommendations may be needed. Clearly, if the period when the patient is NPO waiting for surgery is longer, intravenous glucose will become more important. Often, the first part of the usual morning split formula is given, perhaps using less or no regular or rapid-acting insulin. However, with a surgery time later in the day, there is a longer period of time that the patient is going without eating. Thus, the postoperative dose is often less than the approximately half calculation recommended above for surgery early in the day. If it is close to dinnertime when the surgery is completed, many will recommend giving close to the usual presupper dose, adjusting for actual glucose levels, and then letting the patient eat supper.

However, keep in mind that a patient with type 1 diabetes does need insulin coverage throughout the day. If there is an extended wait for the operating room appointment, glucose levels should be checked every 3 to 4 hours, and small doses of supplemental insulin — regular or rapid-acting this time — should be given if the glucose levels are rising. About 10% of the total daily dose, given as rapid-acting insulin, might suffice.

For Patients Using Physiologic Insulin Replacement Programs

Physiologic insulin replacement programs present additional challenges in calculating doses. A patient's prebreakfast insulin dose may consist of rapid-acting insulin plus coverage by long-acting basal insulin (glargine or detemir) given previously or by the basal of an insulin pump.

The objective of these types of programs is to mimic normal insulin action through the replication of basal and prandial insulin. It is, therefore, still possible to utilize an intermediate insulin dose, or a rapid-acting insulin dose combined with an intermediate insulin dose, as calculated above, or an adjusted bedtime dose of glargine or detemir. As a general rule for calculating the dose, determine the amount of insulin normally working over the first 8 to 12 hours of the day. Use this amount to determine a coverage dose based on one of the formulae above.

All of the above dosing suggestions should be adjusted based on actual glucose levels and the overall clinical status of the patient. Once the patient's condition stabilizes, use of these longer-acting insulins can, and probably should, be resumed.

Intravenous Insulin

Intravenous insulin can also be used in the perioperative period. While perceived by some as more difficult to manage, it has some advantages, particularly for longer procedures. Ultimately, similar levels of control can be achieved with either method, and the success is probably more dependent on the familiarity of the healthcare provider with the use of a particular method than on the method itself.

Threshold for initiation of intravenous insulin infusion therapy:

Perioperative care	>180 mg/dl
Surgical ICU care	>110–180 mg/dl

The advantages and disadvantages of treating with intravenous insulin can be summarized as:

Advantages:

- if the intravenous flow is interrupted which interrupts the glucose infusion, the insulin infusion is stopped also
- useful when the patient is new to insulin therapy and no established dose is known
- useful for prolonged periods when the patient is NPO, or in use with perenteral alimentation programs
- more reliable insulin delivery in cases of peripheral vascular collapse (shock, hypotension)
- useful when emergency surgery is needed in the setting of marked hyperglycemia or ketoacidosis

Disadvantages:

- variable quantity of insulin is given — if the glucose infusion and insulin are stopped, ketogenesis may ensue
- requires close monitoring with bedside testing methods, often during surgery by an OR staff less focused on glucose control than on the surgical procedure itself.

There are a number of protocols recommended for intravenous insulin use. As with injected insulin, none are clearly right or wrong, and hybrids and variations are often used. Insulin dosing should be correlated with glucose infusions. Generally, it has been suggested that 0.25 to 0.35 units of regular insulin per gram of glucose can be used as a rough guide. However, varying degrees of insulin resistance result in insulin infusion doses that can range from 0.5 to 5.0 units per hour. It is through the frequent monitoring and infusion adjustment that the optimal rate can be determined.

While many use this controlled "trial-and-error" manner, some have developed methods and formulas that attempt to be more precise. Joslin Diabetes Center maintains a protocol for management of surgical patients and the latest version of this Guideline, *Guideline for In-Patient Management of Surgical and ICU Patients,* can be found on Joslin's website (www.joslin.org).

Postoperative Management

Glucose

For patients treated with a "split" insulin dose during the perioperative period, it is assumed that they will resume eating relatively soon after surgery. Therefore, they often can resume their preoperative dosing program. However, frequently, modifications are needed based on changes in food consumption, amount of intravenous glucose, and surgical complications, and/or infections.

For those on insulin infusions, once they can again take food by mouth (usually at least 50% of their normally prescribed diet), they will need to be converted back to periodic subcutaneous insulin injections. However, do not stop the insulin infusion too soon, even if the patient is becoming hypoglycemic. Treat the hypoglycemia with glucose. Remember that injected insulin takes some time to begin working, so stop the intravenous glucose only after the injection dose is seen to be having a significant effect. Note that the use of the newer very rapid insulins can shorten this interval.

Though in the past the time needed to process a clinical lab-performed glucose determination made sliding scale dosing inconvenient, today bedside monitors allow instantaneous glucose readings upon which to base the dosing decision.

However, sliding scales must be reviewed daily. Particularly in the perioperative period, numerous clinical changes often take place quite rapidly and can affect insulin requirements. In general, various factors may influence insulin requirements and glucose control in conflicting directions. A list of such **potential influences on glucose control may include:**

- *Tending to promote hyperglycemia*
  - stress: from surgery or other causes
  - excessive intravenous glucose
  - infection: residual or new
  - insufficient insulin doses
  - overeating
  - immobilization and inactivity
- *Tending to promote hypoglycemia*
  - resolution of the stress from surgery or other causes
  - resolution of infections
  - insufficient intravenous glucose
  - failure to reduce insulin doses that had been increased previously
  - undereating (particularly hospital food in relation to "home cooking")
  - increasing activity

Nutrition

Proper nutritional support during the recovery period is important to assure adequate wound healing. Sufficient intake of total calories, as well as protein, vitamins, and minerals must be insured. This is not the time, even for the obese individual, for a low-calorie diet. Review of caloric needs by a registered dietitian can be useful in designing a nutritional support program that is individualized to a patients own needs. For patients who are unable to eat, parenteral nutrition should be considered. Most hospitals have hyperalimentation protocols or teams that can be called upon for help. In such settings, diabetes is often managed by using intermediate insulin injections given every 12 hours to provide a basal insulin supply, supplemented by rapid-acting insulin doses based on bedside glucose determinations. Alternatively, intravenous glucose may be included with intravenous alimentation using protocols similar to those used during surgery.

Status of Cardiac and Renal Functioning

As patients recover from surgery, it is also important to monitor cardiac status as well as renal function. Problems with both of these organ systems may begin with clinical silence initially, but progress to impart an overt clinical impact that can be quite serious.

Educational Opportunity

The in-hospital recuperative period may be useful to address diabetes self-care issues. Once the patient is over the immediate postoperative discomfort, it might be an opportunity for dietary counseling or review from a diabetes nurse educator. The events leading up to hospitalization, particularly if diabetes-related, may make some people profess to be "turning over a new leaf" in their self-care efforts. We all realize that this new approach may be short-lived. Nevertheless, using the recuperative period for some instruction, with focus on behavior modification techniques, might have some impact. Outpatient follow-up of this intervention is essential if the behavior changes are to persist.

Discharge Diabetes Medications

For patients whose treatment intensity was not increased due to preoperative infection or stress, and who were in adequate control prior to surgery, their dose of oral medication or insulin may be returned to preoperative levels once the patient is fully recovered. (This recovery period may persist past the hospital discharge.) On the other hand, permanent or temporary changes might be required due to altered eating habits, changes in physical activity, or any residual infections. Therefore, close follow-up with the diabetes care-provider should be arranged. This is also an excellent time to assess the patient's diabetes regimen and to institute change if this is warranted. Often, if the diabetes is the cause of the patient's need for surgery, then he or she may be more open to recommended changes at this time.

The considerations set out in Table 18-1 should be kept in mind with regard to oral agents and whether or not it is appropriate to restart them.

TABLE 18-1.   Considerations Regarding Discharge Diabetes Medications

Medication		Metabolism/excretion
Metformin	• Contraindicated in heart failure and renal dysfunction (creatinine >1.5 (M) and 1.4 mg/dl (W)) • Hold for iodinated studies. Confirm normal creatinine post-study • Adverse effects — diarrhea, nausea, anorexia	Renal excretion
Thiazolidinediones (pioglitazone, rosiglitazone)	• Contraindicated in class III and IV heart failure • Caution in patients with edema • Avoid in hepatic dysfunction • Adverse effects include increased intravascular volume	Metabolized in liver
Sulfonylureas/ secretagogues	• Risk of hypoglycemia • Adjustment necessary if food intake decreased.	Metabolized in liver Glyburide metabolized to active metabolites — 50% renally excreted

Suggested Reading

Alberti KGMM, Marshall SM, Diabetes and surgery. In Alberti KGMM, Krall LP, eds. The diabetes annual/4. New York: Elsevier, 1988. Alberti KGMM in Rifkin H, Porte D Jr., eds. Diabetes Mellitus: Theory and Practice. New York Elsevier. 1990:626–633.

Furnary AP, Zerr KJ, Grunkemeier GL, et al. Continuous intravenous insulin infusion reduces the incidence of deep sternal wound infection in diabetic patients after cardiac surgical procedures. Ann Thorac Surg. 1999;67;352–60.

Goldman L, Caldera DL, Nussbaum SR, et al. Multifactorial index of cardiac risk in noncardiac surgical procedures. N Engl J Med 1977;297:845–850.

Hirsch, I, et al, *"Practical Management of Inpatient Hyperglycemia,"* 2005, Hilliard Publishing LLC.

Inpatient Diabetes and Glycemic Control: A Call to Action Conference, Consensus Development Conference, American College of Endocrinology, AACE, ADA, February 1, 2006

Pezzarossa, et. al. Perioperative management of diabetic subjects. Subcutaneous versus intravenous insulin administration during glucose-potassium infusion. Diabetes Care 1988;11:52–58.

Wolpert HA, Treatment of Diabetes in the Hospitalized Patient. In: Kahn CR, Weir GC, King GL, Jacobson, AM, Moses, AC, Smith RJ, eds. *Joslin's Diabetes Mellitus.* 14th ed. Philadelphia: Lea & Febiger, 2005: 1103–10.

19

Gender-Specific Issues

Julie Sharpless, MD,
Peter N. Weissman, MD, and
Kenneth J. Snow, MD, MBA

Introduction

Gender issues and sexual function and dysfunction have become more comfortable topics for conversation in the last few decades. This is true in many settings, including the medical office, the television talk show, and even the bedroom itself. For people with diabetes, in particular, the impact of their condition on gender-related issues, including sexual and reproductive function, can be significant, and the need to address these concerns is an important part of the care they seek.

While it is assumed that primary care practitioners are comfortable addressing gender and sexual function issues, people with diabetes have a number of specific concerns outlined herein that must be addressed in detail. In addition, like any other specialized area of medical practice, each practitioner will develop a comfort level with what he or she is willing to treat rather than refer to specialists. The key is that, regardless of a practitioner's individualized plan for either addressing or referring gender-related problems, these issues must become a regular part of the assessment and care plan for all patients with diabetes, male and female.

Women's Health Issues

Several aspects of the female reproductive life cycle are influenced by insulin and therefore present special challenges to the management of the patient with diabetes mellitus. From puberty through childbearing to menopause, women with diabetes may need to make special adjustments in their regimens to maintain tight control as the reproductive hormones change. Conversely, poor diabetes control can impair normal reproductive function. Further, as reproductive hormones wane at menopause, diabetes raises additional issues in the hormone replacement therapy decision.

Menstrual Cycles

There have been numerous studies examining the impact of diabetes on the female reproductive cycle. While it has been suggested that the onset of menarche may be affected by having diabetes, or at least by the quality of glucose control, none have proven a conclusive link. The age-old adage that girls with very poorly controlled diabetes have a delay in the onset of menarche is probably based on the fact that any severe illness suppresses reproductive function.

Menstrual disturbances have been described in women with diabetes, including secondary amenorrhea and oligomenorrhea. Irregular menses are frequently noted in women with diabetes, with up to 60% reporting irregular, missed, or occasional extra periods. When evaluated closely, these menstrual irregularities tend to occur with increasing likelihood with poorly controlled diabetes, as well as lower body weights.

Regular menstrual function requires integrated neuronal and hormonal signals between the hypothalamus, the pituitary, the ovaries and the uterus. In healthy women, neuronal signals in the hypothalamus stimulate the release of gonadotropin-releasing hormone (GnRH), which causes the pituitary to release follicle-stimulating hormone (FSH), and luteinizing hormone (LH), which in turn stimulate the development of eggs and steroid hormones in the ovary. The estrogen stimulates proliferation of the endometrium and feeds back to the hypothalamus and pituitary to control its own production. A single mechanism of impairment in diabetes has not been established, although several organ level abnormalities have been described.

Hypothalamic Amenorrhea (HA)

One of the most clearly described syndromes of menstrual dysfunction in diabetes is hypothalamic amenorrhea (HA). The levels of the gonadotropic hormones LH and FSH are low and result in low estrogen, similar to HA in women who have inadequate nutrition due to excessive exercise or anorexia nervosa. Women with diabetes who experience HA tend to have poor diabetes control and to be underweight. The first approach to these patients is to improve diabetes control, though some small studies show conflict as to the effectiveness of this approach. One must also be aware that there is an increased incidence of eating disorders in women with diabetes, and eating disorders can independently cause HA. Even without overt eating disorders, many young women with diabetes will underdose their insulin as a tool for weight loss without comprehending the long-term consequences of poor control. The risk of complications from diabetes is shown to be significantly increased for patients with diabetes who also have eating disorders

Oligomenorrhea

In insulin-dependent diabetic women with oligomenorrhea, the specific mechanism causing the menstrual disorder is not known, but hormonal changes at each level of the hypothalamic-pituitary-ovarian axis have been identified. The gonadotropins LH and FSH if not normal are low, implying a hypothalamic disorder as in hypothalamic amenorrhea. The pituitary shows increased responsiveness to exogenous GnRH, which is also similar to HA. Another common abnormality is that of the "polycystic ovary syndrome" phenotype, with elevated levels of the androgens, including testosterone and androstenedione. Polycystic ovarian syndrome (PCOS) is the most common endocrine abnormality in young women and may occur in as many as 10%. Polycystic ovarian syndrome is not always associated with clinical signs of hyperandrogenism such as hirsutism or acne, and the free androgen levels in these cases are usually normal/high normal. Rather than an ovarian problem, this is probably due to elevated sex hormone-binding globulin levels stimulated by insulin. PCOS is usually associated with decreased sex hormone-binding globulin (SHBG) leading to preferential elevation of free testosterone.

The measurement and interpretation of both total and free testosterone levels may be complicated by the fact that, in most commercial laboratories, the population on which the "normal" ranges are based may contain a large number of patients who have milder forms of PCOS and therefore have higher than true normal testosterone levels to begin with. This skews the normal range for testosterone/free testosterone to the higher end. The clinical implication of this is that individuals with diabetes and oligomenorrhea may have testosterone/free testosterone levels that are in the high"normal" range.

Free as well as total testosterone should always be measured since low sex hormone-binding globulin levels may lead to lowered total (but not free) testosterone values.

A possible unifying explanation for the finding of oligmenorrhea with or without signs of hyperandrogenism may be the presence of insulin resistance. The vast majority of patients with type 2 diabetes have insulin resistance. However there are many patients with type 1 diabetes who may also have inherited insulin resistance, the genotype for which appears to be very common in the population. Therefore, some insulin dependant (type 1) patients may also have insulin resistance, a cardinal feature of type 2 diabetes. They are insulin dependant and have the auto-immune features of type 1 diabetes but may have features of insulin resistance as well, such as hirsutism, acne, acanthosis nigricans and may have other macrovascular risk factors commonly associated with insulin resistance such as hypertension and dyslipidemia.

Such patients either exhibit a compensatory hyperinsulinemia (type 2 patients) or may require higher amounts of insulin to achieve glycemic control (type 1 patients). In either situation, higher than usual insulin levels stimulate androgen production from ovarian thecal cells.

Fluctuations in Glucose Levels across the Cycle

Women with diabetes who have regular menstrual cycles may note changes in the levels of capillary blood glucose at specific times during the month. For women without diabetes who are non-obese, there is no correlation between glucose tolerance or insulin secretion and the phase of the menstrual cycle. However, in observational studies of women with diabetes, about one-third report noticeable changes in glucose levels related to the phase of the cycle. Most of these women describe higher sugars in the luteal phase, often the week prior to menses. A consistent but much smaller set reports hypoglycemia during this time or with the onset of menses. The mechanism behind these changes has been controversial, perhaps because of the heterogeneity of individual responses. Euglycemic clamp studies in women with type 1 diabetes show no changes in basal or insulin-stimulated rates of glucose production and utilization across the cycle, but under hyperglycemic conditions, glucose uptake is impaired in the luteal phase. Premenstrual symptoms have been correlated only with depression (specifically *not* hypoglycemia) and do not differ from those in women who do not have diabetes

From a clinical standpoint, a decision has to be made whether or not to try to adjust for these pre-menses variations. Often, this decision will be made taking into consideration how close the A1C is to target, how erratic the control is, what degree of effort would be needed to improve the control, and the overall safety of making such an effort. Good self-monitoring blood glucose test records are essential if an attempt to make compensatory treatment adjustments is to be attempted. Patients must keep records of:

- their glucose levels
- insulin doses
- variability of other factors that affect glucose control such as activity and food consumption
- the onset of menses

Keep in mind, that menses may be blamed for a temporary change in glucose control that in reality may be due to some other factor. One study looked at dose adjustment for menstrual variation and did not show an improvement in A1C although, some individual subjects had good responses, so this approach must be aimed at these individuals. If a clear correlation can be made between the premenstrual time period and a systematic variation in the glucose levels, then insulin adjustments may be attempted. It may take a number of months of attempts at changing the dose and careful recordkeeping to document the impact of these changes before a regular routine can be determined.

For women who increase insulin doses during the premenstrual time period, it is important to reduce the insulin quantity again at the time that such a reduction in the insulin requirements is *anticipated*, rather than waiting to see a drop in glucose levels. This drop in the insulin requirement usually occurs with the start of menses. Failure to reduce the dose in time may result in hypoglycemic reactions.

Fertility and Contraception

In women with diabetes and regular menses, fertility is not affected. However, in women with irregular cycles, there are obviously fewer ovulations available for fertilization. Therefore, the first approach for those seeking fertility should be to optimize control, not only to improve ovulation but to protect the fetus from the teratogenic effects of poor control during organogenesis. A further discussion of diabetes control and pregnancy will be found in Chapter 20.

Women with diabetes are also subject to the many problems with fertility and conception that have nothing to do with diabetes. For example, thyroid disease, which is increased in incidence in people with diabetes, can also be a cause of oligomenorrhea and should be ruled out. Polycystic ovarian syndrome (PCOS) is associated with the insulin resistance syndrome and is a frequent cause of menstrual irregularities in women with type 2 diabetes. However, there is no increase in its incidence in women with type 1 diabetes.

Once poor glucose control and these other causes of fertility disorders are ruled out or treated, the remaining causes and treatments are usually the same as for the general population. For example, women with well-controlled diabetes undergoing *in vitro* fertilization have been shown to have the same results as women without diabetes.

Birth Control Pills (BCPs)

Fertility and the planning of conception are uniquely important for women with diabetes due to the need to insure optimal glucose control *prior to conception.* Control is key, as women with well-controlled diabetes have a decreased risk of birth defects (discussed in more detail in Chapter 20).

With the importance of planning pregnancy in conjunction with optimizing glucose control, women with diabetes are often quite interested in how the various birth control methods impact diabetes, and vice versa. Diabetes is not a contraindication for any particular method of contraception, but there are advantages to some types.

Birth control pills (BCPs) are the most popular form of reversible contraception, and have one of the lowest rates of unintended pregnancy, yet many women and their healthcare providers have hesitated to use this method due to a fear that their use will worsen glucose control. However, if the many benefits of pill use are important to the woman, then usually minor adjustments in diabetes treatment will balance out the rare detrimental effect on glucose control.

BCPs may unmask a tendency toward glucose intolerance that was not previously known. In some women who do not have pre-existing diabetes, estrogen-progesterone-containing oral contraceptives induce an impairment in glucose tolerance. Higher-dose estrogen (>50 mcg) produces more glucose intolerance and gonane-derived progestins (norgestrel) produce more hyperinsulinemia. These phenomena are more commonly seen in women with a history of gestational diabetes, a first-degree relative with diabetes, those who are obese, or those who are older. This impairment of glucose tolerance is often reversible in most women within 6 months of discontinuation of BCP use. However, it is less likely to resolve in those with a history of gestational diabetes. In addition, with the growing concern over the impact of the insulin resistance syndrome and its various manifestations, women who develop glucose intolerance while using BCPs should be screened for other disorders such as hypertension and dyslipidemia for this reason among others directly related to BCP use.

In women with pre-existing insulin dependent diabetes, BCPs can also decrease glucose tolerance, and may require small insulin adjustments. Rarely, BCPs can induce hypertriglyceridemia and pancreatitis. In healthy women this is mostly a risk for women with baseline triglycerides greater than 600 mg/dl. Lipid profiles should be monitored because women with poor diabetes control often have elevated triglycerides; however, severe hypertriglyceridemia is a rare side effect and has not been a problem in studies of BCPs in women with diabetes.

Hypertension is an uncommon side effect of BCPs in women without diabetes but merits careful attention in the diabetic population. Sudden development or worsening of hypertension after starting BCPs should be considered a complication of the medication and warrants discontinuation of the BCP. Hypertension due to BCPs is almost always reversible.

Newer progestins (desogestrel, gestodene, norgestimate) may have a reduced risk of hypertension because of anti-mineralocorticoid effects.

Nuisance side effects such as bloating, nausea, or moodiness may be improved by switching formulations of BCPs. However, different formulations have not been shown to ameliorate more serious side effects such as hypertriglyceridemia or hypertension, and an alternative form of contraception is recommended.

Secondary benefits of BCPs include regularization of cycles for women with oligomenorrhea, and estrogenization for women with diabetes and HA. Such estrogenization is essential for women with type 1 diabetes because of their high risk for osteoporosis.

Progesterone-only "mini-pills" have not been studied for their effects on glucose control in women with diabetes, but are of concern for their high risk (~3%) of failure. Depot formulations of progesterone do not fail as frequently but may increase insulin resistance slightly, and may be associated with weight gain in many individuals. Progesterone-only contraceptives are associated with a high incidence of breakthrough bleeding. The major advantages of progesterone contraceptives are that they do not affect blood clotting and depots offer good contraception for a patient who is unable to comply with daily pills (although this situation is uncommon in patients who manage their own diabetes).

Some newer birth control pills contain progestins which may have antiandrogenic properties as well. These are particularly helpful in those patients (type 1 or type 2) who exhibit hyperandrogenic features.

Intrauterine devices (IUDs) do not have any disadvantages specific to women with diabetes. Their failure rate of 3.5% is high and is the same whether or not diabetes is present. IUDs have been shown not to be associated with an increased incidence of infection in women with diabetes. Other barrier methods (i.e., condoms and cervical caps) do not have metabolic side effects but have high failure rates.

Women with diabetes need careful counseling on the risks of unplanned pregnancy and should also be reminded that most of the above forms of contraception fail to protect against contagious diseases.

It must be noted that most investigations into the effects of diabetes on reproductive function have focused on insulin-dependent diabetes because it is common in women of reproductive age and requires such intense clinical attention. However, insulin resistance also has reproductive consequences, in severe forms such as type A insulin resistance with receptor defects, or in milder forms such as PCOs. The changing epidemiology of diabetes in the United States is making the reproductive consequences of the more common insulin resistant diabetes more significant.

Hormone Replacement Therapy (HRT)

Until 2002, debate regarding HRT was focused around the carcinogenic risk of HRT weighed against the potential cardiovascular, skeletal and neurologic benefits of HRT.

Several studies showed an increased risk of breast cancer among HRT users, particularly with estrogen/progestin combinations; other studies failed to demonstrate this increased risk. While unopposed estrogen is associated with endometrial cancer, the use of progestational agents eliminates this risk.

Although not unanimous, a large number of studies which examined the effect of estrogen on endothelial function, biomarkers of vascular inflammation, and other surrogates for cardiovascular disease, showed a beneficial effect. In addition, a number of large population-based epidemiologic studies seemed to indicate a cardiovascular protection associated with HRT. At least one prospective, randomized study — the HERS study — also suggested a cardiovascular protective effect of HRT.

In 2002, however, results of the WHI (Women's Health Initiative), a large NIH study designed to prospectively examine the effect of ERT/HRT on a number of clinical outcomes, were published. These results drastically changed the approach to ERT/HRT, since they indicated no cardiovascular protection and no protection from time-related decreases in cognitive skills. In fact, a subsequent sub-study from the WHI suggested a possible increase in non-hemorrhagic stroke. The study also demonstrated increased breast cancer risk as well.

Although the WHI showed that ERT/HRT was associated with a decrease in colon cancer and osteoporotic fractures, this protection was not felt to be enough to outweigh the lack of CV and CNS protection when balanced against breast cancer risk.

Therefore, since the publication of the WHI results in 2002, estrogen is now ONLY recommended in post-menopausal women for control of estrogen deficiency symptoms. Dosage should be the lowest dose that satisfactorily controls symptoms and should be used for a maximum of five years. It is specifically recommended that ERT/HRT **not** be used for cardiovascular, neurocognitive or skeletal protection.

The WHI results were criticized because although the study set out to examine this issue with respect to ERT/HRT use in recently menopausal women, the average age of the women in the study was in the mid-sixties and time since menopause was 10–15 years. Therefore, atherosclerotic or neurodegenerative changes may have already started and had progressed to a point at which potential protective effects of ERT/HRT were diminished or absent.

Recent publications have suggested that women between the ages of 50–59 and within 5 years of menopause given ERT/HRT may indeed experience protective benefits, and that the adverse experience of older women, further from menopause, may have masked the protective effects in younger women.

As of now, the official recommendation to use ERT/HRT only for symptom control still stands, but modification or qualification of this position may soon appear.

The situation for perimenopausal and postmenopausl women with diabetes remains particularly frustrating and begs clarification. Consider just one dimension of the problem:

- Pre-menopausal women with diabetes appear to have lost their advantage of having fewer CV events than do men.
- Post-menopausal women with diabetes appear to fare worse than males with respect to cardiac disease (occurrence, severity, recovery).
- If estrogen were to help post-menospausal women who have recently experienced menopause and may therefore have little atherosclerosis, ERT/HRT may prove to be good.
- If however, diabetes patients have accelerated atherosclerotic disease, a 50 year old recently post-menopausal woman with diabetes, and with no clinical features to suggest CV disease, may still actually have underlying vascular disease which may have progressed to the point that she is not protected by estrogen.

It is likely that more information will appear within the next few years to guide clinicians in identifying which women, if any, are candidates for ERT/HRT

Osteoporosis

Osteoporosis, like diabetes, is a common condition. Studies that have examined the prevalence of osteoporosis in diabetes patients have generally shown an increase in the condition in type 1 patients. Study results in type 2 patients are more mixed, although favor an increased prevalence in these patients. Some of the variance may be related to numerous factors such as genetics, duration/degree of control, body size, and underlying hormonal imbalances (e.g., elevated testosterone).

Regardless of the etiology, osteoporosis is a concern, particularly in those women with type 1 diabetes. These women should all undergo evaluation for osteoporosis and be counseled about modifiable risk factors. Such modifications include getting appropriate amounts of exercise, taking calcium supplements and vitamin D, and avoiding smoking and excessive alcohol consumption.

Non-pharmacologic treatment of osteoporosis in women with diabetes is similar to that for a patient without diabetes, except in cases in which nephropathy or gastrointestinal complications exist. Renal impairment necessitates evaluation of the parathyroid-vitamin D axis as well as adjustment of medication doses. Gastroparesis, malabsorption or sprue, and diabetic diarrhea can all contribute to osteoporosis by interfering with calcium and vitamin D absorption. These conditions require separate evaluation and treatment. Patients with amputations are at increased risk for osteoporosis because of their limited mobility. Interestingly, while women with type 2 diabetes have fewer vertebral and hip fractures consistent with their higher bone density, the one site at which they have increased risk for fracture is the medial malleolus, which may be due to either obesity or neuropathy. All patients with diabetes who have extensive neuropathy, amputations, orthostatic hypotension or impaired vision are at increased risk for falls and, therefore, fractures. In addition to evaluation for osteoporosis, these patients need counseling on fall prevention, including the use of walkers, nightlights, muscle strengthening exercises and removal of hazards in the house.

Pharmacologic treatment is also the same in women with diabetes as it is in women without diabetes. Bisphosphonates, weekly or monthly, are generally considered to be the treatment of choice. Raloxifene and teraparatide (synthetic recombinant parathyroid hormone) injections are also approved treatments. At this point in time, although ERT/HRT have beneficial skeletal effects, these agents should NOT be given solely as skeletal therapy. If ERT/HRT is, however, given for the appropriate clinical indication, that is, for symptom control, preservation of or possibly increases in bone mass may still occur.

Endometrial Cancer

Diabetes has long been thought of as a risk factor for endometrial cancer. However, the exact nature of the relationship between diabetes and this form of cancer has not been demonstrated clearly. Most study analyses, after controlling for obesity, have demonstrated that having diabetes does increase the risk of endometrial cancer. Nevertheless, one recent study failed to prove that diabetes itself had an *independent* impact on increasing endometrial cancer risk.

It has been speculated that insulin levels might be a risk factor for endometrial cancer, though studies examining the influence of insulin levels in women who do not have diabetes have not universally demonstrated a correlation. Another theory is that the risk results from the additional estrogen exposure that results from increased estrogen exposure resulting from augmented peripheral steroid conversion by body fat. Therefore, one might conclude that many people with diabetes have multiple factors (diabetes, obesity, sedentary lifestyle) that contribute to the increased risk.

It *is* recognized that unopposed estrogen exposure is a major independent risk factor for endometrial cancer. This fact led to a change in the HRT prescription during the 1970s. Women who still have a uterus are given progesterone along with the estrogen to prevent the increased incidence of endometrial cancer that is seen with estrogen alone.

Increased awareness of the risk of endometrial cancer in women with diabetes is quite important, especially if these women also have other risk factors. This cancer may be recognized by the presence of postmenopausal uterine bleeding. Irregular bleeding on or off HRT should be evaluated aggressively in any postmenopausal woman with diabetes.

Sexual Dysfunction in Women

Most of the attention to sexual dysfunction in people with diabetes is focused on males, as the erectile dysfunction that they may suffer is more readily apparent during sexual activity.

Yet, there is probably a female equivalent to male impotency that can affect a woman's sexual function, as well as her level of satisfaction. Whether or not female dysfunction has been investigated less due to its lesser impact on sexual function, because it is a less obvious function to measure, or, as some suggest, because of the prejudices of a male-dominated medical profession, this book will not dare to speculate. However, the practitioner should be sensitive to possible female sexual function issues, as total patient care should address quality of life.

The female equivalent of male erectile dysfunction has been described as a reduction in labial blood engorgement and lubrication. The result may still be successful intercourse from the male perspective, but the woman's satisfaction may not be optimal. As a woman can usually still function sexually, unlike her male counterpart, she may not complain to her physician.

Nevertheless, a caring practitioner may be able to get a sense of some decline in sexual function that can be addressed clinically. Use of a vaginal lubricant, for example, can be of benefit in some cases. Vaginal estrogen preparations improve vaginal tone and lubrication to treat dyspareunia while being only minimally absorbed into the bloodstream. Further, just reassuring a woman that the problem can be due to the diabetes may be helpful to her. And, of course, an understanding of the situation by the sexual partner is also important in restoring the woman's ability to be comfortable with sexual activity. Medications, similar to those used in males, may at some point provide a solution, but are not currently recommended.

Conclusion

In summary, diabetes has diverse effects on reproductive, postmenopausal and sexual health. As with other complications of diabetes, good glucose control may ameliorate some of the problems; others require approaches particular to diabetes. Many of the issues have not been specifically studied and generalizations can only be made from studies of women without diabetes. An appreciation of the unique consequences of diabetes for women will improve healthcare for these patients but also highlights the need for further research.

Male Sexual Dysfunction

Complications affecting the sexual and reproductive function of men with diabetes have long been a dreaded impact of this condition. While these problems do not carry with them the potential for mortality that accompany other complications of diabetes, they significantly affect a man's quality of life, robbing him of a key component of his self-image and, sometimes, his ability to procreate.

The effects of diabetes on the vascular and neurologic mechanisms involved in normal penile function can lead to various forms of sexual dysfunction. In the past, the term "impotence" was used interchangeably with "sexual dysfunction" for all aspects of sexual dysfunction. An NIH Consensus Conference in 1992 recommended that the term erectile dysfunction (ED) be used to described problems relating to erections and defined ED as the inability to achieve or maintain an erection long enough to permit satisfactory sexual intercourse.

Normal Aging Changes

Some men seeking help for presumed ED may only be having normal changes that are part of the aging process. As men age, they lose the ability to achieve spontaneous erections from visual sexual images or sexual fantasy. More direct genital stimulation (foreplay) may still lead to erections, however. In addition, with aging, sexual activity needs to be attempted in a place with minimum distractions. A distraction or loss of focus invites detumescence, as does attempting sexual activity when fatigued.

As penile sensation decreases with age, it may be difficult to differentiate between a problem resulting from the aging process and one that occurs as a result of diabetic neuropathy. While there is less chance of premature ejaculation with age, patients often experience the opposite phenomenon — retarded ejaculation or anejaculation. Continued unsuccessful attempts to produce ejaculation may lead to fatigue and detumescence without achieving orgasm, but with considerable frustration and disappointment. The refractory period, defined as the time from ejaculation to the next penile erection, also lengthens with age, and may be 30 minutes at age 20, but as much as 2 days at age 70.

Normal Penile Physiology

For normal erectile function to occur, both adequate blood flow and appropriate neural stimulation must be present. Sexual stimulation leads to relaxation of the smooth muscle of the corpus cavernosum. As this smooth muscle relaxes, blood flows into the corpus cavernosum causing expansion of the penile tissue. In addition, the expanding tissue of the corpus cavernosum compress the veins that drain the corpus cavernosum tissue. The veins are pressed against the tunica albuginea, the elastic outer membrane of the corpus cavernosum, further increasing intracavernosal pressure and allowing maintenance of an erection. Ejaculation causes a reversal of this process with the contraction of the cavernosal smooth muscle, decreased inflow of blood, and opening of the veins draining the cavernosal tissue. This concept has special meaning to the patient with diabetes who has microneurovascular changes at the medium and small vessel level. In the past, vascular problems meant decreased vascular flow to the penis. While this does occur in men with diabetes due to increased atherogenesis in blood vessels, the more important change occurs in the intrapenile vascular supply. Intrapenile blood supply is highly dependent on neural impulses and chemical mediators that affect intracavernosal smooth muscle and vascular tone.

Erectile Dysfunction (ED)

Pathophysiology of ED

Due to past societal reluctance to address personal sexual issues, the medical community has only recently begun addressing the extent of sexual problems. The recent Massachusetts Male Aging Study, which evaluated nearly 1300 men, found some degree of erectile difficulty in 52% of men age 40 to 70. Studies report the incidence of erectile dysfunction in men with diabetes varying from 27.5% to 75%. As the age of the study population increased, the incidence increased, with up to 95% of diabetic men over the age of 70 having some degree of erectile dysfunction. In men with diabetes under the age of 30, 20% had ED.

For men with diabetes, the incidence of ED seems to be related to age, duration of diabetes, the level of glucose control, and the presence or absence of diabetic complications. Poor glycemic control, as reflected by an elevated HbA1c, and the presence of diabetic complications seem to be associated with an increased incidence of erectile problems. Macrovascular risk factors that often accompany diabetes, such as hypercholesterolemia, hypertension, and smoking seem to also contribute to the risk of ED. For most of these patients, the etiology of the erectile dysfunction seems to be multifactorial.

From a pathophysiologic standpoint, erectile dysfunction is most commonly produced by cavernosal artery insufficiency and autonomic neuropathy. Nearly 90% of all men with diabetes and ED have at least one of these abnormalities as a causative factor, and 40% have both. In addition to structural pathology, changes in chemical mediators in penile tissue are also present. The major chemical mediator of smooth muscle relaxation in the corpora cavernosum is nitric oxide (NO) which is produced by both nonadrenergic and noncholinergic nerve fibers, as well as endothelial cells. Men with diabetes have been found to have a deficiency in NO activity. This reduction in the pharmacologic action of NO is probably a more significant cause of erectile dysfunction than is any decrease in its level that may occur.

Hypogonadism is not uncommon in men with diabetes, and can be another cause of erectile dysfunction. NO synthase activity is decreased in hypogonadism and seems to be related to androgen deficiency. The testosterone levels also appear to be lower when one's control of diabetes is poor. While a study in 1984 (Ficher et al. J Androl 5:8–16.) failed to show a difference in testosterone levels between diabetic men and controls may have been due to the use of total testosterone values and a population that may have been biased toward psychological problems.

Abnormalities in the function of other endocrine glands can also cause erectile dysfunction. Up to one-third of men reporting ED have abnormalities in the production of androgen, prolactin or thyroid hormones. Interestingly, a recent study of 657 men, all 67 years of age, showed a correlation between a low testosterone level and elevations of blood glucose. Many of these men had not previously been diagnosed as having diabetes or glucose intolerance. Another study confirmed the relationship between elevated blood sugars and low levels of free testosterone and DHEA sulfate. These low androgens were also inversely related to insulin concentrations.

Medications that Affect Erectile Function

There are a variety of medications that can affect erectile function. Table 19-1 lists some of the more commonly used medications.

Many older antihypertensive medications, such as reserpine, guanethidine, and hydralazine, had a high likelihood of affecting sexual function. Drugs such as beta-blockers and thiazide diuretics produced similar problems as well. The earlier beta-blockers, like propranolol, caused more difficulties than the more recent ones, such as atenolol. Even the local ophthalmologic beta-blocker, timolol, may affect erections. Many drugs that affect the central nervous system may inhibit sexual function by direct

TABLE 19-1. Commonly Used Drugs that Affect Erectile Function

---

Cardiovascular
    β-blockers (especially propranolol, metoprolol, penbutolol,
        pindolol, timolol)
    Certain α-blockers (clonidine, guanfacine, prazosin)
    α- and β-blockers (labetalol)
    Alpha-methyldopa
    Thiazide diuretics
    Older antihypertensives (reserpine, guanethidine, hydralazine)
        spironolactone
    Digoxin
    Calcium channel blockers (fairly low risk)
Central nervous system-acting drugs
    Antidepressants
    Antipsychotics
    Tranquilizers
    Anorexiants
Allergy-related
    Corticosteroids
    Theophylline
    Bronchodilators
Antifungals
    Fluconazole, ketoconazole, itraconazole
Miscellaneous
    Metoclopramide, flutamide, clofibrate, gemfibrozil
Recreational
    Marijuana
    Alcohol
Nonprescription
    Antihistamines (chlorpheniramine, diphenhydramine,
        chlotrimeton)
    Decongestants
    Cimetidine

action on the central neurological impulses or by the production of pro-lactin.

Many over-the-counter drugs can affect erectile dysfunction as well. Medications such as pseudoephedrine and certain antihistamines such as diphenhydramine and chlorpheniramine are included in this group.

Men with diabetes are not, of course, immune from having perfor-mance anxiety and relationship problems. Among men with diabetes and ED, various studies have shown a predominantly psychogenic cause from less than 10% to over 33%. Clearly, one would imagine that if a man were experiencing early organic ED, the heightened anxiety over performance capabilities could quite possibly result in a psychogenic component as well, and determining whether the organic or the psychogenic compo-nent is the predominant one can be difficult.

Diagnostic Evaluation

History

As part of the evaluation of ED, one should perform a careful history and physical with emphasis placed on a history of sexual and reproductive functions as well as pertinent, related medical history (see Table 19-2). The first issue that needs to be clarified is exactly what the real problem is. Many patients may complain of "impotence," while the primary problem in their ED is decreased libido or ejaculatory problems. When dealing with ED, the duration of the problem and its presentation — whether sud-den or gradual, with or without progression — provides information to suggest a greater or lesser likelihood of organic disease. The presence of nocturnal or morning erections suggests a psychogenic component to the ED, although their absence does not dispute it, since morning erections decrease in frequency as men age.

Since poor blood glucose control increases the likelihood of ED, one must ascertain the patient's glycemic control as well as the presence of di-abetic complications. Concomitant medical illnesses should be identified, with particular attention paid to medications used and the presence of vascular disease.

Psychological Considerations

If possible, the initial interview should be undertaken with the sexual partner present. While this arrangement may not always be either possible or comfortable for the patient, it is useful for the healthcare provider to observe the dynamics between the two. ED can cause, or be caused by, problems in a relationship, and a sense for the presence and predominance of this component of the problem can be useful in determining the course of evaluation and/or treatment.

Significant numbers of impotent men with diabetes will have psychological problems. Various psychometric tests are available to aid in making the diagnosis of these problems, including the *Florida Sexual History Questionnaire*, which can be used in the office setting. It can help discriminate between organic and primary psychogenic etiologies for the ED. If in doubt, or if maneuvers to restore erectile function that seemingly have overcome organic problems have not restored adequate sexual function, referral to a mental health professional with expertise in sexual counseling is often helpful. With the frequency of combined organic and psychogenic impotence, this second component of the problem may not have been adequately addressed when the first component was treated.

Physical Examination

The physical examination that should be performed must seek evidence of both specific disease states relating to sexual function, as well as a more general screening to assess overall health. Of particular importance, however, would be examination for evidence of the following:

- normal virilization
- anatomical changes such as Peyronnie's disease, hypospadias, or past injury
- testicular abnormalities
- diffuse vascular disease
- diabetic neuropathies

Laboratory Measurements

The list of laboratory tests that are needed for a complete evaluation of ED starts with an assessment of overall health, and, in particular for men with diabetes, an assessment of glucose control (HbA1c), and the presence of diabetes-related conditions such as dyslipidemia.

Measuring free testosterone is a specific test that should also be performed and that can help determine the etiology of the problem. In interpreting this measurement, keep in mind that the age of the patient must be taken into account, as free testosterone decreases with age, with a drop of 1.2% per year for men over the age of 40. Also, free testosterone assays can be somewhat unreliable at the low end of normal or when slightly low. Measuring total testosterone by itself in this setting is not helpful. Total testosterone measures the amount of testosterone bound to its carrier protein, sex hormone-binding globulin. Sex hormone-binding globulin levels rise with age, thus binding more testosterone and rendering a measurement of total testosterone inaccurate. One can measure both the total testosterone and the sex hormone-binding globulin. In this way, one can assess the total testosterone and a calculated free testosterone. When levels of testosterone are questionably low, then use of an empiric trial of testosterone therapy may be considered.

When confronted with a patient having a low testosterone level, the next step would be to measure the leutinizing hormone (LH) level to differentiate as to whether the hypogonadism is due to primary testicular

TABLE 19-2. Evaluation of Men with Diabetes and Erectile Dysfunction

History
exact problem
onset
duration
control of blood glucose
complications of diabetes
other medical conditions
medications (prescription and nonprescription)
performance anxiety
relationship problems
health of partner
Physical Examination
blood pressure
cardiovascular examination
neurologic examination
breast examination
genital examination
Diagnostic tests
A1C, free testosterone
Nocturnal penile tumescence and rigidity (for possible psychologic etiology)

failure, in which case the LH level would be elevated, or due to central hypogonadism, in which case the LH level would be reduced.

If the testosterone level is normal in a patient with a normal physical examination, no further laboratory evaluation is needed. However, if testosterone levels are normal but the physical examination is not, showing a decreased testicular volume, Sertoli cell dysfunction should be considered, and an FSH level should be tested. The FSH level would be increased in Sertoli cell dysfunction.

Nocturnal Penile Tumescence and Rigidity Monitoring

If the differentiation between organic and psychogenic ED is difficult to determine using methods described above, measuring nocturnal penile activity may be beneficial. In the last decade, a portable home monitor, the RigiScan, was developed which can measure tumescence and rigidity while the patient sleeps in the privacy of his own home. Patients with organic dysfunction will have a loss of nocturnal erections, with a decrease in both the frequency of nocturnal erections and in their tumescence. Patients with a psychogenic cause of ED may maintain near normal nocturnal erections, which will be measured by the RigiScan. Sleep disorders, including sleep apnea and nocturnal myoclonus, may invalidate the results and patients should be questioned about these beforehand.

Vascular Evaluation

Men with diabetes have a high incidence of vascular disease. Duplex ultrasound after the intracavernosal injection of papaverine or prostaglandin E1 can be used to monitor cavernosal artery pressure. One must be cautious in interpreting these results, however, since decreased blood flow (versus controls) is seen in men with diabetes who have normal erectile function. The more risk factors for arterial insufficiency, such as aortoiliac disease, hypertension and history of tobacco abuse, the greater the chance that intrapenile blood flow is decreased. There is still no good substitute for a good history and examination of the femoral arteries for pulses and bruits for diagnosing vascular disease.

Neurologic Evaluation

The patient's history and physical examination will generally disclose the presence of neuropathy. Patients with severe autonomic neuropathy have an even greater decrease in the intrapenile circulation. Unfortunately, diabetic neuropathy is often a diagnosis of exclusion and other causes must be considered.

Various methods of measuring pudendal nerve function have shown that men with diabetes with ED have abnormal results. One must remember that decreased penile sensation along with decreased conduction velocities are normal aging phenomenon in all men, including those with diabetes. Where the impact of the normal aging process ends and the effects of diabetic neuropathic changes begin may be difficult to determine.

Treatment

Correct What Can Be Corrected

The first consideration in a man who has diabetes and ED is to achieve optimal control of his blood glucose while avoiding hypoglycemia. In addition, if the patient is on a drug that is known to affect erectile function, consider changing the medication if possible to an agent less likely to be a problem. Even if the agent is not the entire cause for the ED, and full function does not resume, the medication may be contributing along with other factors.

Sex Therapy

A qualified therapist should be part of the health team. Not every psychologist has had the training and experience necessary to treat disorders of sexual function. Brief therapy using behavioral methods seems to achieve the best results. For some, performance anxiety needs to be addressed, and in other cases relationship issues may be the dominant issue in need of attention. For some patients who have experienced years of ED, the patient and his partner may have established a pattern of avoidance that must be surmounted. Some older couples may have to be taught about the need for more extended foreplay.

Hormone Treatments

Thyroid disorders, whether caused by an overactive or underactive thyroid, should be treated with appropriate medications. Generally, borderline thyroid levels contribute very little to ED. Nevertheless, some patients with low libido and subclinical hypothyroidism may respond to thyroid replacement therapy. Elevated prolactin levels may respond to the withdrawal of any offending medications. Pituitary tumors may need to be ruled out if prolactin levels are high. Hyperprolactinemia may be treated with the dopamine agonists bromocriptine or pergolide.

Patients with primary gonadal failure need permanent testosterone replacement. Though it may help with libido and erectile problems, testosterone treatment may also correct the deficiency which may cause lethargy, depression, muscle weakness, anemia and osteoporosis. The choice for testosterone therapy is usually a topical gel. Not all men with low testosterone levels and ED will respond to testosterone replacement. In general, the more medical risk factors for ED that are present, the less likely is the response to testosterone replacement alone.

Because testosterone may aggravate a pre-existing prostate cancer, a sample for determination of prostate-specific antigen (PSA) should be drawn before testosterone treatment. One can then check the PSA again after a few months of treatment, then yearly thereafter. Hemoglobin and hematocrit levels should also be checked regularly because of the risk of polycythemia, especially in smokers. A digital rectal examination is also required.

Men with diabetes often have secondary hypogonadism. The central axis may be suppressed from uncontrolled diabetes, multiple medications, alcohol excess or stress. Such patients may also be treated with testosterone directly, but this will further suppress the central axis. One can treat these patients by stimulating the central axis with clomiphene citrate (50 mg three times each week for 1 month and then slowly taper the dose). The response may be better in younger patients and those with fewer medical risk factors.

Medical Therapies

If controlling the blood glucose, changing medications or replacing deficient hormones is not sufficient to re-establish normal sexual function, one must consider other methods (see Table 19-3).

Oral Medication

Sildenafil

Sildenafil, the first PDE5 inhibitor, was released in early 1998. Since then tadalafil (Cialis) and vardenafil (Levitra) have been released. All work through the same mechanism of PDE 5 inhibition. During sexual stimulation, NO is released in the corpus cavernosum which activates guanylate cyclase and results in increased levels of cyclic guanosine monophosphate

**TABLE 19-3. Frequently Used Therapies for Erectile Failure in the Man
with Diabetes**

Nonpharmacologic Therapy
    penile constriction rings
    vacuum tumescence devices
    penile implants
Local Pharmacologic Therapy
    penile injections
    intraurethral suppositories
Oral Therapy
    sildenafil
    tadalafil
    vardenafil
    yohimbine

(cGMP). This causes smooth muscle relaxation in the corpus cavernosum allowing blood to flow in. These agents inhibit phosphodiesterase type 5 (PDE-5), which degrades cGMP. Thus, inhibition of PDE-5 causes an increase in cGMP with subsequent increased vasodilation.

Both sildenafil and vardenafilare are rapidly absorbed with peak serum levels about 30 to 120 minutes after being taken. One should therefore instruct patients to take the medication about 1 hour prior to attempting intercourse and that sexual stimulation (foreplay) is necessary to attain an erection. The duration of action of these agents is about 4–6 hours. Tardalafil is more slowly absorbed, with peak serum concentrations occurring between 1 and 12 hours after being taken, with a duration of action up to 36 hours long.

All 3 agents have been shown to improve erections in up to 80% of patients. Patients with complete or near complete loss of erectile function have a lower response rate. Most common side effects include headache, flushing, dyspepsia and nasal congestion for all 3 agents. The drugs are contraindicated for patients taking nitrates because of the high likelihood of developing significant hypotension.

Sildenafil has been shown to occasionally increase sensitivity to light and to affect blue-green color discrimination because of cross reactivity with PDE6 receptors in the retina. Because tadalafil and vardenafil are less likely to bind to PDE6 receptors, difficulties with blue-green color discrimination, have not been described with these agents.

Direct head to head studies have not yet been performed between these agents and therefore, definitive conclusions about greater efficacy from one drug to another cannot be made.

To date, there have not been adequate studies evaluating the affect of this agent on retinal blood vessels in patients with diabetes. Because of its vasodilatory action, there is some concern over its use in patients with retinopathy, especially those patients with proliferative disease. Therefore, it is important that patients with diabetes undergo a careful ophthalmologic examination by a qualified specialist prior to initiating therapy with sildenafil. That specialist should indicate whether or not the use of this medication would be safe.

The recommended starting dose of sildenafil is 50 mg 1 hour prior to sexual activity. The dosage can be increased to 100 mg if needed or decreased to 25 mg if side effects outlined above occur. A patient should not take more than one dose each day.

Recently, several cases of non-arteritic anterior ischemic optic neuropathy (NAION) have been reported in men using PDE-5 inhibitors. While the majority of cases have been associated with Viagra use, reports have occurred with Cialis and Levitra. This greater frequency in Viagra users probably reflects the greater number of men using this agent. Most, but not all, of these patients had underlying anatomic or vascular risk factors for development of NAION, including a low cup to disc ratio, age over 50, diabetes, hypertension, coronary artery disease, hyperlipidemia and smoking. Given the small number of total events reported, the large number of users of PDE-5 inhibitors, and the fact that risk factors for NAION are also risk factors for ED so that this event occurs in a similar population who do not take these medicines, it is not possible to determine whether these events are related directly to the use of PDE-5 inhibitors, to the patient's underlying vascular risk factors or anatomical defects, to a combination of these factors, or to other unrelated factors. Patients should be informed that there is no firm evidence for a causal link between NAION and PDE-5 inhibitor use but that they should contact their physician immediately if they experience sudden loss of vision whether associated with PDE-5 use or not.

Yohimbine

Yohimbine is a beta-2-blocker derived from the yohimbe tree in Africa. Its usage predates the existence of the FDA and its efficacy is debated. Studies have shown yohimbine to be more effective in psychological impotence. While its overall positive response may be as high as 30%–40%, it is usually much lower in men with diabetes. The starting dose is one 5.4-mg tablet three times a day and it may take 2 weeks to notice an effect. Usually, if there is going to be a response, it will occur in the first month. If there is a response, patients may be able to decrease the dose and eventually only need one or two tablets about one hour before desired sexual activity.

Local Phamacologic Therapy

Intracavernosal Injection Therapy

Intrapenile injection with vasoactive substances has been used for about 20 years. Initially, papaverine was used, but there was a high incidence of penile fibrosis. This fibrosis is decreased when phentolamine is added to the injection solution. The addition of prostaglandin E1 was found to improve the results, with up to 90% of patients responding. Studies have revealed that half of all patients do not continue therapy by the end of 1 year. Infection is uncommon.

Recently, the use of prostaglandin E1 alone has increased. It is the only intrapenile drug approved for use by the FDA. It does not appear to be as effective in diabetic ED (about 50% success rate) as are the mixtures. Acceptance of this therapy has been limited by the patient's willingness to perform intrapenile injections. Penile scarring and priapism are potential complications.

Intraurethral Therapy

Prostaglandin E1 has been formulated into an intraurethral suppository that is absorbed into the corpora spongiosum of the glans penis and migrates rapidly into the corpora cavernosa. Penile or scrotum pain and orthostatic hypotension are rare complications.

Nonpharmacologic Therapy

Constriction Rings

Patients who have no trouble in attaining an adequate erection with foreplay but who lose it prematurely before ejaculation are said to have early detumescence or venous leakage. They do not need medications or devices to produce an erection, but rather something to prevent detumescence. Kits are available with rubber rings of various sizes that can be placed at the base of the penis after a suitable erection has been produced. These can be cumbersome and are relatively expensive. A newer, simplified adjustable latex ring called the *Actis Venous Flow Controller* is available and is simple, safe and inexpensive.

Vacuum Tumescence Devices

Vacuum pumps are plastic cylinders that are placed over the penis. Air is evacuated from the cylinder creating a negative pressure drawing blood into the penis. A ring is placed around the base of the penis to retain the erection. Various models have been developed over the past two to three decades. Satisfactory erections are obtained in about 75% of patients, and about 50% of patients have long-term satisfaction with the resulting sexual function. This method is safe but quite mechanical. As one might imagine, a certain percentage of partners will fail to accept this technique. Younger men and those patients who do not have a long-term relationship may find the technique cumbersome and embarrassing. Yet some couples use the procedure of pumping the device and placement of the ring as a form of foreplay and turn this negative factor into a positive one. Vacuum devices may be useful for men with diabetes who have a significant vascular component and in whom other therapies have had no effect.

Penile Implants

Penile implants were one of the first therapies for ED. There are two basic types. The simpler model is the semirigid rod. The second type, an inflatable rod, has more hardware that is placed in the penis, scrotum, and suprapubic area, increasing the risk of mechanical failure or infection. Earlier models had a high rate of mechanical failure that has decreased significantly with engineering improvements. Satisfaction rates among men with diabetes and their partners vary depending on the study. Preoperative counseling should be given to couples to dispel any unrealistic expectations. With the development of newer therapies, the number of implants performed yearly has substantially decreased.

Approach to Therapy

Because of the variety of therapies available, treatment for ED should be tailored to the patient's complaints, utilizing the therapy most readily accepted by the patient. For patients with venous leakage, a venous flow controller might be the first choice if the patient will accept it, because it is inexpensive and has no side effects.

For those with a significant psychogenic component, counseling along with a PDE5 inhibitor has a high likelihood of working. For the vast majority of patients with diabetes who have a significant neurovascular component as the cause of their ED, one may start with a PDE5 inhibitor. If the drug is contraindicated or unsuccessful, second-line therapy could include either intracavernosal injection therapy or a vacuum tumescence device, as the patient chooses.

When to Refer a Diabetes Patient with ED

After performing the initial evaluation, one may wish to start therapy if the cause of the ED is clear and the physician is comfortable with the use of oral therapy for ED. If the cause is not clear, consultation is probably indicated. If therapy with an oral medication is not successful, one should refer that patient to a specialist for further treatment, unless the physician is quite comfortable with advising the patient regarding the other forms of available therapy.

Ejaculatory Dysfunction

Problems with ejaculation are not discussed as often as problems with erectile function because they often go undetected. Men not seeking to impregnate their partner may not notice the lack of ejaculatory function in many instances, particularly if a condom is not used.

Problems with ejaculation may be grouped into three categories:

- *Anatomic problems,* including both congenital and acquired defects in ejaculatory function
- *Functional problems* including both retarded and premature ejaculation
- *Neuropathic ejaculatory problems,* the category of difficulty often related to diabetes, may occur in about one-third of all diabetic men. The most common problem in this category is retrograde ejaculation due to autonomic neuropathy. With this condition, incompetence of the bladder sphincter leads to ejaculation of the semen in a retrograde manner, back into the bladder.

TABLE 19-4: Commonly Used Drugs that Affect Ejaculatory Function

Antidepressants
> Tricyclics
> Monoamine oxidase (MAO) inhibitors

Antipsychotics
Tranquilizers
Antihypertensives
> Ganglionic blockers
> β-adrenergic blockers

Evaluation

One should perform a history and physical with the emphasis similar to that for ED. Since ejaculation is mostly under adrenergic control, medications that affect the autonomic nervous system (ganglionic blockers) or beta-adrenergic receptor blockers can cause ejaculatory dysfunction. A partial list of these is offered in Table 19-4.

Retrograde ejaculation, when orgasmic function is still present, may often be detected if a man using a condom discovers that no semen is present in the condom after sexual activity. For men with diabetes who have been attempting impregnation, use of a condom with examination of the contents can establish a cause for infertility. The presence of sperm in a post-coital urine sample can also establish the diagnosis.

Generally, if this condition is discovered in the first place, it is unnecessary to treat retrograde ejaculation in the absence of the desire for fertility. Reassurance is often all that is needed. However, if the retrograde ejaculation is preventing a desired impregnation, or if it is accompanied by anorgasmia, then further steps may be warranted.

If the patient is on a medication that can interfere with ejaculation (see Table 19-4), changing the medication may be beneficial. If he is not, then referral to a competent urologist is warranted. Evaluation will begin by looking for any correctable anatomic defects. All other therapies will focus on sperm retrieval for fertility purposes.

Conclusion

If one is a woman with diabetes, there are issues that must be considered from that unique perspective — menstrual dysfunction, the effect of diabetes on fertility, contraception and pregnancy, and hormone replacement therapy, to name a few. It is likely she will be willing, if not eager, to discuss these issues with her primary care provider.

Sexual dysfunction, on the other hand, can be present in both men and women with diabetes. The recent trend toward more open discussion of this problem has resulted in the recognition of the scope of the types of problems among people with diabetes and the development of newer means of treatment.

While sexual dysfunction does not directly lead to much mortality, the morbidity, particularly the psychological morbidity and the impact on quality of life, can be significant. For people with diabetes, a reduction or loss of sexual or reproductive ability added to the other accompanying problems and complications of this condition may further impact their self-image and thus reduce their enthusiasm for self-care.

Medical professionals can provide considerable assistance by just bringing up the subject of sexual function and allowing the patient to know that it can be a problem that accompanies diabetes. Medical professionals sometimes take for granted that people know this fact, though many patients do not. Even if no treatment is desired, it might be a tremendous relief for a patient and his or her partner to know that it is the diabetes that has caused the sexual dysfunction, and not a loss of love or desirability.

Also, the primary care provider should be aware that discussion of sexual dysfunction may be a circuitous or drawn-out process. Bringing up the subject with both partners present may result in a cathartic conversation for both. Conversely, it might be too uncomfortable a topic for them to discuss together. Not uncommonly, the subject may be broached with both present with minimal response. However, if the medical professional senses that there might be more to discuss, asking the partner to leave the room during the physical examination provides a more private setting for the patient to address this issue. Similarly, it may not be until a subsequent appointment that the patient will feel comfortable discussing issues of sexual function.

The clear message that medical professionals must give, perhaps repeatedly, is that the subject of sexual function, and the impact of diabetes on this function, is something that he or she is willing to discuss. The message must be that addressing problems of sexual function is an important component of the care being provided to each patient with diabetes. Then, when the patient is ready to address these problems, the door will have been left open for a useful discussion.

Suggested Reading

GD Braunstein. Impotence in diabetic men. *Mt Sinai J Med* 54:236–240,1987. Drugs that cause sexual dysfunction: An update. *Med Lett* 34:73–78,1992. Feldman HA, Goldstein I, Hatzichristou DG, Krane RJ, McKinley JB. Impotence and its medical and psychosocial correlates: Results of the Massachusetts Male Aging Study. *J. Urol* 151:54–61,1994.

Guay AT. Treatment of erectile dysfunction in men with diabetes. *Diabetes Spectrum* 11:101–111,1998.

Hakim LS and Goldstein I. Diabetic sexual dysfunction. *Endocrinol Metab Clin North Am* 25:379–400,1996.

Lue TF. Erectile Dysfunction. NEJM 2000; 342:1802–13.

Kapoor D, Aldred H, Clark S, Channer K and Jones TH. Clinical and Biochemical Assessment of Hypogonadism in Men with Type 2 Diabetes. Diabetes Care 2007; 30:911–7.

20

Pregnancy and Diabetes

Florence M. Brown, MD, and
Richard S. Beaser, MD

Introduction

There is nothing like pregnancy to motivate a woman to pay extra special attention to her health. During this 9-month period, the life and health of the child is dependent on the mother's health. When diabetes complicates the picture, there are many additional considerations in order to insure the health of the offspring. Yet, the ominous outlook of years past has evolved into one of optimism for the health of both mother and child. This evolution began with the pioneering work of the Joslin Clinic initiated by Dr. Priscilla White decades ago and has continued through succeeding generations of diabetes and obstetrical specialists. Their efforts have made successful pregnancies possible for women with diabetes. However, a successful outcome is not automatic but can only be achieved through careful attention by both the patient and her healthcare team. For the woman with pre-existing diabetes, that effort begins before conception. For the woman who may not have diabetes but is at high risk, it is the vigilance during pregnancy that is crucial. Either way, with proper care, the chances for a successful outcome are great.

Metabolic Changes during Pregnancy

Before discussing clinical aspects of pregnancy and diabetes, it is important to review the metabolic changes that occur in women who become pregnant. As the conceptus grows within the womb, it both metabolizes maternal hormones and makes hormones itself. Its growth also affects maternal metabolism, particularly fuel utilization.

As pregnancy progresses, there is increased insulin resistance, possibly due to increasing levels of placental hormones. Normally, insulin secretion increases to compensate for this insulin resistance, with levels doubling by the third trimester. However, as with someone with type 2 diabetes, if the degree of hyperinsulinemia is relatively insufficient to overcome the insulin resistance, a state of carbohydrate intolerance may result. The insulin secretory deficiency that causes a woman to fail to match the needs imposed by insulin resistance of pregnancy leads to the development of glucose intolerance referred to as "gestational diabetes" (GDM), discussed in more detail below.

Clinically, the manifestations of these changes are related to the degree of insulin secretory insufficiency that a woman may have, ranging from hyperinsulinemia and only minimal relative insufficiency, to an absolute insulin secretory deficiency, resembling type 1 diabetes. In fact, some women may coincidentally develop true type 1 diabetes during pregnancy, which should be determined based on clinical presentation, particularly when the diabetes remains after the pregnancy is completed.

For a woman with GDM, at the time labor begins, the increasing insulin resistance that has occurred over the previous 9 months makes a dramatic reversal. The complete resolution of the need for insulin that can occur in many women with GDM can be quite startling, and certainly cannot be explained by the "exercise" of the uterine and skeletal muscle. Similarly, with a reduction in insulin resistance, insulin requirements for patients with type 1 or type 2 diabetes can fall markedly as well.

In the immediate postpartum period, insulin sensitivity is markedly increased as compared with third trimester levels. For women with pre-existing diabetes, insulin requirements decrease by as much as half of the *prepregnancy* requirement. This is probably due to the sudden drop of levels of placental (and anti-insulin) hormones. Response of maternal growth hormone, an anti-insulin hormone, is blunted as maternal pregnancy hormone levels subside as well. Subsequently, insulin requirements return to their prepregnancy levels.

Gestational Diabetes (GDM)

The American College of Obstetrics and Gynecology lists two separate criteria for the diagnosis of gestational diabetes. The National Diabetes Data Group (NDDG) and the American Diabetes Association's (ADA) "Carpenter and Coustan" criteria are shown below. These criteria are based on the O'Sullivan and Mahan data published in 1964, which defined gestational diabetes based on 2 standard deviations above the mean for normal and correlated it with future maternal risk of of diabetes (50% over the ensuing 20 years at that time). Fetal outcomes were not evaluated in the study. The NDDG criteria were established to take into account measurement changes from whole blood to plasma. The Carpenter and Coustan criteria made additional revisions for changes in the measurement of glucose from the non-specific Somogyi- Nelson to the glucose oxidase method. At the present time, there is insufficient data to determine which criteria best predict adverse fetal outcomes. It is likely that there is a continuum of risk between these 2 criteria but that risk may be so small as to not warrant the significant increase in the number of women diagnosed based on the Carpenter and Coustan criteria. The "Hyperglycemia and Adverse Pregnancy Outcomes" (HAPO) study is designed to the unanswered questions of maternal glycemia, less severe than overt diabetes, and the risk of adverse pregnancy outcome.

The 1997 revisions of ADA diagnostic criteria for diabetes, republished in 2001, say that all pregnant women do not need to be screened. However, women with characteristics putting them at *high risk* for GDM (history of GDM, obesity, glycosuria, family history of diabetes) should be tested for GDM as soon as possible. If testing indicates that they do not have GDM, the ADA recommends retesting between the 24th and 28th week of pregnancy. High risk women who are diagnosed with gestational diabetes in the 1st or 2nd trimester may actually have undiagnosed preexisting type 2 (rarely type 1) diabetes that comes to medical attention in pregnancy. Suboptimal glucose control during the first trimester of pregnancy of these patients is associated with a significant increase in risk for fetal anomalies.

Women with *average-risk* characteristics should just be tested at the 24- to 28-week time frame in the absence of any other indication.

For women with *low risk*, the ADA suggests that no glucose testing is needed. To qualify as low risk, a woman must meet all of the following criteria:

TABLE 20-1. Screening and Diagnosis Scheme for Gestational Diabetes Mellitus

| | Carpenter & Coustan | | | NDDG |
| | 50-g screening test (mg/dl) | 100-g diagnostic test* (mg/dl) | mmol/1 | mg/dl |
Plasma glucose				
Fasting	—	95	5.3	105
1 hour	140	180	10.0	190
2 hour	—	155	8.6	165
3 hour	—	140	7.8	145

*The 100-g diagnostic test is performed on patients who have a positive screening test. The diagnosis of GDM requires any two of the four plasma glucose values obtained during the test to meet or exceed the values shown above.

See *Diabetes Care* 24 (Suppl 1):S77–S79, 2001, American College of Obstetrics and Gynecology: Practice Bulletin. Clinical Management Guidelines for Obstetricians-Gynecologists. No. 30, September 2001.

- < 25 years of age
- normal prepregnancy weight
- member of an ethnic group with a low prevalence of GDM
- no known diabetes in first-degree relatives
- no history of abnormal glucose tolerance
- no history of poor obstetric outcome

Screening: A fasting glucose level >126 mg/dl (7.0 mmol/l) or a casual plasma glucose >200 mg/dl (11.1 mmol/l) is the correct diagnostic threshold for diabetes. If these are met, and confirmed by subsequent testing on another day, there is no need for a glucose challenge. Women who do not reach these diagnostic thresholds but are still average or high risk need further screening.

The usual screening test for GDM is a glucose challenge test (GCT). This screening test consists of the consumption of a 50-gram oral glucose load, followed by a subsequent plasma glucose determination one hour later. The patient does not need to be fasting for this test to be performed. A value of ≥140 mg/dl (7.8 mmol/l) one hour after the 50-gram load is abnormal and is an indication that a full 3-hour oral glucose tolerance test with a 100-gram glucose load should be performed. A cutoff value of

>130 mg/dl (7.2 mmol/1) further improves sensitivity from 80 to 90% and reduces specificity but may be considered in high risk populations. Criteria for positive screening and diagnosis of GDM are listed in Table 20-1.

Treatment of GDM

The goal of treatment for the woman with GDM, as recommended by both the ADA and the American College of Obstetricians and Gynecologists, is a fasting plasma glucose level below 95 mg/dl, and a 2-hour postprandial glucose level of less than 120 mg/dl. ADA technical guidelines for preexisting diabetes (Kitzmiller in press) target fasting glucose 60–99 mg/dl and 1 hour postprandial (close to the peak postprandial glucose) under 130 which are an option for GDM as well.

To reach these goals, the primary focus of treatment should be initiation of a medical nutrition therapy (MNT) program. The design of such a program depends on maternal height and weight and includes adequate calories and nutrients for both maternal and fetal nutrition. For a mother who is not overweight, this usually amounts to about 30 kcal/kg. However, it is estimated that 60% to 80% of women with GDM are obese, with both the obesity and the pregnancy contributing to insulin resistance. Thus, some caloric restriction is necessary. For those women with a body mass index (BMI) >25, the ADA has recommended a 20%calorie restriction, or about 24 kcal/kg (see Fig. 1, Chapter 5).

Physical activity should also be encouraged as an adjunct to MNT to lower maternal hyperglycemia for women who exercised prior to pregnancy. Women who did not previously exercise regularly should not initiate an exercise program for the first time when pregnant, but should be encouraged to walk regularly if allowed by their obstetrician. Exercise, clearly effective in increasing insulin sensitivity in people with type 2 diabetes, seems to be effective in reaching glucose goals for women with GDM as well.

If MNT and exercise do not reduce hyperglycemia sufficiently to reach recommended glucose goals, insulin therapy is needed. The oral antidiabetic medication glyburide has been studied in gestational diabetes with efficacy in mild GDM but without sufficient power to evaluate neonatal outcomes. Some health care providers use glyburide in mild gestational diabetes while others choose not to. Metformin is not sufficiently studied in GDM. It crosses the placenta and may be present in higher concentrations in the fetal circulation than in the maternal circulation. The ongoing randomized MiG study in Australia and New Zealand is designed to compare outcomes using metformin compared to insulin in women with gestational diabetes. Use of this insulin sensitizer should be deferred until these results are available.

The determinant of the need for insulin therapy is usually maternal glycemia, but may also be modified by the assessment of fetal growth. However, fetal growth ultrasounds are not always accurate and normative data for different ethnic populations are not well defined. Design of the insulin treatment program should follow the recommended targets for fasting and postprandial glucose levels. Human insulin is recommended, as it is less antigenic than animal-species insulins, which is important in this setting where insulin cessation postpartum is a strong likelihood, but retreatment with insulin years later is a distinct possibility.

Self-monitoring of blood glucose (SMBG) is strongly recommended for all women with GDM. Initially, all patients should check blood glucose fasting and 1–2 hours after each meal. The 1 hour postprandial glucose is close to the peak glucose following a meal. Daily monitoring to gauge success in reaching glucose treatment goals, as with people who are not pregnant, reflects metabolic control while they are living in their normal routine. Infrequent or random office glucose measurements do not reflect such a real-life measure. Therefore, all women should be taught SMBG skills for use during pregnancy, even if there is a possibility that they will not need these skills after the pregnancy is completed.

Insulin therapy in women with gestational diabetes is targeted to lower the elevated blood glucose levels. To accomplish this, some women will need only bedtime intermediate (NPH) insulin aimed at lowering the fasting glucose. Others may need premeal rapid acting insulin (Humalog, Novolog) only. Others may need both.

Initial insulin doses for such a full insulin program may be estimated using a calculation based on existing pregnant weight at the time the dose is initiated. A total daily insulin dose of 0.5 to 0.7 units/kg. weight can be used to determine the starting dose. Forty percent of the starting dose may be given as bedtime NPH and 20 % may be given as rapid acting insulin premeals. Chapter 10 discusses design of other programs in more detail. In addition, maternal blood pressure and urinary protein should be closely monitored as women with gestational diabetes have a higher incidence of gestational hypertension and preeclampsia.

From an obstetrical standpoint, women with GDM who can achieve adequate glucose control with MNT alone can be managed in a manner similar to the general population. However, when insulin therapy is needed or other complications such as hypertension are present, more careful monitoring is needed. In such cases, fetal testing is often recommended by week 32. For these women, delivery is often recommended at week 38 to 40, similar to women with pregestational diabetes. Macrosomia is a common neonatal risk for the infant of the GDM mother and may lead to birth injury. Therefore, efforts to estimate fetal size are indicated, realizing the inherent inaccuracies in such determinations. Clinical judgment often becomes the determinant on whether a cesarean delivery is or is not indicated.

Pregestational Diabetes — Preparing Women with Type 1 or Type 2 for Pregnancy

Aggressive treatment of women with diabetes who become pregnant was demonstrated early-on to provide beneficial results. Dr. Pricilla White and the Joslin pregnancy program adopted this approach decades ago, and over the last 20 years the evidence has mounted that, in fact, the approach is valid.

A successful pregnancy outcome demands that an aggressive approach to glucose management begin *before* conception. Doing so requires efforts beyond those of a physician alone. Diabetes educators and dietitians are needed to teach the self-care skills necessary for intensive glucose management, and the woman herself must also agree with, and participate in, this aggressive approach.

Unplanned pregnancies often do not allow the needed preconception intensification of therapy that is required, and therefore they may lead to unfavorable fetal outcomes. *All* women with diabetes who are of childbearing potential should be counseled about the recommendations for preconception care, and the use of appropriate contraception until intensification of glucose management has occurred. While the tendency may

be to ignore this advice when pregnancy seems unlikely, it is just such circumstances, when pregnancy might be a surprise, where such counseling
is most clearly needed, but most often overlooked.

Initial Evaluation of a Woman with Diabetes Who Wishes to Become Pregnant

Initial evaluation of a woman with diabetes who wishes to consider becoming pregnant must be multifactoral in scope and multidisciplinary in
its presentation to the patient. (see Table 20-2). Such preconception evaluations must provide assessment of risk and counseling based on these
risks. Women should be informed as to the risks of morbidity or mortality
for themselves and the risks of congenital malformations or death for
their child. The importance of planning the pregnancy should be discussed. Diabetes control issues are often at the core of these preconception
evaluations, and control should be optimized before conception. In addition, the status of existing complications must be reviewed and action
taken to monitor or treat such conditions prior to pregnancy.

The preconception medical evaluation should review diabetes type,
duration, and history, including onset, acute complications such as ketoacidosis, severe hypoglycemia, or infection. Current treatment should be
reviewed, including insulin regimen, self-testing frequency, techniques
and accuracy, and results. Medical nutrition therapy (MNT) should be assessed and reviewed or revised as needed, and the activity level, including formal exercise programs, should be documented.

A careful review of the presence and status of any chronic diabetes-
related complications is important. Specific issues relating to these complications will be discussed below. Concomitant medical conditions and
use of medications, particularly when impacting pregnancy, should be assessed. A menstrual and pregnancy history is also important. Finally, a social assessment should be completed — documenting support systems,
family, cultural, and work environments, and any psychosocial issues that
may be magnified by a pregnancy and childbearing, or may come to bear
on diabetes self-management during pregnancy.

It is important that the basics of diabetes self-care be optimized prior to
conception. Often, educational review sessions are at the heart of such an
effort. In addition to review of techniques such as SMBG listed above, topics for review often include avoidance and treatment of hypoglycemia,

TABLE 20-2. Checklist: Evaluation of a Woman with Diabetes Who Wishes to Become Pregnant

- **Prepregnancy counseling**
  - current medical status
  - risks of pregnancy to mother and fetus
- **Prepregnancy medical evaluation**
  - diabetes history, including a clear identification of diabetes type, duration, and history
  - acute complications history, including history of ketoacidosis and frequency of significant hypoglycemia
  - personal / social / family history
  - menstrual / pregnancy history
  - assessment of maternal glucose control
  - documentation of current treatment
  - self-monitoring frequency, and skills in technique usage and result interpretation
  - current medical nutrition prescription and degree of adherence
  - exercise habits
  - review of presence and status of complications, particular ophthalmologic, renal, and cardiovascular status
  - medication use
  - blood pressure
- **Laboratory screening**
  - A1C
  - serum creatinine
  - urine microalbumin measurement
  - thyroid function testing
  - other testing as indicated by history or physical examination
- **Optimizing prepregnancy diabetes status**
  - educational review focusing on techniques, interpretation and self-management, nutrition, and exercise
  - optimize blood pressure with medications that are safe for pregnancy
  - assess cardiovascular and peripheral vascular status if indicated
  - ophthalmologic evaluation
  - gynecologic evaluation, with pap smear
  - adequate contraception until ready for pregnancy

treatment of hyperglycemia, sick-day management, and details of nutritional therapy, including carbohydrate counting. Utilization of the skills of medical support personnel such as diabetes educators, registered dietitians, and mental health professionals is necessary.

The focus of the patient examination prior to conception should reflect areas of concern for pregnancy-related conditions or complication progression. Such items include, but are not limited to, measurement of postural blood pressures, cardiovascular examinations, documentation of neurologic abnormalities, and assessment of peripheral vascular circulation. A thorough ophthalmologic evaluation is also recommended, as well as a preconception gynecologic examination and pap smear.

The results of laboratory tests are also an important part of the preconception evaluation. Such testing should include the HbA1c, renal function assessment, including screening for microalbuminuria (detailed below), thyroid function testing, and any other tests suggested by items documented on the history of physical examination.

Effects of Pregnancy on Diabetes and Its Complications

When contemplating pregnancy, women with diabetes clearly must take into consideration the effect of that pregnancy on their diabetes and the risk of development and/or progression of its complications. To address this concern it is important to carefully assess the presence or status of existing complications.

These concerns were clear to Dr. Priscilla White decades ago. Early in her career, Dr. White was able to identify factors that increased the risk to the pregnancy. For example, it was known that if diabetes had been preexisting for many years prior to pregnancy, if it was diagnosed at a very young age, or if vascular complications were already present at the time of pregnancy, there was a greater likelihood of a complicated pregnancy with an adverse outcome. It was known also that the risks were less with more recently diagnosed diabetes, diagnosis at an older age, and when there was no evidence of vascular disease.

To assist in the identification of high-risk factors for pregnancy in women with diabetes, Dr. White developed risk categories, now known

TABLE 20-3. White Classification

Gestational diabetes	Abnormal oral glucose tolerance test. Euglycemia maintained by diet alone Diet alone insufficient, insulin required
Class A	Diet alone, any duration or onset age
Class B	Onset age 20 years or older and duration less than 10 years
Class C	Onset age 10-19 years or duration 10-19 years
Class D	Onset age under 10 years, duration over 20 years, background retinopathy, or hypertension (not preeclampsia)
Class R	Proliferative retinopathy or vitreous hemorrhage
Class F	Nephropathy with over 500 mg/day proteinuria
Class RF	Criteria for both Classes R and F coexist
Class H	Arteriosclerotic heart disease clinically evident
Class T	Prior renal transplantation

Reprinted from Hare JW, White P. Gestational diabetes and the White classification. *Diabetes Care* 3:394, 1980

worldwide as the White Classification (see Table 20-3). This classification was first formally used in about 1948. It was later modified by Dr. White and more recently modified again in 1980 by Dr. White in association with Dr. John Hare to include gestational diabetes.

Using the White Classification, except for women in Class A, which represents diet-controlled gestational diabetes, women in all other classes are insulin-treated. A woman should be placed in the lowest (worst) class for which she would qualify. Thus, a 24-year-old women with diagnosis at age 18 would have less than 10 years' duration of diabetes (as in Class B) but would be placed in class C because of diagnosis at age 18. Women with proliferative retinopathy treated with laser photocoagulation or spontaneously remitted are still placed in Class R.

As diabetes and obstetrical management has improved in recent years, leading to better outcomes of pregnancies in women with diabetes, the necessity of strictly classifying women has somewhat lessened. However, the message conveyed by the White Classification — that these key factors can affect risk — should prompt all women with diabetes who are contemplating pregnancy, and their healthcare providers, to think about the risks and prepare for appropriate management. This is even more important for complications particularly sensitive to the effects of pregnancy.

Retinopathy

Retinopathy is one such condition affected by pregnancy. It has long been recognized that diabetic retinopathy may progress during pregnancy. However, there are multiple factors predisposing the patient to this progression, including the level of preexisting retinopathy, duration of diabetes, the level of glucose control, and the existence of hypertension and renal disease.

Therefore, it is strongly recommended that a woman with diabetes who is contemplating pregnancy should have a dilated ophthalmologic examination by an ophthalmologist. This examination will determine the existing level of retinopathy and, thus, the risk of progression. Women with mild nonproliferative retinopathy may experience slight progression but usually return to baseline after delivery. Women with moderate to moderately severe nonproliferative diabetic retinopathy (NPDR) may also experience some exacerbation and subsequent regression postpartum. The presence of severe NPDR is more worrisome and often warrants panretinal photocoagulation prior to the pregnancy. Once proliferative diabetes retinopathy is present, the likelihood of progression to more severe disease is high, but laser surgery can significantly impact such progression and is indicated. Macular edema is also a complication of diabetes in pregnancy occurring more frequently in patients with hypertension, proteinuria and more severe retinopathy. All women with diabetes need close ophthalmology follow up with dilated eye exams approximately each trimester or more frequently if active retinal changes are noted.

Hypertension and Renal Function

Hypertension and renal function. must also be assessed prior to conception. The presence of hypertension and/or renal complications affects gestational outcome, as reflected by the White classifications. Perinatal mortality in Class F (renal disease) can be two to four times as common as in other classes. Early diabetic nephropathy is characterized by hyperfiltration and increased glomerular filtration rate (GFR). The presence of microalbuminuria is often detectable at this stage. As the renal disease progresses, increasing glomerular pressures brought on by the hyperfiltration lead to glomerulosclerosis. This process eventually results in reduced GFR and rising protein excretion. Use of ACE inhibitors has been shown to slow this process.

In pregnancy, there is an increase in GFR and urinary albumin excretion, particularly in the third trimester. Postpartum, many of these changes reverse, and the overall rate of decline that was present preconception seems to be reestablished. However, if the renal function is reduced, there may be a paradoxical worsening of the GFR leading to clinically significant renal impairment that persists after delivery. Therefore, women who have early renal disease should be encouraged to have their children sooner rather than later.

Assessment of renal function prior to pregnancy should include a serum creatinine level and an assessment of urinary protein excretion (spot urine microalbumin level or measurement of 24-hour urinary albumin excretion). If the serum creatinine is ≥ 1.5 mg/dl or the creatinine clearance is <50 ml/min, a recommendation should be made to delay pregnancy until renal function can be stabilized. Renal transplantation may be needed to do so. If renal function is not this severely impaired, progression during pregnancy should not be much greater than if there were no pregnancy. Nevertheless, these parameters should be repeated at intervals throughout the gestational period.

If chronic hypertension is present, aggressive monitoring and treatment is important. However, because of concerns with effects on the developing fetus, ACE inhibitors, angiotensin receptor blockers and diuretics should not be used. The B1 selective beta blocker atenolol should not be used because of its association with intrauterine growth retardation. α-Methyldopa, calcium channel blockers, and labetalol may be used to treat hypertension during pregnancy. Goals of therapy should be to target blood pressure 110–129 mm Hg systolic and 65–79 mm Hg diastolic throughout pregnancy. For women using an ACE inhibitor to treat microalbuminuria in the absence of hypertension, the ACE inhibitor should be stopped prior to conception with no substitution of other medication during pregnancy. They can be resumed after pregnancy, however. For mothers wishing to breastfeed, levels of ACE inhibitors are quite low in breast milk, and nursing for about 3 to 4 months while using ACEIs (especially enalapril and captopril) is considered safe.

The risk of preeclampsia is greater in patients with either hypertension or renal disease (20–30%) compared with a risk of 10 % in women with uncomplicated diabetes and 5% in the general population.

The presence of renal disease or hypertension can also make the progression of retinopathy more likely and may also suggest significant cardiac disease. Therefore, careful screening for and/or monitoring of the status of ophthalmologic and cardiac conditions in the presence of renal impairment becomes all the more important.

Neuropathy

Neuropathy may also be affected by pregnancy. The autonomic neuropathies are most often affected, including hypoglycemic unawareness, orthostatic hypotension, urinary retention, and gastroparesis. However, peripheral neuropathies may also be exacerbated. Aggressive glucose control often helps ameliorate symptoms of neuropathies, but for severe neuropathies, the period of more intense control often must be lengthy before improvement is seen, and often a period of worsening occurs first. Therefore, it is recommended that the presence of these problems should be identified as early as possible before conception and aggressive treatments initiated, centering on improved glucose control.

Symptoms of autonomic neuropathies may resemble symptoms of pregnancy, and the degree to which one or the other is causing a given problem can be unclear. For example, typical "morning sickness" of pregnancy may also be due, in part, to exacerbation of gastroparesis. Such gastrointestinal disturbances may make glucose control more difficult due to erratic food absorption. Metoclopramide may be useful in this setting. Neuropathies of the lower bowel may cause classic symptoms of diarrhea alternating with constipation. Other causes of these symptoms, particularly infections, should be sought. Loperamide treatment may be used if needed.

Similarly, symptoms of bladder neuropathies may exacerbate symptoms of uterine pressure on the bladder. Resulting increased risk of urinary tract infections may lead to further discomfort, risk, and deterioration of control. Routine screening for urinary tract infections is recommended. Orthostatic hypotension may improve during pregnancy because of plasma volume expansion.

Cardiovascular Disease

Cardiovascular disease is usually uncommon in women of the age group who can become pregnant. However, when present, coronary artery disease (CAD) suggests a very significant risk of maternal mortality during pregnancy. As women may defer childbearing until their 30s or 40s, when they may have had type 1 diabetes for many years, the presence of CAD is not surprising. Any women with age greater than 35 years or with diabetes for more than 10 years or with multiple risk factors for coronary disease risk should be screened for the presence of cardiac conditions before conception. Pregnancy is still possible following treatments of coronary occlusions such as bypass surgery and with less risk than if the surgery had not been performed. Yet, the overall risk of maternal mortality still remains higher in these women than those in the general population.

The appearance of nonspecific atypical symptoms of coronary disease such as fatigue, dyspnea on exertion, mid epigastric discomfort, and gastroesophageal symptoms for the first time during pregnancy presents a difficult diagnostic dilemma. The stress echo is the best option for screening patients, as nuclear studies cannot be performed. However, the positive predictive value of stress echo is low for this age group. Referral to a cardiologist for careful clinical monitoring and treatment may be indicated.

Glucose Management during Pregnancy

Glucose control should be optimized before conception. Patients taking oral medications should be switched to insulin. Medical nutritional therapy should have been optimized as well. Preconception targets should be fasting and premeal glucose 80–110 mg/dl, and 1 hour postprandial glucose 100–155 mg/dl. A1C should be < 7%, aiming for normal if possible.

Insulin treatment algorithms should have been developed prior to conception so that they can be "fine tuned" for intensity, manageability, and safety. The prenatal glucose targets are fasting levels of 60 to 99 mg/dl (3.9–5.6 mmol/l), and postprandial glucose levels at 1 hour of 130 mg/dl (<7.8 mmol/l) and at 2 hours of <120 mg/dl (<6.7 mmol/l). A1C goals recommended by the ADA should be within or near the upper limit of normal for the laboratory, or within four standard deviations of the normal mean and preferably as close to normal as possible. In most laboratories the normal range of the A1C is 4–6% representing a mean of 5 ± 2 standard deviations. The preconception target of under 7% and as close to 6% as possible reduces the risk of congenital malformations to close the the risk seen in the general population of approximately 2%. Such goals may need some modification based on practical considerations such as patient safety.

To achieve adequate glucose control in preparation for pregnancy, frequent visits to healthcare professionals are usually needed. Once an appropriate level of control is achieved, it is usually recommended that patients return for documentation of continued optimal control, using the HbA1c, at intervals of between 4 and 8 weeks.

The incidence of unplanned pregnancy in diabetic populations is approximately 50%. By the time patients present with unplanned pregnancies, organogenesis is usually completed, so it is too late to alter the course of birth defects and miscarriages. Nevertheless, rapid optimization of diabetes control is necessary to reduce fetal loss, control excess fetal growth, and decrease the risk of post partum neonatal hypoglycemia. Patients with type 2 diabetes taking oral medications should be switched to insulin as soon as possible.

Once conception occurs, visits to the healthcare team for ongoing management are just as important. In addition to obstetrical management, medical care, focusing primarily but not exclusively on diabetes-related issues, is important to maximize likelihood of a successful outcome. These visits should document that appropriate diabetes self-care is occurring and is successful in maintaining necessary levels of glucose control. Such sessions should include all aspects of the treatment program, their success, patient adherence, and treatment complications. Management of blood glucose should focus on reviews of SMBG technique and patterns, assessment of hypo-and hyperglycemic events, assessment of adherence to MNT and exercise recommendations, and a review of the application and success of the insulin treatment algorithm.

Psychosocial impacts of both the treatment program as well as the pregnancy itself on family, work, self-care behaviors, and even personal finances should be examined. The A1C should be measured. Laboratory monitoring of other areas of concern should occur as well, including assessment of renal, thyroid, or lipid status, as indicated.

Weight Gain

Weight gain is an important factor to measure during pregnancy. Weight assessment should be made using both actual weight and BMI (see Fig. 1, Chapter 5). Current recommendations for weight change are listed in Table 20-4. The degree of weight gain reflects adequacy of nutritional support for both the mother and the developing fetus. In addition, proper weight gain implies that enough carbohydrate is being provided and covered with adequate insulinization. It is important to avoid underinsulinization, which could result in fat metabolism to provide an alternative energy source, resulting in ketone production.

About half of the weight gain during pregnancy is from maternal body enlargement, particularly the growth of tissues that support the growth of the baby. This includes an increase in the blood volume, breast size, and fat stores. The other half of the weight gain is the baby, the placenta, and the amniotic fluid.

Weight increases at varying rates during pregnancy. Only about 2 to 5 pounds will be gained over the first trimester. Subsequently, steady weight gain of about 1 pound per week is recommended. Underweight women should gain slightly more (1.1 pound/week) while overweight women should gain slightly less (0.7 pound/week). Individual variation in these patterns can be expected, yet gradual weight gain is the ideal, with no dramatic increases or plateaus. Any weight loss during pregnancy warrants immediate evaluation.

TABLE 20-4. Weight-Gain Recommendations During Pregnancy

Description	Percent of ideal body weight	BMI (Kg/M²)	Pregnancy weight-gain recommendation
Under-weight	<90%	<19.8	28–40 lb
Normal weight	90–120%	19.8–26.0	25–35 lb
Overweight	120–135%	26.0–29.0	15–25 lb
Obese	>135%	>29.0	at least 15 lb

Medical Nutrition Therapy (MNT)

Even for women who do not have diabetes, nutritional management during pregnancy is appreciated for its importance in the health of the developing fetus. For those who have diabetes, there is the added impact on glucose management. Development of a proper MNT plan is therefore crucial for all women with diabetes who become pregnant. In developing an MNT plan, all the issues that impact on adherence to such a plan in a nonpregnant woman — cultural, psychosocial, and religious issues, lifestyle, daily routine, and finances, work and family schedules, and personal preferences — must be taken into account. Many of the components of an MNT plan for a woman with diabetes reflect general recommendations outlined in Chapter 5.

The daily caloric intake during the first trimester of pregnancy for women with diabetes usually varies between 30 to 38 kcal/kg of ideal prepregnancy weight. It is recommended that this level increase to 36 to 38 kcal/kg of ideal body weight during the second and third trimesters. Actual recommendations vary, and individualization of caloric targets is important. Vitamin and mineral supplements are also recommended and are no different for women with or without diabetes, including strong recommendation for use of folic acid.

In recent years, concerns about the use of substances during pregnancy such as caffeine, alcohol, non-nutritive sweeteners, and tobacco have been raised. Opinions on the use of some of these substances have vacillated in recent times. The issues here are not specific to diabetes, however, and current thinking on the use of these items for all pregnant women would be applicable to those with diabetes. In general, minimizing the use of caffeine to prudent levels is recommended. Alcohol use during pregnancy is not recommended. Among non-nutritive or minimally nutritive sweeteners, aspartame use is probably safe during pregnancy, although no specific levels of use have been established. Saccharin and acesulfame potassium can cross the placenta, but there is no evidence that either causes harm to the fetus.

Of course, tobacco, whether your patient has diabetes or not, or is pregnant or not, is hazardous to her health.

Obstetrical Management

A complete discussion of obstetrical management is beyond the scope of this text. Care is provided by an obstetrician or a maternal fetal medicine specialist. A detailed history and physical is performed. Ultrasound examination is used in the first trimester to establish gestational age, particularly if the date of the last menstrual period is unclear or uterine size does not match dates. A fetal anatomic survey is performed at approximately 18 weeks to identify major congenital malformations. Ultrasound monitoring of fetal growth is followed periodically starting at approximately 28 weeks. Third trimester fetal surveillance using the nonstress test or biophysical profile is used to monitor fetal well being. This has eliminated the need for routine early delivery.

Delivery

In the past, women with diabetes were delivered as early as 4 to 6 weeks ahead of their due date. This early delivery helped prevent the late-stage fetal death that was more common in women with diabetes. At one time, 50% of stillbirths occurred after the 38th week of gestation. However, modern techniques of care and monitoring have reduced these risks. Delivery often occurs at the 38th or 39th week, or even at full term (40 weeks).

Most babies are mature enough to deliver at 38 weeks, and many obstetricians still prefer to deliver at this time. Key to determination of whether the fetus is ready for delivery is the level of fetal pulmonary maturity and the readiness of the cervix. Delay to week 39 or 40 may be recommended if these factors are not optimal. Having diabetes is not, itself, an indication for cesarean section. Indications for cesarean section in a women with diabetes are the same as for women without diabetes. Cesarean delivery may also be recommended in women with significant diabetic retinopathy where the "bearing down" during delivery can increase retinal pressure, increasing the risk of hemorrhage. There is an increased risk of shoulder dystocia with vaginal delivery and providers must be ready to handle this complication in any weight neonate. However, in uncomplicated deliveries, there is no contraindication to natural childbirth, with or without epidural anesthesia.

Insulin requirements usually drop markedly during delivery and in the postpartum period. During the first 2 days postpartum, they may drop below prepregnancy levels, but return to baseline fairly rapidly in most instances. It is common practice to relax aggressive glucose control during this period to avoid significant hypoglycemia.

Breastfeeding

Breastfeeding by women with diabetes does not cause significant problems and is encouraged. It is recommended by most pediatricians. However, nursing may cause a reduction in insulin requirements. Glucose levels should be carefully monitored and women should be especially vigilant for signs of hypoglycemia during the months of nursing. Insulin adjustments may be needed during this period. Snacks taken before nursing may be helpful in preventing hypoglycemia. An increase in caloric intake by about 300 calories per day may also be suggested, and an adequate calcium intake is important.

Conclusion

Pregnancy for women with diabetes is now commonplace. The tremendous implication of that statement upon the quality of life for women with diabetes and their families cannot be underestimated. A chronic disease such as diabetes can impact so many aspects of a so-called normal life, that it is of considerable significance that this once-forbidden part of life has become so mainstream today. While it does take considerable effort for the healthcare team and, in particular, the woman, obviously the rewards are great.

For many women, the experience of conception, pregnancy, and childbearing provides the first life-event that truly motivates them to achieve a higher level of intensity of self-care. Seize the moment! Proper support and encouragement during this period may result in continuation of increased intensity postpartum. To "sell" intensification of self-care for 9 months may have initially been possible due to the finite timeframe of the effort. However, once having experienced the benefits of the more physiologic approach to insulin treatment, many women are willing to continue.

To stay healthy and enjoy their family may also be a strong motivating force!

Suggested Reading

American Diabetes Association, Position Statement on Preconception Care of Women With Diabetes. *Diabetes Care* 27 (Suppl. 1):S76–S78, 2004

American Diabetes Association, Position Statement on Gestational Diabetes Mellitus *Diabetes Care* 27 (Suppl. 1):S88–S90, 2004

Joslin Diabetes Center and Joslin Clinic. Guideline for Detection and Management of Diabetes in Pregnancy. Available online at www.joslin.org

21

Treatment of Children with Diabetes

Elise Bismuth, MD,
Lori M. Laffel, MD, MPH

Epidemiology

The overall prevalence for diabetes in children under the age of 20 in the United States is approximately 1 out of every 523 youth; however there is a wide variation in prevalence according to age and ethnicity. Youth 0 to 9 years old have much lower rates than those 10 to 19 years old; non-Hispanic white youth have the highest prevalence among younger children, while among youth 10 to 19 years old, black youth and non-Hispanic white youth have the highest rates. Recent epidemiologic data show rising incidence rates of *both* type 1 and type 2 diabetes in children, the impact of which will be more fully understood as these children grow to adulthood and are at increased risk of developing the long-term complications of diabetes. Type 2 diabetes is found in all racial/ethnic groups, but generally is less common than type 1, with the exception of American Indian youth.

Type 1 Diabetes

Type 1 diabetes is a multifactorial autoimmune disease characterized by T-cell-mediated autoimmune destruction of the pancreatic beta cells. Its etiology is likely due to a combination of genetic and environmental factors.

Several HLA class II genes have been linked to type 1 diabetes susceptibility, and some have been linked to a reduced risk of diabetes. It is clear that genetic factors alone do not account for the pathogenesis of type 1 diabetes. In fact, 80% of families of children with newly diagnosed type 1 diabetes do not report any family history of the disease, and there is only a 30 to 50% concordance rate in identical twins. It appears that the autoimmune destruction of beta cells in genetically predisposed individuals is triggered by environmental factors that have not yet been fully elucidated. The complex interplay of genetics, environment, and autoimmunity as it relates to the etiology, pathogenesis, and possible prevention of type 1 diabetes is the subject of active ongoing research. The prevalence of type 1 diabetes in the United States is approximately 1 in 2,500 children at age 5 years, to about 1 in 300 children by 18 years of age. The overall incidence for type 1 diabetes in children under 18 years old is 23.9 per 100,000 per year according to a recent report from Colorado.

Worldwide, there is a wide geographic variation in the incidence of type 1 diabetes in children, with about a 400-fold difference between the highest and lowest rates, ranging from an incidence of about 0.1 per 100,000 per year in China and Peru up to about 40.9 per 100,000 in Finland. In the northern hemisphere, the incidence of type 1 diabetes increases in proportion to the distance from the equator, and, in general, there appears to be a higher frequency of new diagnoses during the cooler months of the year. In Mediterranean countries, however, where many different ethnic groups live in close proximity in a temperate climate, the incidence of type 1 diabetes does not follow any particular geographical or seasonal pattern, but rather appears to reflect the distribution of ethnic populations, demonstrating the importance of the differential genetic susceptibility among populations.

The age of peak incidence of type 1 diabetes is gender-specific and coincides with the increased insulin demands of puberty. In general, the highest incidence occurs in the 10-to 14-year-old group and the lowest in the 0-to 5-year-old group for both sexes. Girls are most likely to develop type 1 diabetes between the ages of 10 and 12 and boys between the ages of 12 and 14. White children below the age of 5 years have an incidence rate of type 1 diabetes that is 2 to 8 times higher than the incidence rate in black children, and children below 5 years of age are less likely to display the typical seasonal pattern observed in older children.

In children of all age groups, the overall incidence of type 1 diabetes has been rising over the past few decades. The rising incidence of type 1 diabetes is a global phenomenon, but again with a wide variation among countries and populations. Worldwide, the incidence of type 1 diabetes has increased by an average of 2.8% per year during the years 1990–1999; while in the United States, the overall incidence of type 1 diabetes increased by about 5.5% per year during the same period. Specifically, from 1978 to 2004, the incidence of type 1 diabetes increased by 2.3% per year in the state of Colorado. The increase in incidence was significant for both non-Hispanic white and Hispanic youth.

In a recent study of incidence trends in childhood diabetes across the world, the 0- to 4-year age group displayed the highest annual increase in Europe, North America and Oceania with annual increases of up to 5% per year for those 0–5 years of age.

This trend is also a cause for concern given the challenges associated with diagnosing young children with early symptoms, potentially leading to diagnosis delay and a greater rate of acidosis and coma reaching rates of 30%.

Various antibodies are present in the serum of 80% to 90% of newly diagnosed patients with type 1 diabetes. These include islet-cell antibodies (ICA), insulin autoantibodies (IAA), glutamic acid decarboxylase (GAD) antibodies, and the protein tyrosine phosphatase-like antibodies (IA2/ICA512). These antibodies appear to be *markers* only, as it does not appear that they cause the beta-cell destruction but are a result of it. Furthermore, the presence of these antibodies is not needed to make the diagnosis of type 1 diabetes, nor do these antibodies alone predict that type 1 diabetes will occur. Levels of IAA appear to correlate with the speed of beta-cell destruction and the onset of type 1 diabetes. Those diagnosed with diabetes at less than five years of age have the highest titers of IAAs. Both GAD antibodies and ICA are more prevalent in patients with type 1 diabetes studied before onset or at diagnosis than IAA. In fact, antibody screening among first and second-degree relatives is now an important research tool for type 1 diabetes prevention trials. Identifying the presence of these autoantibodies may be helpful in certain clinical situations in which it is unclear whether the child/adolescent has type 1 or type 2 diabetes, particularly with the current epidemic of childhood obesity and type 2 diabetes in youth (see below).

Type 2 Diabetes

Type 2 diabetes had previously been reported to account for only 2%–3% of all cases of diabetes in children, but recent reports suggest that this number is rising steadily, paralleling the increasing prevalence of obesity in children. Also there is a wide variation among populations. In younger children, type 1 diabetes accounts for about 80% of diabetes, the proportion of type 2 diabetes in older children ranges from 6% for non-Hispanic white youth to 76% for American Indian youth. The earliest systematic study of type 2 diabetes in youth came in 1979 from the Pima Indian population, the ethnic group with the highest documented prevalence of type 2 diabetes in the world (51 per 1000 youth aged 15 to 19 years). On the other hand, the incidence rate of type 2 diabetes in Pima Indian children was 100 in 100,000 person-years in children 5 to14 years of age and 900 in 100,000 person-years in those 15 to 24 years of age. In northwest Ontario, between 1978–1984, the prevalence of type 2 diabetes in Indian children under the age of 16 was 2.5 per 1000, a prevalence higher than that for type 1 diabetes in the white population. In Native American children in Manitoba studied between 1984 and 1990, the prevalence of type 2 diabetes was found to be at least 0.53 per 1000 children 7 to 14 years of age. In Japanese junior-high-school children, the incidence of type 2 diabetes was recently found to be seven times higher than the incidence of type 1 (13.9/ 100,000 vs. 2.07/100,000), and has increased more than 30-fold over the past 20 years, concomitant with increased obesity rates in these children. Type 2 diabetes appears to account for 80% of all cases of diabetes in Japan. A review of patients cared for at a pediatric endocrinology center in Thailand reported the proportion of new cases due to type 2 diabetes rose from 5% to 18% between the periods of 1986–1995 and 1996–1999. The prevalence of overweight children also increased from 5.8% to 13.3% between 1990 and 1996.

A study from Cincinnati, Ohio, was the first to document incidence rates of type 2 diabetes in the pediatric population over an extended period of time. One-third of all new cases of diabetes diagnosed between 1982 and 1995 in the 10 to 19 year-old age group were classified as type 2, giving an age-specific incidence of 7.2 per 100,000 per year. In 1992, type 2 diabetes accounted for only 2% to 4% of all newly identified patients with diabetes under the age of 19, but by 1994, 16% of all new cases in children had type 2 diabetes. In the Cincinnati report, 70% of the children with type 2 diabetes were African-American, whereas only 10% of the type 1 diabetes patients and 14.5% of the general population were comprised of African-Americans.

In contrast to the slight preponderance of males with type 1 diabetes, the sex ratio was remarkably skewed towards females in all of the above reports of type 2 diabetes in children. In the Pima Indian population, the female: male ratio was 2:1, in Ontario Indians 6:1, in Manitoba Indians 4:1, and in the predominantly African-American population in Cincinnati 2:1. Furthermore, the diabetes was invariably related to obesity and occurred at or around the time of puberty.

While the increasing prevalence of type 2 diabetes has been most marked in the African-American population, recent data show that the disease is affecting many ethnic groups, including Mexican Americans, Asians, Caucasians, Hispanics, and Native Americans, and there are similarities in clinical features amongst these groups at presentation.

Risk Factors for Type 2 Diabetes

As one can see, several risk factors tend to be associated with the development of type 2 diabetes: ethnic background, family history of type 2 diabetes, elevated blood pressure, elevated lipid levels and obesity.

These factors are quite similar to those risk factors in adults that would increase risk and suggest a need for screening or diagnostic testing. In addition, the presence of acanthosis nigricans, a relatively common dermatologic condition present in 7% of school-aged children consisting of hyperpigmentation and thickening of the skin in flexural and intertriginous areas, is thought to be a cutaneous manifestation of hyperinsulinism and is present in 60% to 70% of children with type 2 diabetes. In girls, insulin resistance is a component of polycystic ovary syndrome (PCOS) and may play a role in its pathogenesis. Female patients with PCOS are at increased risk for developing type 2 diabetes.

Two other described risk factors for type 2 diabetes in children are supported by the "in-utero programming" hypothesis, which suggests that in-utero programming due to prenatal undernutrition or gestational diabetes causes metabolic and hormonal changes that promote obesity and insulin resistance and increase type 2 diabetes risk in adult offspring. One study demonstrated an increased prevalence of impaired glucose tolerance and type 2 diabetes in patients whose mothers had gestational diabetes in poor metabolic control, leading to the suggestion that fetal and neonatal beta-cell development may be adversely affected by the maternal metabolic environment. Furthermore, in both North American and British populations, low birth weight, as measured by the ponderal index (kg/m^3), has been found to correlate with fasting hyperinsulinemia, insulin resistance, and increased risk for type 2 diabetes in adulthood. The pathophysiologic basis for these associations is not entirely clear. The combination of low birth weight and increasing weight gain in adult middle age increases insulin resistance and the risk for type 2 diabetes. Individuals with the lowest birth weight and the highest prepubertal body weight appear to be at the greatest risk for insulin resistance and type 2 diabetes.

While it is apparent that increasing numbers of children are developing type 2 diabetes, as in adults, the prevalence of this disorder is likely underestimated, given the typical lack of symptoms early in the course of the disease. A recent study screening middle school-aged children identified 2% with prediabetes (impaired fasting glucose or impaired glucose tolerance), and 0.5% with type 2 diabetes.

Thus, the emerging epidemic of type 2 diabetes in children presents a challenge not only to the diabetes specialist but to the primary care provider as well, who plays a pivotal role in screening for risk factors for development of this disease in the general pediatric population. The American Academy of Pediatrics (AAP) and the ADA recommend screening children every 2 years beginning at 10 years of age or at onset of puberty (whichever comes first) if they are overweight (BMI≥95th percentile) and have two or more of the following additional risk factors:

- type 2 diabetes in a first- or second degree relative
- member of a high risk ethnic group — Native American, non-Hispanic black, Hispanic, or Asian American
- signs of insulin resistance (e.g., hypertension, dyslipidemia, acanthosis nigricans, and polycystic ovary syndrome)

Team Approach to Patient Care

Care of children and adolescents with diabetes can be optimized if the primary care provider has referral access to the coordinated efforts of a multidisciplinary team experienced in the management of young patients with diabetes. Ideally, the team complements the efforts of the primary care provider and consists of a pediatric endocrinologist, a diabetes nurse specialist/educator, a dietician, an exercise physiologist, a mental health professional (social worker and/or psychologist), and referral sources for subspecialists such as ophthalmologists, podiatrists, and nephrologists. All members of the team should be trained in the intricacies of diabetes care, its complications, and its impact on the family and on the psychosocial development of the child.

At the core of the healthcare team are the child with diabetes and his or her family, whose goals and concerns provide the framework for planning and implementing the treatment program.

The primary care provider plays a key role in this process. Often more closely involved with the patient and his or her family, the primary care provider can provide crucial perspective on many of the dynamics and processes affecting the outcome of diabetes management efforts. In addition, the primary care provider is on the "front lines," often the first medical professional to see a patient with a diabetes-related complication, or another condition which can impact diabetes care.

Therefore, it is essential that all members of the diabetes team communicate on a regular basis with the child's primary care provider. In addition, either directly or through the primary care provider, key members of the diabetes management team may need to be in communication with others impacting the child's care, including the child's teacher, school nurse, school guidance counselor, and possibly team coach. This collaborative approach to care of the child with diabetes ensures that the patient receives an optimal, individualized diabetes treatment plan, taking into account his or her age, day care or school schedule, eating patterns, personality, temperament, family structure, cultural background, and other medical conditions.

Goals of Treatment

The overall goal of treatment is to reduce the risk of acute and chronic complications of diabetes. Thus, treatment is aimed at lowering blood glucose levels to near-normal values in all patients with diabetes in order to avoid:

- Acute metabolic decompensation due to ketoacidosis in those with type 1 diabetes or hyperosmolar hyperglycemic non-ketotic syndrome in those with type 2 diabetes
- Symptoms of polyuria, polydipsia, fatigue, weight loss with polyphagia, blurred vision, recurrent vaginitis/balanitis
- The development or progression of complications involving the eyes, kidneys, and nerves
- Failure to maintain normal growth and development and a near normal lifestyle

Ultimately, the goals in treating diabetes in children are to relieve the symptoms caused by hyperglycemia, prevent acute complications such as ketoacidosis and hypoglycemic coma, maintain normal growth and development, prevent the long-term complications of diabetes, and promote a sense of physical and emotional well-being. However, to accomplish these goals requires a complex process addressing multiple components of the treatment plan.

The cornerstone of all successful diabetes care is education of the child and the family, a multistage process that begins at diagnosis and continues throughout the patient's life. At initial diagnosis, emphasis is placed on learning the "survival skills" of diabetes management — the fundamentals of insulin injection, self-monitoring, and recognition of symptoms of hypoglycemia. Over the ensuing weeks, as the child's regimen is stabilized and he or she resumes normal activities, the family begins to acquire the skills necessary for long-term care of the child. Education should include factual information about meal planning and insulin action, skill development, problem solving, as well as reinforcement for successes and support for mistakes. Finally, learning to cope with variations in the child's routine, such as dealing with intercurrent illnesses and changing eating patterns, is a constant, interactive learning process in which the family is engaged on a long-term basis.

The basic tools for management of type 1 diabetes in children are essentially the same as those in adults with diabetes, and include delivery of insulin in an effective manner mimicking normal physiology, monitoring blood glucose, attention to meal planning through carbohydrate counting or other means (i.e. exchanges), and balancing an exercise regimen with the treatment plan. A detailed discussion of the approach to treatment of type 1 diabetes can be found in Chapters 9, 10, and 11. As with adults, the theoretical goal of treatment is to restore metabolic function to as near normal as possible while avoiding episodes of severe hypoglycemia. Based on substantial evidence of the relationship between glucose control and diabetic complications, each iteration of standards for those with diabetes along with advances in therapies during the past decade has lowered the target glucose level.

While the results from the Diabetes Control and Complications Trial (DCCT), the main impetus for improving diabetes care, did not enroll subjects under 13 years of age, adolescent patients in the study who achieved good glycemic control with intensive-management had a clear reduction in the development of diabetes complications similar to that seen in adults. Although adolescents in the intensively managed group had a higher frequency of hypoglycemic episodes, there were no long-term neurocognitive consequences or adverse effects on quality of life seen in this population. Hence, the DCCT study group recommends intensive therapy with the goal of achieving near-normal glycemic control as the treatment of choice for patients with type 1 diabetes who are 13 years of age or older.

However, in young children, who otherwise may be somewhat protected from microvascular complications during the prepubertal years, and in whom severe hypoglycemia may impact neurocognitive function more so than in older children, glycemic goals become age-specific. In addition, most children younger than 6 or 7 years of age are unable to recognize and respond adequately to hypoglycemic symptoms due to their lack of cognitive capacity. The age-specific glycemic goals recommended by the ADA for children <6 years of age, 6–12 years of age (prepubertal), and 13 years of age (or pubertal) to adulthood appear in Table 21-1. The current ADA position does **not** recommend tight glycemic control for children under the age of 2 years, and great discretion should guide its use in toddlers and preschoolers child.

It is important to note, however, that no matter what the target blood

TABLE 21-1. Glycemic Control Goals Recommended by the ADA for Youth with Diabetes

Age	Plasma Blood Glucose Goal Range		
	Before meals	Bedtime/ overnight	A1C
Toddlers and preschoolers (<6 years)	100–180	110-200	<8.5 (but >7.5 %)
School age (6–12 years)	90–180	100–180	<8%
Adolescents and young adults (13–19 years)	90–130	90–150	<7.5%

- *Goals should be individualized and lower goals may be reasonable based on benefit-risk assessment*

- *Blood glucose goals should be higher than those listed above in children with frequent hypoglycemia or hypoglycemia unawareness*

- *Postprandial blood glucose values should be measured when there is a disparity between preprandial blood glucose values and A1C levels.*

Copyright © 2007 American Diabetes Association, from Diabetes Care®, Volume 30, Suppl.1, 2007; S4–S41. Reprinted with permission.

glucose or A1C may be for a particular patient, the **process** of achieving that outcome — that is, frequent blood glucose monitoring and attention to the interplay of diet, physical activity, and insulin doses — should be emphasized to all families and patients alike. *Parent monitoring of blood glucose before each meal and before bedtime and supervision of insulin administration are necessary parts of the diabetes treatment plan for any child with diabetes.*

As with adults, individualization of the treatment program is important for children. While in highly motivated families, close monitoring of blood glucose and administering multiple insulin injections using dosage adjustment algorithms are fairly routine, in other families, simplification of the regimen may be the only key to successful management. Thus, while keeping the general therapeutic principles in mind, the clinician must also tailor the goals of treatment to the needs and capabilities of each individual patient and family.

Insulin Therapy in Youth with Diabetes

Insulin type, the mixture of insulins in the same syringe, site of the injection, and individual patient response differences can all affect the onset, peak, and duration of insulin activity. In general, insulins used in children are rapid-acting insulin analogs, short-acting (regular) insulin, intermediate-acting insulin (NPH), and long-acting insulin analogs. These insulins are delivered by syringe, or in some cases, by a pen or pump. Children with diabetes often require multiple daily injections of insulin, using combinations of rapid-, short-, intermediate-, or long-acting insulin before meals and at bedtime to maintain optimal blood glucose control. Important factors to consider in choosing an insulin regimen include blood glucose monitoring frequency, the child's individual temperament, the number of daily injections the family can perform, the need for flexibility in meal planning, the family's schedule, and support systems in school or daycare.

Insulin requirements are usually based on body weight, age, and pubertal status. Children with newly diagnosed type 1 diabetes usually require an initial total daily dose of 0.5–1 units/kg; in general, the younger the child, the lower the dose.

Insulin Therapy in Young Children

Young children are often exquisitely sensitive to insulin; hence, insulin requirements are often small in infants, toddlers, preschoolers and school-aged children with type 1 diabetes. The typical starting regimen consists of two or three injections per day, combining human intermediate-acting (NPH) or long-acting analog (glargine or detemir), and rapid-acting analogs at a total daily dose of about 0.5-unit/kg.

Rapid-acting insulin analogs such as lispro, aspart, or glulisine, with very rapid onset and shorter duration of action as compared to regular insulin, are generally used instead of regular insulin. This type of insulin peaks sooner after the meal, and more closely resembles the action pattern of endogenous insulin. It also can be administered shortly before, or even after, the child eats and may allow for more flexibility in dosing children with erratic eating patterns, a particular benefit for very young children who are highly selective eaters. Use of these rapid-acting analogs has decreased the rate of hypoglycemia associated with intensive treatment, and has given patients and families more flexibility with meal planning by eliminating the need to give regular insulin 30 minutes prior eating or having to coordinate a meal time with the peak activity of an intermediate-acting insulin such as NPH. However, one must be careful to avoid too precipitous a drop in blood glucose, so caution must be exercised in prescribing rapid-acting analogs to small children, and blood glucose monitoring before and after administration of rapid-acting analogs may be necessary, at least initially. Diluents for insulin lispro and apart are available from the manufacturer for clinical use, and are particularly useful in young children who may require less than 2 units of insulin per injections or extremely small doses given at 0.1 or 0.25 unit increments. The smallest available syringe ($\frac{1}{4}$ cc, $\frac{3}{10}$ cc, or $\frac{1}{3}$ cc) and highest gauge (31G) needle are recommended for young children; some syringes have $\frac{1}{2}$-unit marking. Needleless jet injectors are seldom used, as they have not been shown to decrease emotional or physical trauma to the child, and there is potential for very rapid insulin action and resulting hypoglycemia with these devices. Injector devices such as insulin pens are particularly useful for caretakers of the child who tend to give injections less frequently (such as a grandparent or babysitter) or for those who are afraid of needles. New insulin pens can dose insulin at 0.5-unit increments, again useful for very young children.

Families of young children may elect physiologic insulin replacement programs at onset with once daily long-acting analog use along with prandial rapid-acting analogs. However, many young children begin with a more traditional injection program with a bi-daily NPH (before breakfast and before supper or bedtime) and bi-daily rapid insulin analog use before breakfast and supper. For the traditional NPH program, two-thirds of the total insulin dose is typically given in the morning before breakfast and one-third as a predinner dose. Each of the doses is usually divided in a 2:1 ratio of intermediate acting insulin and rapid-acting analogs, with adjustments made based on at least four blood glucose measurements per day, with the goal of attaining preprandial blood glucose levels between 100 and 180 mg/dl (or lower based on individual goal) and blood glucose levels at or above 80 mg/dl at 2:00 to 3:00 AM. The morning NPH insulin usually provides the lunchtime coverage. Often, insulin algorithms, or sliding scales, are used to adjust the rapid-, short-acting insulin dose. Algorithms should be individually designed for the child by an experienced diabetes clinician, and complicated regimens should be avoided so as not to overwhelm the family.

One potential problem with twice-daily injections is the possible occurrence of hypoglycemia in the middle of the night, followed by fasting hyperglycemia in the morning. This may occur because the peak of the predinner intermediate-acting insulin coincides with the time of minimal insulin requirement, in the middle of the night. Subsequently, insulin levels are at a nadir toward the end of the sleep cycle, a time that basal insulin requirements begin to increase in the early morning. Thus, the tendency for blood glucose levels to rise before breakfast (dawn phenomenon) may be compounded by the release of counterregulatory hormones in response to hypoglycemia occurring earlier during the middle of the night (Somogyi phenomenon). For these reasons, NPH is often administered at bedtime rather than before supper. Another potential problem with the conventional two-dose regimen is high pre-dinner blood glucose, despite normal or low prelunch values. This usually occurs due to the afternoon snack, which is given at the time when the morning intermediate-acting insulin is waning. To obtain better insulin coverage in the late afternoon, an extra dose of rapid-acting analogs can be added before lunch or before the afternoon snack.

Parents should be reminded that children's insulin requirements are not fixed and continue to change as the child grows and develops; thus, periodic re-evaluation is necessary. Also, children's activity level and eating patterns are notoriously variable, and dose adjustments are often necessary on a day-to-day basis as well as on a more long-term basis throughout childhood and adolescence.

Preparing and injecting insulin are adult responsibilities, and young children should not be pushed into handling their own insulin injections until they are physically and psychologically mature enough to do so, and at that point, parental supervision is advised. Over time, "normalization" of injections by using distraction techniques, such as injecting insulin to a young child while he or she is watching television or playing a game, helps to make a child feel less "singled out" or "different" from other family members. In addition, giving the child as much control as possible, such as in choosing the site for the injection, may be helpful when conflicts arise at injection time.

Insulin pumps are often used in young children with success (see section covering pump therapy). Good glycemic control can be accomplished with multiple daily injections of insulin or with pump therapy in young children.

Insulin Therapy in Older Children and Adolescents

As noted previously, the standard of care based on the DCCT is to achieve near-normal blood glucose levels in order to prevent or delay the development of the chronic complications. This goal remains difficult to achieve for many patients, however, the approach using intensive insulin therapy in the older child and adolescent compared with younger children is well accepted although challenging. The central nervous system of the younger child, age 7 or less, is particularly vulnerable to severe, recurrent hypoglycemia. Therefore, glycemic goals must be based on the child's attained age and be subject to change as the child grows older. Initially, prevention of hypoglycemia is paramount in order to avoid brain injury.

For the child age seven or less, blood glucose goals of 100 to 180 prior to meals may be acceptable. As the child attains school age, preprandial goals are lowered to 80–180 or even lower, tailored to the individual patient and family needs. In the young child, total daily insulin dosage may be .5 U/kg per day or less, while in the school-aged child the daily dosage is generally 0.7 to 1 U/kg per day. The insulin resistance that accompanies the period of pubertal growth and development adds to the daily insulin requirements such that growing adolescents may need 1 to 1.5 U/kg per day of insulin. See Table 21-2 for the usual daily dosages of insulin shortly after diagnosis.

A multiple daily insulin regimen will generally be required in the older child and adolescent in order to achieve the recommended glycemic goals, and most youth now receive a minimum of three injections per day

TABLE 21-2. Usual Subcutaneous Daily Insulin Dosages

	non-DKA presentation	s/p DKA presentation
Type 1 diabetes		
Child — prepubertal	0.25–.5 U/kg per day	0.5–0.75 U/kg per day
Adolescent — pubertal	0.5–.75 U/kg per day	0.75–1.0 U/kg per day
Type 2 diabetes		
Adolescent	20–40 U/day*	—

* Often administered as intermediate insulin as starting dosage, depending on level of hyperglycemia at presentation.

DKA = diabetic ketoacidosis.

in order to achieve the glycemic goals recommended by the ADA. Basal/bolus insulin therapy is often the preferred treatment modality. However, a modified split-mixed insulin regimen may be used. This includes a mix of rapid-acting analog and intermediate-acting insulin given prebreakfast, rapid-acting analog before the evening meal, with intermediate-acting insulin administered at bedtime. In addition, the growing child may benefit from an extra injection of rapid-acting analog midday, either before lunch or before an afternoon snack. The outdated twice-daily, mixed-split insulin regimen provides peaks of insulin levels at usual meal times but requires consistent timing for both meals and snacks. While many children experience regularity in their school schedules, the hurried pace of our current era has pushed the limits of consistency, even for children. Many schools have varying lunch periods, and physical education may be limited. Thus, with the push for optimal glycemic control and intensive therapy, insulin administration in school is now a common occurrence.

The goal of insulin replacement therapy is to emulate the physiologic fluctuations of insulin released from the normally functioning pancreas. Exogenous insulin cannot replace perfectly the normal insulin secretion pattern, which combines continuous basal insulin release with additional bursts of insulin in response to prandial elevations of blood glucose levels. The basal and meal-related insulin requirements each account for approximately 50% of the total daily insulin needs. Basal insulin requirements can be met with administration of long-acting insulin administered once or twice daily; mealtime insulin needs are best met by administering premeal rapid-acting analogs. Thus, increases in plasma insulin levels will then accompany the rise of blood glucose that follows the ingestion of carbohydrate-containing meals and snacks. Two long-acting insulin analogues are now available and designed to replace basal insulin secretion. Insulin glargine is an almost peakless insulin, with duration of action of 20–24 hours. Usually it is given at bedtime, although administration at other times of the day may result in similar levels of coverage and glycemic control. In some patients, insulin glargine may not last 24 hours, thus requiring the dose to be divided into two daily injections. Insulin glargine is a clear insulin that cannot be mixed in the same syringe with other insulin preparations, necessitating separate injection for rapid-acting analog administration. Thus, a multiple daily injection program, a so called basal/bolus regimen, uses insulin glargine in combination with a rapid-acting insulin analog and has been associated with fewer hypoglycemic events, particularly nocturnal events, when compared to NPH insulin use. Studies have demonstrated equivalent glycemic control in children receiving glargine and NPH, however, children who received glargine had fewer events of severe hypoglycemia. Although frequently used, insulin glargine is not currently approved for pediatric patients under the age of six years. To date, observational studies demonstrate short-term safety and effectiveness in this age group. Insulin detemir is the newest long-acting insulin analog approved by the Food and Drug Administration (FDA) in June 2005. Insulin detemir is associated with reduced risk of hypoglycemia, weight loss, and improved glycemic control when compared to NPH insulin in adults with type 1 diabetes. It has less variability in absorption than NPH and may have a shorter duration of action than glargine, occasionally requiring twice daily administration in some individuals. Insulin detemir is not yet FDA approved for pediatric use.

Glycemic goals recommended by the ADA include an A1C of <7.5%, preprandial capillary blood glucose of 90 to 130 mg/dl, and bedtime capillary blood glucose of 100 to 140 mg/dl. These goals are difficult to achieve for many youth during childhood and adolescence due to continued growth and developmental changes, compounded by many psychosocial changes and challenges. Because two or three doses of mixed rapid-acting analog with intermediate-acting insulin generally cannot maintain A1C levels within the target range for the majority of pediatric diabetes patients, recommendations support moving toward a basal/bolus insulin regimen for most patients, especially after the honeymoon period. Basal/bolus therapy can consist of injections of long- and rapid-acting analogs, or, continuous subcutaneous insulin infusion delivered by insulin pump (CSII). Greater flexibility results from provision of multiple daily injections, combined with carbohydrate counting and dosage selection using insulin-to-carbohydrate ratios and correction dosages. This is a beneficial therapeutic regimen for many middle school and high school students. At Joslin Clinic, temporal trends in pediatric type 1 diabetes management show that intensified type 1 diabetes management was accompanied by improved A1C, stable body mass index, and decreased severe hypoglycemia.

Pump Therapy

An alternative means to achieve optimal control is by insulin pump therapy. Use of this intensive therapeutic modality is growing rapidly in the pediatric population. There is no best predetermined age to initiate insulin pump therapy. Currently, there are fewer young children than preadolescents and adolescents using insulin pump. Children and teens comprise the most rapidly growing group of patients using the pump. Nonetheless, it is important to consider a number of issues when contemplating initiation of insulin pump treatment for a child or adolescent. The determination of the bolus dosing and the actual programming requires that the user have achieved a certain level of cognitive development. Thus, pump use in children is generally reserved for patients and families who can handle the extra burden that this intensive therapeutic modality warrants. Adult support at both home and school is essential for success with all diabetes management but especially with pump treatment until the child is able to manage the diabetes independently.

Factors to consider in initiating pump therapy include the age and insulin requirement of the child, frequency of blood glucose monitoring, level of parental involvement/supervision, insurance coverage, ability to understand and implement carbohydrate counting, daily schedule of meals and activity; family expectations of insulin pump therapy, and the overall impression of the patient's/family's reliability. It is best that pump therapy in youth be initiated with the aid of a multidisciplinary diabetes team. Pump use requires intensive education, careful monitoring, and ongoing evaluation by medical professionals familiar with pump use. The dynamic of insulin action when delivered by an insulin pump differs from that of injected insulin, often impacting treatment decisions. Unrecognized pump failure can result in ketosis within a few hours.

Nevertheless, as centers with pump expertise may be a distance from where many patients live, increasingly primary care providers are required to know enough about pump use to troubleshoot problems as well as to adjust pump use during times of illness. This book and other materials on pump use can be helpful. However, consultation should be sought with the regional diabetes management team, perhaps by phone or e-mail, when problems arise or if management becomes difficult. As with adults, all patients using a pump should have sick-day protocols written down and ready for use, as well as an "off-pump" injection plan developed, "just in case."

There are several insulin pumps available on the market with numerous features: size, weight, water resistance, type of battery, volume of insulin reservoir, basal rate and bolus increments, number of basal rate profiles, temporary basal rate programming, bolus duration, bolus calculator, insulin on board features, display screens, alerts/alarms, software capabilities, integrated blood glucose meter, ease of use, and choice of color. Pump products change constantly, and medical personnel familiar with current pump models and features can assist with selection recommendations. Details of pump use are outlined in Chapter 11.

The insulin pump has numerous possible advantages including improved or equivalent glycemic control without increased hypoglycemia through a more physiologic delivery of insulin, greater flexibility in timing and size of meals, ability to deliver very small insulin doses in very young or insulin-sensitive children, better matching of insulin delivery with food intake, and improved or equivalent quality of life. Potential disadvantages include pump failure with the possibility of hyperglycemia and ketoacidosis, weigh gain, and the necessity at always being attached to the pump. Several research studies have demonstrated insulin pumps to be a safe and effective mode of insulin delivery in older children and adolescents. Over the last few years, the same conclusion has been reached with respect to insulin pump therapy in very young children (less than 6 years of age). In addition, insulin pump therapy appears to be a durable way to treat children and adolescents with diabetes. One study found that more than 80% of pediatric patients maintained pump therapy after a mean of 3.8 years, with avoidance of the expected deterioration of glycemic control that usually accompanies childhood and adolescence.

Therapy of Type 2 Diabetes in Youth

The goals of treatment for youth with type 2 diabetes include achieving and maintaining near-normal glycemic control, improving insulin sensitivity and secretion, identifying and treating, if necessary, co-morbidities, such as hypertension, dyslipidemia, and nonalcoholic fatty liver disease, and preventing vascular complications of type 2 diabetes. The macrovascular risk factors such as hypertension and dyslipidemia, when found in a younger individual, have an even greater potential to significantly shorten life than when they are found in an older person, because these complications get a "head start" with their damaging effects. Based upon the evidence for adults, strict glycemic control is recommended for children and adolescents with type 2 diabetes, defined as maintaining an A1c <7% and a fasting plasma glucose level (FPG) of <126 mg/dl (6.99 mmo/l).

The initial treatment of type 2 diabetes in youth depends on the clinical presentation. Severe hyperglycemia with hyperosmolar hyperglycemic nonketotic syndrome (HHNS) requires emergency management similar to that for diabetic ketoacidosis. Even after recovery from the acute condition, insulin will likely be needed as ongoing therapy in patients presenting with HHNS. Other patients who are not ill at diagnosis can be initially treated with medical nutrition therapy and exercise (see sections below). Unless there is successful weight loss, most patients will require some form of drug therapy. Currently, insulin and metformin are the only agents approved by FDA for the treatment of type 2 diabetes in children; other agents including sulfonylureas and short-acting secretagogues (repaglinide and nateglinide) have been used to treat pediatric patients. Pharmacologic therapy is initiated in patients who fail to achieve glycemic control three months after the initiation of lifestyle modifications and in patients who are symptomatic at presentation (e.g., polyuria and polydypsia), including those with ketosis.

Indications for initial treatment with insulin include dehydration, ketosis, acidosis, and hyperglycemia $\geq$200 mg/dl and/or an A1C >8.5%. Because patients with type 2 diabetes are insulin resistant, the insulin dose required to restore glycemic control after severe metabolic decompensation may be as high as 2 UI/kg/day. Re-evaluation is necessary as insulin may be tapered with introduction of an oral agent following improvement in metabolic control. Other patients may begin oral agents along with nutrition therapy and exercise. The consensus statement of the ADA recommends that metformin should be the first oral antidiabetes medication used in pediatric patients with type 2 diabetes. Metformin should not be used in patients with known renal disease, hepatic disease, hypoxemic states, severe infections, alcohol abuse, or with radiocontrast material. Liver function studies are needed before beginning metformin treatment. In addition, patients of childbearing age should be cautioned that metformin may normalize anovulatory cycles in patients with polycystic ovary syndrome, a common condition in adolescent females with type 2 diabetes. A further discussion of the use of these antidiabetes medications can be found in Chapter 8. The starting dose for metformin is 500 mg daily with escalation of dosages up to 1000 mg bi-daily over a few weeks. Patients must be cautioned to take metformin with meals to avoid adverse gastro-intestinal effects, particularly involving diarrhea.

In some patients, metformin and lifestyle modifications fail to maintain adequate glycemic control. These patients require additional therapy. Options include insulin therapy or an additional antidiabetes medication, such as a sulfonylurea; or a short-acting insulin secretagogue such as nateglinide or repaglinide, or an α-glucosidase inhibitor. If daily insulin is added to metformin, a long-acting insulin analog (insulin glargine or insulin detemir) can be administrated. These insulin analogs deliver basal insulin and decrease the risk of nocturnal hypoglycemia compared to intermediate-acting insulin (NPH). The starting dose is usually about 0.2 UI/kg/day. Frequent blood glucose monitoring should be encouraged, with a goal of achieving fasting blood glucose levels of < 126 mg/dl. Clinical trials have evaluated the efficacy of different treatment regimen in adults. However, similar data are lacking in children and adolescents. A randomized pediatric trial, called the TODAY study, is now being conducted to determine the efficacy of different treatment regimens for pediatric type 2 diabetes.

Frequency of contact with the primary care provider or healthcare team will depend on the therapeutic response to treatment, but should occur at least quarterly and more often when therapies are being altered. Similar to the treatment of type 1 diabetes, teaching and care by a multidisciplinary team (including an endocrinologist/diabetologist, a nurse educator, a dietitian, and a mental health professional) provide the most ideal setting for the patient and family to acquire the knowledge and skills needed for successful diabetes management. Family involvement is essential to initiate and support the lifestyle changes required in the management of a pediatric patient with type 2 diabetes. Weight reduction resulting from decreased caloric intake and increased energy expenditure improves glycemic control. These lifestyle modifications are crucial components for the successful management of childhood type 2 diabetes and should be initiated in all patients with this disorder.

Monitoring Diabetes Control: General Guidelines for Children and Adolescents

All children and adolescents and their families should receive comprehensive self-management training. Self-monitoring of blood glucose (SMBG) is necessary in order to achieve any of the treatment goals outlined above. Frequency of monitoring should be individualized to the patient's needs but should be recommended at various times of the day. There is a good correlation between frequency of monitoring and glycemic control. Multiple pre- and postprandial blood glucose measurements should be done each day to determine patterns of hypoglycemia and hyperglycemia and to provide data for insulin dose adjustments. Special attention should be addressed to the pre-school and early school-aged child who may be unable to identify and self-report episodes of hypoglycemia. Safe management of these children requires more frequent blood glucose monitoring. A statement of the ADA on care of youth with diabetes published in 2005, recommends testing at least four times a day, and periodically testing post-prandial, before- and after-exercise, and nocturnal glucose levels. Newer technologies are now allowing near continuous blood glucose monitoring. These technologies will provide detailed information about blood glucose fluctuations: extent, duration, and frequency of hyper- or hypoglycemia, relationship of excursions in blood glucose to certain activities or foods, and trend data to help the individual predict and possibly prevent periods of hyper- or hypoglycemia. These devices may hold promise for improved assessment of metabolic control, and one such device is approved for use in pediatric patients ages 7 years old and up.

During periods of acute illness, monitoring frequency should be increased to at least four to six times daily in order to avoid metabolic decompensation such as DKA. Patient training of sick-day management can provide the education needed to prevent or treat severe hyperglycemia and ketosis. Comprehensive ongoing diabetes education, along with access to a 24-hour diabetes help-line, helps prevent metabolic decompensation and DKA in children and adolescents with diabetes. Sick-day rules should be reinforced periodically, especially at the start of the school year and during flu season when illness is more common. New technologies like blood ketone monitoring and real-time continuous glucose sensing may provide opportunities to prevent or reduce the occurrence of DKA in youth with diabetes with potential cost savings.

Children and adolescents with diabetes, especially those treated with insulin, should wear a bracelet, necklace, or tag at all times that identifies them as having diabetes.

Nutrition Education

While often considered by patients the most difficult part of the diabetes treatment regimen, nutrition therapy is an integral component of any management program. Appropriate meal planning enables patients of all ages to optimize glycemic control by matching the injected/infused exogenous insulin with their usual eating and activity habits. Nutrition also contributes to various medical outcomes such as blood glucose levels, lipid levels, blood pressure, renal function, and normal growth and development in children.

As with adults, nutrition therapy for children and adolescents with diabetes must be individualized, provide appropriate nutrition for growth, and match the individual's and family's lifestyle. New nutrition recommendations from the ADA provide increased flexibility. As a member of the diabetes treatment team, a registered dietitian provides nutrition education and counseling. Patients/families with newly diagnosed type 1 diabetes should begin nutrition therapy as soon as the patient is medically stable following the diagnosis. Nutrition follow-up should be incorporated into the patient's continuing medical care every 3 to 6 months in very young children and every 6 to 12 months in older youth.

General nutrition goals are:

- maintain glycemic control goals by balancing food with insulin and activity
- achieve optimal lipid levels
- provide adequate calories for maintaining or attaining acceptable weight for adolescents and normal growth and development rates for children
- prevent and treat acute and long-term complications of diabetes including optimal nutrition for cardiovascular risk factor reduction

Consistency of food intake, especially carbohydrates, is important for the rare child or adolescent who is on fixed insulin regimens and does not adjust premeal insulin dosage. For these youth, carbohydrate, protein, and fat contents of meal plans have to be individualized to achieve optimal metabolic control. There is some evidence that total carbohydrate content of meal and snacks is most important in determining the postprandial glucose response and, thus, in determining the premeal insulin dosage. Youth with multiple daily injection therapy or pump therapy have to be able to adapt their premeal rapid-acting analog dosage to the content of carbohydrate of the meal. The carbohydrate counting method derives from the 1994 ADA Nutrition Recommendation Guidelines, which state the total *amount* of carbohydrate, not the *type* of carbohydrate, impacts glycemic control. There is intermittent interest in the impact on blood glucose levels of the quality of the carbohydrates in the ingested foods, measured as the glycemic index (see Chapter 5).

Advanced carbohydrate counting is used by most of the youth/ families using basal/bolus regimen or insulin pump therapy. An older approach to meal planning used by some youth, is to use the exchange method using food choice lists, which consist of lists of six different exchange groups: bread/starch, milk, meat, fruit, vegetable and fat.

The nutritional requirements of children with diabetes do not differ from those of healthy children. Therefore, nutrient recommendations are based on the needs of healthy children and adolescents. Nutrition therapy requires a caloric and macronutrient prescription. General guidelines for calculating daily calorie requirements are set out in Table 21-3. Protein intake of 10% to 20% is adequate for the general population. The Recommended Dietary Allowance (RDA) for protein ranges from 2.2 gm/kg per day for infants to 0.9 gm/kg per day for adolescent males through age 18 years. Individuals, particularly adolescent males, who exercise and lift weights often, may need additional protein intake, which should be provided in foods rather than as protein supplements or drinks. Carbohydrates and fat should respectively provide 45 to 65% and 30% of the total calories. The National Cholesterol Education Program (NCEP) recommends that persons over 2 years of age limit fat intake to <30% of calories with <10% derived from saturated fat intake. Dietary cholesterol should be limited to <300 mg/day.

Physical Activity Program

The use of physical activity is an important part of the treatment of diabetes. Regular aerobic exercise:

- improves blood glucose control by increasing tissue sensitivity to insulin
- reduces dosage of insulin

TABLE 21-3. Guidelines for Calculating Daily Calorie Requirements

Age	Calorie requirements
0–12 yr	1,000 kcal for 1st yr + 100 kcal/yr over age 1 yr
12–15 yr	
Female	1,500–2,000 kcal + 100 kcal/yr over age 12 yr
Male	2,000–2,500 kcal + 200 kcal/yr over age 12 yr
15–20 yr	
Female	13–15 kcal/lb (29–33 kcal/kg) desired body weight
Male	15–18 kcal/lb (33-40 kcal/kg) desired body weight

Adapted from Nutrition in Medical Management of Insulin-dependent (type I) Diabetes. American Diabetes Association, 1994; pp 57–66.

- reduces cardiovascular risk factors
- serves as an important adjunct for a weight maintenance or a weight reduction diet to promote weight loss
- improves psychological well-being, quality of life, and reduces stress

Stress reduction may have secondary benefits in improving glycemic control by improving adherence with the overall diabetes treatment regimen. The main risk of exercise in the pediatric population is hypoglycemia. Insulin doses may need to be adjusted to avoid this (see below). Exercise involving Valsalva-like movements and high intensity and activity associated with rapid movements of the head may increase the risk of hemorrhage in patients with diabetic proliferative retinopathy, an unusual outcome for pediatric patients.

Self-monitoring of blood glucose (SMBG) before and after exercise is crucial. Physical activity can lower blood glucose levels for patients with normal blood glucose levels or those with moderate hyperglycemia. With extreme hyperglycemia, exercise can exacerbate a hypoinsulinemic state and blood glucose values may actually rise. It is best to avoid exercise in the presence of ketones and/or if blood glucose levels are >300 mg/dl and to treat the ketonemia (ketonuria)/hyperglycemia first. If blood glucose levels are <100 mg/dl prior to exercise, patients should eat a carbohydrate snack to avoid hypoglycemia. Patients should be alert to the symptoms and signs of hypoglycemia during exercise and for several hours thereafter. Patients should have a source of rapidly absorbable carbohydrate (such as glucose tablets or glucose gel) readily available during and after exercise to treat hypoglycemia.

Many healthcare providers suggest avoiding injecting insulin into limbs that will be actively exercised during the time that subcutaneous absorption is expected to occur. Exercise increases the rate of insulin absorption from affected limbs. Insulin doses may need to be decreased on the day of exercise. The amount of decrease necessary varies from patient to patient and is highly individualized. In general, however, mild to moderate exercise may require decreases in the pre-exercise doses of about 20% for rapid-acting insulin and 10% for intermediate-acting insulin. Heavy exercise may require decreases of 30% to 50% for rapid-acting insulin and 20% to 35% for intermediate-acting insulin. It is difficult to make adjustments in long-acting analog for exercise because of its long length of action. For patients treated with insulin pump therapy, temporary basal rates can help manage exercise-related glycemic excursions. Some youth disconnect their pumps for short periods of exercise, generally no more than 1–2 hours. The child may need to bolus a fraction (~50%) of the soon-to-be-missed basal insulin prior to disconnecting from the pump.

Adequate fluid intake is extremely important to avoid dehydration. Alcohol and high doses of salicylates can potentiate exercise-induced hypoglycemia and should be avoided. It is important that activities be chosen that the patient enjoys and finds convenient in order to ensure ongoing participation.

Co-Morbidities In Youth with Diabetes

Nephropathy

The first manifestation of diabetic nephropathy is microalbuminuria, an elevated albumin excretion rate (AER). The presence of persistent microalbuminuria, defined by AER of 20–199 mcg/min, documented in two out of three samples, predicts the future progression to gross proteinuria. Annual screening for microalbuminuria should be initiated once the child is 10 years of age and has had diabetes for 5 years. Confirmed, persistently elevated microalbuminuria should be treated with an ACE inhibitor titrated to normalization of microalbumin excretion if possible. Children may display elevations in urinary albumin excretion related to orthostatic changes; repeating the microalbumin measurement in a first morning sample is recommended.

Hypertension

Hypertension is a common co-morbidity of diabetes, which, in adults, is associated with development of both microvascular and macrovascular disease. Blood pressure determination, using an appropriately sized cuff and with the patient relaxed and seated, should be part of every diabetes physical examination. Hypertension is defined as an average systolic or diastolic blood pressure (measured on at least 3 separate days) ≥95th percentile for age, sex, and height percentile. If elevated blood pressure persists, non-diabetes-associated causes of hypertension should first be excluded. ACE inhibitors are the initial treatment of hypertension in the setting of pediatric diabetes.

Dyslipidemia

Cardiovascular disease, cerebrovascular disease, and peripheral vascular disease resulting from atherosclerosis are leading causes of morbidity and mortality in adults with type 1 diabetes. Factors contributing to atherosclerosis in children and youth, in addition to elevated plasma lipid concentrations, include smoking, hypertension, family history of heart disease and diabetes. If there is a family history of hypercholesterolemia, a history of a cardiovascular event before age 55 years, or if the family history is unknown, screening should proceed in children >2 years of age with a fasting lipid profile following diagnosis (after glucose control has been established), and repeated every five years. Borderline (LDL≥100–129 mg/dl) or abnormal (LDL≥130 mg/dl) values should be repeated for confirmation. If family history is not of concern, the first lipid profile should be performed at puberty. For children with diabetes diagnosed at a pubertal age, a fasting lipid profile should be performed at the time of diagnosis and repeated every five years. Initial therapy of elevated fasting lipid levels consists of optimization of glucose control and medical nutrition therapy; the addition of pharmacologic lipid-lowering agents is strongly recommended for LDL≥160 mg/dl for 6 months or longer.

Retinopathy

Retinopathy is usually not recognized before 5–10 years of diabetes duration. Hypertension, poor metabolic control, presence of albuminuria, hyperlipidemia, smoking, duration of diabetes, and pregnancy all confer increased risk of developing retinopathy. Early identification can lead to appropriate treatment and prevention of loss of vision. The first ophthalmologic examination should be obtained once the child is 10 years of age and/or has had diabetes for 3–5 years. After the initial examination, annual routine follow-up are advised. Often, upon school entry at ages 5 to 6 years, children undergo routine eye examination and this provides an opportunity for education about eye health in the setting of diabetes.

Associated Auto-Immune Conditions

The most common autoimmune disorder associated with type 1 diabetes is autoimmune thyroid disorder, with a prevalence of 17%. Patients with thyroid autoimmunity may be euthyroid, hypothyroid, or hyperthyroid. Hyperthyroidism alters glucose metabolism, potentially resulting in deterioration of metabolic control. Subclinical hypothyroidism has been associated with an increased risk of symptomatic hypoglycemia and with reduced linear growth. Patient with type 1 diabetes should be screened for autoimmune disease shortly after diabetes diagnosis with thyroid antoantibodies and TSH dosages. The presence of thyroid autoantibodies (antithyroid peroxidase and antithyroglobulin) identifies patients at increased risk for thyroid autoimmunity. If TSH is abnormal, thyroid function tests with free T4 can be measured. Thyroid function tests should be also obtained at any time clinical thyroid dysfunction is suspected and in any patient who has thyromegaly.

Patients with type 1 diabetes have a five- to ten-fold increased risk for celiac disease, an immune-mediated disorder that causes malabsorption of nutrients, compared with the general population. In addition to the digestive symptoms of malabsorption, symptoms of celiac disease in patients who also have diabetes may include unpredictable blood glucose levels, unexplained hypoglycemia, and deterioration in glycemic control. Patients with type 1 diabetes should be screened for celiac disease around the time of diagnosis, and subsequently with growth or weight failure, gastroenterological symptoms, or anemia, using assays for IgA to transglutaminase (the more specific) and possibly endomysial autoantibodies, with documentation of normal serum IgA levels.

Adjustment and Psychiatric Disorders

Diabetes is a risk factor for adolescent psychiatric disorders. Compared with adolescents without diabetes or with other chronic conditions, adolescents with diabetes have a three-fold increased risk of psychiatric disorders, with rates as high as 33%. These disorders include major depression (~27.5%) and generalized anxiety disorder (18.4%), rather than psychiatric behavioral disorders. Routine annual screening of psychosocial functioning, especially depression and family coping, should be considered. Youth with difficulties achieving treatment goals or with recurrent DKA should also be screened for psychiatric disorders and eating disorders. Some studies have found rates of both anorexia and bulimia to be higher in youth with type 1 diabetes, while others suggest that adolescents with diabetes are at no higher risk for eating disorders than peers without diabetes. Any adolescent who has poor metabolic control and has recurrent hospitalizations for DKA should be screened for eating disorders by an experienced mental health professional.

Conclusion

The saying that "there is more to pediatrics than just treating small adults" is quite true for the management of diabetes. Many of the habits, goals and attitudes established during childhood diabetes management continue into adulthood and are reflected in a lifetime of diabetes self-care. Thus, treating a child with diabetes can also be thought of as providing the foundation for the treatment of an adult with diabetes. Yet issues of growth and maturation can be reflected in diabetes self-care habits, as diabetes self-care requirements can impact growth and maturation, intensifying the challenges for practitioner, patient and parents. Technological advances now offer patients, families, and healthcare providers new approaches to managing pediatric diabetes with the potential for improved glycemic control and preserved quality of life. The challenge is for all youth with diabetes to get off to a good start!

22

Diabetes in the Older Adult

Medha N. Munshi, MD,
Elizabeth Blair, MSN, APRN,
BC, CDE, and Ramachandiran
Cooppan, MD

Introduction

Treatment of the older adult with diabetes is in many ways no different from treatment of the younger patient. The primary goal is to improve the quality and quantity of life by preventing and/or slowing the onset and progression of the microvascular (retinopathy, nephropathy), macrovascular (coronary, cerebral, and peripheral vascular), and neuropathic (sensory and autonomic neuropathy) complications associated with diabetes. Evidence suggests that poor glycemic control may synergistically interact with other age-related pathology to accelerate diabetic complications, and that optimizing glucose control as well as decreasing other risk factors will decrease the risk for the development of acute and chronic complications associated with diabetes.

At the same time, it is important to consider the "larger picture" with regard to older adults who may have other co-existing medical conditions, multiple medications (polypharmacy), physical disabilities and sometimes limited life expectancy. These conditions may act as barriers to their ability to perform self-care. The risk of hypoglycemia is an important issue in this population as even a mild episode of hypoglycemia can result in falls and injury for older adults.

Diabetes mellitus in older patients is usually type 2, but it can also be type 1. With better treatment of infection and hypertension, and with recent progress in cardiovascular therapy, many patients with type 1 diabetes are living into their 70s with duration of disease of 30 to 40 years. Thus, some people in the older age groups who have diabetes are those with type 1 that were diagnosed much earlier in life. It is crucial to exercise continued vigilance in monitoring their glucose control, screening for and treating early signs of complications and helping them control cardiovascular risk factors.

Pharmacologic treatment of older patients with diabetes often goes beyond familiarity with the use of oral antihyperglycemic medications and insulin and extends to medications to treat coronary heart disease (CHD), hyperlipidemia, hypertension, neuropathy, and more. Moreover, older adults with diabetes are at higher risk of developing co-morbidities like cognitive dysfunction, depression, urinary incontinence, persistent pain, and falls. This combination of conditions, also known as "geriatric syndrome," leads to problems with polypharmacy and functional disabilities. Therefore, familiarity with the patient, the patient's support system, other co-existing medical illnesses as well as his or her view of illness, health and aging will help the provider and the patient decide on an appropriate diabetes treatment plan.

Treatment Goals

Type 2 diabetes can go undiagnosed for years, giving the development of complications a "head start." This, along with increasing life expectancy, puts the older adult at increased risk, over time, for developing complications associated with diabetes. The "conservative" approach with regard to maintaining glucose levels — an approach that often targets levels as high as the low to mid-200s as being acceptable upper limits — in order to avoid symptoms of hypoglycemia or hyperglycemia, or because type 2 diabetes is "mild" diabetes, will further increase the risk of complications. On the other hand, treatment goals are different in a healthy, functionally active older adult in their 70's than one in their 90's, as life expectancy is an important consideration.

In addition, the population of older adults with diabetes is heterogeneous. Some older adults have diabetes of long duration and resultant complications and physical disability, while others may have newly diagnosed diabetes with few co-morbidities, requiring different considerations in accordance with the patient's ability to comply with treatment goals. Certainly the chronically ill, institutionalized patient with a short life expectancy does not require aggressive glucose control but does require adequate control to prevent dehydration, symptoms of hyperglycemia or hypoglycemia, to prevent weight loss and to facilitate healing. Targeting a glucose level in the 200 mg/dl range will prevent such symptoms. However, in the otherwise *healthy* older patient with diabetes, current Joslin Guidelines recommend a preprandial glucose of 80 to 120 mg/dl. Treatment adjustment should occur if the glucose level is less than 80 mg/dl or greater than 140 mg/dl. The goal for the bedtime glucose level is 100 to 150 mg/ dl. Treatment adjustment should occur if the glucose level is less than 100 or greater than 160 mg/dl. The general goal for the A1C is less than 7%.

Hypoglycemia is a major barrier to achieving glycemic goal in an older patient with diabetes. Presenting symptoms of hypoglycemia in older adults can be primarily neuroglycopenic (dizziness, confusion, weakness, etc.) rather than adrenergic (tremors, sweating, palpitation, etc.) and subsequently may remain undiagnosed. Even mild episodes of hypoglycemia can lead to fall and injury, increased risk of cardiovascular or cerebrovascular events or worsening of cognitive dysfunction. In a frail older adult with multiple medical problems, risk of hypoglycemia may outweigh benefits of tight glycemic control. Targets should be adjusted upwards for such patients, and particularly those with a history of recurrent or unrecognized hypoglycemia and for patients of very advanced age.

Screening for and Diagnosing Diabetes

Individuals age 45 years and older should be screened for diabetes, as outlined in Chapter 2. If the screening glucose level is normal, it should be repeated every three years. Testing should be initiated *earlier* or carried out *more frequently* for patients at higher risk for developing diabetes. The recommended screen is a fasting serum glucose. If a fasting glucose cannot be obtained, a random glucose level can be done. If the random glucose value is 160 mg/dl or more, further evaluation is necessary with either a fasting glucose level or an OGTT (oral glucose tolerance test). Diabetes can be diagnosed if the patient, on two separate occasions, has a fasting level of ≥126 mg/dl *or* a 2-hour value on an OGTT of ≥200 mg/dl *or* a random glucose level ≥200 mg/dl associated with symptoms of hyperglycemia.

The ADA's reliance on a fasting plasma glucose may be problematic with regard to older patients, as they tend to have more postprandial hyperglycemia early in the disease, which could be a reflection of early first-phase insulin secretory defects that can lead to type 2 diabetes. Thus, a diagnosis may be missed if the fasting glucose is used as the only screening test. In fact, an OGTT may be needed to make the early diagnosis of diabetes in high risk older patients or in patients with fasting glucose value between normal and diabetic range.

Because many older people have physiological changes in renal and hepatic function, they may not have the typical symptoms associated with diabetes. Infections, neuropathic pain, and failure to thrive may be the only clues to consider the diagnosis. This is especially so in the nursing home population. Diabetic neuropathy can present as painful distal polyneuropathy or as amyotrophy. This latter condition is associated with proximal muscle wasting, weakness and weight loss. It is seen mainly in the older patient with diabetes and needs to be recognized. In many cases, a work-up for malignant disease is undertaken because of the profound weight loss that can occur. The presence of an autonomic neuropathy can affect bladder and bowel function and lead to supine hypertension and orthostatic hypotension. These varied neuropathic manifestations of diabetes affect the quality of life of the patient and also become important when considering medication use for other diseases as well as for the neuropathy. For example, the use of tricyclic antidepressants for painful neuropathy can cause drowsiness and dry mouth and can worsen orthostasis and constipation.

Older adults with diabetes also have increased risk of common geriatric conditions such as cognitive dysfunction, depression, chronic pain, urinary incontinence, falls and functional disabilities. When assessing the patient in this age group, it is important to screen for common geriatric syndrome as recommended by the American Geriatric Society. Additional evaluation during clinical assessment with history and physical examination may include:

- nutritional assessment with special emphasis on unintended weight loss
- functional assessment including gait and balance evaluation
- psychological assessment including screening for cognitive function and depression
- chronic pain assessment

Co-existing medical conditions:

Cognitive dysfunction — Both type 1 and type 2 diabetes are assotciated with increased risk of cognitive dysfunction. Subtle decline in cognitive function may remain unrecognized by family as well as healthcare providers. Older patients with these conditions may have difficulty understanding instructions and following complicated diabetes regimen. These patients are at increased risk of hypoglycemia and resultant morbidities. Brief screening tests like the MMSE and the clock drawing test can be useful in screening for cognitive dysfunction. Older patients presenting with deterioration of glycemic control and/or frequent episodes of hypoglycemia should be screened for cognitive dysfunction before nonadherence is assumed.

Depression — Older adults with diabetes are at higher risk of developing depression when compared to an age-matched control group. The treatment of depression may increase compliance and glycemic control along with overall quality of life for older adults. Screening tools like the Geriatric Depression Scale may help identify depressed patients because older adults are less likely to volunteer such information,

Functional disabilities and falls — Older adults with diabetes have a higher risk of functional disabilities. They may have difficulty performing activities of daily living (bathing, toileting, eating, dressing, and grooming) as well as instrumental activities of daily living (traveling, shopping, using the telephone, managing finances, doing housework, and taking medications). Individuals with these disabilities may require assistance from other caregivers or family members to implement tasks such as home glucose monitoring, giving insulin injections, meal preparation and following a physical activity regimen. Consulting with a social worker may help establish a support network for such patients.

Falls, especially the ones resulting in injury, are also more common in older adults. The etiology of falls for the elderly with diabetes is multifactorial and includes conditions such as functional disability; gait and balance difficulty; loss of vision and/or hearing; complications of diabetes, such as peripheral or autonomic neuropathy; or other co-existing medical conditions like arthritis. Even a mild episode of hypoglycemia in a frail individual can result in falls and injury. Patients who are afraid of falling are usually reluctant to follow physical activity recommendations. Referral to an exercise physiologist and a supervised program for physical activity may help such patients lower their risk of falling.

Urinary incontinence and chronic pain — Increased risk of urinary incontinence in older patients with diabetes, especially women, is also multifactorial in etiology. The contributing factors include increased frequency of UTI, vaginal atrophy and/or infection and complications of diabetes like autonomic neuropathy leading to neurogenic bladder or fecal impaction. These conditions can be exacerbated by uncontrolled diabetes causing polyuria. Urinary incontinence frequently remains undiagnosed because women do not volunteer the information. Identifying and treating this condition may improve the quality of life for such women.

Chronic pain is also more prevalent in older adults with diabetes. Chronic pain can be secondary to co-exisisting conditions or complications of diabetes such as neuropathy. Pain is considered to be a fifth vital sign by many experts and evaluation and management of pain is recommended to improve the overall quality of life for older adults.

Diabetes in the Older Adult: Not Always Type 2

Once diabetes is diagnosed, the provider needs to decide if the patient has type 1 or 2 diabetes. *Typically,* the type 2 patient is obese, over 40 years of age and has a gradual onset of symptoms of hyperglycemia. Due to the gradual onset of symptoms and delays in seeking healthcare, older adults may present with markedly elevated glucose levels, profound dehydration (worsened by the older adult's decreased thirst sensation), impaired sensorium and a lack of ketones. This life-threatening state is known as a hyperosmolar hyperglycemic state (HHS). These patients require immediate hospitalization for hydration, short-term insulin therapy and the correction of the precipitating event. Precipitating events include use of glucocorticoids, peritoneal dialysis, infection or an acute event such as an MI or CVA.

The patient with type 1 diabetes is *typically* under 40 years of age, lean, has a rapid onset of symptoms, and may have ketonuria. However, type 1 diabetes can occur at any age and can occur in the obese patient. The onset of symptoms of hyperglycemia in the older adult with type 1 may occur in the typical, rapid fashion. However, quite often they develop more slowly and without ketonuria, making an accurate diagnosis difficult. Although some patients will seemingly achieve glycemic goal initially using oral treatments, ultimately, and over varying time frames, these patients may not maintain optimal control and may progress to insulin therapy. If the older adult is experiencing a rapid onset of polyuria, polydypsia, polyphonies, and weight loss associated with an elevated glucose level, the provider must also consider a secondary underlying diagnosis such as pancreatic cancer or other illness. Similarly, if a person with previously well-controlled type 2 diabetes develops marked elevations in glucose levels without a change in program adherence, other underlying pathology as well as secondary oral therapy insufficiency need to be considered.

Nutrition

The foundation for treating type 1 and type 2 diabetes is a plan for medical nutrition therapy, an exercise program, and an SMBG program. The patient should be seen by a dietitian to assess nutritional needs. It is important to remember that older adults are at increased risk of unintentional weight loss, which puts them at increased risk of morbidity and mortality. Other barriers to consider before formulating nutritional therapy plans are long-term dietary habits, the impact of the use of multiple medications, changes in taste perception, difficulty obtaining appropriate food and/or the ability to prepare or cook it, and financial constraints. As finances affect the food choices of many older adults, a dietitian can help maximize the patient's "nutrition dollar" as well as establish a nutrition plan that can minimize glucose excursions, decrease risk factors such as elevated lipids and help maintain or achieve a reasonable weight. *Ideally,* to limit glucose excursions, the patient should have meals and snacks spaced throughout the day. If the patient is treated with insulin, snacks should coincide with the peak time of insulin action.

The use of the food pyramid is often a good starting point to review healthy eating habits. Explaining portion control of carbohydrates and fats rather than eliminating foods, as well as considering current eating habits, may help increase program adherence (see Chapter 5).

Other nutritional issues arise in long-term treatment facilities where malnutrition is a common problem. With this comes dehydration and increased risk for infection and bedsores. These patients present greater challenges with nutritional needs because of changes in taste as well as differences in food preferences and cooking. In the setting of chronic care, the current trend is to distribute the carbohydrate throughout the day, using some portion in all meals as well as snacks, allowing consistency in the diet on an ongoing basis and avoiding the effect on blood glucose of large loads of carbohydrate. This makes for better diabetes control in this particular setting.

Physical Activity

Physical activity remains an important component of health maintenance for most adults, as it can effectively lower glucose levels in patients with type 1 and 2 diabetes. It also has well-documented cardiovascular, peripheral vascular, weight control and lipid benefits. Further, older patients may have an increased risk for osteoporosis, and weight-bearing exercises can help maintain bone density. Muscle strengthening and conditioning can also improve gait and balance and lower the risk of falls in elderly patients. Since regular physical activity has so many benefits, it is important to encourage patients to participate in a regular program.

A program of strenuous physical activity should be initiated only after the completion of a complete history and physical exam. The assessment should include an electrocardiogram and a stress test if a rigorous exercise program is planned, as the presence or absence of complications will influence the design of the program. Patients with diabetes are at risk for CHD characterized by atypical angina, due in part, to autonomic neuropathy. A baseline EKG should be done and an ETT, often using thallium, should be strongly considered. In most older adults gradual activity like walking, as tolerated, can be prescribed safely without additional investigations.

If the patient is suspected of having had undiagnosed diabetes for a considerable period of time, he or she is likely to have some degree of peripheral sensory neuropathy. Moderate to severe neuropathy can effect proprioception and balance and contribute to the development of structural foot deformities. Long-term diabetes also increases the risk for peripheral vascular disease with claudication, which may limit exercise duration. As patients with active proliferative retinopathy may precipitate a hemorrhage with strenuous activity, input from an ophthalmologist will be needed. The severity of retinopathy, neuropathy, peripheral vascular disease, and CHD will influence the choice of physical activities. For many older adults, starting with chair exercises or a brief daily walk is an appropriate low-stress activity. Chair exercises may also be recommended for patients who are at increased risk of falls or are afraid of falling.

It is necessary to have a careful understanding of the effects of exercise on blood glucose, especially in relation to the medication being used for glucose control. This is very important when insulin is being used for control, because hypoglycemia may occur, either during the exercise, immediately after, or up to 6 to 8 hours later. Therefore appropriate dose adjustment is needed if the patient plans to engage in a regular program. See Chapter 6 for a detailed discussion of physical activity.

When starting a physical activity program, the principles of daily foot care should be reviewed with the patient. Wearing supportive, properly fitting shoes, moisturizing dry feet, as well as checking the feet daily for signs of friction or pressure, will help decrease the risk of foot injury, ulceration and potential foot infection.

Monitoring

SMBG should be taught to all patients with diabetes. The results help both the patient and the provider assess the effectiveness of treatment. Co-existing medical conditions like cognitive dysfunction, visual impairment, arthritis and low dexterity should be taken in to account before counseling older adults about self-monitoring. Devices such as talking meters for the visually impaired and large meters for patients with arthritis should be considered in such instances.

Glucose goals should be shared with the patient and a plan created if goals are not achieved. The frequency of glucose checking will be influenced by the intensity of the program, finances, the patient's cognitive and physical abilities and resulting adherence. In many cases, checking the fasting and presupper or bedtime glucose levels is adequate. Block testing may be helpful, where patients check glucose levels at a lower frequency most of the time, and then choose two to four consecutive, typical days per month to check more intensively, perhaps up to four to six times daily, to get a better sense as to the patterns. In more intensive programs, premeal, 2 hours after meals and bedtime checking is needed most days. Chapter 3 has more details on monitoring programs.

Pharmacotherapy

When medical nutrition therapy, physical activity, weight loss and lifestyle changes no longer control the blood glucose or allow the patient to meet his or her goals, consideration has to be given to the use of hypoglycemic therapies. Broadly, there is a choice between non-insulin antidiabetes medications, most, but not all of which are taken orally, and insulin injections. Most physicians and patients prefer to use the orally administered medications as the first-line therapy, which is appropriate provided the patient does not have absolute insulin deficiency and/or significant glucotoxicity, requiring insulin treatment.

An occasional patient with new-onset type 1 diabetes in this age group will need insulin from the outset. Those patients with type 2 diabetes who are very symptomatic or have significant hyperglycemia and glucose toxicity (glucose >350–400 mg/dl) at presentation will need insulin initially to establish control. In these cases it may be possible to later change the patient to an oral antidiabetes medication once the glucose levels are controlled and the effects of glucose toxicity have resolved.

In choosing treatment, especially the oral medication, care must be given to a number of factors such as renal and hepatic function, use of other medications, concomitant illnesses, and the goals set for the individual patient. The patient's mental status and living circumstances are also important factors to be assessed. Complicated treatments are bound to fail — and may even cause harm — if the patient cannot follow the instructions given.

Antidiabetes Medications

The selection of antidiabetes medications has been the subject of much attention recently with the growing list of available drugs. Recently developed medications target specific defects in the glucose metabolic axis and may work through previously untargeted mechanisms. One new medication, exenatide, must be given by injection, similar to insulin. A detailed discussion of the use of these medications can be found in Chapter 8. Most of the information therein is applicable to older people with diabetes requiring such treatments.

When choosing an antidiabetes medication for use in an older patient, there are several factors to consider. One is the risk of hypoglycemia. This complication of therapy may be annoying to a younger individual, but it is often more dangerous in an older person due to the resulting physiologic stress impacting other conditions, the potential for falls leading to injury, exacerbation of dysfunction from previous strokes, and reduced visual acuity and mental capacity leading to functional difficulties, particularly while driving. Not all antidiabetes medications have the same risk of causing hypoglycemia, and a review of the details outlined in Chapter 8 should be used in guiding selection.

A common approach to treatment is the use of combination therapies, including the newer combination tablets. Combination treatments, in theory, will achieve better control using two or more medications. A lesser amount of each medication is needed and multiple pathophysiologic abnormalities are addressed. Careful balancing of medication dosing can reduce the risk of hypoglycemia. In addition, the use of the pre-set combination tablets improves adherence and also reduces the risk of dosage errors.

Other important treatment risks to consider when selecting medications for older individuals include potential adverse drug effects, drug-to-drug interactions, costs and program adherence related to dosing frequency.

There are seven classes of antidiabetes medicastions now available for use in diabetes. These include the sulfonylureas (both first and second generation), biguanides (e.g., metformin), α-glucosidase inhibitors (e.g., acarbose and miglitol), meglitinides (repaglinide), the thiazolidinediones (rosiglitazone and pioglitazone), the D-phenylalanine derivatives (nateglinide), and the incretin mimetics (the injectable exenatide, and another class likely to be on the market shortly, the DPP-IV inhibitors). Each class of drugs has unique actions and variable dose responses that should be understood. These drugs are discussed more fully in the chapter on pharmacotherapy of type 2 diabetes (see Chapter 8). A few points about their use in this older age group are worth making, however.

When advising the older patient regarding oral medications, it is still a good principle to start with a low dose and gradually increase to the effective therapeutic level. This approach will avoid overmedication and also reduce the number of adverse reactions and potential drug interactions. Most elderly patients have postprandial hyperglycemia, especially in the early stages of their diabetes. In these cases, a drug that works to address this abnormality, such as a short-acting insulin secretagogue repaglinide or nateglinide, or an α-glucosidase inhibitor (e.g., acarbose or miglitol) might be a reasonable choice. The gastrointestinal side effects of the latter class, however, may limit usefulness in the older patient. Starting with a small dose and making slow dose increases can improve tolerance to these drugs. The advantage of repaglinide and nateglinide is that they are taken just before a meal, and if there is a delay or the patient does not want to eat, then the drug is either given later or held if no calories are ingested. These short-acting medications are given before each meal. Therefore, if a meal is skipped or added, a dose of the medication can be skipped or added, respectively. The dose may also be adjusted if a patient has a variable appetite. This approach is especially useful in frail nursing home patients with variable food intake. These two medications are not chemically related to sulfonylureas, therefore they can be used instead of a sulfonylurea in the setting of a sulfa allergy. However, these drugs cost more than a generic sulfonylurea and need frequent administration by the patient, increasing the likelihood that a dose will be forgotten.

The longer-acting sulfonylureas can also be used with older patients, as long as one is cognizant of the main concern, that of hypoglycemia. This is lessened when smaller doses can be used and titrated to the individual's need such as with low-dose glipizide GITS, glimepiride, and the smaller doses available in the tablets of glyburide in combination with metformin. In general, one should remember that the elderly patient may not exhibit the typical signs of hypoglycemia, and the diagnosis can be missed. Similarly, they may take longer to recover from mental status changes caused by hypoglycemia.

When using metformin, care must be taken to measure the serum creatinine before starting the drug. The problem with creatinine measurements in this age group is that persons with small muscle mass can have normal or high normal levels and still have significant renal dysfunction by more formal testing. Close monitoring of serum creatinine is recommended in older adults who are started on metformin therapy. Lactic acidosis is a rare complication with metformin use, but there is a very high mortality when it occurs. If patients are carefully selected, excluding those with renal or hepatic dysfunction, pharmacologically treated CHF, or severe lung disease, this can be a good therapy for the overweight, dyslipidemic patient. In some patients, metformin can be associated with weight loss that can be severe, and care must be taken to monitor for this, especially in the non-obese patient. Metformin can be used if the fasting plasma glucose is 200 to 300 mg in an obese and dyslipidemic patient.

The thiazolidinediones are a class of oral antidiabetes medications that increase insulin sensitivity. The two thiazolidinediones that are available, pioglitazone and rosiglitazone, appear to be safe with liver function monitoring even in older patients. This group of drugs does not pose risk of hypoglycemia, making them an excellent choice for older patient with high risk of hypoglycemia and its complications. However, these medications do cause fluid retention, and are contraindicated in people with New York Heart Association Class 3 or 4 cardiac status. And, keep in mind that the fluid retention can also lead to congestive heart failure even if there is no pre-treatment diagnosis. While not a contraindication to use, this concern does lead to the suggestion that cardiac function should be monitored, particularly around the time of drug initiation and titration. Also, at this writing, a meta-analysis of rosiglitazone use is suggestive of increased cardiovascular risk, a risk not apparent with pioglitazone. It is expected that ongoing FDA review and study will clarify this concern in the near future.

The incretin-mimetic medication, exenatide, is useful for older individuals as well, provided they are able to self-inject twice daily (see Chapter 8). It does have a tendency to promote weight loss, which may be useful in the overweight individual. The DPP-IV inhibitors, are oral incretin mimetics but without as much weight loss potential. These agents do not cause hypoglycemia and are weight neutral, making them attractive for use in older patients.

It is now clear that most patients with type 2 diabetes will benefit from the initiation of combination therapy sooner rather than later. The most

important factors in making choices will be the degree of β-cell dysfunction as well as current renal and hepatic function. Multiple combinations
are available to use, and the choice depends on the individual patient and
the goals set for control. Details on the different combinations are presented in the chapter on therapies for type 2 diabetes (see Chapter 8). In
using combination treatments in the elderly patient, care must be taken to
balance the advantages of multidrug therapy with the disadvantages of
treatments with multiple drugs requiring dosing throughout the day, as
many older patients can have a problem with polypharmacy and adherence to therapy.

Insulin

When antidiabetes medication therapies no longer can achieve the degree
of blood glucose control that is desired, insulin therapy will be needed. In
using insulin with older patients, we should not compromise the approach, based on age alone. Some patients will need multiple injections,
especially those with long-standing type 1 diabetes. While hypoglycemia
is a serious issue, it can be handled by setting realistic goals for control.
The availability of premixed insulin, pen devices, and other injection aids
can help facilitate the process in those patients with dexterity or visual
problems. It is important to assess timing of meals with insulin peak action, because meals can be late and hypoglycemia can be a problem.

Insulin treatment has to be individualized and monitored carefully
with regular follow-up to make changes before serious problems occur.
For older patients, adding a bedtime dose of basal insulin can be a good
way of initiating insulin therapy in cases of inadequacy of therapy using
antidiabetes medication. Similarly, those who had avoided the complex
physiologic basal/bolus programs might now accept them and benefit
from their flexibility since they can use basal insulin at bedtime and
premeal rapid-acting insulin delivered by a pen device. Details on insulin
therapy are presented in Chapters 9 and 10.

It is important to remember that an older adult's ability to manage a
complicated insulin regimen may change with increasing age or worsening overall health. Physical and/or mental capacity may decline over a
period of time and therefore the benefit/burden of tight glycemic control,
especially with a complicated regimen, should be periodically assessed in
older adults.

Screening for and Treating Complications Associated with Diabetes

People, including those who have diabetes, are living considerably longer. Although it is important to consider life expectancy of an individual before formulating treatment goals, many older adults are healthy and would benefit from risk factor management and preventive strategies for complications of diabetes.

Retinopathy should be screened for at the time of diagnosis of type 2 diabetes and after 3 to 5 years of having type 1 diabetes. If retinopathy is diagnosed at the time diabetes is diagnosed, assume the patient has had diabetes for at least 6 to 10 years. In addition to an ophthalmologic evaluation and the vision-saving potential of laser surgery, optimal glucose and blood pressure control can slow the progression of retinopathy. If retinopathy is noted, one should also look for the presence of nephropathy, another microvascular complication.

The earliest sign of nephropathy is microalbuminuria. All patients should be screened for microalbuminuria at the time of diagnosis of type 2 diabetes and after 5 years of type 1 diabetes. The progression of nephropathy in type 2 diabetes is slower than in type 1. Optimal treatment of type 1 patients with microalbuminuria, with or without hypertension, includes optimal glucose and blood pressure control and the use of ACE inhibitors. Studies clearly show the renal protective effects of adding an ACE inhibitor. Because of the slower progression of microalbuminuria to nephropathy in type 2 diabetes, the use of an ACE inhibitor in the normotensive patient has not been well substantiated. However, the results of the HOPE trial give added impetus to aggressive treatment (see Chapter 14). If micro-albuminuria progresses or hypertension develops, an ACE inhibitor should be added. Use caution, however, if the patient is on a potassium-sparing diuretic or on potassium supplement. Changing the diuretic or decreasing or discontinuing the potassium supplement may be necessary. More frequent monitoring of renal function test and serum potassium level is recommended for older adults when such changes in regimen or doses are made. Details on these issues can be found in Chapter 14.

The presence of microalbuminuria is also a marker for CHD. As noted previously, the older adult should have a baseline EKG. The value of an

ETT in all older patients is not clear. Treatment of CHD includes optimal glucose and blood pressure control, smoking cessation, exercise and reduction of lipid levels. Poor glycemic control is an important predictor of CHD. Due to the altered coagulation state found in patients with diabetes, unless there are contraindications, daily aspirin should be recommended for patients with evidence of macrovascular disease or with macrovascular risk factors.

Lipids should also be evaluated. Elevated lipids are associated with an increased risk for CAD and are an independent risk factor for retinopathy in the elderly. Current Joslin Clinical Guidelines recommend an LDL of less than 100 mg/dl, or even lower in high risk individuals (see Chapter 15). Target levels for LDL have been decreasing in recent years as the benefits of aggressive lipid therapy have become known.

Keep in mind that management of diabetes that includes treatment of hyperglycemia and risk factor management, as discussed above, puts older patients at risk of polypharmacy. These medications in addition to treatment for other co-existing medical conditions may overwhelm older patients and increase their risk for medication side-effects, renal-hepatic dysfunction and drug interactions. There is also evidence that for older adults, as the number of medications increases, the patient's ability to comply with a medication regimen decreases. This should be kept in mind when deciding overall goals for older adults and their medication list should be kept current and reviewed at each visit.

Conclusion

Diabetes is a complex disease with far-reaching implications for the patient. As the person with diabetes ages, treatment decisions become more complex especially, in the setting of concomitant illness. The healthcare provider must look beyond "just" the glucose level and continue to screen for and treat complications and risk factors associated with diabetes. In addition, co-existing conditions like cognitive dysfunction, depression and physical disabilities should be identified so that the best management plan that patients can follow can be formed. Achieving the best glycemic control without putting the patient at risk of hypoglycemia can be a good strategy for establishing treatment goals in this age group. One needs to remember that learning new skills may be difficult for older patients because of other disease processes, so for some patients, giving them small, simple steps to follow may be better. Group classes are also useful, as is involving family members and caretakers in the process. Also, poor eyesight and changes in dexterity are important issues to these patients and must be addressed in order to make treatment a success.

All that being said, many older patients are very motivated, able and willing to participate in their care, and their chronological age becomes less of a factor in treatment design. We are living longer and healthier, and the calendar should not override good clinical judgment in developing an individualized approach for each patient.

Suggested Reading

Samos L, Roos B. diabetes mellitus in older persons. *Medical Clinics of North Am* 1998; 82(4):791–801.

The Diabetes Control and Complications Trial Research Group. The effect of intensive treatment of diabetes on the development and progression of long term complications in insulin-dependent diabetes mellitus. *New England J Med.* 1993; 329:977–986.

American Diabetes Association. Implication of the United Kingdom Prospective Diabetes Study. *Diabetes Care* 2001; 242 (Supp. 1):S28–S32.

American Diabetes Association. Standards of Medical Care in Diabetes — 2006. *Diabetes Care* 29:S4–S42, 2006.

Morleey, J. The elderly type 2 diabetic patient: special considerations. *Diabetic Medicine.* 1998;15 (4):S41–S46.

Brown, A. F., et al., *Guidelines for improving the care of the older person with diabetes mellitus.* J Am Geriatr Soc, 2003. 51(5 Suppl Guidelines): p. S265–80.

23

Psychological Issues in the Treatment of Diabetes

Barbara J. Anderson, PhD, CDE and
Abigail K. Mansfield, MA

Introduction

The treatment of diabetes involves more than just correction of metabolic abnormalities and extends beyond the prevention of this condition's feared complications. People with diabetes have a chronic disease, one that will be with them for the rest of their lives, and one that they cannot easily ignore for any extended period of time. Every aspect of their lives is intertwined with the treatment of their disease.

Not surprisingly, the impact of diabetes on the psychological status of a patient, as well as the impact of a patient's mental health on his or her diabetes, must be addressed as an important component of the treatment of diabetes. Failure to do so will potentially reduce the efficacy of other metabolically focused treatment modalities and negatively impact the quality of life for the patient.

This chapter traces the mental health needs of people with diabetes throughout the lifecycle of their condition, beginning with diagnosis and extending through the many years of treatment. It is incumbent on all healthcare professionals who interact with a person having diabetes to be cognizant of the patient's mental health needs and to forge supportive relationships with that individual. Such relationships, in turn, can foster healthy behaviors.

One must also recognize that there are obstacles to diabetes care and self-management. Often, the primary care provider is best equipped to recognize such obstacles and to work with patients to overcome them effectively. On occasion, help from mental health professionals may also be needed to assist in addressing the needs of these individuals, to provide support and intervention to address both the impact of diabetes on the psyche and the influence of the psyche on the diabetes.

Diagnosis and Ongoing Support

Supporting Patients through the Crisis of Diagnosis

The diagnosis of diabetes is a period of crisis for many individuals and their families. Patients and family members face two complex and often conflicting tasks — to begin grieving the loss of health and a spontaneous lifestyle and to learn the complex new language and skills involved in managing diabetes. The discovery of a chronic illness can trigger strong emotions and stir up existing emotional problems. For this reason, it is important to screen patients carefully at diagnosis to identify the following:

Patient's developmental stage: Determine the expected developmental tasks for the patient's stage in the life cycle (see Table 23-1).

Patient's coping style: Determine how patient and family members have handled other medical crises.

Mental health history of patient/family members: Ask about current or past mental health diagnoses, especially depression, anxiety disorders, and learning problems. Find out if the patient is currently receiving, or has received, mental health treatment.

Current life stresses that are potential psychosocial barriers to effective diabetes management: Screen for financial problems, other health/ mental health problems, health insurance problems, educational/

learning problems, a recent move, job stresses, marriage and family conflicts, etc.

Previous exposure and experience with diabetes: Many patients and families only know out-of-date "horror stories" based on older family members or friends who suffered from diabetes complications. Assess how a patient's experiences with diabetes may impact his or her adjustment to it.

Emotions Commonly Seen at Diagnosis

Sadness. Feelings of sadness are very normal at diagnosis, as patients and family members begin the necessary process of mourning the loss of health. Typical behaviors include crying, withdrawal, lack of interest in sleeping or eating, and anger at healthcare providers or hospital staff. When these feelings and behaviors last more than a month, the patient should be referred to a mental health professional who is familiar with diabetes and depression.

Anxiety. Feelings of distress, anxious thoughts, and increased worrying are also commonly seen at diagnosis. Patients and family members may pace, talk fast, ask the same questions over and over, seem unable to concentrate and learn, and express concern over every decision that is made about treatment. If this level of anxiety persists for more than a month, the patient should be referred to a mental health professional who is skilled in treating patients with diabetes and anxiety disorders.

Denial. Many patients and family members initially show feelings of disbelief about the diagnosis of diabetes or try to minimize the reality of its onset. These efforts to deny the diagnosis are very normal initially, but if denial continues, it can interfere with effective learning and disease management. It is important for healthcare providers to be straightforward about the diagnosis. Especially when a patient is diagnosed with type 2 diabetes, providers should *not* state that the patient has "borderline diabetes" or "a touch of sugar" or the "mild kind" of diabetes.

Sensitive pacing of information to be learned is another important strategy for preventing denial. Many patients become overwhelmed in dealing with their grief and the new medical language and technical skills that they must learn immediately. It is important to be realistic about what patients are expected to learn and master at diagnosis. Focusing on "sur-

TABLE 23-1. Development and Diabetes

When working with patients with diabetes, it is very important to keep their developmental stage in mind. What follows is a table that charts normal developmental stages and how diabetes may impact these stages. Bear in mind that individuals age differently, so while we have listed approximate ages for each stage, the ages and stages, and life events may not fit all individuals.

Stage of Development	Normal Tasks of Development	Implications and Tasks for Diabetes Management
Childhood 0–11 years	Develop bond with parents. Develop sense of self, test bond with parents. Learn to make own choices. Socialize with others outside of family. Feel secure outside home. Fit-in with peers.	Learn to work as a team around diabetes tasks, with parents shouldering most of the responsibility. Attention to diabetes care will have to be balanced with the need to be like other children and to do what they're doing.
Adolescence 12–18 years	Explore autonomy within context of safety. Develop core values. Begin development of sexual orientation and identity.	Teens with diabetes will need to have support with diabetes tasks as they explore independence and autonomy. The need for parent-teen inter-dependence and continual support with diabetes tasks is strong.
Young Adulthood 19–29 years	Develop intimate relationships. Develop professional identity. Further develop sexual orientation and identity, especially for women.	Tell colleagues, friends and lovers about diabetes. Negotiate physical intimacy within the context of diabetes. Maintain support for diabetes care in a culture that glorifies independence and self-sufficiency.
Adulthood 30–65 years	Sustain intimate relationships and continue professional development. Parenting.	Incorporate diabetes care into intimate relationships. Continue to receive support for diabetes care. Prioritize diabetes self-care even when other family members and children need attention and care. This may be especially difficult for women.
Older Adulthood 65+ years	Transition to retirement. Establish new roles and activities Develop compassion towards parents and children. Tolerate physical and cognitive changes of the aging process. Discover meaningful purpose for the remainder of life.	Identify barriers to self-care—i.e., can patient see well enough to draw up insulin or dose oral medications? When necessary, make small, incremental changes in diabetes care routine. For some people, adulthood and older adulthood may involve adjusting to some of the long-term complications of diabetes.

vival skills" at this stage will help many patients become more quickly engaged in learning to manage their disease.

Guilt and Blame. Guilt and blame are negative feelings that can hinder a patient's ability to cope and family members' capacity to make lifestyle adjustments. Feeling guilty is a very common response to the diagnosis of both type 1 and type 2 diabetes. With regard to type 2 diabetes, there is a common misconception that solely the person's eating habits, especially eating too many sweets, caused diabetes. If this misconception is not addressed at diagnosis, the patient may feel guilty and/or family members may blame the patient or themselves for the disease. The ramifications of guilt and blame can undermine the crucial support networks that are integral to effective and sustained diabetes care. Thus, it is important for primary care providers to foster support by encouraging patients and family members to look forward, not backward.

When a person is diagnosed with type 1 diabetes, it is very important to make three points clear to the patient and family:

1. Type 1 diabetes is caused by an interaction of genetic predisposition factors and environmental trigger factors.
2. Nothing the patient and/or parents did caused the diagnosis of type 1 diabetes.
3. Although researchers are investigating the prevention and causes of type 1 diabetes, currently there is no way to prevent it.

Doctors and healthcare providers can help support patients through the crisis of diabetes by being aware of the aforementioned responses to the disease, and by being sure to:

- screen the patient/family for depression, anxiety, and learning problems
- identify psychosocial barriers to effective diabetes management in the patient's environment
- provide straightforward information about the diagnosis and a realistic discussion of disease management, addressing patient/family concerns and questions
- pace information so that patient/family do not become overwhelmed

- inform the patient about new advances in treatment of diabetes and prevention of complications
- normalize initial feelings of sadness, denial or anxiety
- refer to a mental health provider familiar with diabetes if strong emotions persist for one month beyond diagnosis

Supporting the Person with Diabetes after Diagnosis

It is imperative that all patients have consistent and reliable social, medical, and emotional support, both at diagnosis and beyond. Paradoxically, American cultural values such as independence and self-sufficiency often prove to be detrimental when applied to diabetes management. Such expectations of independence and self-sufficiency contribute to a dynamic in which the person with diabetes is completely alone with his or her disease. Sadly, this dynamic in turn leads to diminished attention to diabetes care. There is a great deal of research that shows that patients who have strong support networks adjust better to life with diabetes, both physically and emotionally, than those who do not.

In addition, because diabetes care demands a great deal of time and energy both in the doctor's office and at home, two sources of support are important: medical and family support. Patients need strong medical support to help :

- know how/when/why to check blood glucose levels and administer medications
- learn about sick-day management, sliding scales, exercise, carbohydrate counting and meal planning, weight loss, and reduction of other risk factors to good health
- problem-solve around the broad range of questions that all new patients inevitably have about lifestyle, behavior change and safety

In the same way that patients benefit from a cooperative approach to medical care, so too do they benefit from a supportive approach to diabetes care outside of a medical setting. A life-long condition that demands daily energy and attention, diabetes is not a "do-it-yourself" disease. People with diabetes need support from family members and friends for all of the following reasons:

- to help with the timing and work of daily diabetes tasks like giving insulin, taking medication and checking blood glucose
- to recognize and respond to the signs of severe low blood glucose and extreme high blood glucose
- to listen to and support the person with diabetes through the highs and lows that predictably come with adjusting to life with a chronic disease

Diabetes requires involvement and support from medical personnel, family and friends. No one with diabetes should be expected to "go it alone."

Avoiding "Miscarried Helping"

Support from family and friends helps patients cope with the complex disease of diabetes and its management; likewise, primary care providers can help families help the patient. But without specific guidance from medical providers, family members who mean well and try to help often achieve precisely the opposite. Misguided attempts at helping often result in undermining patients' sense of control or competence in diabetes management. "Miscarried helping" is the term that describes family involvement that becomes destructive and undermines the patient's attempts at healthy diabetes self-care. The overall goal in encouraging families to help the patient is to provide help that feels positive and supportive to the patient (see Table 23-1) "Miscarried helping" happens when the support attempts of family members (or friends) fail because they are excessive, untimely, or inappropriate. Examples of "miscarried helping" include:

- *second-guessing* or arguing with the patient about his or her management decisions ("if only you had checked your blood glucose, you would have known you were low")
- *blaming* the patient for making an unhealthy choice (saying "should you be eating that?" just as the patient bites into a donut)

Often when family members have unrealistically high expectations for the patient's blood glucose levels, weight loss, or self-care behavior, the help they provide tends to "blame and shame" rather than support the patient.

TABLE 23-2. Steps to Prevent "Miscarried Helping" and Teach Positive Family Involvement

Step 1	Encourage your patient to bring in a family member(s) for education about diabetes in general.
Step 2	Listen to the family's fears, worries, and past experiences with diabetes. Influenced by out-of-date information about diabetes, many family members are convinced the patient will develop complications.
Step 3	Educate the patient and family to have realistic and appropriate expectations concerning blood glucose levels and self-care behavior. Avoid perfectionism.
Step 4	Model positive helping by directly asking your patient how and when his or her family members could be of help.
Step 5	When serious family communication problems and family stress are present, refer the patient and family to a family therapist who is knowledgeable about family interaction and chronic disease. Encourage patients to address the complex problems that negatively impact diabetes management in this context.

Fostering a Supportive and Open Provider-Patient Relationship

The provider-patient relationship plays a pivotal role in effectively managing diabetes. Although research has shown that both doctors and patients believe that discussing emotional well-being is important, most often, *neither doctors nor patients raise the issue.* Since physical and emotional health are linked, and because emotional well-being has a direct impact on patients' capacity for self-care, healthcare providers must address emotional health. They can begin to do so by raising the following issues at each medical visit:

- Ask about the emotional impact of diabetes.
- Invite patients to talk about their negative feelings about diabetes.

The primary characteristic of a good provider-patient relationship is open, trusting communication. Healthcare providers can help foster good communication with patients:

- Encourage patients to bring a written list of questions they would like to have answered by the end of the visit. Work through the list together. If time does not allow for all questions to be answered, work with the patient to prioritize and get the most important questions answered before the end of the visit.
- Avoid blame and criticism. Focus instead on positive steps the patient is already taking or is ready to take.

In addition to forging supportive and trusting relationships with patients, it is important for providers to be aware of some of the practical obstacles to successful diabetes treatment that many patients face. Below is a list of such obstacles.

Cost. Diabetes supplies may not be affordable if patients do not have health insurance; doctor visits may be too expensive, and/or transportation to and from appointments may also be a barrier.

Timing. Many patients have difficulty finding time in their daily routines for diabetes tasks. In addition, taking time off from work for regular healthcare appointments may be especially problematic for some patients.

Assertiveness. Many patients do not know how to take advantage of the resources their healthcare team has to offer. The idea of asking questions, and making sure that the answers are clear, is foreign to many patients.

Work and School Environments. Not all patients have an educated or supportive work or school environment in which diabetes tasks can be easily attended to without embarrassment.

Preventing Burnout

Diabetes can be a heavy load to carry, for both patients and family members. Often, people with diabetes come to feel discouraged and overwhelmed by all of the responsibilities that come with managing diabetes, especially when expectations for blood glucose values or self-care behavior are unrealistic. These feelings can lead to "diabetes burnout," which can be dangerous because burnout makes engagement in healthcare management tasks and general self-care impossible.

Some common symptoms of burnout are:

- feeling helpless, irritable, hostile
- feeling chronically depleted and lacking energy and motivation for diabetes care
- feeling overwhelmed and defeated by diabetes
- feeling unmotivated and/or unwilling to change
- having strong negative feelings about diabetes
- seeing healthcare providers infrequently
- feeling alone with diabetes care

Below are some steps primary care providers can take to help patients who are struggling with burnout (adapted from Polonsky, 2002. See *Suggested Reading* at end of chapter.):

- Help patients to recognize the signs of diabetes burnout (see list of symptoms above).
- Establish a strong, collaborative relationship with patients.
- Negotiate treatment goals with patients, with an emphasis on being realistic. *Make sure goals are concrete and achievable.*
- Pay attention to strong, negative feelings about diabetes. Your best "first response" is to listen well, and not to jump in to solve patients' problems for them.
- Optimize social and family support.
- Engage patients in active problem solving. The patient may need help articulating the problem. Or the patient may have a solution, but need help articulating or implementing it.

One of the most important things providers can do in working with patients who suffer from burnout is to allow patients to talk about their negative feelings and, above all, to foster open and trusting communication. Keeping the door open to medical care is imperative.

Major Psychological Obstacles to Diabetes Care

Thus far, we have given attention to promoting supportive relationships and behaviors. Unfortunately, even in the context of supportive familial and provider-patient relationships, patients sometimes come up against major psychological obstacles to diabetes care. The following sections address some of these obstacles.

Alcoholism and Addictions

Addictions and alcoholism have important implications for diabetes care because they severely limit the capacity of a person with diabetes to attend to daily self-care tasks such as blood glucose monitoring, insulin injections, and taking oral medications. In addition, maintaining daily structure and keeping medical appointments is often problematic for people with an active addiction. Healthcare providers can help patients to identify addictions and/or substance abuse patterns, and can provide resources and referrals for treatment. It is critical that doctors maintain open and respectful relationships with people struggling with substance abuse or dependence.

Substance Use as Self-Medication

Unfortunately, one of the most common myths about substance abusers is that they are disreputable people. In fact, people who abuse alcohol and/or drugs are almost always abused, anxious, or depressed. People who use drugs and/or alcohol as a coping mechanism may be trying to escape from any of the following feelings or situations: current or past physical or emotional abuse, professional or interpersonal stress, financial stress, emptiness, depression, anxiety, loneliness, hopelessness, grief or anger.

Screening

Screening for substance abuse should be a standard part of a medical interview. Ask patients about routine alcohol and drug use (e.g., how many drinks do you have each day) If patients report using alcohol or drugs frequently, ask if them if they believe this is causing problems for them. If they answer affirmatively, make referrals (see "Intervention and Support" below). Finally, if you believe a patient may be struggling with alcohol or drug use, raise the issue yourself. State what you see and why you believe that what you are seeing is a problem, but avoid statements like "you're an addict" or "you're an alcoholic."

The following commonly used acronym, CAGE, may be helpful in screening for substance abuse:

Cut Down — have you ever tried to cut down on your alcohol/drug use?

Annoyed — have you ever gotten annoyed by someone's criticism of your drug/alcohol use?

Guilty — have you ever felt guilty about your use of alcohol/drugs?

Early — have you ever felt as though you had to use alcohol/drugs early in the Day?

Diabetes-Specific Implications

The obvious and important diabetes-specific problem with substance abuse is that its impact on self-care capability usually prevents patients from achieving optimal glucose control. For people with diabetes, this can be extremely dangerous, and may lead to severe low blood glucose levels or, conversely, elevated levels leading to diabetic ketoacidosis or hyperosmotic coma.

When severe, addictions can prevent an individual from achieving any semblance of control at all, and efforts to concurrently control the glucose levels and the addictive behavior may lead to failure and frustration on both fronts. In such extreme situations, it may be necessary to temporarily abandon all efforts at improving glucose control beyond survival management, and directly address the addiction first. While seemingly sidetracking efforts to improve metabolic control, this approach may ultimately achieve better success sooner than struggling with both together and achieving neither.

Insulin syringes can be a source of anxiety for people with substance abuse problems. For a recovering drug addict, syringes often represent intense shame. Using insulin syringes for diabetes care can trigger memories of using drugs or shooting up, or can feel like "back-sliding." It is important to validate feelings that come up with the use of insulin syringes and also to remind patients that within the context of diabetes, using syringes is about self-care, not drug abuse.

Intervention and Support

- Keep a list of local Alcoholics Anonymous and Narcotics Anonymous meetings handy to give to patients when necessary.
- Familiarize yourself with local drug and alcohol treatment programs.
- Keep a list of drug and alcohol detoxification centers on hand and

offer to call to reserve a spot for patients who are ready to go, but need help getting there.

- Encourage patients who are trying to stop using alcohol or drugs to take advantage of their social supports whenever possible. Recovery from addiction is not a "one person show."

Eating Disorders

Women with diabetes are close to twice as likely to develop an eating disorder than women without diabetes, and about one-third of all women taking insulin struggle with "subclinical" symptoms of eating disturbances, such as restrictive eating, a preoccupation with weight and shape, feelings of guilt after eating specific foods, and misuse of insulin for weight control (Jones, et al, 2000. See *Suggested Reading* at end of chapter). As in the population at large, women are more vulnerable to the diagnosis of eating disorders than are men. Clinically diagnosable eating disorders such as anorexia nervosa and bulimia nervosa, as well as more "subclinical" disturbances of "disordered" eating attitudes and behaviors present a serious risk to the patient with diabetes. It is well-documented that eating disorders and "disordered eating" are associated with poor metabolic control, problems in adherence, and increased rates of microvascular complications in women with diabetes. Therefore, it is important for primary care providers to understand how to identify an eating disorder or "disordered eating" in a patient with diabetes, as well as how to work with the patient and family to prevent the development of an eating disorder secondary to the diagnosis of diabetes.

As a Cultural Phenomenon

Dieting, preoccupation with weight, and striving for the thin body ideal are common among girls and women in American culture today. This obsession with thinness is apparent in the media and in advertising. Recent studies have revealed that more than 50% of 9-and 10-year-old girls are already dieting and trying to lose weight. It is important to keep this cultural perspective in focus when working with women who have diabetes. In addition, a range of other variables such as genetics, individual temperament, self-esteem, and family interaction all contribute to the development of eating disorders.

Some female patients may be struggling with an eating disorder at the time of diagnosis of diabetes. Moreover, specific aspects of diabetes and its treatment (e.g., weight gain associated with the start of insulin treatment or improved metabolic control, and dietary restraint as a method of metabolic control) may cause feelings of deprivation and accentuate the drive for thinness that accompanies eating disturbances.

Early Warning Signs of Eating Disorders

(Adapted from Goebel-Fabbri et al, 2002. See *Suggested Reading* at end of chapter)

- An unexplainable elevated hemoglobin HbA1c in a patient knowledgeable about diabetes may indicate the patient is cutting back on insulin to control weight by purging calories from the body through the urine.
- Frequent diabetic ketoacidosis (DKA) may be caused by omission of insulin. Patients with serious eating disorders may learn how to avoid hospitalization for DKA by giving themselves only enough insulin to stay out of the hospital.
- Anxiety and avoidance surrounding being weighed may indicate an eating disorder.
- Bingeing with food or abusing alcohol frequently occur along with an eating disorder.

Prevention of Eating Disorders — Steps for Primary Care Providers

- Ask female patients of all ages directly about body and weight dissatisfaction. Keep in mind that many women experience dissatisfaction with their weight due to media images and cultural messages. Respect the patient's feelings about her weight and educate the patient who has unhealthy or inappropriate weight goals.
- Ask new patients directly about past or current struggles with eating or weight. Clearly, diabetes in the context of an established eating disorder is a risk factor, and the patient should be asked about past or current treatment. If the patient is currently seeing a therapist for eating issues, this therapist needs to become part of the diabetes team and be educated about how diabetes adds to the risk of an existing eating disorder.
- Nutritionists on diabetes teams need to be up-to-date and emphasize healthy eating, not rigid dieting. *The goal of a diabetes meal plan is*

flexibility, not restriction. Collaborate with the patient to set realistic weight goals.

- Be realistic; avoid perfectionism. Avoid setting unrealistic blood sugar goals or expectations for perfect self-care behaviors. Help patients to avoid self-blame by modeling realistic expectations for their blood sugars and behavior.
- Allow patients to express their negative feelings about having diabetes. Make it clear that it is normal for patients to occasionally feel burdened or discouraged by the diabetes regimen.
- Avoid transferring all the responsibility for diabetes care to preadolescent patients. Positive family involvement provides important support for the challenges of managing diabetes during adolescence.

Intervention and Support

Individual Therapy	Because eating disorders constitute a major risk factor in diabetes, it is important to identify therapists (psychologists, social workers, psychiatrists) who are comfortable treating patients with diabetes *and* an eating disorder.
Inpatient Treatment	Severe eating disorders, especially anorexia nervosa or chronic insulin omission, are life-threatening, and the patient may require an admission in an inpatient eating disorders unit. Identify one that has experience in the treatment of patients with eating disorders and diabetes.
State and National Agencies	If it is difficult to identify local inpatient or outpatient intervention resources, contact the state medical society, the state diabetes association, IAEDP (International Association of Eating Disorder Professionals), or AABA (American Anorexia and Bulimia Society).

Depression

The term depression has at least two different meanings. First, people may say they feel "depressed" when they are having a bad day or temporarily "feeling blue." However, these short-lived drops in mood are very different from the psychiatric diagnosis of depression, a serious and often life-threatening chronic mental disorder as identified in the *Diagnostic and Statistical Manual of Mental Disorders*, 4th Ed. This depression, called major depression, is diagnosed on the basis of both *mental symptoms* (e.g., sadness, inability to concentrate) *and physical symptoms* (e.g. fatigue, appetite changes, change in sleep patterns) that continue for an extended period of time and interfere with people's work and family functioning.

The incidence of major depression in the general population is about 5% to 8%. *Research has shown that Major Depression is about three times more common in people with diabetes than in the general population.* Depression occurs equally often in type 1 diabetes and type 2 diabetes — in about 15% to 20% of patients. Similar to the higher incidence of major depression in women in the general population, Major Depression occurs more frequently in women with diabetes than in men with diabetes (Lustman. See *Suggested Reading* at end of chapter.). Although major depression is more common in patients with diabetes, diabetes does not necessarily cause depression. In fact, the complex interaction of genetic, psychological, and physical factors which likely cause major depression in people with diabetes is not yet precisely known. However, it is well documented that major depression impacts negatively on patients' abilities to cope with diabetes emotionally and to carry out the self-care tasks that living with diabetes requires.

Researchers and clinicians studying major depression in persons with diabetes have identified three important issues:

1. **Distinguishing depression from hyperglycemia** — The symptoms of major depression and the symptoms of chronic hyperglycemia are often very similar (e.g., lethargy, fatigue, poor concentration, changes in appetite and sleep patterns). Therefore, it can be very difficult to diagnose depression in a person who simultaneously has chronic high blood glucose levels.
2. **Depression and its implications for self-care** — Living with diabetes often brings with it a broad range of diabetes-related distresses. It has been reported that the following diabetes-specific stressors occur frequently in patients with diabetes and can interfere with effective self-care (Polonsky et al, 2002. See *Suggested Reading* at end of chapter.):
   - not having clear and concrete goals for diabetes care
   - feeling discouraged and/or overwhelmed with the diabetes regimen

- feeling scared when thinking about having and living with diabetes
- uncomfortable interactions concerning diabetes with family, friends, or acquaintances who do not have diabetes
- not knowing if the moods or feelings they are experiencing are related to blood glucose levels
- feeling constantly concerned about food and eating
- worrying about the future and the possibility of serious complications
- feelings of guilt or anxiety when they get off-track with their diabetes management
- feeling unsatisfied with their relationship with their diabetes physician
- feeling that diabetes is taking up too much mental and physical energy every day
- coping with complications of diabetes

3. **Depression and its relationship to diabetes complications** — Major depression has been identified as a risk factor for the development of complications of diabetes. In addition, major depression can also occur secondarily to the complications of diabetes. The onset of a long-term debilitating complication of diabetes, such as visual impairment or painful neuropathy, represents another "loss" for the person who has diabetes. Some patients feel very discouraged and angry that their hard work and diabetes management efforts did not protect them from debilitating complications. Other patients, however, may feel guilty and think that complications are the direct result of their inadequate self-care.

Support and Intervention

Because of the high prevalence of Major Depression among persons with diabetes, the range of diabetes-related stressors which face patients, and the connection between Major Depression and diabetes complications, it is critical for primary care providers to have a sense of the available treatments for Major Depression — psychotherapy and medication.

- Psychotherapy, which targets the symptoms of depression, is different from general supportive counseling. One system of psychotherapy that has been proven to be a useful treatment for persons who struggle with depression is cognitive-behavioral therapy. In addition, there are several new antidepressant medications (selective serotonin reuptake inhibitors or SSRIs) on the market that are effective and have minimal side effects.

- It is important for primary care providers to refer their depressed patients to competent therapists in their local area. Make referrals to a qualified therapist (social worker, psychologist, or psychiatrist) who has experience in treating depression and in working with persons with diabetes, with therapy or medication. In addition, primary care providers should be aware of the inpatient psychiatric facilities in their local area that have experience with patients who have both depression and diabetes
- Some patients with major depression will require an inpatient psychiatric hospitalization in order to receive the level of treatment needed when depression becomes severe and life-threatening.

Anxiety Disorders

Anxiety disorders, which are the most frequently diagnosed psychiatric disorder in the general population, represent a spectrum of behaviors from anxiety and avoidance behavior, to panic and phobic behavior, to obsessive and compulsive behaviors. As with depression, we commonly think of being "anxious" as part of coping with new or difficult parts of everyday life. However, anxiety disorders are diagnosed when:

- the anxiety or worry the person experiences is unrealistic or excessive
- it extends over a 6-month period
- behavior is characterized by symptoms of motor tension (trembling, twitching, feeling shaky, restlessness, and easy fatigability) and autonomic hyperactivity (shortness of breath, palpitations, accelerated heart rate, sweating, cold clammy hands, dry mouth, dizziness or lightheadedness, nausea, diarrhea, flushes or chills, frequent urination, and trouble swallowing)

Anxiety Disorders and Diabetes

Anxiety disorders can complicate living with diabetes and its management in the following four ways:

1. *Confusion between anxiety and hypoglycemia* — The symptoms of autonomic hyperactivity listed above, which are part of a serious anxiety disorder, *overlap almost completely with the symptoms of hypoglycemia.* This can make it very difficult for a person with diabetes to differentiate between feelings of anxiety and symptoms of low blood sugars, which should receive immediate treatment.

2. *Exacerbation of pre-existing injection/blood testing anxiety* — There are several aspects of the diabetes treatment regimen that may be sources of extreme anxiety for some patients. For example, individuals who have been extremely anxious during routine injections or blood tests may develop symptoms of a severe panic disorder when faced with injecting insulin or pricking a finger to monitor blood sugar levels. At this point it is important for the primary care physician to make a referral to a mental health professional skilled in helping persons with anxiety disorders and diabetes.

3. *Fear of hypoglycemia* — The most common and potentially damaging source of anxiety for patients with type 1 diabetes, as well as for patients with type 2 diabetes taking blood glucose-lowering medication, is fear of hypoglycemia. Patients who are extremely anxious about low blood glucose levels will understandably strive to keep their blood glucose levels at a constantly higher target range than that recommended by their diabetes healthcare team. Behavioral scientists who study fear of hypoglycemia emphasize that it is not surprising that many patients experience fear and anxiety about hypoglycemia and its embarrassing consequences and have identified four groups of diabetes patients at high risk for fear of hypoglycemia (Gonder-Frederick, Cox, and Clarke, 1996. See *Suggested Reading* at end of chapter.):

   - newly-diagnosed patients who have not yet learned that they can deal effectively with hypoglycemia
   - patients who have had a recent or past traumatic episode of hypoglycemia
   - patients who are overly anxious in other areas of their lives
   - parents of children who have experienced severe hypoglycemia or episodes of serious low blood glucose in their children.

4. *Outside stresses and other externally caused sources of anxiety* — An acute state of anxiety (such as caused by serious stresses) can trigger neuroendocrine responses leading to hyperglycemia. Thus, anxiety

disorders can affect blood sugars directly through physiological pathways, as well as indirectly by interfering with the learning and execution of diabetes management skills.

Support and Intervention

Primary care providers need to be familiar with the treatments available for anxiety disorders: psychotherapy and medication for generalized anxiety disorders, and Blood Glucose Awareness Training for severe fear of hypoglycemia.

- **Psychotherapy and Medication.** Sometimes symptoms of anxiety disorders, such as fatigue, sleep problems, difficulty concentrating, and irritability, are similar to those of Major Depression. Thus it is important to refer patients struggling with these symptoms to a mental health professional (social worker, psychologist, or psychiatrist) who has experience working with people with diabetes. There are several newer medications for treating anxiety in the context of therapy which are effective and not as habit-forming as older anti-anxiety medications.
- **Blood Glucose Awareness Training (BGAT).** A group of psychologists and behavioral scientists at the University of Virginia have developed a behavioral treatment program which improves a patient's ability to recognize, avoid, and treat hypoglycemia. This program is designed for patients who have lost their awareness of the symptoms of low blood glucose and/or patients who have a profound fear of low blood glucose . To identify the BGAT program in your local area, you can contact the University of Virginia Health Behavioral Medicine Center in Charlottesville, VA.

Conclusion

Support from medical personnel and family members is crucial in promoting and maintaining diabetes care. Primary care providers can foster this support by building strong relationships with their patients that attend to the emotional aspects of diabetes as well as the medical ones. They can also help families to provide support for the person with diabetes. Finally, primary care providers play a pivotal role in screening, diagnosis and referral when serious psychological barriers to mental and physical health arise.

Suggested Reading

American Psychiatric Association. Diagnostic and Statistical Manual of Mental Disorders, 4TH ed. Washington, DC., American Psychiatric Association, 1994.

Goebel-Fabbri AE, Fikkan JL, Connell A, Vangsness L, Anderson BJ. Identification and treatment of eating disorders in women with type 1 diabetes mellitus. *Treatments in Endocrinology.* 2002; 1 (3): 155–162.

Gonder-Frederick L, Cox DJ, Clarke WL. Helping patients understand, recognize and avoid hypoglycemia. In B. Anderson & R. Rubin (Eds.) *Practical Psychology for Diabetes Clinicians.* American Diabetes Association, Alexandria, VA; 2002, 113–124.

Jones JM, Lawson ML, Daneman D, Omsted MP, Rodin G. Eating disorders in adolescent females with and without type 1 diabetes: cross sectional study. *British Medical Journal* 2000; 320:1563–1566.

Lustman PJ, Griffith LS, Gavard JA, Clouse RE. Depression in adults with diabetes. Diabetes Care 15: 1631–1639, 1992.

Lustman PJ, Singh PK, Clouse RE. Recognizing and managing depression in patients with diabetes. In B. Anderson and R. Rubin (Eds.) *Practical Psychology for Diabetes Clinicians.* American Diabetes Association, Alexandria, VA; 2002, 229–238.

Peyrot M. Recognizing emotional responses to diagnosis. In B. Anderson and R. Rubin (Eds.) *Practical Psychology for Diabetes Clinicians.* American Diabetes Association, Alexandria, VA; 2002, 211–218.

Polonsky, WH. Understanding and treating patients with diabetes burnout. In B. Anderson and R. Rubin (Eds.) *Practical Psychology for Diabetes Clinicians.* Alexandria, VA: American Diabetes Association, 2002, 219–228.

24

Diabetes in Culturally Diverse Populations: Facing the Challenge in Clinical Practice

Enrique Caballero, MD

Introduction

All individuals share biological, psychological, spiritual, and social elements. At the same time, all are different enough in some or most of these elements to make each person unique. An evident and closer share of genetically transmitted physical characteristics, history, nationality, religion, language, traditions, and cultural heritage gives the basis to our integration in races or ethnic groups. *Race,* defined as a group of persons who come from the same ancestor, refers primarily to genetically transmitted physical characteristics, whereas ethnicity is a broader concept that relates to large groups of people classified according to common racial, national, tribal, religious, linguistic, or cultural origin or background. Therefore, ethnicity alludes to a perceived cultural distinctiveness, expressed in language, music, values, art, styles, literature, family life, religion, ritual, food, naming, public life, and material culture.

A good example to distinguish race from ethnicity is the nature of the Latino or Hispanic population. The term *Latino* or *Hispanic* represents ethnicity, not race. Racially speaking, Latinos have 3 possible genetic back-

grounds: white, African American, and/or Native American. These genetic backgrounds are seen in any possible combination among Latinos,
creating a very heterogeneous group. However, Latinos have multiple
shared linguistic, traditional, and cultural values.

Multicultural, multiethnic and multiracial societies define our world.
Although white Americans account for three-quarters of the United States
population, increasing numbers of other racial and ethnic groups contribute to making many cities a true mosaic of heterogeneous cultures. The
minority groups with the highest numbers of people in the United States
are Latinos/Hispanics, African Americans, American Indians, Alaska Natives, Asian and Pacific Islanders, Southeast Asians, and Arabs. Most of
these groups will continue to increase at a higher rate than the non-
Hispanic white population. Table 24-1 shows the current and projected increase in the distribution of the U.S. population by race and ethnicity according to the US census data.

Unfortunately, minority groups have lagged behind in their healthcare
when compared to the predominant group in the United States, a similar
situation to that occurring in many other countries around the world. The
Institute of Medicine, a private, nonprofit organization that provides
health policy advice under a congressional charter granted to the National Academy of Sciences, reported that when comparing the white
population and minority groups in the U.S., there are clear healthcare disparities for many health outcomes, including several related to diabetes
care. In general, minorities receive a lower quality of diabetes care than do
white Americans. It is important to mention that these disparities are not
accounted for only by level of access to care, socioeconomic status, age,
stage of presentation, or existing comorbidities. Further, they can be
found in multiple heath care settings (e.g., managed care, public, private,
teaching, and community centers). Other elements contribute to this phenomenon; in a healthcare system that is often not oriented to cultural differences, multiple patient- and provider-based factors collide At the same
time that providers work toward improving the lives of *all* people with diabetes, fundamental questions emerge: How can healthcare providers improve the quality of diabetes care given to people who belong to a different racial/ethnic group and, thus, culture from their own? How to
implement effective strategies in diabetes care when the health care system allows for very limited time for the patient-doctor interaction?

The objective of this chapter is to raise awareness among health care
providers about the most common biological, social and cultural factors

TABLE 24-1. Current and Projected Percentage of the U.S. Population by Race and Ethnicity from The Year 2000 to 2050.

	2000	2010	2020	2030	2040	2050
TOTAL	100.0	100.0	100.0	100.0	100.0	100.0
white alone	81.0	79.3	77.6	75.8	73.9	72.1
black alone	12.7	13.1	13.5	13.9	14.3	14.6
Asian alone	3.8	4.6	5.4	6.2	7.1	8.0
all other races 1/	2.5	3.0	3.5	4.1	4.7	5.3
Hispanic (of any race)	12.6	15.5	17.8	20.1	22.3	24.4
white alone, not Hispanic	69.4	65.1	61.3	57.5	53.7	50.1

that may influence the development of type 2 diabetes, progression of the disease, and adherence to treatment plans in patients from culturally diverse populations. Identifying these elements is the first step toward developing effective clinical practice strategies.

Type 2 Diabetes in Culturally Diverse Populations: Genes or Culture?

Whereas the prevalence and incidence rates for type 1 diabetes in minority populations have been reported to be equal to or lower than the rates for whites, the rates for type 2 diabetes and its complications have been consistently reported higher in minority groups. Type 2 diabetes is a heterogeneous disease that results from the combination of a genetic predisposition and environmental factors.

Biological Factors

Many studies have shown that these minority groups have a strong genetic predisposition for the development of type 2 diabetes. The "thrifty gene" theory has emerged as a possible explanation for this genetic tendency to develop diabetes. This theory, first proposed by J.V. Neel in 1962, suggests that populations of indigenous people who experienced alternating periods of feast and famine gradually adapted by developing a way to store fat more efficiently during periods of plenty to better survive famine. However, this genetic adaptation has now become detrimental since food supplies are more constant and abundant, leading to an increased prevalence of obesity and type 2 diabetes in certain populations. A significant amount of research has been devoted to identifying the precise nature of the "thrifty gene or genes," but unfortunately, no uniform genes across ethnic groups have been identified to fully support this theory. In a broad view, type 2 diabetes is characterized by a dual abnormality, decreased ability of insulin to promote glucose uptake in peripheral tissues (insulin resistance) and a decreased insulin production by the beta cells in the pancreas (beta cell dysfunction). Several studies have now shown some biological differences among various racial and ethnic groups that may contribute to increase the risk for type 2 diabetes and/or its course. Most studies have shown that Latinos/Hispanics, African Americans, Asian Americans, Native Americans, South East Asians, and Arabs have lower insulin sensitivity (higher insulin resistance) than whites. These differences have been shown in youngsters from some of these racial and ethnic minorities, such as Hispanic American and African American children, even after adjustment for differences in body fat. In addition, the associated compensatory responses to increased insulin resistance may differ across these ethnic groups, suggesting that the underlying pathology of diabetes may indeed vary in high-risk ethnic subpopulations.

Another biological difference is related to the degree and type of abdominal obesity in some of these populations. Abdominal obesity plays a major role in the development of type 2 diabetes and cardiovascular disease. In particular, visceral fat is related to insulin resistance and endothelial dysfunction. Most of the minority groups in the U.S., except African Americans, tend to accumulate more visceral fat than whites, at any degree of obesity. Whereas we still need to better understand the mechanisms that lead to differential fat accumulation, in any given racial/ethnic group, increased levels of intra-abdominal or visceral fat leads to multiple metabolic and vascular derangements. Although African-Americans seem to have lower visceral fat levels than whites, their risk for type 2 diabetes is higher, most likely due to genetically determined insulin resistance in peripheral tissues and in some, a rapid decline in beta cell function. Other consistent biological differences between African Americans and whites have been identified, such as higher rates of hypertension and better lipid profiles. Interestingly, whereas lower visceral fat content and better lipid profiles are certainly beneficial for any population, the strong genetic tendency to insulin resistance and high hypertension rates among African Americans seem to predominate to increase the rates of type 2 diabetes and cardiovascular outcomes in this high risk group.

In some other groups, such as Asian Americans and South East Asians, significant insulin resistance and, thus, the risk for type 2 diabetes may be present at body mass index levels that could be considered normal or slightly increased according to standards applied to the general white population. For instance, a BMI of 24 is considered normal among whites, while it is considered to be in the overweight range for Asians.

Environmental or Acquired Factors

Environmental factors have undoubtedly contributed to increase the risk for obesity and diabetes in these populations. The best data to support this concept comes from the multiple studies that have found that the rates for type 2 diabetes and obesity are significantly higher in some minority groups in the U.S. compared to those in the same racial and ethnic groups in their country of origin. The common elements of "Westernization" that increase the risk for obesity, diabetes and related diseases include a diet higher in total calories and fat but lower in fiber and less need to expend energy because of labor-saving devices. In addition, particular aspects of preferred foods and lifestyle practices in each of these groups certainly play a role in the development of diabetes and its treatment. Cultural factors that influence some of these lifestyle aspects will be discussed in more detail in other sections of this chapter.

Diabetes-Related Complications

Unfortunately, minority populations not only more frequently develop type 2 diabetes, but also experience higher rates of diabetes-related complications than their white counterparts. Consistent data have emerged from multiple studies showing higher rates of retinopathy, nephropathy, peripheral vascular disease, leg amputations and cardiovascular disease among many of these groups. For some complications, like chronic kidney disease, some specific factors, such as very high rates of hypertension in African Americans, partially explain these differences. However, it is still unclear whether certain biological factors consistently increase the risk of complications in minorities. Some recent data suggests that glycemic control is particularly poor in some of these groups. The National Health Examination Survey Study has shown higher glycohemoglobin (A1C) levels among Hispanics, represented by Mexican Americans and in African Americans when compared to the white population. Clearly, poor glycemic control contributes to increased risk of diabetes-related complications.

Social and Cultural Factors

Some of the most relevant social and cultural factors that influence the development and/or course of type 2 diabetes in culturally diverse populations are listed in Table 24-2. These factors have been arranged in alphabetical order, not in order of importance. Some important factors may therefore be included in another category for simplicity. The primary purpose of the list is to help healthcare providers address multiple factors in the day-to-day management of patients with type 2 diabetes.

Acculturation

Culture refers to the behavior patterns, beliefs, arts, and all other products of human work and thought, as expressed in a particular community. *Acculturation* refers to the adoption of some specific elements of one culture by a different cultural group. For immigrants to the United States, it relates to the integration of multiple preferences and behaviors from mainstream culture. No uniform instrument to assess acculturation exists. Self-identification, behavior, and language skills are common elements that may allow classification of individuals into the above categories. Many reports consider language preference a good estimate of the degree of acculturation of any given individual. Whereas conflicting results exist in the literature as to whether high acculturation translates into better or worse

TABLE 24-2. Main Factors To Be Considered in a Culturally Oriented Clinical Encounter and/or Education Program for Diabetes Patients from Diverse Racial and Ethnic Groups.

Acculturation	Knowledge about the disease
Body image	Language
Cultural awareness	Myths
Depression	Nutritional preferences
Educational level	Other forms of medicine (alternative)
Fears	
General family integration and support	Physical activity preferences
Health literacy	Quality of life
Individual and social interaction	Religion and faith
Judgment about the disease	Socioeconomic status

health care behaviors, some reports point to the fact that groups with low acculturation are more likely to be without a routine place for health care, have no health insurance, and have lower levels of education. These factors are clearly related to health care outcomes. At the same time, a high acculturation level can also be associated with higher rates of diabetes, perhaps through the adoption of a more "diabetogenic" lifestyle, that is, by eating higher portions of foods richer in carbohydrates and fats and becoming more sedentary. It is also true that the acculturation process can lead to the adoption of a healthier lifestyle. Ultimately, individuals choose what behaviors and preferences to adopt. Healthcare providers should openly ask patients about behaviors that they have adopted from mainstream culture.

Body Image

The concept of ideal body weight may vary among individuals within and across racial and ethnic groups. Although it would be erroneous to assume that some people prefer to be overweight, the ideal weight that people have conceptualized may be different. In some groups, like Hispanics, African Americans, some American Indian tribes, and in some Arab groups, being robust and slightly overweight has been considered equivalent to being well nourished and financially successful. Children are often encouraged to "eat well" and finish their entire meal. For some groups, achieving a higher socioeconomic status translates into the possibility of eating more, not necessarily eating better. As an example, a study in African American women with type 2 diabetes showed that most participants preferred a middle-to-small body size but indicated that a middle-to-large body size was healthier. They also said that a large body size did result in some untoward social consequences. When discussing weight-loss strategies, it is therefore crucial that clinicians ask patients about their personal goals.

Cultural Awareness

It is important for both the patient and the healthcare provider to develop *cultural awareness*. Being aware of how our own culture influences our thoughts, beliefs and behaviors, and respecting the fact that others may see the world in a completely different way, is the first step towards good personal interactions. *Cultural competence* is defined by the American Medical Association as the knowledge and interpersonal skills that allow healthcare providers to understand, appreciate, and work with individuals from cultures other than their own. It involves an awareness and acceptance of cultural differences, self-awareness, knowledge of the patient's culture, and adaptation of skills.

Although no randomized clinical trial has been conducted to demonstrate that diabetes control and/or complication rates are improved by a group of healthcare providers with higher cultural competence compared with a group with a lower level, it seems clear that cultural competence can lead to a much more pleasant and productive healthcare provider–patient interaction. In the field of diabetes, it may be particularly relevant because disease control is greatly determined by effective lifestyle and behavior modification. The need to improve the skills of healthcare providers in the area of cultural competency has become increasingly recognized. At this writing, two states — New Jersey and California — require physicians to obtain some annual continuing medical education (CME) credits in programs that address cultural aspects in healthcare. It is antici-pated that more states will join the effort to disseminate information on how to improve the lives of people with diabetes from various cultures, and for some time, the Joslin Diabetes Center Professional Education de-partment has provided CME programs to address this need.

Unfortunately, many healthcare providers blame the patient for not fol-lowing a treatment plan. It is disappointing to hear many professionals refer to patients as *noncompliant*. Although it is true that some patients may not adhere to their treatment plan, perhaps it is fairer and more help-ful to say: "I have not found the best way to interact with my patient so that some specific behavioral changes occur." It is common to create ste-reotypes in clinical encounters. However, creating a stereotype about a patient based on his or her racial/ethnic or cultural background is likely to endanger the clinical encounter. It is helpful to be aware of the most common cultural aspects that may influence diabetes care in any particu-lar cultural group, but a productive clinical encounter must focus on a particular *patient's* characteristics and preferences.

Of course, it would be helpful if patients also raised their own cultural awareness. Patients should feel comfortable receiving their healthcare from a provider with a cultural background different than his or her own. This may present more of a challenge, but it may happen naturally as the result of a better and more culturally-oriented interaction with healthcare providers.

Keep in mind that *all* people have cultures. Cultural issues are not just limited to groups that we commonly identify as "minorities." From this perspective, it is commonplace, rather than the exception, that people re-ceive care from those who have different cultural backgrounds from their own. Thus, every provider who has the opportunity to treat patients from any culture other than his or her own must make the effort to be aware and sensitive to the impact of culture on the process of medical care if the impact of that care is to be optimized.

Depression

Depression is frequently associated with diabetes. In addition, it is a pow-erful predictor of poor health diabetes related outcomes. Multiple factors may account for this association, including low socioeconomic status, lack of family and social support, and sense of isolation, many of which are more common in some ethnic groups, particularly those that have immigrated to the United States. In addition, ethnicity is also related to worse glycemic control, which is related to worse clinical outcomes that may exacerbate depression. Therefore, a vicious cycle that includes diabetes and depression is very common among patients with diabetes from culturally diverse populations. The presence of depression also influences adherence to any diabetes treatment plan. Some immigrants to the United States may be more likely to develop stress and depression because of the need to live in, and adapt to, a completely different social and cultural environment. A recent study showed that Puerto Rican elders in Massachusetts are significantly more likely to have physical disability, depression, cognitive impairment, diabetes, and other chronic health conditions than non-Hispanic white elders living in the same neighborhoods.

Depression is one of the most frequently missed diagnoses in clinical practice. Health- care providers should become familiar with various ways of assessing the presence of depression in their patients. Although specific scales are useful in assessing depression in specific cultural groups, some general approaches may also be useful in regular clinical encounters. For instance, specific questions such as: "Have you felt depressed or sad much of the time this past year?" may provide insight into whether a patient may be depressed.

Educational Level

Some data shows that a higher education level may be related to better diabetes-related outcomes. For instance, the association of educational level with either type 2 diabetes or cardiovascular disease (CVD) was examined in a sample of second-generation Japanese American men living in King County, Washington. Men with a technical school education showed higher frequencies of both diseases compared with men with any college education or high school diplomas. The association of educational level with risk of type 2 diabetes was not explained by other factors, such as occupation, income, diet, physical activity, weight, insulin, lipids, and lipoproteins, whereas the association with CVD was explained in part by the larger average body mass index (BMI), higher total and very-low-density lipoprotein, triglycerides, and lower high-density lipoprotein

(HDL), and HDL-2 cholesterol observed in men with technical school educations compared with the other men. Therefore, a low educational level may not be the direct cause of worse outcomes in patients with type 2 diabetes, but rather a "marker" of multiple socioeconomic and cultural factors that may influence adherence to treatment and the course of the disease.

It is recommended that healthcare providers take into consideration patients' educational level when implementing any educational activity, whether in a regular clinical encounter or through a group diabetes education program, since it may lead to the identification of other important social and cultural factors that may influence diabetes care.

Fears

Patients may have multiple fears that may influence their adherence to a diabetes treatment plan. Many patients fear the presence of type 2 diabetes and its complications. This fear, expressed by a sense of hopelessness, may be due to lack of adequate information about the disease. On the other hand, in some patients, a sense of fear may lead to a more responsible attitude towards the disease and improve self-management behavior.

Another common fear in patients with type 2 diabetes, particularly in some ethnic groups, is related to the consequences of medications. For instance, insulin use is considered by many as a treatment of last resort that equals the development of severe diabetes-related complications, such as going blind and ultimately dying of the disease. It is perceived as basically a death sentence and decreases patients' likelihood of following a good treatment plan. This concept may be more prevalent in some groups. Our own experience in the Latino Diabetes Initiative at Joslin Diabetes Center confirms that this fear is common among Latinos. In a recent analysis of our data, approximately, 43% of new patients to our program thought that insulin causes blindness and 25% were not sure whether this was true or not. The basic implication of fear on diabetes care is quite obvious. Before prescribing medicine, health care providers should openly ask patients if they have any particular fears about taking insulin or any other diabetes medication. As an anecdotal experience, a few years ago I saw a patient who, according to notes by his primary care physician, had been taking insulin for several years. When referred to us for uncontrolled diabetes, one of my first questions to him was: "Are you taking your insulin injections?" He openly said to me: "Claro que no, doctor!" (Of course not, doctor!) "No quiero quedarme ciego por usar la insulina" (I don't want to get blind from taking insulin!). Unfortunately, and as happens frequently with many patients, he had already developed severe complications. Both his legs were amputated within a year, and he died of a cardiovascular event within two years. A very simple question before starting a patient on insulin can be the first step to overcoming this common fear to insulin. Among Asian Americans, the effect of substances in the body may be referred to as "cold" or "hot." Sometimes, medications that produce "hot" reactions may not be well accepted. For instance, some patients may associate these reactions to those of hypoglycemia, due to the accompanying adrenergic burst. It is thus imperative to ask and address these issues with the patients.

General Family Integration and Support

Although family is important for virtually all human beings, the level of closeness and dependence between family members may differ in various populations. In general, some groups such as Latinos, Arabs, Asian Indians, and others often exhibit a collective loyalty to the extended family or group that supercedes the needs of the individual. This loyalty may provide pros and cons in diabetes care. The benefit is that more members in any given family may provide support to the patient. Some reports suggest that structural togetherness in families is positively related to diabetes quality of life and satisfaction among patients with diabetes.

The downside is that it is more difficult for some patients to make their own decisions. Nevertheless, suggesting that the patient bring along family members to the clinical encounters may be a good start towards addressing this factor. Inviting relatives to group education activities has been reported as a successful strategy in several cultural groups.

Health Literacy

Health literacy is defined as the degree to which individuals have the capacity to obtain, process, and understand the basic health information and services they need to make appropriate health decisions. Knowing a language is not a guarantee of high health literacy, although it certainly plays a role. Limited health literacy, common in patients with both type 1 and type 2 diabetes, has been associated with worse diabetes outcomes. A particular association that may influence the development of specific diabetes outcomes is that of health literacy with diabetes self-management behaviors, as assessed in a population of patients with type 2 diabetes. Self-management behaviors can be improved in people with low, as well as high, health literacy. Furthermore, a recent study showed that self-efficacy was associated with self-management behaviors across Asian/Pacific Islanders, African Americans, Latinos, and white Americans with various degrees of health literacy.

Ideally, specific low-health-literacy patient education programs and materials should be developed for each racial and ethnic group. Healthcare providers should evaluate their patients' health literacy levels when implementing a DM education program or even when providing regular patient education materials. There are various ways to evaluate health literacy. A common instrument used for this purpose is the test of functional literacy in adults. The reader may want to become familiar with this instrument as a starting point to formally evaluate patients' health literacy.

Individual and Social Interaction

Every individual has a unique character and personality and different approaches to interacting with other people. There is no right or wrong about how various cultures approach this issue. Each group may just be different. For instance, many Latino patients expect to develop a warm and personal relationship with their physicians. This type of patient-physician relationship would be characterized by interactions that occur at close distances and emphasize physical contact, such as handshakes, a hand on the shoulder, and even hugging under certain circumstances. Some Latino patients with diabetes may erroneously think that their healthcare provider does not care about them if they do not experience this type of interaction. Even though healthcare providers cannot switch behaviors as they interact with patients with diverse backgrounds and cultures, keeping in mind that certain groups prefer particular approaches may facilitate clinical encounters and help establish a more trusting and effective relationship with patients. The ability to adapt one's own approach and behaviors to the perceived needs of a patient is a very useful clinical skill.

Judgment and Beliefs about the Disease

Every social group shares beliefs about health and illness. Groups and individuals may have a particular diabetes explanatory model of illness. Knowledge and understanding of these health beliefs and explanatory models are essential for effective clinical encounters and education programs. Some beliefs related to the development of diabetes include heredity, eating sweets, stress, emotional instability, and, sometimes, even an acute episode of fear or anxiety.

A recent study explored some health-related beliefs and experiences of African Americans, Hispanic/Latinos, American Indians, and among people with diabetes. The investigators found that many participants attributed their loss of health to the modern American lifestyle, lack of confidence in the medical system, and the general lack of spirituality in modern life. Interestingly, participants recommended improvements in the areas of health care, diabetes education, social support, and community action that emphasized respectful and knowledgeable health care providers, culturally responsive diabetes education for patients and their families, and broad-based community action as ways to improve diabetes care and education programs.

Health care providers should explore beliefs about the development and course of diabetes with their patients. A simple question to start with is: "Why do you think that you developed diabetes?" This initial evaluation may guide the clinician as to which important factors to address with that patient.

Knowledge about the Disease

Patients' knowledge of diabetes is usually associated with self-management behaviors but not necessarily or directly associated with diabetes-related outcomes. However, because improving self-management behaviors is likely to lead to better diabetes control and, hence, a lower risk of diabetes complications, general knowledge of diabetes will continue to be an important aspect of diabetes education programs. Culturally oriented programs should focus on improving patients' knowledge of diabetes that can specifically help them improve those self-care management behaviors that may be more problematic in specific population groups. Specific culturally oriented programs to improve self-management behaviors are necessary.

Language

The most obvious cultural barrier in a clinical and educational encounter is the inability to communicate in the same language. It may limit the patient's ability to ask questions, to verbalize important information and concerns, and to establish a natural and spontaneous relationship with the healthcare provider. Language has been shown to affect clinical outcomes and may be a serious barrier to effective patient care.

In general, patients prefer healthcare providers who have a similar ethnic background. It may improve compliance and follow-up. However, there is currently a pronounced discrepancy between the number of physicians who can communicate in both English and an additional language and the number of non-English-speaking patients. For instance, in 1999, Latino physicians accounted for ~3.3% of practicing physicians in the United States; however, 13.9% of the patient population is of Latino origin. Therefore, the use of interpreters is necessary. A word of caution is necessary concerning the common circumstance in which a family member acts as an interpreter during routine clinical encounters. The advantage to this is that the family member may be able to provide additional helpful information to the healthcare provider. The disadvantage is that the family member may not be objective about translating all information, may not put aside his or her emotional attachment to the patient, and may communicate only what he or she considers important.

Healthcare providers should find the best translating option(s) for their patients. Although speaking the same language facilitates the clinician-patient interaction, other elements (e.g., trust, genuine interest and honesty) have no language barriers.

Myths

Myths, which are generally not explicit and are usually interwoven with values and beliefs, are common in patients with diabetes. Such myths include those related to why diabetes has occurred or why it has taken a specific course. In some groups, a clear link with faith and religion is present. There are many possible myths — that diabetes occurs from eating a lot of sweets, is the result of destiny, is caused by lack of faith, or is punishment for a particular action. Certain myths and fears have developed in relation to insulin use. Healthcare providers should ask patients about possible myths and be respectful of patients' answers. Understanding what myths patients believe can help clinicians develop specific strategies to dispel them.

Nutritional Preferences

Humans are biologically adapted to their ancestral food environment, in which foods were dispersed and energy expenditure was required to obtain them. The modern developed world has a surplus of very accessible, inexpensive food. Unfortunately, this food is usually rich in carbohydrates and saturated fats. Minority populations in the United States have a high risk of developing type 2 diabetes, partly due to a strong genetic predisposition. Because more people are incorporating unhealthy foods in their regular meals, eating continuously larger portions, and not engaging in regular physical activity, rates of obesity, type 2 diabetes, and CVD are rising.

Although similarities between racial and ethnic groups exist, different groups have different food and nutritional preferences. In fact, foods may be so diverse that considerable discrepancies may exist in subgroups within each general racial/ethnic group, such as in Asians (e.g., Japanese, Chinese, Korean, Hawaiian) or Hispanics/Latinos (e.g., Caribbean, Mexican American, Central American, and South American). Food preferences even vary by country or region in each of these subgroups. For instance, food preferences in Venezuela may differ from those in Colombia, and those in the Dominican Republic may differ from those in Puerto Rico.

Food is usually at the core of family and social interaction. It is certainly worthwhile addressing this aspect in detail with the patient with diabetes. Clinicians must identify local educational resources to help their patients receive culturally oriented medical nutrition therapy. Bicultural dieticians are an excellent resource for physicians. In addition, patient education materials in this important area of nutrition may be identified through national organizations such as the American Diabetes Association, the National Institutes of Health, and the National Diabetes Education Program. Some specific programs, such as the Latino Diabetes Initiative and the Asian American Initiative at Joslin Diabetes Center, can also provide some helpful information.

Other Types of Medicine (Alternative)

Many patients with diabetes combine alternative and traditional medicine. Alternative medicine has long been part of most cultures throughout the world. The most common forms of alternative medicine are herbs, chiropractic care, yoga, relaxation, acupuncture, ayurveda, biofeedback, chelation, energy healing, Reiki therapy, hypnosis, massage, naturopathy, and homeopathy. A recent report showed that of 2472 adults with diabetes included in the study, 48% used some form of alternative medicine. Interestingly, this study found that the use of alternative medicine was associated with increased likelihood of receiving preventive care services and increased emergency department and primary care visits. This association does not necessarily represent causality. In other words, alternative medicine use may represent a factor that leads to a more proactive healthcare behavior and use of conventional medical services in adults with diabetes; conversely, high use of conventional medical services may lead to increased use of alternative medicine. Information on the effect of alternative medicine on diabetes care is starting to emerge. For instance, a recent study showed that yoga may have a positive influence on blood glucose and lipid levels in a short period of time in some patients with diabetes. Obviously, more research on alternative medicine use in patients with DM is needed. Health care providers should not forget to ask patients if they are using any form of alternative medicine. This question should be asked in a sensitive and respectful manner so that patients do not feel threatened or embarrassed.

Physical Activity

Physical-activity preferences may vary among racial and ethnic groups. For instance, older white Americans may prefer jogging or going to the gym; older Latinos may prefer activities such as walking or dancing. When prescribing an exercise program for a patient, physicians and patients should discuss preferred physical activities to enhance a higher chance of continuity.

Further research is needed to identify attitudes toward, and barriers to, physical activity in specific ethnic and racial groups. This type of research may help the development of community culturally-oriented programs that, in combination with the availability of accessible facilities and transportation options, may motivate people from certain racial/ethnic populations to engage in regular physical activity.

Quality of life

Type 2 diabetes has significant adverse effects on health-related quality of life. The effect of diabetes on reducing health-related quality of life has also been evaluated and confirmed in multiethnic populations. Some factors, such as family structure and support, may improve quality of life in patients with diabetes, as shown in a study of African Americans.

Although a patient's quality of life is difficult to routinely assess in clinical practice, health care providers should try to explore how diabetes and its complications have affected a patient's quality of life. Quality of life clearly influences patients' behavior, receptiveness to treatment, and adherence to a treatment plan.

Religion and Faith

Religion and faith influence daily life. Religious traditions are expressions of faith in, and reverence for, specific conceptions of ultimate reality. They express one's place in, and relation to, this reality. Ultimate reality may be known as God, Allah, Atman, Nirvana, or by many other names, and it is understood and experienced differently by each religious tradition. The forms of faith and reverence may be expressed and experienced through sacred stories, sacred symbols and objects, sacred music, art and dance, devotion, meditation, rituals, sacred laws, philosophy, ethics, calls to social transformation, relationship with spirits, and healing.

Some of these expressions may affect the health care arena. In diabetes care, a clear example of one important influence is the fasting during the daylight hours that Muslims practice during one month each year. This practice requires the healthcare provider to show cultural sensitivity and understanding by adjusting any treatment strategies during this time.

For a healthcare provider to address the topic of religion and faith, two sets of skills are indispensable. The first involves cultivating self-awareness and reflecting on the components of one's own identity. The second involves learning strategies for talking with patients about this topic and for responding to what patients say.

Socioeconomic Status

Poverty influences not only the development of type 2 diabetes, but complications of diabetes as well. A recent study showed that family poverty accounts for differences in diabetic amputation rates of African Americans, Hispanic Americans, and other persons aged ≥ 50 years. Place of birth and time in the United States are factors closely related to socioeconomic status, and these two factors may have a direct effect on specific diseases.

For instance, The Multi-Ethnic Study of Atherosclerosis, a population-based study of coronary calcification assessed through a CT scan in a large number of non-Hispanic white Americans, non-Hispanic blacks, Hispanics, and Chinese residing in the United States, found that not being born in the United States was associated with a lower prevalence of calcification in blacks and Hispanics after adjustment for age, sex, income, and education. Years in the United States was positively associated with prevalence of calcification in non-US-born Chinese and non-US-born blacks. Low education was associated with a higher prevalence of calcification in white Americans but a lower prevalence of calcification in Hispanics. US birth and time in the United States were also positively associated with the extent of calcification in persons with detectable calcium as revealed in the scan.

These differences did not appear to be accounted for by smoking, BMI,

LDL and HDL cholesterol, hypertension, and diabetes. Therefore, multiple socioeconomic and acculturation factors in various racial and ethnic groups seem to be related to the development and progression of various metabolic and vascular conditions. From a practical perspective, healthcare providers should always consider their patients' socioeconomic status when understanding the presence of various disease processes and when implementing any treatment plan.

Conclusion

Multicultural societies exist throughout the world. Many clinicians routinely provide healthcare to people from different racial/ethnic and cultural groups. Some of these groups have a particularly high risk of developing certain diseases, including type 2 diabetes. Providing high-quality care to any group of patients with diabetes continues to be a challenge in the United States, as it is in most areas in the world. Because multiple medical, social, and cultural factors influence the development and progression of type 2 diabetes, management of patients becomes even more challenging if healthcare providers cannot identify and address the many contributing factors.

The standards of diabetes care apply to every individual with this disease and should continue to be the core of every clinician's practice. However, improving health care providers' cultural competence may help improve the quality of care provided to minority groups, and may ultimately reduce healthcare disparities. Increased cultural competence may also improve patient-provider trust and communication, as well as help patients adhere to prevention and treatment plans.

Index

Note: Entries followed by "f" indicate figures; "t" tables.